Physical Therapy in Acute Care

A CLINICIAN'S GUIDE

Editor

Daniel Malone, MPT, CCS

Cardiovascular & Pulmonary Team Leader
University of Pennsylvania Health System
Hospital of the University of Pennsylvania
Department of Rehabilitation Medicine
Philadelphia, Pennsylvania

Assistant Editor

Kathy Lee Bishop Lindsay, MS, PT, CCS

Manager, Emory HeartWise^SM Risk Reduction Program
Adjunct Faculty, Emory University School of Physical Therapy
Atlanta, Georgia

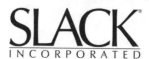

SLACK

INCORPORATED

Delivering the best in health care information and education worldwide www.slackbooks.com

ISBN-13: 978-1-55642-534-9

Published by: SLACK Incorporated
                       6900 Grove Road
                       Thorofare, NJ 08086 USA
                       Telephone: 856-848-1000
                       Fax: 856-853-5991
                       www.slackbooks.com

Contact SLACK Incorporated for more information about other books in this field or about the availability of our books from distributors outside the United States.

Library of Congress Cataloging-in-Publication Data

Physical therapy in acute care : a clinician's guide / edited by Daniel Joseph Malone, Kathy Lee Bishop Lindsay.
    p. ; cm.
  Includes bibliographical references and index.
  ISBN-13: 978-1-55642-534-9 (pbk. : alk. paper)
  ISBN-10: 1-55642-534-1 (pbk. : alk. paper)
  1. Physical therapy. 2. Critical care medicine. I. Malone, Daniel Joseph. II. Lindsay, Kathy Lee Bishop.
  [DNLM: 1. Acute Disease. 2. Physical Therapy Modalities. WB 460 P5783 2006]
  RM700.P4736 2006
  615.8'2--dc22
                            2005037379

Printed in the United States of America.

Last digit is print number: 10   9   8   7   6   5   4   3   2

ABOUT THE EDITORS

The physical therapy career of Daniel J. Malone MPT, CCS is highlighted by 15 years of acute care and cardiopulmonary practice and achieving specialist certification by the American Board of Physical Therapy Specialists. Since graduating from Temple University in 1992, Dan has been employed by the University of Pennsylvania Health System where his career has spanned all services from critical care to long-term care. His current position at the Hospital of the University of Pennsylvania is the Cardiovascular & Pulmonary Team Leader where he provides a leadership role for the Department of Rehabilitation Medicine for staff education, research, staff and program development, and quality improvement initiatives pertaining to cardiovascular and pulmonary therapy service lines.

Academically, Dan has coordinated the acute care and cardiovascular and pulmonary coursework for regional physical therapy programs including Hahnemann University, Neumann College, the University of Medicine and Dentistry of New Jersey and Arcadia University. He continues as an adjunct faculty member, providing lectures and laboratory guidance on the examination and interventions for patients with cardiopulmonary diseases and impairments at Arcadia University.

Dan is active in the Cardiovascular and Pulmonary Section of the APTA, serving as program chair for the past five years as well as being an elected member of the nominating committee. Additionally, he has served as a member of the Specialization Academy of Content Experts and the Standard Setting Committee for the Cardiovascular and Pulmonary specialization examination.

In addition to his clinical practice, Dan is pursuing a PhD in physiology with an emphasis in acute lung injury in the School of Medicine at Temple University.

DJM

Kathy Lee Bishop Lindsay, MS, PT, CCS has been passionate about cardiopulmonary physical therapy for over 25 years. She became a board certified cardiopulmonary specialist in 1993 and renewed her certification in 2003. She graduated from the University of Vermont in 1982 with a BS and received her advanced Masters in physical therapy from the Institute of Health Professions at Massachusetts General Hospital in 1991. Her realm of practice was grounded in acute care starting at a small community hospital in northeast Pennsylvania. She started the pulmonary rehabilitation program and then moved to Boston to attend graduate school as well as to work at Massachusetts General Hospital where she became a Senior Cardiopulmonary Physical Therapist. In 1993, she became the

Cardiopulmonary Clinical Team Leader for the University of Pennsylvania Medical Center and provided mentoring and staff development. In 1996, her position expanded to include the title of Clinical Director for the Cardiac Rehabilitation Program. Kathy Lee has been manager of the Emory HeartWise^{SM} Risk Reduction Program in Atlanta since 2000. This program provides wellness and prevention to the community as well as Emory Healthcare and University employees.

Academically, Kathy Lee has instructed and coordinated cardiopulmonary classes at North Eastern University in Boston; Allegheny University; Beaver College (now Arcadia University), Widener University, and Luzerne County Community College in Pennsylvania; University of Medicine and Dentistry in New Jersey; and Emory University in Atlanta. She has been a guest speaker on airway clearance as well as diabetes locally and nationally. She has spoken at the Combined Section Meeting as well as presenting poster and platform presentations. She has also been a moderator and a presenter at the North American Cystic Fibrosis Conferences and presented a poster at ACSM on the relationship of heart rate and perceived exertion altered by severity of Parkinson's disease. Her published chapters include "Physical Therapy Interventions: Practice Pattern C" in Cardiopulmonary Physical Therapy, by DeTurk and Cahalin; "Rehabilitation for the Pediatric Patient with Pulmonary Disease" in Pulmonary Rehabilitation: Guidelines for Success, Third Edition, by Hodgkin JE, Celli BR, and Connors GL; and "Pulmonary Rehabilitation in the Intensive Care Unit" in Pulmonary Rehabilitation, by Fishman AP.

Kathy Lee has participated in the Cardiovascular and Pulmonary Standard Setting Meeting and has been an ABPTS writer for the specialty exam, chairman of the nominating committee for the Cardiopulmonary Section, and recently served on the Board of Directors for the Georgia Chapter of the Cystic Fibrosis Foundation.

KLBL

Contents

ACKNOWLEDGMENTS

As noted in the preface, acute care physical therapy demands skill and resolve to focus on the impairments and functional capabilities of the individual in order to maximize patient outcomes. This book also required the skills and resolve of many dedicated people. It is with sincere gratitude that I thank Kathy Lee, my HUP colleagues—Colleen and Heather ("Could you check those references?"), Joe ("Big Daddy"), Lora (you'll always be "LB"), Esther and Robin ("How about another appendix?"), and our additional contributors—Zoher, David, and Christy. I also want to acknowledge my new friends from SLACK—Carrie, Jenn, and John. Thanks for the opportunity. Your flexibility, guidance, and patience were greatly appreciated. Most importantly, I need to thank my wife, Margie. Your patience and support allowed this project to be completed. Now, I'll balance the budget. No, I guess that's really not a good idea. Let's take the boy for a walk, together.

"We make a living by what we get, we make a life by what we give."

—Sir Winston Churchill

DJM

Over the years practicing in the acute care setting, I have had many mentors: Colleen Kigin, Terri Hoskins Michel, Meryl Cohen, Cindy Zadai, Mica Rie, and the list goes on. I have always been challenged not to accept tradition, but to strive for the best and often times to take the path not typically accepted to help a patient transition from the intensive care unit to home. The culture of the acute care therapist has changed drastically over the past three decades: the length of stay, the acuteness of the patients, the co-morbidities, the technology, not to mention the financial hurdles of the hospital setting and the cost of recovering from a catastrophic injury. The first time I walked into an intensive care unit, all eyes were on me and wondered what a PT was doing in the ICU. Now I know beyond any doubt, PT needs to start early, be aggressive, and be on the team that successfully progresses the patient through the acute care stay to discharge.

I want to thank each of my patients, each of my mentors, each of the wonderful friends that I have gained from working in so many different acute care facilities, and my family for teaching me to have such passion and desire to give all of myself. I also want to thank the contributors to the book as well as Dan Malone who is not only a true friend but has been the steady hand in completion of the text. Last but not least to my husband, Jack, and our boys, Sandy and Snow, you have been the most patient with me as this book has come to fruition from idea to actual pages.

KLBL

Contributing Authors

Joseph Adler, MS, PT

Senior II Physical Therapist
Center Coordinator of Clinical Education
University of Pennsylvania Health System
Hospital of the University of Pennsylvania
Department of Rehabilitation Medicine
Philadelphia, Pennsylvania

Esther H. Bae, MPT

Staff Physical Therapist
University of Pennsylvania Health System
Hospital of the University of Pennsylvania
Department of Rehabilitation Medicine
Philadelphia, Pennsylvania

Kathy Lee Bishop Lindsay, MS, PT, CCS

Manager, Emory HeartWise[SM] Risk Reduction Program
Adjunct Faculty, Emory University School of Physical Therapy
Atlanta, Georgia

Colleen Chancler, PT, MHS

University of Pennsylvania Health System
Hospital of the University of Pennsylvania
Department of Rehabilitation Medicine
Philadelphia, Pennsylvania

Heather Dillon, MSPT, NCS

Senior II Physical Therapist
University of Pennsylvania Health System
Hospital of the University of Pennsylvania
Department of Rehabilitation Medicine
Philadelphia, Pennsylvania

Christy F. Ehlers, PT, CWS

Emory University Hospital
Coordinator, Wound Management Specialist and
Cardiopulmonary Team Coordinator
Atlanta, Georgia

David Fichandler, MSPT

Therapy Manager
Mount Sinai Medical Center
New York, NY

Zoher F. Kapasi, PT, PhD

Associate Director and Associate Professor
Division of Physical Therapy
Department of Rehabilitation Medicine
Emory University School of Medicine
Atlanta, Georgia

Daniel J. Malone, MPT, CCS

Cardiovascular & Pulmonary Team Leader
University of Pennsylvania Health System
Hospital of the University of Pennsylvania
Department of Rehabilitation Medicine
Philadelphia, Pennsylvania

Lora Packel, MS, PT

Coordinator of Cancer Rehabilitation
Hospital of the University of Pennsylvania
Assistant Professor
Physical Therapy
University of the Sciences in Philadelphia
Philadelphia, Pennsylvania

Robin Stott-McNulty, MPT

Senior Physical Therapist
University of Pennsylvania Health System
Hospital of the University of Pennsylvania
Department of Rehabilitation Medicine
Philadelphia, Pennsylvania

PREFACE

The ability to effectively treat patients across the broad spectrum of acute care is one of the most interesting and challenging aspects of the physical therapy profession. Acute care physical therapy demands skill and resolve to focus on the impairments and functional capabilities of the individual. The physical therapist and physical therapist assistant must consider the pathophysiology of disease and the impact of medications while utilizing the benefits, but not impeding the physiologic monitoring and patient-support equipment. Therapists will often participate in patient-centered rounds that can include representatives from physician groups, nursing, nutrition, speech pathology, respiratory and occupational therapy, performance improvement, and even spiritual counseling. Often, the PT is making clinical judgments that impact discharge planning after only one patient interaction. The work is demanding, challenging, and at times disheartening, but the rewards in clinical development and positive patient outcomes abound.

Physical Therapy in Acute Care: A Clinician's Guide evolved from a bulleted list of diagnoses and procedures to a narrative text attempting to highlight the breadth and complexity of hospital-based physical therapy services. The authors understand that it is impossible to compile all diseases, disorders, diagnostic tests, and medical/surgical procedures, as well as provide a comprehensive portrayal of physical therapy examination procedures and therapeutic interventions, into one text due to the evolving nature of hospital-based practice. However, all attempts have been made to incorporate the most relevant information pertaining to this dynamic field of physical therapy practice.

Physical Therapy in Acute Care: A Clinician's Guide is organized by organ system preceded by the common universal topics of examination and discharge planning, common medical diagnostic tests, and patient support equipment. Complications of bed rest and the ubiquitous issues of immunity and infection control are also reviewed. Each organ system chapter begins with a brief description of pertinent anatomy and physiology followed by the most common diseases and disorders associated with the described system. This should provide the reader with an understanding of the basic physiologic mechanisms underlying normal organ function contrasted with the pathophysiology of disease. Following the didactic information, the impact of these conditions on physical therapy examination and therapeutic interventions is provided and highlighted by the inclusion of real-life case studies. A section called Pharmacological Information is included at the end of each disease/disorder chapter that outlines standard medications and their respective side effects to aid in the evaluation of patient presentation and responses to therapeutic interventions. The *Guide to Physical Therapist Practice* is integrated throughout the text, and the published literature is used to support the described physical therapy practice. However, as all acute care therapists know, there is a paucity of acute care physical therapy research, and this should challenge us all to contribute to this body of evidence. *Physical Therapy in Acute Care: A Clinician's Guide* should serve as a reference to benefit the novice practitioner and the student as well as more experienced clinicians practicing in an evolving acute care environment.

FOREWORD

My first paid job as a licensed physical therapist was a staff position in a 1,000-bed academic medical center. At the time of my interview, there were openings on the outpatient orthopedic and inpatient rehabilitation teams, practice areas in which I had performed the majority of my clinical training while I was a student. By the time I started work 3 months later, however, those openings had been filled, and I was assigned to the acute care team. Upon learning of this change, I told my supervisor "I hope you know what you're doing, because I'm not sure that I do!" This lack of confidence stemmed from my limited exposure to hospital practice, both in terms of clinical experience and didactic content. Textbooks and other references of the time focused on medical and nursing care, not on the physical therapy management of acutely ill patients. *Physical Therapy in Acute Care: A Clinician's Guide* is the resource I wish I had back then!

Eighteen years later, this textbook will be just as useful for me. As a full-time faculty member, my clinical practice opportunities are less frequent. Meanwhile, advances in technology and pharmaceuticals have revolutionized the medical and surgical management of hospitalized patients at the same time that financial and regulatory pressures have accelerated the discharge planning process. I could not step into an intensive care unit now and rely solely on my past experience to safely and effectively manage critically ill patients. Given the opportunity to return to this environment, *Physical Therapy in Acute Care: A Clinician's Guide* will be the resource to which I will turn to refresh and update my knowledge of acute care practice.

Readers like me will find everything they need in this textbook. Chapters 1 through 5 describe the context of the acute care setting and the physical therapist's role within it. Of particular importance is the ubiquitous challenge of preventing or reversing the deleterious effects of prolonged bed rest. The remaining chapters focus on each organ system, providing a review of fundamental knowledge about anatomy, physiology, and pathophysiology while also describing contemporary medical and surgical management of the most common diseases and disorders. A compendium of the most relevant pharmacology also is included. Physical therapy practice is discussed in extensive detail following the patient management model defined by the *Guide to Physical Therapy Practice.* Commonly used tests and measures are described along with interpretive guidelines in easy-to-read table format. Available evidence pertaining to physical therapy examination and treatment techniques is reviewed throughout. Finally, each chapter contains a patient case study illustrating the application of all of this information to practice.

In effect, *Physical Therapy in Acute Care: A Clinician's Guide* represents many textbooks combined into one resource. Daniel Malone, MPT, CCS and Kathy Lee Bishop Lindsay, MS, PT, CCS, clearly have invested an enormous amount of time, energy, and brain-power to make this book possible, and their efforts have paid off. Of course, I am not surprised by this result, as I have had the pleasure of observing their level of professional commitment and talent at numerous meetings and conferences. These individuals are active, evidence-based clinicians who work in myriad ways to promote and advance physical therapy practice. Students, new graduates, vintage practitioners like me, and—most importantly—patients, will benefit from their latest, although not last, contribution. Bravo!

Dianne V. Jewell, PT, PhD, CCS, FAACVPR
Assistant Professor
Virginia Commonwealth University
Department of Physical Therapy
President, Cardiovascular, & Pulmonary Section—APTA, Inc

ACUTE CARE PHYSICAL THERAPY EXAMINATION AND DISCHARGE PLANNING

Daniel J. Malone, MPT, CCS
Joseph Adler, MS, PT

INTRODUCTION

This chapter will introduce the examination process for the acute care patient and will expose the clinician to concepts that comprise the discharge planning process that will serve a complex population in a demanding health care environment. For example, consider a 55-year-old business executive who suffered an acute onset of chest pain followed by an emergent coronary artery bypass graft surgery to the 78-year-old anorexic patient with advanced diabetes, renal disease, and failure to thrive who is noncompliant with his medical care. Each of these scenarios triggers a mental image or a set of hypotheses, but the examination process allows the physical therapist to confirm, refute, or generate new hypotheses relating to the basis of impairments and functional limitations encountered. Although the hypotheses pertaining to these two patients differ, there are many shared elements of the physical therapy examination that the acute care practitioner should consider. This chapter will elucidate these common elements and provide clinicians' views on the examination process as they relate to the patient/client management process. Additional examination and interventions of the acutely injured or medically compromised patient are beyond the scope of this chapter, but can be found in the organ system chapters that follow. A model for the discharge planning process will be presented, and a case scenario, based on a real patient, will be used to highlight patient/client management in the acute care setting. This case study format will follow in subsequent chapters.

EXAMINATION

History

As noted in the *Guide to Physical Therapists Practice*,[1] the elements of patient/client management include examination, evaluation, diagnosis, prognosis (including plan of care), interventions, and outcomes. Examination of the acute care patient, as with all patients, includes three major categories:

1. History
2. Review of systems
3. Specific tests and measures

History is a systematic gathering of data—from both past and present—related to why the patient/client is seeking the services of the physical therapist. Patients in the hospital rarely request therapy services, but other health care practitioners or institutional guidelines have reasoned that therapy services are beneficial in the ongoing care of the patient.

While reviewing the history, the patient's chief complaint or primary reasons for the hospitalization are important to note. The data from the history allow the clinician to hypothesize about impairments and functional limitations that are commonly related to medical conditions and impacted by sociodemographic factors or personal characteristics.[1]

Common Data Generated from a Patient/Client History

General Demographics

Gender, ethnicity, religious beliefs, and language barriers are important considerations when working and communicating with the patient, the patient's family, and primary caregivers. Certain religious and cultural beliefs might limit a patient's acceptance of medical care by a therapist of a different gender. Language barriers often create misunderstanding or limited understanding of complex medical issues and care. Social roles of the patient may dictate specific goals for therapy (eg, homemaking responsibilities in Amish women from Lancaster County, Pennsylvania).

Social History

Resources and cultural beliefs of the family must be identified and acknowledged. Resources can include family and community support and financial or insurance assets. When the current hospitalization ends, the patient may not be independent with activities of daily living (ADLs) or instrumental activities of daily living (IADLs) (Table 1-1). The clinician determines and provides recommendations regarding the minimal frequency and duration of social supports (family/friends) required for safe discharge. The physical therapist/physical therapist assistant must determine if the assistance available successfully meets the needs of the patient. An individual can safely be discharged to home, although he or she may require assist for various ADLs/IADLs with an adequate support network. Clearly, the extent of social resources provides greater flexibility during the discharge planning process.

Living Environment

The patient's current living environment is the hospital. Often this environment is an overwhelming experience for the patient, the patient's family members, and caregivers until the equipment becomes more familiar. Therapists should be accustomed to all monitors, equipment, supplies, and alarms that are utilized in the present care of the patient. Not understanding the indications,

---

Table 1–1
ACTIVITIES OF DAILY LIVING AND INSTRUMENTAL ACTIVITIES OF DAILY LIVING

ADLs

- Eating
- Bathing
- Grooming
- Dressing
- Bed mobility (rolling, supine<>sit)
- Transfers (sit<> stand, toilet/ commode, bed<> chair)

IADLs

- Cooking
- Shopping
- Housekeeping
- Balancing a checkbook
- Driving a car
- Ability to use public transportation

---

precautions, and potential negative impact associated with physiologic monitoring and patient support equipment can lead to untoward events and undermines the therapist–patient/client relationship.

Additionally, the therapist must understand the discharge options for the patient. Will the patient be returning to his or her primary residence or will the patient have an option of residing with a family member? One needs to consider the discharge environment with special emphasis on stairs, bathrooms, and potential space and access requirements for home hospital equipment (eg, wheelchairs/beds/mechanical ventilators/intravenous infusion). Determination of the discharge destination will enable appropriate goal setting and therapeutic intervention.

General Health Status

The patient's functional mobility prior to admission is important to understand. This knowledge will help determine specific goals of therapy. Special emphasis on prior ability to perform the ADLs of bathing, dressing, grooming, and household or community ambulation can be a guide to the general aerobic capacity of the patient. Scales that are useful may include the Borg Scale of Rating Perceived Exertion (RPE) or the New York Heart Association Functional Classification System (NYHA) shown in Table 1–2. These scales will help determine the intensity of limiting symptoms during functional activities. The general health status of the primary caregiver must be assessed to ensure proper care for the patient upon discharge since this individual may assume much of the burden of care. Cognition, memory, and safety awareness are important factors affecting the discharge plan. Again, a significant social support network increases flexibility for discharge planning if impairments are noted in neurocognitive status.

Social/Health Habits

Social and health habits provide useful information regarding the type of living arrangements and environment into which the adult will be discharged upon recovery. This information may signal the need for other consults to maximize a patient's healthy outcome. For example, smoking, alcohol, or other drug history may be an indication for referral to smoking cessation or drug/ alcohol rehabilitation. While hospitalized, a social work consultation is appropriate for frequent admissions related to medical noncompliance due to financial hardship, inadequate social support, and poor living environment. A nutritionist can assist the patient with progressive weight loss or gain and provide valuable information for dietary management of many disease processes. Education on lifestyle modification may be beneficial for the patient and the caregivers to facilitate a healthier living environment.

Family History

Health status of the primary caregivers can have an impact on the provision of optimal care when the patient is discharged to home. Functional limitations of the patient or dependence on devices such as mechanical ventilation can create a large physical and psychological burden of care that caregivers are unable to manage. Early recognition of these issues assists in appropriate discharge management.

Medical/Surgical History

The medical/surgical history represents information of critical importance that will be available in the patient's medical chart and from other caregivers and family members. Of particular importance to the physical therapist are disorders or complications within the pulmonary, cardiovascular, integumentary, neuromuscular, and musculoskeletal systems. The "chronicity" of the medical/ surgical issues and comorbid conditions will provide further information for the physical therapist regarding prognostication for outcomes and the duration of the episode of care.

Current Conditions/Chief Complaints

What is the current concern that has led to the request for physical therapy, and is this an initial episode or a reoccurrence? Is the patient hemodynamically stable, and is it safe to participate in therapy? What are the current therapeutic interventions being provided by other health care providers? Has the patient been receiving any type of positioning, mobilization, exercise, or airway clearance? Has the patient been on bed rest? Why? How long? Are there any weightbearing, activity, or position restrictions? Will hemodynamic (heart rate [HR] blood pressure [BP]) parameters limit therapy? What are the patient/family expectations for this episode of care and for continued care upon discharge? The answers to these questions allow the therapist to gain insight into the patient's activity patterns and tolerance preceding this episode of care. Obviously, the greater the duration of hemodynamic instability or bed rest, the more deconditioned the patient will be regardless of medical or surgical history. The physical therapist uses this data to continue hypothesis generation and prognostication.

Functional Status and Activity Level

As mentioned in the section General Health Status, determining the patient's prior level of function may temper expectations regarding optimal exercise tolerance throughout the episode of care. For example, if the patient could only

Table 1–2

COMMON SCALES FOR PERCEIVED EXERTION, ANGINA, DYSPNEA, AND CLAUDICATION

Borg Scale for Rating Perceived Exertion:

6	No exertion	0	Nothing at all
7	Extremely light		
8		0.5	Very, very light
9	Very light		
10			
11	Light	2	Light
12			
13	Somewhat hard	3	Moderate
14			
15	Hard (heavy)	5	Heavy (strong)
16			
17	Very hard	7	Very heavy
18			
19	Extremely hard	9	
20	Maximal exertion	10	Very, very heavy (maximal)

New York Heart Association Functional Classification System:

I: No limitations on physical activity; ordinary physical activity not resulting in symptoms.

II: Slight limitation on physical activity; no symptoms at rest, but symptoms possible with ordinary physical activity.

III: More severe limitations; patient usually comfortable at rest; clinical manifestations with usual physical activities.

IV: Inability to carry out any physical activity without producing symptoms; symptoms often present at rest.

Angina Scale:

0	No angina
+1	Light, barely noticeable
+2	Moderate, bothersome
+3	Severe, uncomfortable
+4	Most severe pain ever experienced

(continued)

Table 1–2 (continued)

COMMON SCALES FOR PERCEIVED EXERTION, ANGINA, DYSPNEA, AND CLAUDICATION

Five-Grade Dyspnea Scale:

0	No dyspnea
1	Mild, noticeable
2	Mild, some difficulty
3	Moderate difficulty, but can continue
4	Severe difficulty, cannot continue

Claudication Scale:

0	No claudication pain
1	Initial, minimal claudication pain
2	Moderate, bothersome pain
3	Intense pain
4	Maximal pain, cannot continue

Adapted from:
ACSM's Guidelines for Exercise Testing and Prescription. 6th ed. Philadelphia, Pa: Lippincott Williams & Wilkins; 2000.
Borg GA. Psychophysical basis of perceived exertion. *Med Sci Sports Exerc.* 1982;14: 377–387.

ambulate household distances secondary to shortness of breath (SOB), community ambulation of several blocks is not a realistic goal. Comparison of the current and prior functional status in relation to the duration of the hospitalization will enable the physical therapist to prognosticate on the rate and extent of functional return that will influence discharge planning.

Medications

Pharmacological interventions are a mainstay of medical and surgical management. Therapists must consider the impact of medications on the patient's hemodynamic profiles at rest and with activity, as well as determining the potential connection between medication side effects, mental status, and neuromuscular complaints. Side effects are symptoms that occur as a consequence of drug administration. These effects are unrelated to the intended action of the drug, and it must be remembered that unwanted side effects do not only occur at toxic doses, but may commonly occur at therapeutic levels of the desired medication.

Following each organ system chapter is additional information regarding common medications prescribed to patients. Although not an exhaustive listing, the information may guide therapist practice and assist with patient assessment and tolerance to therapeutic interventions.

Other Clinical Tests

Extensive hospital derived data can be accessed, but the utility of this expansive data is somewhat difficult to determine. Laboratory data may not be routinely reviewed by many acute care clinicians, but this is inattentive practice. Laboratory values provide information that may help in determining the patient presentation and clinical responses observed during the examination or follow-up interventions. For example, a patient with anemia may present with complaints of (c/o) SOB and perceived reduction in exercise capacity that can be partially explained by this abnormality in the complete blood cell (CBC) count. The patient with cancer who has low white blood cell numbers, leukocytopenia, should not be scheduled for therapy in a gym setting due to impaired immune defense and infection risk. Laboratory data guide intervention appropriateness, intensity, and duration, and the astute acute care clinician must consider this readily available information for appropriate care. Additional information can be found in Chapter 2.

EVALUATION, DIAGNOSIS, AND PROGNOSIS

Systems Review

The systems review is a gross examination, or "quick check," to provide baseline information and identify the existence of other health problems to be considered in the diagnosis, prognosis, and plan of care. The accumulated data may trigger referral to other health care providers or necessitate further consultation with the current health care team if unsuspected or occult pathologies and impairments are discovered.

Cardiovascular/Pulmonary

The cardiovascular and pulmonary review should include BP and pulse rate determination, respiratory rate (RR), and perceived level of dyspnea or exertion at rest and with activity as described in Tables 1–2, 6–11, and 7–7. If patients are attached to a telemetry system, interpretation of HR and heart rhythm is standard practice (see Chapter 6, Monitoring Information). Pulse oximetry is indicated if the patient presents with any gross indications of cyanosis, history of hypoxemia or respiratory difficulties, complains of (c/o) SOB, or is diagnosed with cardiac or pulmonary disease. The hospitalized patient will likely be monitored extensively and most vitals signs (VS) will be available to the therapist from nursing documentation and telemetry monitors. However, information obtained prior to the therapist's arrival is not a substitute for current, direct monitoring of VS. The therapist should familiarize him- or herself with the patient's status over the prior 12 to 24 hours to determine hemodynamic and respiratory trends and current stability. The medical record may not be up-to-date, and conferencing with the nursing staff will provide valuable and timely information regarding the patient's current status.

Since therapeutic exercises are universally prescribed for hospitalized patients, the therapist must record and understand the cardiopulmonary responses at rest and during activity to determine the presence of hemodynamic and respiratory stability and activity tolerance.

Integumentary

Patients may have fragile skin due to medications (eg, corticosteroids), poor nutrition, and prolonged bed rest. Areas of skin break down, ecchymosis, and pressure sore development should be noted. Hospital acquired integumentary lesions can be avoided with frequent position and postural changes, especially out of bed (OOB) activities. Evaluation of the body habitus may elicit suggestions for beds, chairs, mattress, cushions, or mobility aids (eg, walkers, trapeze, rails) that enable more frequent position changes and patient comfort. Integumentary lesions are potential sites for infection and certainly can limit patient outcomes and prolong the length of stay. The physical therapist should examine incisions and new or old scars and determine the healing status of the wounds (see Table 15–1). Is there any evidence of infection at the site? Indwelling lines and tubes need to be considered during interventions and may influence a patient's mobility. Specific precautions should be adhered to throughout the course of therapy as noted in Chapter 3.

Musculoskeletal

Ascertain gross muscle tone and range of motion (ROM). Contractures/soft tissue limitations are common, unfortunately, in the hospitalized patient, particularly the bed bound mechanically ventilated or critically ill patient. In addition to the extremities, considering the head and neck region in this assessment is important. Patients are often positioned facing the mechanical ventilator to avoid traction on the tubing. The patient may develop limitations in cervical and upper extremity (UE) ROM toward the vicinity of the ventilator. Lower extremity (LE) ROM needs to be considered for the patient to successfully transfer and initiate gait activities while UE ROM will influence ADL performance (eg, bathing, dressing). Identify any chest wall asymmetries that may be associated with surgical incisions/pain, neuromuscular disease, prior thoracic trauma, or orthopedic conditions (scoliosis). These limitations will certainly influence the patient's breathing pattern. Finally, assessment of functional strength will provide direct evidence regarding the potential needs for mobility training and requirements for ambulatory aids.

Neuromuscular

Determination of neuromuscular status is key in the acute care patient. Initial signs of neuromuscular dysfunction may not be apparent until the patient attempts to move. Often the physical therapist is the first health care provider to mobilize or observe the patient's mobility. Gross motor strength, movement patterns, sensation, and proprioceptive testing provide insight into the neuromuscular integrity of the patient. Occult abnormalities should trigger the need for a further medical consultation and more specific physical therapy examination procedures (Tables 1–3 through 1–5; see Chapter 9). Focal deficits discovered during the examination should lead to more specific or focused diagnostic testing (eg, myotome/dermatome testing in the patient with spinal cord injury).

Table 1-3

DEEP TENDON REFLEX TESTING

Deep Tendon	Spinal Level	Grade
Biceps	C5 and C6	0 (No response)
Brachioradial	C5 and C6	1+ (Sluggish/diminished)
Triceps	C6, C7, and C8	2+ (Active/expected/normal)
Patellar	L2, L3, and L4	3+ (More brisk than expected, slightly hyperactive)
Achilles	S1 and S2	4+ (Brisk, hyperactive, intermittent or transient clonus)

Adapted from Seidel HM, Ball JW, et al. *Mosby's Guide to Physical Examination.* St. Louis, Mo: Mosby, Inc; 2003.

Communication, Affect, Cognition, Language, and Learning Style

The level of patient's consciousness and arousal will affect language, learning, and ability to make needs known. Arousal and alertness can be impaired due to sedatives, anxiolytics, narcotics, and other medications. Artificial airways such as endotracheal or tracheostomy tubes can alter and influence communication. Uses of alternative communication devices such as letter boards or electrolarynx are indicated to promote effective communications.

Tests and Measurements

Specific tests and measurements employed by the physical therapist will be determined by information gathered during the systems review process. Frequently used tests/measures are provided in the individual organ system chapters. Common tests and measures that are generally performed during the physical therapy examination are discussed below.

Aerobic Capacity and Endurance

The typical manner of testing aerobic capacity and endurance in adults involves some type of exercise stimulus such as cycle ergometry or treadmill testing. The hospitalized patient does not usually undergo such extensive testing, but must be examined in some other manner. Exercise testing for the patient who has recently experienced an acute myocardial infarction (MI) or electrocardiogram (ECG) abnormality may be the exception. Therapists often challenge and monitor aerobic capacity and endurance through assessment of VS responses and patient's perceived exertion with common ADLs including bed mobility, sit-to-stand transfers, ambulation, toileting, and bathing. Structured assessments can include the 6-minute walk test (6MWT), shuttle tests, or step testing. The therapist should record the patient's VS prior to therapy and

Table 1-4
CRANIAL NERVE TESTING

CN #	Name	Function and Description of Technique	Examination Findings in Common Diseases/Disorders
I	Olfactory	Smell, the ability to smell is tested by asking the person to identify items with very specific odors (such as soap, coffee) placed under the nares.	Lesion symptoms: Loss of sense of smell (**anosmia**) if bilateral. May result from head injury.
II	Optic	Vision and detection of light by the pupil, the patient is tested by reading an eye chart. Detection of objects or movement from the corners of the eyes tests peripheral vision. Confrontation and extinction tests visual fields.	Lesion symptoms: Unilateral damage produces ipsilateral blindness; bilateral damage produces bilateral blindness.
III	Oculomotor	**Extraocular eye movements** (eye upward, downward, and inward). **Pupillary reflex:** Narrowing (constriction) or widening (dilation) of the pupil in response to light. **Convergence:** Medial movements of eyes to an object at close range. The upper eyelid is observed for drooping (**ptosis**).	Lesion symptoms: Loss of medial rectus and unopposed lateral rectus muscle function results in eyeball deviation outward (**lateral strabismus**); may cause double vision (**diplopia**); involuntary back and forth motions (**nystagmus**); ipsilateral ptosis may be present.
IV	Trochlear	Extraocular movements. The ability to move each eye downward and laterally is tested by asking the person to follow a target.	Lesion symptoms: Loss of superior oblique muscle function results in difficulty moving eyeball down and laterally creating a **vertical**, **medial strabismus**; nystagmus may be present.

	Nerve		
V	**Trigeminal**	Facial sensation and chewing; facial sensation is tested using a pin and cotton swab or finger. Clenching the teeth and opening the jaw against resistance tests strength and movement of jaw muscles. The **blink (corneal) reflex** is tested by touching the cornea of the eye (eg, cotton wisp).	Lesion symptoms: Ipsilateral loss of sensation of the head, face, and inner oral cavity; weakness of muscles of mastication make chewing difficult and jaw may deviate ipsilaterally (eg, trigeminal neuralgia).
VI	**Abducens**	Side-to-side (lateral) eye movement.	Lesion symptoms: Loss of lateral rectus muscle function results in difficulty moving eyeball laterally creating a **medial strabismus**; diplopia and nystagmus may be present.
VII	**Facial**	Facial expression (smile, open the mouth and show teeth, close eyes tightly) and taste in the front two thirds of the tongue (eg, sweet [sugar], sour [lemon juice], salty [salt], and bitter [aspirin]).	Lesion symptoms: Decreased taste of anterior tongue; decreased corneal reflex; decreased facial movements (eg, Bell's palsy).
VIII	**Vestibulo-cochlear**	Hearing (tuning fork) and balance (walk a straight line/heel-toe walking/Romberg test).	Lesion symptoms: Auditory—Deafness or ear ringing (**tinnitus**); vestibular—decreased balance, vertigo and/or nystagmus may be present (eg, acoustic tumor, vestibular neuritis).

(continued)

Table 1–4 (continued)
CRANIAL NERVE TESTING

CN #	Name	Function and Description of Technique	Examination Findings in Common Diseases/Disorders
IX	**Glosso-pharyngeal**	Swallowing, gag reflex, and speech. The patient is asked to swallow; say "ah-h-h" to check the movement of the palate and uvula (the small, soft projection that hangs down at the back of throat). A tongue blade is touched to the back of the throat to evoke the gag reflex. The person is asked to speak to check the voice for hoarseness.	Lesion symptoms: Loss of gag and swallowing reflex; difficulty with swallowing (**dysphagia**) enhancing aspiration risk.
X	**Vagus**	Swallowing, gag reflex, and speech; control of muscle in internal organs (including the heart). Because cranial nerves IX and X control similar functions, they are tested together.	Lesion symptoms: As above; tachycardia, air hunger (**dyspnea**), slurred speech (**dysarthria**), and hoarse voice (**dysphonia**).
XI	**Accessory**	Neck ROM and shoulder shrugging against resistance.	Lesion symptoms: Dysphagia; weakness for shoulder elevation ipsilateral cervical flexion/extension and contralateral rotation.
XII	**Hypoglossal**	Tongue movement (stick out the tongue and observe for deviation to one side; assess symmetry of movement from side to side and observe for tongue atrophy or weakness.	Lesion symptoms: Ipsilateral deviation/atrophy of tongue, dysarthria, and dysphagia

Adapted from:
Guttman SA. *Quick Reference Neuroscience for Rehabilitation Professionals*. Thorofare, NJ: SLACK Incorporated; 2001.
Seidel HM, Ball JW, et al. *Mosby's Guide to Physical Examination*. St. Louis, Mo: Mosby, Inc; 2003.

Table 1–5		
SIGNS OF UPPER MOTOR NEURON AND LOWER MOTOR NEURON LESIONS		
Sign	*UMN Lesions*	*LMN Lesions*
Weakness	Yes	Yes
Atrophy	No (however, may accompany disuse)	Yes
Fasciculations	No	Yes
Reflexes	Increased	Decreased
Tone	Increased	Decreased

Reprinted with permission from Blumenfeld H. *Neuroanatomy Through Clinical Cases.* Sinauer Associates Publishers; 2001.

Table 1–6	
BODY MASS INDEX (KG/M²)	
18.5 or less	Underweight
18.5 to 24.9	Normal
25.0 to 29.9	Overweight
30.0 to 34.9	Obesity Class I
35.0 to 39.9	Obesity Class II
40 or greater	Obesity Class III/Severe Obesity

determine the physiologic responses as the therapy session proceeds. Normal exercise physiology must be kept in mind while realizing that the patient who has been admitted to the hospital can present with abnormal responses. Therefore, the therapist expectations need to be guarded. For example, a resting RR of 28 breaths per minute in the normal population may be uncommon, but this tachypnea may be seen with the patient who is recovering from respiratory failure due to reduced lung compliance and resultant limited tidal volumes (V_T). This RR is an attempt to maintain adequate minute ventilation and is not by itself a contraindication to therapy. The work of breathing is elevated as a substantial amount of the patient's oxygen consumption is being utilized for quiet respiration. The therapist should expect limitations in breathing reserve, altering exercise capacity, and modify the intensity of therapeutic interventions.

Anthropometric Characteristics

Measures of body dimensions in adults most commonly include weight and body mass index (BMI) (Table 1–6). However, BMI and body weight alone do not define the patient's body habitus or nutrition status. Additionally, laboratory

Table 1–7
GRADING EDEMA

Scale	Depression (cm)	Description
1+ (Trace)	Slight	Barely perceptible
2+ (Mild)	0.0 to 0.6	Skin rebounds <15 seconds
3+ (Moderate)	0.6 to 1.3	Skin rebounds in 15 to 30 seconds
4+ (Severe)	1.3 to 2.5	Skin rebounds in >30 seconds

Adapted from:
Perloff JK. *Physical Examination of the Heart and Circulation.* 3rd ed. Philadelphia, Pa: WB Saunders Co; 2000.
Seidel HM, Ball JW, et al. *Mosby's Guide to Physical Examination.* St. Louis, Mo: Mosby, Inc; 2003.

studies, including serum albumin and prealbumin, measure nutrition status (see Chapter 2 and Table 2–15). These values are used to evaluate interventions, define nutritional outcomes, and monitor trends.

Edema in the hospitalized adult is likely due to congestive heart failure, nutritional deficits, liver and/or renal dysfunction, fluid overload, and inactivity. Edema can limit joint ROM, cause pain, and impair ADL performance. Edema can be assessed by circumferential or volumetric measurements and is frequently graded as noted in Table 1–7.

Obesity is associated with diabetes mellitus, coronary heart disease, obstructive sleep apnea/obesity hypoventilation syndrome, hypothyroidism, and many other metabolic disease processes (see Chapter 11, Surgical Information, and Tables 11–21 and 11–22). Obesity can independently limit the patient's mobility leading to abnormalities of the integument and cardiopulmonary systems. Creativity and appropriate bariatric equipment are required to successfully initiate antigravity and OOB activities (see Tables 11–24 through 11–27).

Alternatively, cachexia is also prominent in long-standing disease, and impaired nutrition status is associated with poor outcomes. Critical illness results in metabolic consequences including hypermetabolism and hypercatabolism. These terms refer to increased energy expenditure and destruction of existing tissues. The sum of these effects is a rapid depletion of body tissue stores and critical protein elements leading to reduced protein synthesis, enhanced protein breakdown, and malnutrition. Nutrition dysfunction can lead to muscle wasting, reduced respiratory and peripheral muscle strength and endurance, increased rates of infection, increased mortality, and reduced pulmonary function, and certainly impact physical therapy plans of care.

Arousal, Attention, and Cognition

The degree of patient arousal, attention, and cognition will impact the interventions chosen for the patient. For example, your patient requires airway clearance, but is unable to participate in the therapy session due to reduced arousal associated with a medication side effect. The airway clearance modality of choice would be chest percussion/vibration and positioning since the patient cannot actively participate in the intervention. Additionally, arousal, attention, and cognition modify the patient's ability to safely perform ADLs or IADLs providing powerful data that influence the discharge plan.

Cognition is defined as the act or processing of knowing, including awareness, memory, and judgment, and cognitive abilities are frequently assessed through a mental status examination.

Arousal is defined as a state of responsiveness to stimulation or action or of physiologic readiness for activity. The patient's level of arousal and cognition is assessed throughout the examination and subsequent treatment sessions, and frequent descriptors are provided in Table 1–8. Therapists frequently determine orientation by asking the patient his or her name, current location, month/day/year, and reason for admission. Asking patients to repeat your name and discipline, which was provided at the beginning of the interaction, challenges short-term memory. Having patients repeat number sequences assesses immediate recall. Asking patients to recall past personal (confirmed by third parties) or historical events assesses long-term memory. Attention, an important aspect of task completion while performing ADLs, is the selective awareness of the environment or selective responsiveness to stimuli. Spelling "world" backward or counting by twos to 20 determines attention or "stick-to-itiveness." Formal determination of mental status can include specific instruments such as the Glasgow Coma Scale (GCS) or Mini-Mental State Examination (MMSE) (see Table 9-5). These tools incorporate grading systems and standardized norms, but do not provide information on specific areas of loss. For example, a score of less than 24 on the MMSE signifies cognitive impairment warranting further evaluation.

Mental status function might fluctuate throughout a hospitalization due to medication side effects, sleep deprivation, depression secondary to bed rest, or a multitude of potential causes. Clinical judgment and screening tools provide valuable data that can assist with determining alterations in status as well as determining proper therapeutic interventions and appropriate discharge recommendations.

Assistive and Adaptive Devices

Assistive and adaptive devices are implements and equipment used to aid patients/clients in performing tasks or movements (eg, walkers, canes, wheelchairs [see Table 8.14], long-handled reachers, splints, percussors). Certain equipment may be necessary due to medical or surgical management (eg, orthotic, splints [see Tables 8–10 through 8–14 and Table 9–20]), and the therapist's job is to optimize mobility within the constraints of the prescribed device. The physical therapist should assess the patient's safety and determine if the use of assistive and adaptive devices "enables" or "disables" task completion. Determining the patient's prior, present, and future utilization of assistive and adaptive devices can prevent ordering duplicate or unnecessary equipment for discharge. Therapists need to be fiscally aware of the costs associated with assistive and adaptive devices and realize that many patients may not have adequate insurance coverage for durable medical equipment (DME). Therapists will need to

Table 1–8

DESCRIPTORS OF LEVELS OF ALTERED CONSCIOUSNESS OR COGNITIVE FUNCTION

Disorientation: Beginning loss of consciousness (LOC); disorientation to time, place; impaired memory; loss of self-recognition.

Lethargy: Limited spontaneous movement or speech; easy arousal with normal speech or touch; may or may not be oriented to time, place, or person.

Obtundation: Mild to moderate reduction in arousal with limited response to the environment; falls asleep unless stimulated verbally or tactilely; answers questions with minimal responses.

Somnolence: The patient is roused by various stimuli and makes appropriate motor and verbal responses.

Stupor: A condition of deep sleep or unresponsiveness from which the person may be aroused or caused to make a motor or verbal response only by vigorous and repeated stimulation; response is often withdrawal, grabbing at stimulus or patient may be combative.

Coma: No motor or verbal response to the external environment or to any stimuli; even noxious stimuli such as deep pain or suctioning; no arousal to any stimulus. **Semicoma** describes the organized withdrawal to painful stimuli or similar responses to persistent tactile stimuli.

Confusion: Loss of ability to think rapidly and clearly; impaired judgment and decision making.

Delusion: A false belief brought about without appropriate external stimulation and inconsistent with the individual's own knowledge and experience.

Psychosis: A mental disorder where alterations in personality and emotional state, and irrational behaviors and thinking are of psychogenic origins (ie, without clearly defined physical cause or structural alteration in the brain). Hallucinations and delusions are often present.

Illusions: The misinterpretation of sensory input, shadows, noises, odors, bodily sensations, etc.

Hallucination: Subjective sensory perceptions that may occur in any of the sensations (auditory, visual, gustatory [taste], olfactory [smell], tactile).

Compulsion: Repetitive acts that a person feels driven to do.

Obsession: Repetitive thoughts that enter the patient's mind that the patient is unable to control (eg, thoughts of aggression, sexual thoughts).

Ruminations: Repetitive or continuous speculations; often circular and abstract.

Indecision: The inability to make up one's own mind.

Adapted from Huether SE, McCance KL. *Understanding Pathophysiology.* St. Louis, Mo: Mosby-Year Book Inc; 1996.

investigate ways (eg, contact DME companies, consult social work) to provide necessary equipment for those with limited insurance or financial resources.

Circulation (Arterial, Venous, Lymphatic)

Circulation is the movement of blood through organs and tissues to deliver oxygen and nutrients while removing waste products. The cardiovascular system provides the motive force and conduits for distribution and drainage of cellular products and byproducts maintaining homeostasis. Abnormalities discovered during the chart review and history, patient reports of limited cardiopulmonary endurance or reserve associated with mobility dysfunction, or abnormalities discovered during the cardiovascular and pulmonary portion of the systems review may elicit a more thorough investigation of the circulatory system. Common tests performed include measurements of HR and heart rhythm, BP, and the palpation and description of edema and pulses as noted in Tables 1–7 and 1–9. The physical therapist should include ratings of perceived exertion or descriptions of claudication as noted in Table 1–2. Further descriptions of cardiovascular measurements can be found in Chapter 6 (see Table 6–6 and Monitoring Information) and Chapter 15 (see Table 15–2).

Cranial and Peripheral Nerve Integrity

The cranial nerves are 12 pairs of nerves exiting directly from the brain to various parts of the head, neck, and viscera. The peripheral nerves include the spinal nerves and their efferent and afferent components. Abnormalities identified during the history and chart review and/or musculoskeletal and neuromuscular components of the systems review (eg, impaired motor function/weakness, altered sensation, abnormal movement patterns) prompt specific testing. Common measurements of nerve integrity includes deep tendon reflexes as noted in Table 1–3 and cranial nerve testing as outlined in Table 1–4. Sensory testing often includes light touch (eg, cotton swab or finger), sharp versus dull (eg, safety pin), and joint position sense. Sensory testing should be performed bilaterally. Classification of ascending and descending spinal tract and UE and LE motor and sensory nerve root distributions (eg, dermatome/myotome) can be found in Chapter 9.

Environmental, Home, and Work Barriers

Environmental, home, and work barriers refer to the physical impediments that keep patients/clients from functioning optimally in their surroundings. Much of this information is gathered during the review of the patient's history (see Living Environment), and the results of specific tests and measures (eg, aerobic capacity, assistive and adaptive devices, gait/locomotion/balance) will guide the plan of care to optimize the patient's functional independence and to ease the caregiver's burden of care. Additionally, the therapist will provide patient/family education on modification to the discharge environment (eg, grab bars, shower chair, removal of throw rugs, lighting) that will enhance patient/client safety and mobility. Goals to overcome environmental, home, and work barriers may warrant the referral of the patient to another level of care post discharge.

<u>Table 1–9</u>

GRADING PULSES

- UE: Carotid artery (medial and inferior to angle of the jaw)/ brachial artery (medial to biceps tendon)/radial artery (medial and ventral side of wrist)
- LE: Femoral artery/popliteal artery (popliteal fossa with knee bent and patient in prone)/dorsalis pedis artery (medial side of dorsum of foot)/posterior/tibial artery (inferior to medial malleoli)

Scale	Description
4+	Bounding
3+	Full, increased
2+	Normal
1+	Weak, thready
0	Absent

Adapted from:
Perloff JK. *Physical Examination of the Heart and Circulation*. 3rd ed. Philadelphia, Pa: WB Saunders Co; 2000.
Seidel HM, Ball JW, et al. *Mosby's Guide to Physical Examination*. St. Louis, Mo: Mosby, Inc; 2003.

Gait, Locomotion, and Balance

Gait is the manner in which a person walks and may be characterized by difficulty initiating or stopping the gait cycle, rhythm and cadence, stance, step length, speed and distance, posture, trunk and arm movements, stability, and observation of involuntary movements during walking (eg, spasticity/genu recurvatum). Locomotion is the ability to move from one place to another. Ideally, therapists typically observe the gait pattern with the patient walking toward and away from the observer. However, safety and guarding of the patient, especially with changes of direction and turns, may necessitate standing next to the patient. Tests of locomotion may include the Timed Up and GO and the 6-minute walk test. Balance is the ability to maintain the body in equilibrium with gravity both statically and dynamically. In the acute care setting, balance is frequently assessed using the Berg Balance Assessment, Romberg Test, Functional Reach, and/or Tandem Gait (heel-toe walking a straight line). The various tests used to assess gait, locomotion, and balance provide the physical therapist with objective information regarding fall risk and the abilities to independently perform ADLs and IADLs. This information also provides evidence for the prescription of specific assistive and adaptive devices as noted above, and is critical when determining the discharge plan.

Integumentary Integrity

Integumentary integrity refers to the intactness of the skin and the ability to promote immune defense (barrier to microorganisms), provide sensory feedback and organ protection, maintain fluid status and thermoregulation (conservation and dissipation of heat), and synthesize vitamin D. As a component of the systems review, examination of the integument should be standard practice in the acute care setting. Examination of sensation, incisions, bony prominence and pressure points, and indwelling lines is critical in reducing infection risk and wound development. Chapter 15 (see Table 15–1) provides a more detailed description of wound care examination.

Motor Function (Motor Control and Motor Learning)

Motor function is the ability to learn or demonstrate the skillful and efficient assumption, maintenance, modification, and control of voluntary postures and movement patterns. Examination procedures commonly include tests of dexterity and coordination including rapid rhythmic alternating movements (eg, turning palms over and back, touch thumb to each finger in sequence) and accuracy of movements (eg, finger-nose, heel up/down alternate LE shin [heelshin test]). Functional tests may include buttoning a shirt, tying shoes, or performance tests such as the timed up and go test. Motor function provides valuable information regarding ADL/IADL performance and patient safety.

Muscle Performance

Muscle performance is the capacity of a muscle or a group of muscles to generate forces. Strength is the muscle force exerted by a muscle or a group of muscles to overcome a resistance under a specific set of circumstances. Power is the work produced per unit of time or the product of strength and speed. Endurance is the ability for a muscle to sustain forces repeatedly or to generate forces over a period of time.

Similar to tests and measures of nerve integrity and motor function, impairments and functional limitations identified during the history and chart review and/or musculoskeletal and neuromuscular components of the systems review (eg, impaired motor function/weakness, abnormal movement patterns) should trigger specific testing of muscle performance. The most common test is manual muscle testing, but additional procedures may include functional tests such as repeated transfers (floor<>stand, sit<>stand), stair climbing, self-care activities (eg, grooming, dressing, bathing), physical performance tests and timed activity tests, and electrophysiologic testing. While performing specific tests of muscle performance, keep in mind signs of an upper versus a lower motor neuron lesion as noted in Table 1–5 as well as the potential impact of bed rest and immobility (see Chapter 4) and medication side effects (eg, corticosteroids). Focal weakness or weakness patterns (eg, hemiplegia) discovered during the physical therapy examination should lead to consultation with the medical team.

Orthotic, Protective, and Supportive Devices and Prosthetic Requirements

Orthotics and protective and supportive devices are implements and equipment used to support or protect weak or ineffective joints or muscles and serve to enhance performance. Common acute care orthotic devices include braces, casts, shoe inserts, and splints. Protective devices include braces, cushions, and

helmets. Supportive devices include compression garments, abdominal binders, neck collars, serial casts, and slings. Physiologic support devices include
mechanical ventilation and supplemental oxygen, and the physical therapy
management of these devices is described in Chapter 3. Common orthotics and
protective and supportive devices are described in Chapter 8 (see Tables 8–10
through 8–14) and Chapter 9 (see Table 9–20).

Prosthetic requirements are the biomechanical elements necessitated by the
loss of a body part, and a prosthesis is an artificial device used to replace a
missing part of the body. Frequently, the physicians and the patient's medical or
surgical presentation determine the provision of specific orthotics, protective and
supportive devices, and prostheses. Patients rarely are prescribed a prosthesis in
the acute care setting after a recent amputation. However, the physical therapist
may need to evaluate a previously prescribed prosthetic device for a patient who
is admitted to the hospital for issues that may or may not pertain directly to the
residual limb. In all cases, the physical therapist/physical therapist assistant provides valuable patient and family education; objective measurement and training regarding the successful care, alignment, and fit of all equipment; and the
benefits, safety, and potential modifications of existing equipment to enhance
patient/client management and optimize outcomes.

Pain

Pain is a disturbed sensation that causes suffering or distress and is frequently encountered in the acute care population. Pain can be viewed as adaptive and maladaptive. Adaptive pain refers to pain that is mainly a protective
mechanism for the body where the individual reacts to remove the pain stimulus (eg, weightbearing on a recent LE fracture). Maladaptive pain is that which
interferes with normal physiologic processes leading to further impairments,
functional limitations, and disability (eg, chronic pain leading to prolonged
bed rest). Pain arises from stimulation of free nerve endings, nociceptors, by
mechanical (pressure, deformation), chemical (histamine, potassium, bradyki-
nin), or thermal (cold/heat) stimuli. Somatic pain includes superficial and deep
pain. Superficial pain is defined as pain at the body surface, while deep pain
arises from muscle, joints, bones, and connective tissues. Visceral pain originates from internal organs and is typically related to ischemia, deformation,
infection, and inflammation.

Therapists should assess the intensity, quality, location, and duration of
all patient c/o pain, especially pain resulting in functional limitations. Pain
scales provide an objective measurement of pain intensity and may provide
valuable information to guide therapeutic interventions (Figure 1–1). Pain
management is an important consideration to maximize patient interactions
and often involves coordinated management with the medical/surgical and
nursing personnel.

THE DISCHARGE PLANNING PROCESS

As stated previously, the data from the physical therapy examination allows
the clinician to hypothesize about impairments and functional limitations,
thereby creating an efficacious plan of care with goal-directed interventions.
Common considerations and interventions are provided in subsequent chapters

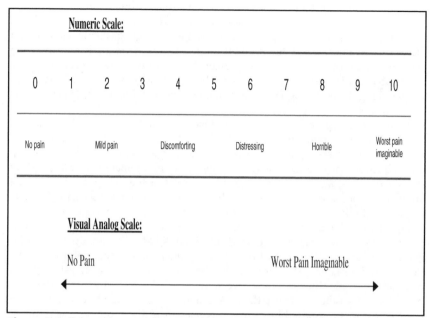

Figure 1–1. Pain scales.

organized by organ system. However, common to all physical therapy intervention is the goal to transition the patient to the next level of care while minimizing functional limitations and disabilities. Included within this challenge is the provision of appropriate discharge recommendations. Therapists must make decisions on assistive devices, appropriate levels of continued inpatient rehabilitation, and whether or not the patient is "safe" to go home. These recommendations are sought not only by patients and their families but also the medical, surgical, nursing, social work, and case management teams. For the new or inexperienced clinician this can be a daunting and often confusing process. The following section highlights pertinent factors that the physical therapist must consider in making effective and reasonable discharge recommendations.

The acute care therapist must appreciate the pressure under which hospital-based medical care functions. Physicians are required, by their daily documentation, to justify "why" the patient requires ongoing hospital-based care. When that care is completed the patient is generally considered medically stable and ready for discharge from the hospital. Prior to this point, a plan should be in place to transition the patient to the next level of appropriate care whether that is home, inpatient rehabilitation, or some other suitable setting. The physical therapy examination should answer several questions related to previous function, current medical and functional status, and future discharge destination, as noted in the section Patient/Client History, to adequately guide the therapist's thought process. To formulate realistic short- and long-term goals the therapist needs information on the patient's prehospital level of function. An example would be to establish ambulation goals for someone who was assisted in bed to wheelchair and commode transfers secondary to a chronic medical condition. This information is vital, but often not readily available for a number of reasons. Patients may be poor historians or unable to speak (language barriers should not affect this issue as hospitals are often required to provide medical translation services) or family members or caregivers who can provide information may not be able to attend therapy sessions. In these instances the therapist is charged with making the best prognosis possible given the information that is attainable and knowable.

Critical information required by therapists to formulate goals and recommendations is at what point the medical/surgical team considers the patient ready for discharge. When the medical status of the patient changes, discharge plans are frequently amended, but with knowledge of approximate hospital length of stay the therapist will be better able to prognosticate achievable goals. What is not attainable in one session, such as stair climbing with a nonweightbearing LE, may be possible in the 3 days required to complete a course of intravenous antibiotics.

Acute care therapists collect data from the patient examination that cover many areas including current level of cognition, ROM, strength, cardiovascular and pulmonary function, sensation, and integument status (see History, Systems Review, and Tests and Measurements). The data from these areas establishes a hospital-based baseline and may give some indication as to the mobility of the patient. Physical therapists use the data generated, clinical and personal experience, and evidenced-based literature to generate the discharge plan as outlined in Figure 1–2. However, no simple formula exists that directly relates a given level of strength or degree of ROM to a functional ability. This is one of the challenges that leads to the difficulty associated with the discharge planning process. For example, a physical therapist receives an emergent consult to evaluate a patient who was admitted 4 days prior. The physician and case manager for the patient inform the therapist that after a procedure the following morning, the patient will be ready for discharge from the hospital. Where the patient goes, they say, is dependent on the physical therapist's recommendations. These critical recommendations are complicated by the fact that the physical therapist's decision is based on the findings of one patient/client interaction, and knowing that the emphasis on hospital-based care is to transition the patient to a less costly, but appropriate environment. The patient, an independent community dwelling elder woman, is admitted with dehydration and hypokalemia and presents with weakness, balance dysfunction, and currently requires minimal assist with mobility. The therapist validates the social history and assesses social supports and determines that home discharge is reasonable even though the patient requires minimal assist with transfers and ambulation. The patient's impairments are a manifestation of her fluid and electrolyte imbalances, and it is anticipated that the patient will return to her prior level of function rapidly with correction of these abnormalities. When the therapist assesses the impact that impairments in ROM, endurance, strength, airflow, and hemodynamics have on functional limitations, he or she must determine whether or not the observed deficits are related to a premorbid condition, or are newly acquired as a result of an acute medical condition or hospitalization. Chronic conditions that negatively influence mobility are generally not aggressively addressed in the acute care environment. This information assists the physical therapist to prognosticate on

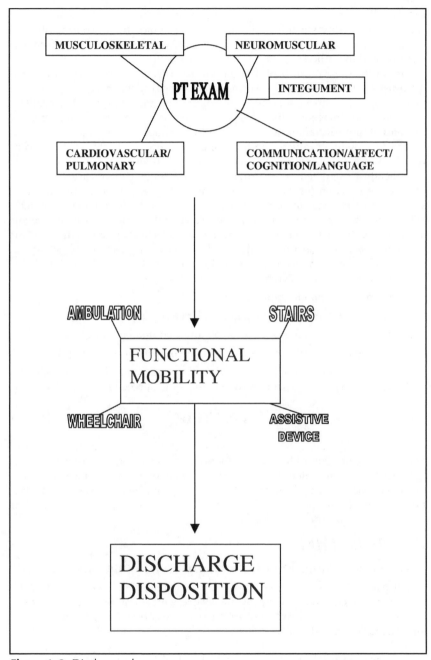

Figure 1–2. Discharge plan.

the rehabilitation potential and determine the discharge plan. A therapist must consider this reality when linking impairments to mobility in consideration of discharge recommendations. Figure 1–3 is provided to assist in the discharge decision-making process.

One of the great rewards of being a physical therapist is observing or assisting a patient with seemingly insurmountable impairments become more independently mobile through accurate diagnosis and interventions that facilitate a mutually advantageous discharge plan. The acute care physical therapist, in response to a physician order, must examine a patient, assess multiple aspects related to mobility, evaluate those findings, and prognosticate what interventions, if any, are required to achieve both short- and long-term goals. The acute care therapist is challenged to provide this efficacious patient care while integrating the function (or dysfunction) of multiple organ systems, medical and surgical interventions, and the physical demands of the hospital environment. When a patient has mobility dysfunction related to the current hospitalization or a chronic condition, the medical/surgical team looks to the physical therapist for recommendations regarding posthospital discharge disposition. Typical questions the physical therapist must respond to are:

- Is the patient safe to go home?
- Is inpatient rehabilitation required?
- How much therapy can the patient tolerate per day?
- If the patient is going home what adaptive equipment must be ordered?
- Is home physical therapy necessary or are outpatient services appropriate?

The previous information, the following case study, and subsequent chapters of this text will enable the acute care practitioner to succeed in this endeavor.

CASE STUDY

A 78-year-old female, Mrs. Carter, was admitted from the emergency room after her daughter found her on the floor of her apartment. Mrs. Carter was on the floor for approximately 15 hours. After evaluation in the emergency department, she is admitted to the hospital for medical management of severe dehydration, presumed syncope, and ECG changes. Two days after admission, a physical therapy consult is ordered because of her fall.

Patient/Client History

General Demographics/Social History/Living Environment

The patient lives alone in a third floor apartment with a working elevator. She has two daughters who visit approximately every other day. She reports that her apartment is on one level and there are four steps to enter the apartment building and a handrail on both sides.

General Health Status/Family History

Patient appears overweight and denies smoking or alcohol use. She does not consider herself active but states "I get along all right by myself." Her hobbies

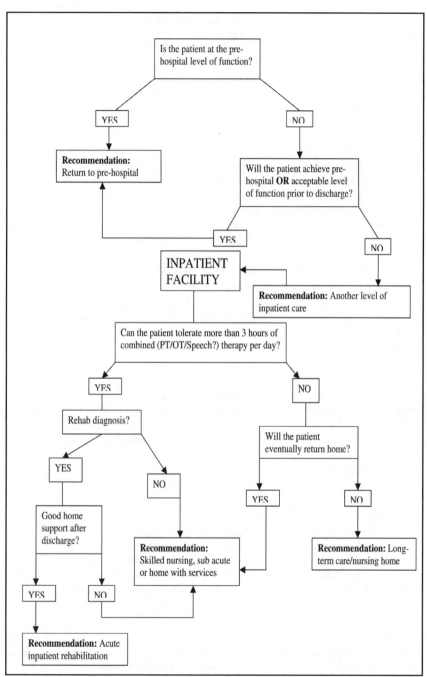

Figure 1–3. Discharge plan decision-making flow chart.

include being active in her church and knitting. Her family history is unremarkable and unrelated to the current condition.

Medical/Surgical History

The patient is diagnosed with noninsulin dependent diabetes mellitus (NIDDM), hypertension (HTN), and acute renal failure (ARF). She takes Glipizide (Glucotrol) for her diabetes and Metoprolol (a beta blocker) for HTN. Surgical history is noncontributory.

Current Conditions/Chief Complaints

The patient is status post falling at home. There was no LOC. Injuries diagnosed upon arrival to the hospital include a left flank hematoma, dehydration, and her resting ECG reveals atrial fibrillation with a ventricular response of approximately 100 to 110. She was transferred to the general care ward on 2 liters of oxygen via nasal cannula, with a foley catheter and a right UE intravenous catheter. Her activity status is OOB as tolerated and full weightbearing (FWB).

Functional Status and Activity Level

Prior to admission the patient was independent with all aspects of mobility, ADLs, and IADLs without the use of an assistive device except for food shopping and paying her bills. Her daughters assist her with shopping, financial management, and cleaning the apartment. She reports being able to walk approximately two blocks before she feels fatigued.

Other Clinical Tests

Clinical laboratory data upon admission is normal except: CBC reveals an elevated hematocrit 51% and leukocytosis (elevated white blood cells [WBC]) 13,500/–mm^3. The electrolyte/chemistry panel reveals an elevated sodium (Na$^+$) 152 mEq/L, fasting blood glucose of 201 mg/dL, and creatinine of 1.8 mg/dL.

Systems Review

Cardiovascular/Pulmonary

Resting BP is 108/78, HR 108 (atrial fibrillation per telemetry), pulse is weak/thready (1+) and irregularly irregular, and SpO$_2$ 97% on 2 liters per minute (lpm). Breath sounds are diminished bilateral bases, and otherwise clear to auscultation (CTA). After sitting at the edge of the bed, standing and transferring to a bedside chair, her vital signs are: BP 102/68, HR 146, SpO$_2$ 94%. Patient reports feeling fatigued but denies lightheadedness. Vital signs return to baseline after 10 minutes.

Integument

Mrs. Carter appears overweight and there are no observed sores or skin lesions. She has been wearing pneumatic compression stockings on both LEs

Musculoskeletal

Gross examination of bilateral upper extremities (BUEs)/lower extremities (LEs) reveals strength of 5/5 and active range of motion (AROM) appears within normal limits (WNL).

Neuromuscular

Sensation to light touch and gross proprioception are intact throughout. Patient reports "tingling" sensation of her distal bilateral lower extremities (BLEs). She reports this is "the way it's been for several years."

Communication, Affect, Cognition, Language, and Learning Style

Mrs. Carter is awake, alert, and oriented to person, place, and time. She reports feeling anxious about moving because of the fear of falling again. Her primary language is English.

Tests and Measures

Aerobic Capacity and Endurance

As noted above, the patient demonstrated a significant HR response to standing at the bedside with minimal change in BP or SpO_2.

Assistive and Adaptive Devices

Patient was assisted into a standing position with use of a rolling walker. The physical therapist was not going to use a walker initially, but Mrs. Carter requested a mobility aid because she is afraid. The patient was able to assist with bed mobility by grabbing the bedrails. The nursing staff has ordered a bedside commode.

Gait, Locomotion, and Balance

The patient required minimal assistance to transition from supine<>sitting at the edge of the bed and minimal assistance to complete the sit<>stand transfer and maintained abbreviated standing with a rolling walker and supervision. A gait assessment was not performed at this time due to her dramatic HR and blunted BP responses with standing and transferring from the bed>chair.

Pain

Mrs. Carter c/o discomfort along her left flank and using a visual analogue scale she reports the pain is 3/10 pain at rest (aching) and 4/10 (sharp) with moving. Subjectively, she states it's "not too bad" and the pain diminishes with rest.

Evaluation

The patient is an elderly female currently hospitalized secondary to a fall at home. The etiology of the fall is multifactorial. She has been admitted with a medical history including dehydration, atrial fibrillation, and diabetes mellitus. These processes can increase her risk of falling due to reduced blood volume and a decreased cardiac output with resultant hypotension. Additionally, sensory changes are noted in BLE. She denies fainting or a LOC but did report feeling "funny" for several hours prior to the fall.

Diagnosis

The patient presents with mobility impairments related primarily to atrial fibrillation (AF) with a rapid ventricular response and a blunted BP response. She reports moderate pain with movement. Her laboratory values confirm the renal insufficiency, resolving dehydration and diabetes (now insulin dependent). Her neuromuscular, musculoskeletal, and integumentary examination is unremarkable except for the sensory deficits. Recommended treatment pattern 6A: primary prevention/risk reduction for cardiovascular/pulmonary disorders.[1]

Prognosis

The patient will most likely return to independent mobility status with improved rate control of her atrial fibrillation, expansion of blood volume, and correction of abnormal electrolytes. These factors should improve her BP responses with activity. Per nursing, she requires supervision for the pharmacological management of her medical conditions. Social work has initiated nursing home placement while the family decides on discharge options. The patient will receive physical therapy two to three times a week with short-term goals of increasing OOB tolerance and decreasing level of assistance required for bedside mobilization, transfers, and ambulation. Interventions included ADL training (eg, bed mobility, transfers, toilet and gait training, wheelchair management), assistive and adaptive device training (eg, walker, reacher), therapeutic exercise (eg, UE/LE AROM and resistive exercises), education on use of blood sugar monitoring, bedside ROM exercise program, and review of prescribed medications.

Reexamination

Patient received a fluid bolus and she was encouraged to increase her free water consumption after the first physical therapy session secondary to mild orthostasis and readjustment of her cardiac medications. Reexamination the following day revealed a supervision level of assistance for OOB activities and ambulating 75 feet with an appropriate vital sign response including an elevation in HR, BP, and stable SpO_2 without complaint of cardiopulmonary symptoms.

Outcomes

The patient was treated for 3 days including the initial physical therapy examination. At this point she was independent with a rolling walker and she was discharged to her elder daughter's home. No physical therapy follow-up was recommended.

CHAPTER REVIEW QUESTIONS

1. What are the elements of the patient/client management as outlined in the *Guide to Physical Therapist Practice*?

2. What impact does the previous function, current medical and functional status, and future discharge destination have on the physical therapy examination?

3. What is the benefit of knowing the social and health habits of the patient when formulating the treatment plan?

4. Describe an algorithm that would assist the therapist in the discharge decision-making process.

5. What elements are involved in deciding if the patient is safe to go home?

REFERENCES

1. Guide to Physical Therapist Practice. 2nd ed. *Phys Ther.* 2001;81:9–744.

BIBLIOGRAPHY

Huether SE, McCance KL. *Understanding Pathophysiology.* St. Louis, Mo: Year Book Inc; 1996.

Jette AM. Physical disablement concepts for physical therapy research and practice. *Phys Ther.* 1994;74:380–386.

Rothstein JM, Echternach JL, Riddle DL. The Hypothesis-Oriented Algorithm for Clinician II (HOACII): a guide for patient management. *Phys Ther.* 2003; 83:455–470.

Seidel HM, Ball JW, Dains JE, Benedict GW. *Mosby's Guide to Physical Examination.* 5th ed. St. Louis, Mo: 2003.

CLINICAL LABORATORY VALUES AND DIAGNOSTIC TESTING

Daniel J. Malone, MPT, CCS
Lora Packel, MS, PT

Laboratory testing, sonagraphy, radiology, and nuclear imaging provide the medical and surgical practitioner with the information required to correctly diagnose, plan interventions, and monitor therapies provided to the patient. Although physical therapy practitioners rarely order specific diagnostic tests, the results will influence therapeutic interventions and the prognosis of our clients. The goal of this chapter is to present the most common laboratory testing and diagnostic examination procedures encountered by the acute care therapist and provide a background on the normal homeostatic mechanisms that form part of the foundation of diagnostic decision making. We will also describe common abnormalities and provide information on how perturbations influence the provision of physical therapy services.

Although a complete description of laboratory and diagnostic testing is beyond the scope of this text, additional information regarding organ- and disease-specific laboratory and diagnostic testing is included in the proceeding chapters of the text. Additionally, the reader should utilize many of the listed references for enhanced descriptions and supplementary information.

BLOOD CHEMISTRY TESTING

The survival of cells in the body is contingent upon tight regulation of electrolyte concentration and pH. Alterations in electrolytes, acid-base status, and fluid balance disrupt cellular functioning, impairing organ function, and can potentially lead to death.[1] The physical therapy practitioner must understand the mechanisms for maintenance of homeostasis as well as understand the pathophysiologic consequences associated with alterations of this dynamic environment. Fluid, electrolyte, and acid-base status are constantly disrupted, but the human body has extensive physiologic mechanisms to preserve homeostasis. Blood chemistry testing identifies many chemical blood constituents, and repeated testing is used

Table 2–1
COMMON SCREENING PROFILES

Group Heading	Routine Tests
Electrolyte panel (lytes)	Sodium (Na^+), potassium (K^+), chloride (Cl^-), carbon dioxide (CO_2), pH
Metabolic panel	Na^+, K^+, Cl^-, CO_2, glucose, blood urea nitrogen (BUN), creatinine
Kidney function	BUN, creatinine, creatinine clearance, glucose, calcium, CO_2
Liver function/hepatic panel	Total bilirubin, alkaline phosphatase, aspartate aminotransferase (AST), gamma glutamyl transferase (GGT), lactate dehydrogenase (LDH), prothrombin (PT), total protein, albumin
Cardiac markers (MI/CHF) (see Table 2–17)	Chemistry panel, cardiac troponins, creatine kinase (CK), MB, beta-type natriuretic peptide (BNP), C-reactive protein (CRP), homocysteines
Lipid panel (see Table 2–18)	Cholesterol, high-density lipoprotein (HDL), low-density lipoprotein (LDL), very low-density liproprotein (VLDL), triglycerides
Complete blood count (CBC) (see Tables 2–12 and 2–13)	Red blood cells (RBC), hemoglobin (Hb), hemotocrit (Hct), platelet count, white blood cells (WBC) and WBC differential

Adapted from Fischbach FT, Dunning MB. *A Manual of Laboratory and Diagnostic Tests.* Philadelphia, Pa: Lippincott Williams & Wilkins; 2004.

to establish patterns of abnormalities. Tests are diverse and can be grouped into "profiles," or tests that screen for certain conditions, or routine automated tests that screen the integrative organ systems of the body, termed standard panels, as listed in Table 2–1.

Fluid Balance/Body Water

The adult human body is composed of approximately 60% water (H_2O), and total body water (TBW) is primarily distributed in three compartments throughout the body as noted in Figure 2–1. These compartments include the intercellular (40%) and extracellular (20%). The extracellular fluid (ECF) compartment is further divided into the intravascular and interstitial compartments. The capillary walls of the blood vessels separate the blood plasma or the intravascular fluid volume (5%) from the interstitial (15%) fluids.[2] The interstitial fluid surrounds the cells of the tissues and organs of the body.

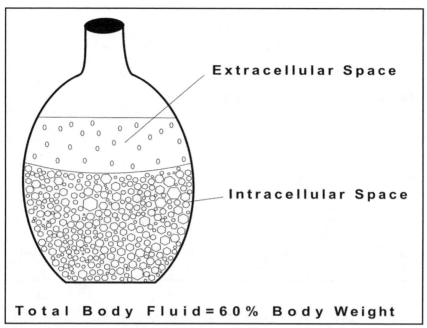

Figure 2–1. Fluid compartments. (Reprinted with permission from Baumberger-Henry M, *Fluids and Electrolytes*. Sudbury, Mass: Jones and Bartlett Publishers; 2004. Available at: www.jbpub.com.)

Osmosis and hydrostatic pressures primarily govern the movement of fluid between the body compartments. Osmosis is the movement of fluids across a semipermeable membrane. Fluids move from an area of high concentration to low concentration (concentration gradient). Hydrostatic pressure in the body refers to the pressure that a fluid exerts on a vessel wall. Water moves freely between the body fluid compartments, and the movement of water across cell membranes is due to hydrostatic pressures and osmotic pressures derived from the concentrations of ions of the body. The major ions of the body are potassium (K^+), sodium (Na^+), bicarbonate (HCO_3^-), chloride (Cl^-), calcium (Ca^{++}), magnesium (Mg), phosphate (P), and bicarbonate (Table 2–2). The intracellular fluid (ICF) compartment is maintained by the function of the Na^+–K^+ pumps embedded in the cell membrane. The action of this pump results in high concentrations of K^+ intracellularly and high concentrations of Na^+ extracellularly. The extracellular compartment is primarily a function of the concentrations of Na^+, HCO_3^-, and Cl^- and is regulated by kidney function.[2]

Movement of fluid across the capillary membrane is essential for the delivery of gasses (O_2 and CO_2) and nutrients. Movement is summarized by the Starling equation:

$$\text{fluid movement} = K_f[(P_c - P_i) - (\pi_c - \pi_i)]$$

Forces that promote the movement of fluid out of the intravascular compartment include vascular hydrostatic pressure (P_c) and interstitial oncotic/osmotic

---

Table 2–2
MAJOR CATIONS/ANIONS

	Extracellular	*Intracellular*
Cations	Na$^+$: 135 to 148 mEq/L Potassium: 3.5 to 5.3 mEq/L Calcium: 8.5 to 10.5 mg/dL; 4.5 to 5.5 mEq/L Magnesium: 1.8 to 2.7 mg/dL	Na$^+$: 10 to 14 mEq/L Potassium: 140 to 150 mEq/L Calcium: <1 mEq/L Magnesium: 40 mEq/L
Anions	Bicarbonate: 23 to 27 mEq/L Chloride: 98 to 106 mEq/L Phosphate: 2.5 to 4.5 mg/dL Proteins: 16 mEq/L Albumin: 3.5 to 5.5 mg/dL	Bicarbonate: 7 to 10 mEq/L Chloride: 3 to 4 mEq/L Phosphate: 40 to 85 mEq/L Proteins: 54 mEq/L

Adapted from Baumberger HM. *Fluids and Electrolytes.* Thorofare, NJ: SLACK Incorporated; ·2004.

---

pressures (π_i). Forces that promote the movement of fluid into the vasculature include interstitial hydrostatic pressures (P_i) and intravascular oncotic/osmotic pressures (π_c). Normally the forces promoting fluid efflux from vessels is greater at the arterial end of a capillary bed, while the forces promoting influx of fluid into the vasculature are higher at the venous end of the capillary network as noted in Figure 2–2. It is important that the physical therapy practitioner understand that alteration of these forces can result in many pathophysiologic sequlae of various diseases and disorders that are common to acute care practice as outlined in Table 2–3. Examples include pulmonary edema in congestive heart failure (CHF) (↑ vascular hydrostatic pressure promoting fluid efflux), ascites in liver failure (↑ vascular hydrostatic pressure, ↓ production of plasma proteins [albumin] decreasing intravascular osmotic pressures), or dehydration related to burns (↑ capillary permeability [↑ K_f]).[1]

Electrolyte Balance

The balance of electrolytes in the body is important for basic functioning including nerve conduction, muscle contraction and relaxation, cardiac rhythm and conduction, bone health, blood coagulation, and maintenance of proper fluid balance in the body. The balance of electrolytes and water is primarily under the control of the renal system although it is influenced by the neurologic, endocrine, gastrointestinal (GI), and musculoskeletal systems. Electrolyte disorders are among the most frequent and challenging problems facing acute care practitioners resulting in significant morbidity and mortality.[3]

Sodium (Na$^+$) is the principal positively charged electrolyte, or cation, of the extracellular compartment and is the primary determinant of the ECF volume.[4] The balance between body water and sodium are closely linked due to their osmotic relationships. Kidney function determines Na$^+$ concentrations, and

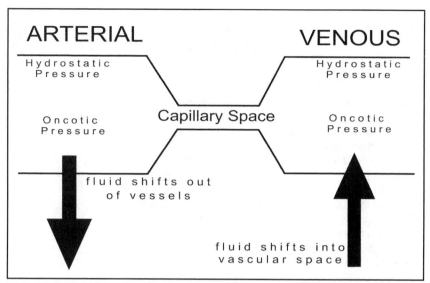

Figure 2–2. Fluid homeostasis. (Reprinted with permission from Baumberger-Henry M, *Fluids and Electrolytes.* Sudbury, Mass: Jones and Bartlett Publishers; 2004. Available at: www.jbpub.com.)

renal handling of Na^+ and H_2O is influenced by sympathetic tone, hormones including aldosterone ($\uparrow$ renal H_2O absorption), antidiuretic hormone (ADH or vasopressin) ($\uparrow$ renal H_2O excretion), and atrial natriuretic factor (ANF) ($\uparrow$ renal H_2O excretion) and medications, most notably diuretics ($\uparrow$ renal H_2O excretion).[3] The most common manifestations of Na^+ imbalance are neurologic symptoms including confusion, seizures, and coma as noted in Table 2–4. **Hyponatremia,** low Na^+ (<135 mEq/L), is more common in hospitalized elderly, and is associated with decreased Na^+ intake, excessive H_2O intake, increased Na^+ loss due to vomiting/GI suctioning/diarrhea/burns, excessive diuretic therapy, CHF, liver disease, and hormonal imbalances including hyperaldosteronism and syndrome of inappropriate ADH secretion (SIADH).[1,4,5] Common manifestations of hyponatremia include muscle weakness and twitching, confusion, headache, nausea, malaise, and fatigue.[1] **Hypernatremia,** excess Na^+ (>147 mEq/L), may result from dehydration or limited water intake or increased Na^+ intake with normal fluid volumes. Hypernatremia is also associated with surgery and febrile illnesses.[4] Elevated Na^+ concentrations draw water out of cells resulting in intracellular dehydration. Patients with normal fluid intake may have symptoms of **hypervolemia** (excess fluid in the extracellular spaces), including elevated BP, weight gain, venous distention, edema, and muscle weakness. Hypernatremia resulting from decreased water intake leads to **hypovolemia** creating postural hypotension, tachycardia, weak pulses, and confusion.

Potassium (K^+) is the most abundant cation within the intracellular fluid compartment. The major force that maintains K^+ inside cells is a negative voltage provided by the cell membrane $Na^+ – K^+$ pump.[2,6] This pump removes Na^+ and promotes the influx of K^+ against the respective concentration gradient,

Table 2-3
FLUID STATUS

Fluid Overload/Hypervolemia

Common Causes:
Excess intake:
- Excess IV fluids
- Hypertonic fluids
Inadequate Output:
- CHF
- Cirrhosis
- Renal insufficiency and failure/ nephrotic syndrome
- Hyperaldosteronism
- Low dietary protein
- Steroid use

Manifestations:
- Pitting peripheral edema
- Shortness of breath
- Anasarca
- Bounding pulse/jugular venous distension (JVD)
- Hypertension
- Tachycardia
- Moist crackles

Fluid Deficit/Dehydration/Hypovolemia

Common causes:
Limited oral intake:
- CVA, dementia, neglect
Excess Loss:
- Vomiting, diarrhea, nasogastric suction
- Diabetes mellitus, diabetes insipidus
- Burns
- Excessive sweating

Manifestations:
- Dry mucus membranes
- Poor skin turgor
- Postural hypotension/hypotension
- Tachycardia
- Tachypnea
- Oliguria
- Altered mental status

therefore requiring energy in the form of ATP. K^+ leakage out of the cell maintains the resting membrane potential that is of paramount importance for skeletal, cardiac, and smooth muscle contraction as well as nerve and cardiac action potential conduction. K^+ balance is important for normal functioning of multiple organ systems (Table 2–5). The major hormones promoting a shift of K^+ into cells are insulin and the catecholamines, norepinephrine and epinephrine. Long-term regulation of K^+ balance is under direct control of the kidneys.

Hypokalemia, low K^+ <3.5 mEq/L or potassium deficiency, usually occurs due to loss of body K^+, reduced intake, or increased cellular uptake. Cellular uptake of ECF K^+ results from alkalosis (hydrogen $[H^+]/K^+$ exchange) and excessive insulin administration. Reduced K^+ intake is associated with malnutrition. Loss of body K^+ occurs with diarrhea, vomiting, and GI drainage tubes. Enhanced renal excretion of K^+ lowers the body stores. Renal K^+ losses occur due to excessive aldosterone secretion, low plasma magnesium that stimulates renin and aldosterone release, and kidney diseases that increase renal flow rates and inhibit Na^+ reabsorbtion.[1] Hypokalemia creates hyperpolarization of cells.

Table 2–4
ELECTROLYTES: SODIUM

Hypernatremia (Na+ >147 mEq/L)

Common causes:
- Hypovolemia/poor water intake
- Excess Na+ intake/hypertonic IV solutions
- Severe vomiting
- CHF
- Renal insufficiency and failure
- Cushing's syndrome
- Diabetes insipidus

Manifestations:
- Irritability/agitation
- Seizure, coma
- Hypotension
- Tachycardia
- Weak, thready pulse
- Decreased urine output

Hyponatremia (Na+ <135 mEq/L)

Common causes:
Hypovolemic:
- Diuretic use
- GI loss
- Burns/wound drainage
- Adrenal insufficiency

Hypervolemia:
- Hypotonic IV fluids
- CHF
- Cirrhosis
- Renal failure
- SIADH (syndrome of inappropriate antidiuretic hormone)

Manifestations:
- Headache
- Lethargy, confusion
- Absent/diminished reflexes
- Seizures, coma
- Nausea/vomiting
- Diarrhea

Hypovolemic Hyponatremia:
- Poor skin turgor
- Dry mucus membranes
- Orthostatic hypotension/tachycardia/ weak pulse

Hypervolemia Hyponatremia:
- Hypertension, tachycardia
- Pitting edema

As potassium moves out of the cells, to correct ECF hypokalemia, the membrane potential becomes more negative. This decreases the excitability of cells, necessitating greater stimuli for formation of action potentials. The clinical manifestations of hypokalemia include muscle weakness and conduction abnormalities including delayed repolarization. The most common dysrhythmias include sinus bradycardia, atrial tachycardia, atrioventricular block, and ventricular tachycardia and fibrillation.[1]

Hyperkalemia, elevated K+ >5.5 mEq/L, is rare due to efficient renal excretion and cellular uptake. Common causes of hyperkalemia include enhanced K+ intake combined with renal insufficiency, and shifts of K+ from the ICF to the ECF due to cellular damage, hypoxia, acidosis, insulin deficiency, muscle damage including crush injuries and burns, and medications including heparin, potassium sparing diuretics, nonsteroidal anti-inflammatory drugs (NSAIDs),

---

Table 2–5
ELECTROLYTES: POTASSIUM

Hyperkalemia (K+ >5.5 mEq/L)

Common Causes:
Impaired excretion:
- Renal failure
- Metabolic acidosis, diabetic ketoacidosis (DKA)
- Addison's disease
- Potassium-sparing diuretics, NSAIDs, ACE inhibitors

Excessive intake:
- Oral potassium supplements
- Blood transfusions
- Excessive IV administration

Manifestations:
- Muscle weakness, flaccid paralysis
- Paresthesias
- Bradycardia, heart block, venticular fibrillation
- Cardiac arrest

Hypokalemia (K+ <3.5 mEq/L)

Common causes:
Excessive loss:
- Diarrhea, vomiting
- GI losses/nasogastric suction
- Diuretics
- Cushing syndrome, steroid use

Inadequate intake:
- Malnutrition/restrictive diets
- Alcoholism
- Inadequate IV replacement

Manifestations:
- Extremity weakness
- Hyporeflexia
- Paresthesias
- Leg cramps
- ECG changes (ST depression, T wave inversion, U waves), dysrhythmias, cardiac arrest
- Hypotension
- Diminished bowel function, constipation, abdominal distension, paralytic ileus

---

angiotensin converting enzyme (ACE) inhibitors, and beta blockers.[3–5] Hyperkalemia produces partial depolarization (hypopolarization) of cell membranes, reducing the overall negative intracellular voltage making it harder to bring a cell to threshold. This can manifest in many ways including muscle weakness and cardiac conduction abnormalities including sinus bradycardia and potentially ventricular fibrillation and cardiac arrest.[1,5]

Calcium (Ca++) ions play major roles in bone formation, cell division and growth, blood coagulation, muscle contraction, and release of neurotransmitters.[2] The majority of calcium, 99%, is stored in bone and teeth, while the remainder is found in two forms: ionized or free Ca^{++} and calcium bound to albumin. Serum levels of free Ca^{++} are normally 4.5 to 5.5 mEq/L and total Ca^{++} levels are 8.5 to 10 mg/dL.[7,8] The amount of Ca^{++} absorbed by the GI tract, the amount of the Ca^{++} excreted by the kidneys, and Ca^{++} mobilized from bone determine total body calcium. Ca^{++} homeostasis is determined by the integrated regulation of

Ca^{++} flux in the GI, renal, and skeletal systems, determined by the interactions of three hormones: parathyroid (PTH) hormone ($\uparrow$ ECF Ca^{++}), calcitonin ($\downarrow$ ECF Ca^{++}), and calcitriol/vitamin D ($\uparrow$ ECF Ca^{++})[7] (see Chapter 10).

Hypercalcemia may result from hyperparathyroidism, cancers involving bone, PTH-like secreting tumors, sarcoidosis, and respiratory acidosis. Common symptoms of hypercalcemia include drowsiness, fatigue, weakness, lethargy, nausea, and constipation.

Hypocalcemia is loss or efflux of Ca^{++} from the ECF and is associated with hypoparathyroidism, respiratory alkalosis, limited Ca^{++} intake, rhabdomyolysis, chronic renal insufficiency, malignancy, and disorders that impair GI absorption including vitamin D deficiency and pancreatitis (Table 2–6).[1,7] Patients with hypocalcemia will show signs of enhanced neuromuscular excitability resulting in tetany accompanied by muscular twitching and potentially convulsions. Common symptoms include numbness, tingling, fatigue, and hyperreflexia.[7] Additionally, patients may complain of abdominal cramping and hyperactive bowel sounds. ECG abnormalities include a prolonged QT interval potentially enhancing the risk of developing a life-threatening dysrhythmia.[1]

Phosphate is necessary for bone formation, and 85% of the body's stores are within the skeletal system. The remainder of phosphate is necessary for acid-base balance and the storage and transfer of energy. Normal phosphate levels are 2.4 to 4.8 mg/dL and abnormalities in serum phosphate are usually inversely related to calcium levels. **Hyperphosphatemia** is associated with renal failure and uremia, hypocalcemia, hypoparathyroidism, and chemotherapies. Symptoms typically reflect the simultaneous hypocalcemia. **Hypophosphatemia** is associated with hypercalcemia, hyperparathyroidism, possible complications of diabetes management, mental status changes, bone and muscle pain, neuromuscular irritability, seizures, and tremors (Table 2–7).[7]

Chloride (Cl^-) is the major anion of the ECF and its movements within the fluid compartments are primarily tied to Na^+ to maintain electroneutrality. Additionally, it is important for fluid balance and acid base status. **Hypochloremia**, chloride concentrations <104 mEq/L, usually results from GI loss including severe vomiting and diarrhea, burns and acidosis, and is often associated with hyponatremia.[1,5] **Hyperchloremia**, elevated chloride >110 mEq/L, is associated with hypernatremia, dehydration, hyperventilation, and anemia (Table 2–8).[1,5]

Magnesium is the fourth most abundant cation in the body and is primarily concentrated in bone and muscle (Table 2–9). It is essential for the use of adenosine triphosphate (ATP) for energy and is necessary for the action of numerous enzyme systems including carbohydrate metabolism, protein synthesis, and muscular contraction. Normal serum levels of magnesium are 1.8 to 2.7 mEq/L and account for only 1% of total body stores. Magnesium is obtained in the diet and absorbed through the GI tract, and the kidneys primarily regulate its concentration in the body. **Hypomagnesemia** (<1.8 mEq/L; symptoms <1.0 mEq/L) resembles hypocalcemia with patients presenting with increased neuromuscular excitability, hyperactive deep tendon reflexes, and tetany.[5] Hypomagnesemia is observed in chronic alcoholism, eating disorders, and may be associated with increased urinary excretion as seen with diabetic crisis. **Hypermagnesemia** (>2.7 mEq/L) is relatively rare, but occurs in the aged and critically ill patients

---

Table 2-6
ELECTROLYTES: CALCIUM

Hypercalcemia (Ca++ >10.5 mg/dL or <5.5 mEq/L)

Common causes:

Excessive Intake or Release:
- Calcium antacids/supplements
- Bone destruction (eg, tumor/ immobilization/bed rest/ trauma/multiple fractures)
- Excess vitamin D
- Cancer (lung, breast, ovary, prostate, GI, leukemia)

Inadequate Excretion:
- Renal failure
- Thiazide diuretics
- Increased parathyroid hormone
- Hypophosphatemia

Manifestations:
- Ventricular dysrhythmias/bradyarrythmias/heart block/asystole
- Stupor/coma
- Lethargy
- Muscle weakness
- Diminished reflexes
- Constipation
- Nausea, vomiting
- Renal calculi

Hypocalcemia Ca++ <8.5 mg/dL or <4.5 mEq/L)

Common causes:

Inadequate Intake:
- Alcoholism
- Poor dietary intake
- Limited GI absorption/chronic diarrhea

Excessive Loss:
- Hypoparathryoidism
- Renal failure
- Hyperphosphatemia
- Pancreatitis
- Laxatives

Manifestations:
- Anxiety, confusion, irritability
- Seizures
- Cardiac dysrhythmias (eg, prolonged QT interval)
- Fatigue
- Numbness/tingling
- Hyperreflexia
- Muscle cramps/tetany

---

and is frequently encountered in patients with renal insufficiency and failure.[4,5] Patients may present with lethargy, dysarthria, hypoactive deep tendon reflexes, and hypotension.

Acid-Base Balance

Acid-base balance describes the equilibrium in ECF between substances that release H^+ ions (acids) and those capable of accepting H^+ (alkalines or bases). The concentration of H^+ is described by pH in an inverse relationship; the greater the pH, the less H^+ in the ECF.[2,9] Virtually all cells, tissues, and organs of the body are sensitive to pH, and life cannot exist outside of a range of body fluid pH from 6.8 to 7.8.[2] Acids and bases are ingested in the diet or produced by cellular processes and metabolism continuously. However, the body has developed

Table 2–7

ELECTROLYTES: PHOSPHATE (2.4 TO 4.8 MG/DL)

Hyperphosphatemia (<2.4 mg/dL)

See Hypocalcemia.

Hypophosphatemia (>4.8 mg/dL)

See Hypercalcemia.

multiple buffering mechanisms that maintain pH in a narrow range. Buffers act like a sponge and absorb excess acids (H$^+$ ions or base [OH])without significant changes in pH. Common endogenous buffers include bicarbonate, hemoglobin, phosphate, and plasma proteins. Ultimately, the respiratory and renal systems maintain the acid-base status of the body. For example, increased ventilation (hyperventilation) will lower arterial carbon dioxide, which increases the pH; decreased production of renal bicarbonate due to kidney disease will result in metabolic acidosis.

Acid-base imbalances can be either acidosis or alkalosis and may be of respiratory, metabolic, or mixed origin (Tables 2–10 and 2–11).[1,5] **Acidosis** is either a loss of base or excess acid, while **alkalosis** is either excess base or loss of acid. Respiratory-initiated imbalances are compensated by the kidneys by producing more acidic or basic urine, and metabolic abnormalities are compensated by the respiratory system by varying the rate and depth of breathing.[1]

Normal arterial **carbon dioxide (CO_2)** is 35 to 45 mmHg (torr) and is the primary regulator of ventilation. A rise in CO_2 stimulates the central chemoreceptors of the medullary respiratory center resulting in an increase in ventilation and subsequent reductions in the **partial pressure of arterial CO_2 ($PaCO_2$)**. Arterial CO_2 <35 mmHg due to increased alveolar ventilation is termed **hyperventilation** and is commonly associated with nervousness, anxiety, panic, pain, pregnancy, and pulmonary emboli. Elevated pH associated with a reduced Pa CO_2 is termed **respiratory alkalosis** and patients will present with dizziness, confusion, paresthesias, and potentially convulsions and coma.[1,9] Common causes of elevated CO_2 due to reduced alveolar ventilation, **hypoventilation**, are obstructive lung diseases (emphysema, chronic bronchitis, asthma flare), pneumonia, thoracic or abdominal surgery, kyphoscoliosis, respiratory insufficiency, sleep apnea, head trauma, anesthesia, and depression of the respiratory center related to oversedation or anesthetics, alcohol, and drug use, specifically barbiturates. These conditions may lead to a reduced pH, **respiratory acidosis**, and an elevation in $PaCO_2$. Common manifestations of respiratory acidosis include restlessness followed by lethargy, muscle twitching, tremors, convulsions, and coma.[1,9]

The primary metabolic buffer is bicarbonate, HCO_3^-, and its excretion and reabsorption is dictated by renal function. **Metabolic acidosis** is a deficit of HCO_3^- and is associated with renal failure and uremia, diabetic ketoacidosis, lactic acidosis, diarrhea, and hypoxia. Loss of normal metabolic acids, specifically gastric acids induced by severe vomiting, can lead to **metabolic alkalosis**.

Table 2–8
ELECTROLYTES: CHLORIDE (104 TO 110 MEQ/L)

Hyperchloremia (>110 mEq/L)

Common causes:
Increased intake/exchange:
- High salt diet without water
- Hypertonic IV solutions
- Metabolic acidosis

Decreased Loss:
- Hyperparathyroidism
- Hyperaldosteronism
- Renal failure

Manifestations:
- Lethargy/reduced level of consciousness
- Weakness
- Edema
- Tachypnea, dyspnea
- Hypertension/tachycardia

Hyperchloremia (<104 mEq/L)

Common causes:
Decreased intake:
- Low salt diet
- Water intoxication

Increased Loss:
- Diuresis
- Excessive vomiting/nasogastric suction/ileostomy/diarrhea

Manifestations:
- Agitation/irritability
- Hypertonicity/hyperreflexia
- Cramping/twitching/tetany

Other causes of this base excess include hyperaldosteronism and diuretics. Patients may present with weakness and muscle cramps, hyperreflexia, tetany, confusion, convulsions, and dysrhythmias including atrial tachycardia.

LABORATORY TESTS AND MEASURES

Hematology Studies

Blood is a specialized connective tissue consisting of cells and plasma. The plasma, the fluid component of blood, contains the plasma proteins, lipids, vitamins, amino acids, and hormones.[10] The **complete blood count (CBC)** evaluates the different cellular components of blood including the RBC, WBC, and platelets (PLT). The CBC is a simple blood draw from a peripheral vein. A CBC with differentials breaks down these cells to look more closely at their component parts. Erythrocyte indices include the mean corpuscular volume, MCV, and mean corpuscular hemoglobin (Hb) concentration, MCH. WBC differential includes the five types of WBCs including neutrophils, eosinophils, basophils, lymphocytes, and monocytes.

To understand the CBC, one must first start with an overview of hematopoesis, or the formation of the blood cells. In adults, hematopoesis begins in the bone marrow and certain components mature in the thymus gland. All blood cells

Table 2–9
ELECTROLYTES: MAGNESIUM (1.8 TO 2.7 MEQ/L)

Hypermagnesemia (>2.7 mEq/L)

Common causes:
Increased intake:
- Increased intake with antacids, lithium, magnesium sulfate medications

Decreased loss:
- Renal failure
- Adrenal insufficiency
- Leukemia
- Hyperparathryoidism
- Dehydration

Manifestations:
- Diaphoresis/warm, flushed appearance
- Nausea/vomiting
- Drowsiness/lethargy
- Weakness/flaccidity
- Diminished deep tendon reflexes
- Hypotension/bradycardia/heart block

Hypomagnesemia (<1.8 mEq/L, Symptoms <1.0 mEq/L)

Common causes:
Decreased intake:
- Alcoholism
- Eating disorders (bulimia/anorexia)
- Hyperalimentation

Increased loss:
- Diuresis
- Primary aldosteronism
- DKA
- Medications: aminoglycosides, amphotericin, cisplatin

Manifestations:
- Neuromuscular irritability/hyperrelfexia/tremors/twitching/spasticity
- Seizures
- Nystagmus
- ECG changes:
  - ➤ Prolonged PR/QT intervals and QRS complex, flattened T waves
  - ➤ Ventricular dysrhythmias (PVC, VT, VF), supraventricular tachycardia (SVT)
- Emotional lability

develop from a pleuripotent stem cell. This stem cell, as it matures, differentiates and is committed to one of three cell types: RBC, WBC, or PLT.

The erythrocyte or RBC's primary functions are the delivery of oxygen to tissues, the uptake of cellular metabolic byproducts, specifically CO_2 and H^+, and maintenance of acid-base balance. Normal RBC values vary depending on the type of sample, age, and sex. Generally, the RBC count, or erythrocyte count, is performed to calculate indices, the MCV (RBC size) and MCH (Hb content) for further classification of specific anemias.[11] The **hematocrit** (hct) is a measurement of the percentage of whole blood occupied by cells. Normal hct is 42% to 52% for males and 36% to 48% for females.[11] RBCs contain Hb, an iron-containing protein, which has a strong affinity for oxygen. Normal hemoglobin concentrations for adult males are 14 to 18 g/dL and for females 12 to 16 g/dL. A single RBC contains four Hb molecules, and when fully saturated, can carry four molecules of oxygen for a total oxygen content of approximately 20 mL/dL of blood.[12] RBCs last 120 days in the bloodstream and are removed by macrophages

Table 2–10	
ACID-BASE/ARTERIAL BLOOD GAS ANALYSIS	
Acid/base balance (pH)	7.35 to 7.45
Partial pressure of oxygen (PaO_2)	80 to 100 mmHg
Partial pressure of carbon dioxide ($PaCO_2$)	35 to 45 mmHg
Bicarbonate (HCO_3^-)	22 to 28 mEq

in the liver and spleen. Hypoxia due to pulmonary disease, heart failure, severe anemia, or altitude may upregulate RBC production in response to the production of the hormone **erythropoietin** made by the kidneys. Erythropoietin signals the stem cells to produce more RBCs thus increasing the body's capabilities of delivering oxygen.

Polycythemia, the compensatory increase in RBC production, may be relative due to a reduction of plasma volume as seen in dehydration, severe vomiting, or fluid loss due to extensive burns, or may be absolute, due to enhanced bone marrow production of RBC, **polycythemia vera.**[11] **Anemia**, a decrease in the number of erythrocytes, low hemoglobin concentrations, or both is demonstrated by a reduced hct, Hb concentration, and erythrocyte count. Anemia is generally classified as:

- Hypoproliferative anemia due to defective red cell production (eg, deficiencies in iron [microcytic/hypochromic anemia], folate, vitamins B12 [pernicious anemia] or B6, bone marrow failure [aplastic anemia])
- Anemia due to loss of RBC (eg, trauma, hemorrhage, GI bleeding)
- Hemolytic anemia resulting in excessive RBC destruction (hemolysis)[13]

As the primary function of RBCs is to deliver oxygen to tissues, low levels can certainly impact a person's ability to participate in therapy. Therapists should reduce the intensity and duration of exercise programs to accommodate for lower levels of hemoglobin as noted in Table 2–12. Therapists should monitor for signs and symptoms of hypoxia such as:

- Chest pain/pressure
- Dizziness
- SOB or DOE
- Muscle cramping

Polycythemia is usually well tolerated, but therapists should consider the associated increased viscosity of blood increasing myocardial oxygen demand in those patients with cardiac disease and the potential reduced peripheral blood flow in patients with vascular disease.

WBCs', or **leukocytes',** primary function is to fight infection. If a CBC with differential is ordered, you will receive information on the five types of WBCs including neutrophils, eosinophils, basophils, lymphocytes, and monocytes as outlined in Table 2–12.

Table 2–11
ACID-BASE DISORDERS

Respiratory Acidosis
(pH <7.35, PaCO$_2$ >45 mmHg, HCO$_3^-$ normal or >27 mEq/L)

Common causes:
- Obstructive airways disease
- Thoracic trauma/incision pain
- Medication/drug overdose

Manifestations:
- Irritability, lethargy
- Headache
- Tremors
- Muscle twitching
- Vertigo
- Tachycardia
- Peripheral vasodilation

Respiratory Alkalosis
(pH >7.45, PaCO$_2$ <35 mmHg, HCO$_3^-$ normal or >27 mEq/L)

Common causes:
- Pain
- Fever
- Hyperthyroidism
- Meningitis
- Brain tumor
- Psychogenic

Manifestations:
- Convulsions
- Coma
- Numbness/tingling
- Lightheadedness/dizziness
- Sweating
- palpitations

Metabolic Acidosis
(pH <7.35, PaCO$_2$ normal or <, HCO$_3^-$ <23 mEq/L)

Common causes:
- Chronic diarrhea
- Shock/sepsis
- Trauma
- DKA (diabetic ketoacidosis)
- Renal failure/uremia

Manifestations:
- Stupor/coma
- Headache
- Malaise/fatigue
- Weakness
- Decreased cardiac contractility/ decreased cardiac output
- Dysrhythmias
- Hyperkalemia

Metabolic Alkalosis
(pH >7.45, PaCO$_2$ >normal or <, HCO$_3^-$ >27 mEq/L)

Common causes:
- Severe vomiting/nasogastric suction
- Excessive use of antacids
- Diuretics
- Hypokalemia
- Hyperaldosteronism

Manifestations:
- Seizures
- Confusion
- Neuromuscular irritability/ hyperreflexia/tingling
- Tetany
- Respiratory insufficiency

Table 2–12
COMMON HEMATOLOGY STUDIES

Blood Component and Indices	Normal Values	Common Abnormalities/ Diseases/Disorders
RBCs	• Men: 4.2 to 5.4 x 10^6/mm^3 • Women: 3.6 to 5.0 x 10^6/mm^3	**Anemia:** ↓ RBC, Hb, and/or Hct Normal MCV: hemolytic anemia, posthemorrhagic anemia, aplastic anemia
• Mean corpuscular volume (MCV)	• 84 to 99 μm^3	↓ MCV: microcytic anemia (eg, iron deficiency, chronic disease)
• Mean copuscular hemoglobin (MCH)	• 5 to 25 pg/cell	↑MCV: macrocytic anemia (eg, vitamin B12 deficiency, intrinsic factor deficiency, ileal
• Mean corpuscular hemoglobin con-centration (MCHC)	• 20 to 30 g/dL	resection, pancreatic disease, neoplastic disease, hyperthy-roidism, alcoholism)
Hematocrit (Hct)	• Men: 42 to 52% • Women: 36 to 48%	**Polycythemia** (↑ RBC): renal cancer, hepatocellular cancers, lung disease, altitude
Hemoglobin (Hb)	• Men: 14 to 17.4 g/dL • Women: 12 to 16 g/dL	↑ **Hb:** COPD, CHF, polycythemia, altitude
WBC • Neutrophil		**Leukocytosis:** WBC >11,000/ mm^3
	• 4 to 10,000/ mm^3	• Infection, leukemia/ myeloproliferative disorders, malignant neoplasms, trauma/surgery
• Basophil	• ~50% of WBC; 3000 to 7000/ mm^3	**Leukopenia:** WBC <4,000/mm^3
• Eosinophil	• 0 to 1% of total WBC; 15 to 50/ mm^3	• Viral infections, chemo-therapy, aplastic anemia **Neutropenia:** <40% or <1800/ mm^3;
• Monocyte	• 0 to 3% of total WBC; 0 to 0.7 x 10^9/L	• Stem cell disorders/over-whelming bacterial or viral infections, ionizing radiation,
• Lymphocyte	• 3% to 7% or total WBC; 100 to 500/mm^3	hypersensitivity reactions

(continued)

Table 2–12 (continued)		
COMMON HEMATOLOGY STUDIES		
Blood Component and Indices	*Normal Values*	*Common Abnormalities/ Diseases/Disorders*
Platelets	• 25% to 40% of total WBC; 1500 to 4000 cells/mm^3 • 140 to 400 x 10^3/mm^3	**Thrombcytopenia:** <140 x 10^3/mm^3 • Idiopathic thrombocytopenia purpura, anemias, CHF, renal insufficiency, sepsis, prosthetic heart valve, hemorrhage, acute/chronic myelogenous leukemia, drug interaction **Thrombocytosis:** >400 x 10^3/mm^3

Granulocytes

- **Neutrophils**: Kill bacteria by phagocytosis and make up 58% of WBC.
- **Eosinophils**: Kill parasites and play a role in allergic disorders. Eosinophils comprise 2% of WBCs.
- **Basophils:** Play a role in some allergies, are responsible for the release of histamine and heparin, and are approximately 1% of WBCs.

Agranulocytes

- **Monocytes**: Differentiate into **macrophages** in tissues and ingest bacteria by phagocytosis. Monocytes are found primarily in the liver, spleen, lungs, and lymph nodes and are responsible for destroying old or damaged cells in the body. Monocytes make up 4% of WBCs.
- **Lymphocytes**: Consist of T lymphocytes and B lymphocytes.
  - o **T lymphocytes** are responsible for cell-mediated immunity. They begin their maturation in the bone marrow and complete differentiation in the thymus gland.
  - o **Helper T** cells help orchestrate the immune response via the use of cytokine messengers. These cells stimulate B cells to form antibodies, stimulate production of cytotoxic T cells, and activate macrophages.
  - o **Cytotoxic T** cells release chemicals that break open cells and kill organisms.
  - o **Memory T** cells preserve a memory of previous antigens. When that antigen is reintroduced into the body, memory T cells accelerate the immune response and direct antibodies specific to the offending bacteria/virus.

- o **Suppressor T** cells modulate the intensity of the immune response.
- o **B lymphocytes** are responsible for humoral immunity by producing antibodies. B cells make up 33% of WBCs.

A high WBC count, **leukocytosis,** can indicate infection, inflammation, or rapid abnormal proliferation of WBC as seen in leukemia. A low WBC, **leuko-penia**, indicates a compromised immune system as a result of chemotherapy, radiation, or hematologic disorders. Exercise intensity and duration may need to be modified or withheld during fever depending on the clinical stability of the patient. If a patient has a low WBC, take caution to avoid infectious exposures. Hand washing, wearing masks, and cleaning exercise equipment will help prevent infections.

Platelets

Platelets (PLT) are cytoplasmic fragments of megakaryocytes in the bone marrow. PLT are an essential component of hemostasis, the arrest of bleeding, and initiate the clotting mechanism (Figure 2–3).[10] PLT adhere to disruptions of the endothelial lining of a wound and to each other, forming a platelet plug. PLT release multiple vasoactive substances that promote the aggregation and activation of other PLT to increase the size of the platelet plug. Factors from the blood plasma, PLT, and damaged blood vessels promote the sequential activation of approximately 13 plasma proteins, giving rise to a polymer, fibrin, that forms a network of fibers trapping red cells, leukocytes, and PLT to form a blood clot, or thrombus.[10,12] Many of these factors require calcium for activation. The blood clotting cascade is composed of an intrinsic and an extrinsic pathway, which both converge to produce fibrin as outlined in Figure 2–3.

Normal platelet values in adults are 140 to $400,000/mm^3$ as noted in Table 2–12. **Thrombocytopenia,** or platelet count below $140,000/mm^3$ of blood, can result from:

- Decreased production of PLT (eg, bone marrow depression/leukemia, cytoxic drugs)
- Increased destruction of PLT (eg, **idiopathic thrombocytopenia purpura [ITP]**), DIC, drug reaction (eg, penicillin, digoxin, sulfonamides)
- Aggregation of PLT in the microvasculature (eg, **thrombotic thrombocytopenic purpura [TTP]**)[1,10]

Patients with thrombocytopenia are at an increase risk for bleeding and may present with petechia, epistaxis, purpura, and menorrhagia.[1] Physical therapists treating patients who are thrombocytopenic should take precautions to avoid activities that might cause bruising or loss of balance and falls as noted in Table 2–13. Closer monitoring for bleeding and bruising during all activities may be important. Caution should be taken when prescribing resistive exercise or weight training in the person with low PLT to avoid intramuscular bleeding. Finally, avoidance of valsalva is important, as small blood vessels in the eyes and nose may burst causing bleeding.

Thrombocytosis is defined as a platelet count greater than $400,000/mm^3$ and is commonly encountered as a response to stress, infection and inflammation, trauma, exercise, and ovulation. This may also be encountered as a consequence

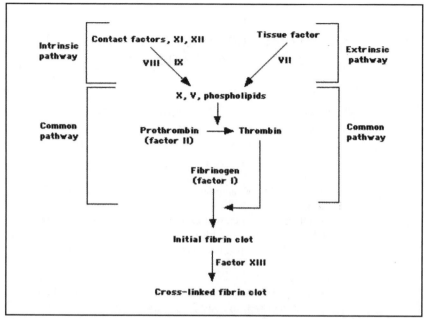

Figure 2–3. Simplified diagram of clotting cascade highlighting the clotting factors of the intrinsic, extrinsic, and common pathways. (Adapted from Rose BD, ed. *UpToDate*. Wellesley, Mass: UpToDate; 2006.)

of splenectomy, rheumatoid arthritis, and cancer.[1] Thrombocytosis may be associated with increased thrombus formation and paradoxically an increased risk of bleeding.[11]

There are simple blood tests to determine the functioning of the clotting cascade and to pinpoint specific deficiencies for a targeted treatment as noted in Table 2–14. **Bleeding time** measures platelet functioning by determining the time it takes for a blood clot to form from a punctured capillary. The duration of bleeding depends on the quantity and quality of PLT and the ability of the vessel to constrict. Normal bleeding time is 3 to 10 minutes and bleeding after 15 minutes is highly significant. **Prothrombin time (PT)** tests the functioning of the extrinsic system of the clotting cascade. Specifically, it evaluates the efficacy of fibrinogen (which converts to fibrin to stabilize the clot), PT (converts to thrombin), Factor V, Factor VII, and Factor X.[6] If any of these factors are malfunctioning, the PT will be prolonged, indicating that blood will take longer to clot. The PT is measured by taking venous blood and adding substances to initiate the extrinsic pathway of the clotting cascade. The time it takes to form a clot, measured in seconds, is the PT. Normal PT is 11 to 13.5 seconds.

The **partial thromboplastin time (PTT)** is another test to determine the efficacy of the clotting cascade and is often ordered in conjunction with the PT. This test evaluates the clotting factors found in the intrinsic and common pathways.[6] The PTT is drawn from venous blood similar to the PT. This blood is then separated into plasma and cells. Substances are added to the vial that

Table 2-13

HEMATOLOGY: BLOOD VALUES AND COMMON PHYSICAL THERAPY CONSIDERATIONS

Component   Values and Considerations

Hemoglobin   **Normal**
- Men: 14 to 17.4 g/dL
- Women: 12 to 16 g/dL

Subnormal values:
Anemias
>10 g/dL: therapy as indicated; no distinct precautions
8 to 10 g/dL:
- Anticipate poor cardiopulmonary reserve/limited endurance
- Monitor vital signs closely
- Patient symptoms: Exercise intolerance/DOE/tachycardia/pallor

<8: g/dL
- Therapy may be contraindicated; blood transfusion probable
- <5 g/dL: Leads to heart failure and death

Elevated values:
- 20 g/dL: Increased blood viscosity leading to capillary blockage and tissue ischemia

Platelets   **Normal**
- 140 to 400 x 10^3/mm^3

Subnormal values:
Thrombocytopenia: <10 x 10^3/mm^3
50 to 140 x 10^3/mm^3:
- Low intensity progressive resistive exercise (PRE) and aerobic exercise (no- to minimal grade/elevations)

30 to 50 x 10^3/mm^3 (50 x 10^3/mm^3 typically not associated with spontaneous bleeding)
- AROM exercise, walking ad lib

<20 x 10^3/mm^3:
- Risk of spontaneous bleeding, petechia, ecchymosis, and prolonged bleeding time
- Therapy may be contraindicated/minimal AROM
- No brushing of teeth

Elevated values
Thrombocytosis: >400 x 10^3/mm^3
- No distinct recommendation; note paradoxical increased risk of bleeding

(continued)

Table 2–13 (continued)

HEMATOLOGY: BLOOD VALUES AND COMMON PHYSICAL THERAPY CONSIDERATIONS

Component	*Values and Considerations*
WBC	**Neutropenia:** <40% or <1800/mm³
• Neutrophil	• ↑Infection risk; patient should wear mask outside room
• Basophil	• PT/PTA should wear mask of respiratory infection
• Eosinophil	• No fresh fruit/flowers
• Monocyte	**Leukopenia:** WBC <4,000/mm³
• Lymphocyte	**Leukocytosis:** WBC >11,000/mm³

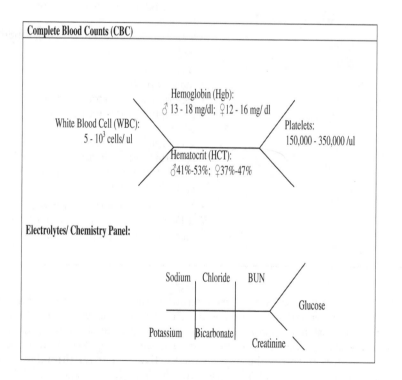

Complete Blood Counts (CBC)

Hemoglobin (Hgb):
♂ 13 - 18 mg/dl; ♀ 12 - 16 mg/dl

White Blood Cell (WBC):
5 - 10³ cells/ ul

Platelets:
150,000 - 350,000 /ul

Hematocrit (HCT):
♂ 41%-53%; ♀ 37%-47%

Electrolytes/ Chemistry Panel:

Sodium   Chloride   BUN

Glucose

Potassium   Bicarbonate   Creatinine

Table 2–14

HEMOSTASIS AND COAGULATION

Normal Values	*Common Abnormalities/Diseases/ Disorders*
Platelet count: 140 to 400 x 10^3/ mm^3 **Clotting time:** 3 to 10 minutes **PT:** 11 to 13.5 seconds **PTT:** 30 to 45 seconds **APTT:** 25 to 40 seconds **INR** **D-Dimer**	↑ **PT:** • Malabsorption • Vitamin K deficiency • Patient is on coumadin (disrupts vitamin K which is essential for the activity of Factors VII, IX, X) • Deficiencies in Factors V, VII, X, fibrinogen or PT • Hepatitis/cirrhosis/hepatic dysfunction (liver produces many of the clotting factors) • Disseminated intravascular coagulation (DIC) ↑ **PTT:** • Malabsorption • Hemophilia A (Factor VIII deficiency) • Hemophilia B (Factor IX deficiency) • Cirrhosis • Von Willebrand's disease • Heparin therapy (increases action of Antithrombin III which inhibits multiple clotting factors) • Therapy contraindicated if PT/PTT values >2.5 reference range due to bleeding risk; need to check institution guidelines

activate the intrinsic pathway of the clotting cascade. The time that it takes to form a clot, measured in seconds, is the PTT and normal values are 30 to 45 seconds. The test may also be done with a substance to shorten the clotting time, allowing test results to be read in less than 1 hour. When an activator is used for this purpose, the test is called **activated partial thromboplastin time (APTT)**, and normal APTT is between 25 to 40 seconds. The **INR,** or **International Normalization Ratio,** is used to correct for differences in the laboratory reagents used to test the prothombin time by various institutions. **D-Dimers** are produced by the action of plasmin on cross-linked fibrin and their presence in the blood confirms that clotting has occurred. Blood tests for D-Dimers are used to screen for deep vein thrombosis (DVT), pulmonary emboli (PE), and disseminated intravascular coagulation (DIC).

The PT, PTT, and INR are tests also used to monitor the dosage of anticoagulant therapies such as heparin and coumadin. These medications are often prescribed to treat and prevent blood clot formation from mechanical valves, dysrhythmias, and deep vein thromboses. Physicians may prescribe anticoagulant therapy such as heparin and designate that the PTT be 1.5 to 2.5 times the normative values. Therapists should consider bleeding risk when treating patients with impaired clotting (eg, cerebral vascular accidents [CVA]) or enhanced clotting (eg, PE/DVT) and review institutional guidelines regarding specific policies and procedures outlining activity restrictions.

Proteins, Protein Metabolites, Enzymes, and Pigments

Amino acids are the building blocks of **proteins** that are the most abundant compounds found in the serum. Proteins function as enzymes, detoxifying agents, antibodies, hormones, buffers, and energy sources. Serum proteins consist of albumin, globulins (alpha$_1$, alpha$_2$, beta, and gamma) and fibrinogen, and the remainder consists of hormones, enzymes, complement, and lipid transporters. Protein metabolites are the byproducts of protein catabolism or degradation. **Enzymes** are proteins that catalyze or increase the rate of chemical reactions within cells enabling normal physiologic processes. Different cells of the body produce different enzymes catalyzing specific biochemical reactions. The **bile pigments** are waste products of heme degradation, initiated by the breakdown of erythrocytes, the RBCs. Detection of organ and tissue specific enzymes, protein, protein metabolites, and pigments allows for precise diagnosis and monitoring of therapeutic interventions. Standard values and common abnormalities are presented in Tables 2–15 and 2–17.

Cardiac and Skeletal Muscle Enzymes and Proteins

Creatine kinase (CK), also termed **creatine phosphokinase (CPK)**, is found in high concentration in skeletal and cardiac muscle and in smaller concentration in brain tissue. CK is used as a specific index of injury to myocardial and skeletal muscle. Leakage of these enzymes is associated with dying cells and is used in determining myocardial infarction, myocarditis, inflammatory muscle disorders, rhabdomyolysis, muscular dystrophies, and trauma. CK occurs in multiple forms and can be further subdivided into three isoenzymes to enhance testing specificity. **CK-BB** is found in brain and neural tissue, **CK-MB** is found in heart muscle, and **CK-MM** is found primarily in skeletal muscle.

Troponins are proteins associated with the contractile apparatus of muscle. Cardiac troponins are unique proteins of cardiomyocytes that are released into the serum following myocardial injury and infarction. These proteins are highly specific to heart tissue and are a useful test for monitoring myocardial damage (Table 2–16).

Lactate dehydrogenase (LDH) catalyzes the conversion of lactic acid to pyruvic acid, which then enters the Kreb's or tricarboxylic acid (TCA) cycle resulting in energy (ATP) formation. LDH is found in most cells of the body, limiting its specificity to detect tissue abnormalities. However LDH is present in five tissue-specific isoenzymes enhancing diagnostic accuracy.

B-type natriuretic peptide (BNP) and **atrial natriuretic peptide (ANP)** are hormones secreted by the heart due to pressure or volume overload. BNP is a

Table 2–15
PROTEINS, PROTEIN METABOLITES, AND TRACE ELEMENTS

Component	Normal Values	Common Abnormalities
Ammonia (NH_3)	15 to 56 µg/dL	↑ NH_3: Liver disease/cirrhosis, renal disease, GI infections/hemorrhage, total parenteral nutrition (TPN)
Blood urea nitrogen (BUN)	6 to 20 mg/dL	↑ BUN: CHF, DM, MI, urinary tract obstruction, burns, cancer ↓ BUN: Liver failure, malnutrition, SIADH
Creatinine (Cr)	0.9 to 1.3 mg/dL	↑ Cr: Renal dysfunction, nephritis, urinary tract obstruction, muscular dystrophy, myasthenia gravis, rhabdomyolysis, hyperthyroidism, CHF, acromegaly, dehydration
Bilirubin	0.3 to 1.0 mg/dL	↑ Bili: Liver disease (cirrhosis, hepatitis), bile or hepatic duct ostruction (obstructive jaundice), pernicious anemia, sickle cell disease, CHF
Albumin (Alb) and Prealbumin	3.5 to 4.8 g/dL 19 to 38 mg/dL	↓ Alb: Acute/chronic infections and inflammation, cirrhosis/liver disease, nephrotic syndrome, Crohn's disease, burns, starvation/malnutrition, thyroid disease
Iron (Fe)	Men: 65 to 175 µg/dL Women: 50 to 170 µg/dL	↓ Fe: Iron deficiency/malabsorption, blood loss/hemorrhage, SLE, RA, chronic infections
Transferrin	250 to 425 mg/dL	↓: Malnutrition, burns, chronic infections, liver disease, renal disease

more sensitive marker of heart failure severity due to a wider range of plasma concentrations in normal versus patients with heart failure.

C-reactive protein (CRP) is an abnormal protein produced by the liver that is elevated in the blood of individuals after trauma, bacterial infections, inflammation, surgery, and neoplastic proliferation. CRP is used to monitor inflammatory processes and diseases including systemic lupus erythematosus (SLE) and postoperative infections. Additionally, elevated CRP values are used to screen for cardiovascular risk as well as predict future cardiovascular events such as CVA or MI.

Homocysteine is an amino acid that is an intermediate of the metabolic pathway to synthesize cysteine from methionine. Homocysteine measurements are

Table 2–16

CARDIAC AND SKELETAL MUSCLE ENZYMES AND HORMONES

		Peak	*Release*	*Decline*	*Common Abnormalities*
Myoglobin	<55 ng/mL				↑ CK/DC-MB: Acute MI, peri-surgical MI, unstable angina, myocarditis
CPK • **CK-MB**	0 to 120 ng/mL • 3 ng/mL; 0 to 3%	3 to 6 hrs	1 to 2 days	3 to 4 days	
Troponin • **Cardiac troponin I** • **Cardiac troponin T**	< 0.4 ng/mL • <0.35 ng/mL • <0.2 ng/mL	3 hrs 3 hrs	7 to 10 days 10–14 days		↑ Troponin: Acute MI, unstable angina, Myocarditis.
LDH	140 to 280 U/L	1 to 2 days	8 to 14 days		
AST and SGOT	Men: 14 to 20 U/L Women: 10 to 36 U/L	8 to 12 hrs	3 to 4 days		↑ AST: MI, hepa-titis, cirrhosis, dermatomyositis, polymyositis, cerebral infarc-tion, trauma, PE, gangrene, hemolytic anemia
ANF and BNP	20 to 77 pg/dL <100 pg/dL				↑ ANP/BNP: CHF, heart disease with elevated filling pressures, volume overload, parox-ysmal atrial tachy-cardia
CRP	<8 mg/L				↑ CRP: Elevated cardiac risk/atherosclerosis (CAD)

(continued)

Table 2–16 (continued) CARDIAC AND SKELETAL MUSCLE ENZYMES AND HORMONES				
	Peak	Release	Decline	Common Abnormalities
Homocysteine	4 to 17 μmol/L			↑ Homocysteine: Elevated cardiac risk/atherosclerosis (CAD) ↓ Homocysteine: Folic acid/folate deficiency, homocystinuria

used to assess risk for coronary artery disease (CAD) and thromboses, anemia and abnormalities in folate, methionine, and vitamins B_6 and B_{12} metabolism.

Hepatic Enzymes

Aspartate aminotrasferase (AST) (also termed **serum glutamic-oxaloacetic transaminase [SGOT]**) is an enzyme present in tissues of high metabolic activity including the liver, skeletal, and cardiac muscle. This enzyme is released into the circulation following cellular damage or death (see Table 2–16).

Alanine aminotransferase (ALT) and **gamma glutamyl transferase (GGT)** are also found primarily in the liver. The major amino acid precursor to produce glucose is alanine, and ALT catalyzes the chemical reaction that creates pyruvate from alanine for gluconeogenesis. GGT is important in the transport of amino acids into the cells of the intestines and kidneys. These enzymes are commonly monitored in hepatitis, cirrhosis, and drug therapy to determine the extent of hepatocellular damage.

The liver produces **alpha-1 antitrypsin (AAT)** and it functions to neutralize elastase, which breaks down elastic fibers. Elastic fibers are an important component of many organs, especially the bronchioles and alveoli of the lungs. AAT deficiency is associated with enhanced elastase activity, damaged elastic fibers, loss of lung recoil, and the development of early onset emphysema.

Pancreatic Enzymes

Amylase/Lipase

Amylase is an enzyme important for the conversion of starch to glucose. It is produced primarily in the salivary (parotid) glands and pancreas. **Lipase** is produced by the pancreas and is vital for fat digestion and absorption. Triacylglycerols are the major fat of the human diet, and the major enzyme that digests these fats is pancreatic lipase. Amylase and lipase are normally secreted

Table 2–17 CARBOHYDRATES AND KETONE BODIES; INSULIN AND GLUCAGON; DIABETES CRITERIA			
	Normal	*Prediabetes*	*Diabetes Mellitus*
Insulin	• 0 to 35 μIU/mL		
Glucagon	• 20 to 100 pg/mL		
Blood glucose	• 70 to 110 mg/dL		
Urine glucose	• 1 to 15 mg/dL/24 hours		
Fasting glucose test	• <110 mg/dL	• 110 to 200 mg/dL	• >126 mg/dL
Oral glucose tolerance test (OGTT)	• <140 mg/dL	• 140 to 200 mg/dL	• >200 mg/dL
Hemoglobin A1c	• 4% to 6.7% of total Hb		• >8.1% of total Hb
Blood ketones			
• **Acetone**	• <2 mg/dL		
• **Beta-hydroxy-butyric acid**	• 0.21 to 2.81 mg/dL		
• **Acetoacetic acid**	• <1 mg/dL		
Urine ketones	negative		

into the small intestine, and laboratory monitoring is common to determine the presence and impact of therapy for pancreatitis. Normal serum amylase is 25 to 125 U/L and lipase is 10 to 140 U/L.

Proteins and Protein Metabolites

Transferrin/Ferritin

Transferrin, a glycoprotein formed in the liver, regulates iron absorption and functions as a transporter of serum iron, which is toxic. Iron (Fe^{3+}) comes from the diet or the breakdown of RBCs, and transferrin transports Fe^{3+} to the bone marrow for hemoglobin synthesis or to the spleen, liver, and bone marrow for storage as **ferritin**. Tranferrin and iron concentrations are used in the assessment of iron-deficiency anemia, thalassemias, and hemochromatosis (see Table 2-15).

Ammonia

Amino acid nitrogen forms **ammonia** that is converted to **urea** and readily excreted in the urine. Ammonia is toxic to the body, impacting acid-base balance and neurologic functioning, and is usually excreted rapidly. However, serum levels may rise due to renal disease, hyperalimentation therapy, and hepatic dysfunction leading to hepatic encephalopathy (see Table 2-15).

Creatinine

Creatinine excretion each day is constant and depends on the body muscle mass. The serum concentration of creatinine is the most useful indicator of renal function, specifically the glomerular filtration rate (GFR). A rise in serum creatinine is assumed to result from decreased excretion of this protein metabolite in the urine, and the extent of the rise is directly related to the severity of the pathologic process involving the kidneys.

Blood Urea Nitrogen

Urea forms in the liver from the breakdown of proteins and amino acids, and urea excretion varies with dietary protein intake, metabolic state of the body, and the presence of disease. **Blood urea nitrogen (BUN)** is used to measure renal excretory capacity and estimate protein catabolism and/or tissue necrosis.

Albumin/Prealbumin

Albumin (ALB) and **prealbumin (PAB)** are tests used to analyze nutrition status. ALB is the primary protein for maintaining the colloid osmotic pressure in the vascular and extravascular spaces and is, therefore, vital to fluid distribution, as noted previously. Decreased serum level of ALB leads to peripheral edema and potentially hypotension. Serum levels of ALB and transferrin may be used as indicators of the degree of protein malnutrition. However, ALB has a half-life of approximately 21 days and does not provide an accurate estimate of recent nutrition status. PAB is the preferred marker of nutrition status due to its short half-life, approximately 2 days, while ALB is slower to respond to a patient's recent change in nutrition status.

Carbohydrates and Ketone Bodies

Carbohydrates (CHOs) are the largest source of dietary calories in the typical American diet, and the primary CHOs consist of starch, a polysaccharide of multiple glucose molecules; lactose, a disaccharide of glucose and galactose; and sucrose, a disaccharide composed of glucose and fructose. Polysaccharides and disaccharides are converted to monosaccharides by digestive enzymes and absorbed via specific cell membrane transporters in the GI tract. **Glucose**, the body's major energy source, is principally obtained from the diet but can also be synthesized from certain amino acids. CHOs, stored in limited quantities in the liver and muscle as **glycogen**, provide a major source of energy via ATP production for the majority of metabolic processes, sparing protein breakdown, function as a primer for fat metabolism and are a necessary fuel for the central nervous system. Glucose metabolism is governed by the inverse actions of the pancreatic hormones, insulin, and glucagon (see Chapter 10). **Insulin** promotes the cellular absorption of glucose, production of hepatic and skeletal muscle glycogen, muscle protein synthesis and amino acid storage, and synthesis of triglycerides in adipose tissues. **Glucagon**, which is secreted during periods of fasting or low blood glucose, stimulates glycogen breakdown (**glycogenolysis**) and glucose formation from protein and fat (**gluconeogenesis**) and stimulates lipolysis of adipose tissue resulting in the formation of fatty acids and glycerol. Monitoring of blood glucose provides insight into the metabolism of CHO and is one of the most commonly performed laboratory tests of the acute care setting.

Fasting plasma glucose test is the measurement of plasma glucose after a 12- to 14-hour fast. The **oral glucose tolerance test (OGTT)** is the most sensitive method of evaluating borderline cases of diabetes mellitus and is based on the fact that the insulin response to a large oral glucose dose is almost immediate with a return to normal levels within 3 hours.

The OGTT and fasting glucose provide information regarding the immediate plasma levels of glucose but provide limited information regarding the long-term management of blood glucose concentrations. Another test, the **glycosylated hemoglobin test** or **hemoglobin A_{1C} (Hb A_{1C})** is used to monitor the effectiveness of diabetes therapy. Hemoglobin, like other proteins, may be chemically modified by the addition of carbohydrates in a process termed glycosylation. The addition of glucose to heme occurs spontaneously over the lifespan of RBCs in proportion to the blood glucose concentration. Therefore, Hb A_{1C} is an indicator of the extent to which the blood glucose level has been elevated over the preceding 2 to 3 months.

Ketones or **ketone bodies** are three substances—acetone, beta-hydroxybutyric acid, and acetoacetic acid—synthesized in the liver resulting from the metabolism of fatty acids. Ketones are formed when fatty acid levels are elevated in the blood, as seen in fasting, starvation, high fat, low carbohydrate diets, and lack of insulin function. Normally, ketones are completely metabolized by extrahepatic tissues so that negligible amounts enter the urine. However, when carbohydrate metabolism is disturbed, fats and proteins become predominate fuel sources resulting in enhanced ketone formation. The result is excess ketones in the blood, **ketonemia**, the potential to develop **ketoacidosis**, and the eventual appearance in the urine, **ketonuria**. Monitoring of ketone bodies is common in uncontrolled diabetes mellitus, alcoholism, malnutrition, and metabolic acidosis.

Table 2–17 lists normal values for plasma glucose, insulin, and glucagon and diagnostic criteria for diabetes mellitus.

Bilirubin is the breakdown product of hemoglobin that is transported to the liver and primarily excreted in the bile. Bilirubin is found in the serum, and small amounts are present in the urine as **urobilinogen** (see Table 2–15). **Hyperbilirubinemia**, or elevated bilirubin levels, usually indicate hepatic damage, biliary obstruction, or hemolytic anemia, and the deposition of bilirubin in tissues produces the yellow appearance of jaundice.

Lipids and Lipoproteins

Lipids, also called fats, can be categorized into simple, compound, and derived forms. The simple lipids consist primarily of triglycerides, the major fat of the diet as well as the major storage form of fat in tissues. Compound lipids include the phospholipids and glycolipids, which are components of cell membranes, and the lipoproteins such as very-low density (VLDL), low density (LDL), and the high-density lipoproteins (HDL). The lipoproteins, the combination of plasma proteins with triglycerides, allow the transport of fat in the blood. Specifically, HDL transports cholesterol in the periphery to the liver, while LDL and its precursor VLDL carry cholesterol synthesized in the liver to the peripheral cells of the body. The apolipoproteins A and B are specific surface proteins on the lipoprotein molecules. HDL and LDL maintain cellular cholesterol balance and are important markers of cardiovascular risk assessment (Table 2–18). Derived lipids include the fatty acids used for energy production and steroids that are components of hormones, bile acids, and vitamin D.

Cholesterol and lipid testing are measures that evaluate the risk for cardiac disease including atherosclerosis and CAD. Additionally, cholesterol and lipid measurements are used in the assessment of thyroid, renal, and liver function and diabetes mellitus.

Common Diagnostic Tests

The following section will describe the mechanistic principles behind several common diagnostic tests. These descriptions are a general overview to provide the therapist with an understanding of how these devices and procedures promote an accurate diagnosis or promote safe and competent patient care. Additional procedures are described in the organ system chapters that follow.

Ultrasonagraphy

Ultrasonagraphy, sonogram, or **ultrasound** is a noninvasive procedure for visualizing soft tissue structures of the body. High frequency sound waves from a transducer are directed at a structure or organ. The sound waves are reflected back to the transducer producing a structural image on a monitor providing information characterizing the position, size, shape, and nature of the organ.

The **Doppler effect** is used during sonography to provide information about the presence, quality, and changing nature of the circulation. Sound waves strike moving RBCs and reflect back allowing direct listening and recording of blood flow patterns including direction, velocity, and magnitude of flow. For example, narrowed blood vessels produce high velocities, indicating possible stenosis or vasospasm or potential arteriovenous malformations.

Duplex scans are the combination of anatomic imaging of blood vessels and hemodynamic information provided by Doppler ultrasound. Duplex scans provide information regarding the direction, pulsatile nature, and resistance of blood flow.

Common sonographic and duplex procedures include:
- Echocardiography/transesophageal echocardiography (TEE)/Doppler echocardiography to evaluate the cardiac structures and blood flow through the chambers and valves
- Upper/lower extremity duplex scans to evaluate arterial and venous blood flow
- Abdominal sonograms to evaluate soft tissue organs (hepatobiliary, pancreas, kidneys, spleen, aorta/other large abdominal vessels, and lymph nodes)

Table 2–18
COMMON LIPIDS AND CARDIOVASCULAR RISK

	Cardiac Risk	*Common Abnormalities*
Cholesterol	High >240 mg/dL Borderline: 200 to 239 mg/dL Desirable: <200 mg/dL	↑ **cholesterol:** High cholesterol diet, hypothyroidism, chronic renal disease, alcoholism, obesity ↓ **cholesterol:** Myeloproliferative disease, malabsorption syndrome/malnutrition, severe burns, chronic anemias, hyperthyroidism
Triglycerides (Tg)	High: 200 to 499 mg/dL Borderline: 150 to 199 mg/dL Optimal: <150 mg/dL	↑ **Tg:** Liver disease/alcoholism, pancreatitis, renal disease, MI ↓ **Tg:** Malnutrition, malabsorption, hyperthyroidism, hyperparathyroidism, COPD.
LDL	Optimal: <100 mg/dL Above optimal: 100 to 129 mg/dL Borderline: 130 to 159 mg/dL High risk: 160 to 189 mg/dL Very high risk: >190 mg/dL	↑ **LDL:** High cholesterol/high fat diet; DM, chronic renal disease/nephrotic syndrome, hepatic obstruction, multiple myeloma ↓ **LDL:** Hyperthyroidism, chronic anemias, acute stress (burns, illness)
HDL	Normal: 35 to 65 mg/dL Goal: >60 mg/dL Increased risk: <40 mg/dL	↓ **HDL:** DM, chronic renal failure/nephrotic syndrome

Adapted from Adult Treatment Panel III at http://www.nhlbi.nih.gov.

- Head and neck sonograms to evaluate pathologies of the thyroid/PTH glands, assess carotid and vertebral arteries and cerebral blood flow

Endoscopy

Endoscopy is an invasive procedure that provides direct visualization of internal body structures by means of a lighted lens system, or fiberoptic, attached to either a rigid or flexible tube. Separate ports allow the administration of drugs, suction, and insertion of lasers, brushes, forceps, or other instruments for excision or tissue sampling. Examples of common endoscopic procedures include the following:

- Arthroscopy to examine the interior of a joint
- Bronchoscopy to examine the airways
- Laparoscopy to examine the intra-abdominal and pelvic cavities
- Cystoscopy to examine the lower urinary tract

Radiography

X-rays are short-wavelength electromagnetic vibrations that are absorbed or deflected as they pass through matter. The density of the matter or tissue will determine the degree of absorption allowing the differentiation of various body structures. Dense tissues will appear white, while air-filled regions will appear black.

X-ray studies are usually used for more dense structures, but the additions of **contrast agents** of varying densities are used to further differentiate tissue especially hollow viscera. Contrast agents are generally described as radiopaque, or high absorption, resulting in no transmission of x-rays onto the film, or radiolucent which allow partial transmission of the x-rays. Contrast agents may by injected or administered orally or rectally. Contrast agents are not benign and the risk of allergic reactions can range from simple nausea to severe anaphylaxis. X-rays produce a two-dimensional image in a gray scale and superimposed structures may create odd appearing lines, shadows, or apparent structural abnormalities. X-rays are often termed by the radiographic view that describes the direction of the beam entry and exit. For example, an anterior-posterior (A-P) view implies the beam entered the patient anteriorly and exited posteriorly, a lateral view is from the side while an oblique view is on an angle.

Fluoroscopy

Fluoroscopy uses a continuous stream of x-rays and the direct viewing of the image on a fluorescent screen to view real-time movement of anatomic structures or contrast material through anatomic structures. The image clarity is typically limited, but this modality is often used for central line placement and assessment of diaphragm function, digestive tract motility, or swallowing dysfunction.

Angiography

Angiography involves the injection of a contrast medium into the vasculature to allow radiographic examination. Angiography is used to detect aneurysms, arteriovenous malformation (AVM), thrombosis, vasospasm, and narrowing or occlusion of suspect vessels. Angiography is a diagnostic tool commonly used to assess the coronary circulation, the carotid and vertebral vessels, and cerebral circulation.

Digital subtraction angiography (DSA) uses fluoroscopic imaging before and after injection of contrast material, angiography, to remove or "subtract" common features from the two images. Common features "subtracted" include bone and soft tissue providing an enhanced image of the vasculature. DSA is used to visualize the intracranial and carotid vessels, aorta and visceral organ vessels, and other peripheral vessels.

Computed Tomography

Computed tomography (CT scan) or **computerized axial tomography (CAT scan)** combines multiple x-ray beams and computer-based calculations to determine the different absorption patterns of soft tissues providing delineation of minor differences in tissue densities. The image is displayed in cross-section or "slices" without superimposing structures. A **spiral CT** employs a continuous "corkscrew" scan pattern that allows the reconstruction of a three-dimensional image. Use of contrast media can further accentuate differences in tissue densities, providing a more accurate description of the anatomy.

Magnetic Resonance Imaging

Magnetic resonance imaging (MRI) uses a superconducting magnet to polarize protons, the positively charged nucleus of H^+ atoms and a radio-frequency signal that is pulsed through the H^+ atoms causing them to become energized or knocked out of alignment and resonate. The H^+ atoms will eventually reestablish the previous equilibrium and the decay of the resonation signal is monitored by sensors and recorded and processed by computer. The greater the concentration of protons in a tissue, the greater the resonance and longer decay time allowing the computer to construct an image. For example, tissues that contain a lot of water, and therefore, a high concentration of H^+, have high signal strength and are detected more readily than tissues with little water such as adipose tissue. MRI allows multiplanar scanning and allows contrast-free three-dimensional imaging.

Nuclear Medicine Imaging

Nuclear medicine imaging includes **single photon emission computed tomography, SPECT,** and **positron emission tomography, PET**. These diagnostic modalities study the function of organs of the body through the use of a radiopharmaceutical that incorporates a radioactive label, or radioisotope, and a pharmaceutical, or substrate, that is specified for the organ or tissue of interest. The radiopharmaceutical chosen for tagging are those that are biologically active and will remain in the organ to be studied long enough to produce a usable image but with relatively short half-lives to minimize radiation to the patient's tissues. The radiopharmaceutical is inhaled, ingested, or injected, and the target organ or tissue takes up the radiolabeled substrate. The radioisotope emits gamma rays allowing the target organ to be scanned by a camera providing quantitative and qualitative physiologic data.

Electrodiagnostic Studies

Electrophysiology (EP) studies are invasive tests for the diagnosis and treatment of supraventricular and ventricular dysrhythmias, syncope, and sick sinus syndrome. The EP studies measure cardiac electrical conduction system activity through solid electrode catheters that are guided via fluoroscopy through the venous system to the right atrium and ventricle. In addition to measuring baseline electrical activity, the EP catheters may be used to pace the heart in an attempt to induce the suspected dysrhythmia.

Electromyography and Nerve Conduction Studies

Electromyography (EMG) and **nerve conduction studies (NCV)** measure the functional state and structural integrity of the lower motor neurons to discriminate between myopathy and neuropathy. Conventional EMG uses concentric or monopolar electrodes, while needle EMG involves the percutaneous insertion of a needle electrode into the desired muscle. EMG records the electrical activity of selected muscle fibers at rest, during voluntary contraction, and/or in combination with electrical stimulation.

NCV studies involve the application of an electrical stimulus to a nerve of interest with the recording of the action potentials a known distance from the point of stimulation, allowing computation of the conduction velocity.

Tests of repetitive motor nerve stimulation are intended to distinguish disorders of neuromuscular junction transmission, presynaptic, or postsynaptic failure as the cause of weakness.

Electroencephalogram and Evoked Potentials

Electroencephalograms (EEGs) measure and record the electrical impulses from the brain cortex. Electrodes are attached to areas of the patient's scalp and brain waves are recorded. Common waveforms include the following:

- Alpha waves (frequency of 8 to 11 Hz; occur in the wakened state)
- Beta waves (13 to 30 Hz; associated with anxiety, depression, and sedatives)
- Theta waves (4 to 7 Hz; common in frontal and temporal regions of children and young adults)
- Delta waves (0.5 to 3.5 Hz; common in children and sleep)

Waveforms are evaluated for symmetry, amplitude, distinct patterns, and observation for transient discharges and responses to stimulation. Common indications for an EEG include epilepsy and seizure activity, focal brain abnormalities including tumor, abscess, or hemorrhage, as well as various diseases including Parkinson's and Alzheimer's.

Evoked potentials evaluate the integrity of visual, somatosensory, and auditory nerve pathways by measuring the brain's electrical responses to specific stimulation.

CHAPTER REVIEW QUESTIONS

1. What are the benefits of laboratory testing, sonagraphy, radiology, and nuclear imaging for the physical therapist in the acute care setting?
2. What test is used to monitor the effectiveness of diabetes therapy?
3. What physiologic mechanisms maintain the components of the intracellular compartment? The ECF compartment?

4. What are three factors that influence a loss of body K^+?

5. What are clinical symptoms of decreased extracellular potassium (hypokalemia)?

REFERENCES

1. Huether SE, McCance. *Understanding Pathophysiology*. St. Louis, Mo: Mosby-Year Book; 1996.
2. Koeppen BM, Stanton BA. *Renal Physiology*. St. Louis, Mo: Mosby, Inc; 2001.
3. Ackril P, France MW. Common electrolyte problems. *Clin Med.* 2002;2:205–208.
4. Luckey AE, Parsa CJ. Fluid and electrolytes in the aged. *Arch Surg.* 2003;138: 1055–1060.
5. Crutchlow EM, Dudac PJ, MacAvoy S, et al. *Pathophysiology*. Sudbury, Mass: Jones and Bartlett; 2002.
6. Ravel R. *Clinical Laboratory Medicine*. 6th ed. St. Louis, Mo: Mosby-Year Book Inc; 2004:86–88.
7. Bushinsky DA, Monk RD. Electrolyte quintet: calcium. *Lancet.* 1998;352: 305–311.
8. Bove LA. Restoring electrolyte balance: calcium & phosphorus. *RN.* 1996; 59:47–52.
9. Horne C, Derrico D. Mastering ABGs. *AJN.* 1999;99:26–32.
10. Kierszenbaum AL. *Histology and Cell Biology*. St. Louis, Mo: Mosby, Inc; 2002.
11. Abramo L, Alexander IM, Bastien D, et al. *Professional Guide to Diagnostic Tests*. Philadelphia, Pa: Lippincott Williams & Wilkins; 2005.
12. Junqueira LC, Carneiro J. *Basic Histology Text and Atlas*. 10th ed. New York, NY: McGraw-Hill Co; 2003.
13. Hand H. Blood and the classification of anaemia. *Nursing Standard.* 2001; 15:45–55.

BIBLIOGRAPHY

Chen MY, Pope ML, Ott DJ. *Basic Radiology*. New York, NY: Mc-Graw-Hill Co; 1996.

Fischbach FT, Dunning MB. *A Manual of Laboratory and Diagnostic Tests*. Philadelphia, Pa: Lippincott Williams & Wilkins; 2004.

Halperin ML, Kamel KS. Electrolyte quintet: potassium. *Lancet.* 1998;352:135–140.

Johnson EW, Pease WS. *Practical Electromyography*. Baltimore, Md: Williams & Wilkins Co; 1997.

Marks DB, Marks AD, Smith CM. *Basic Medical Biochemistry*. Philadelphia, Pa: Lippincott Williams & Wilkins; 1996.

McArdle WD, Katch FI, Katch VL. *Exercise Physiology: Energy, Nutrition, and Human Performance*. Philadelphia, Pa: Lippincott Williams & Wilkins; 2001.

Mettler RA, Guibereau MJ. *Essentials of Nuclear Imaging*. Philadelphia, Pa: WB Saunders Co; 1991.

PHYSIOLOGIC MONITORS AND PATIENT SUPPORT EQUIPMENT

Daniel J. Malone, MPT, CCS

Physical therapy has taken a greater role in providing examination and interventions in the acute care and critical care settings.[1] Physical therapists may be intimidated to provide care in the intensive care unit (ICU) due to the tenuous pathophysiologic state of the patient and the overwhelming nature of the physiologic monitors and support equipment attached to the patient. The use of life support and monitoring equipment; the prescription of sedative and paralytic agents; and the presence of pain, malnutrition, and sleep deprivation further complicate the patient's presentation, leading to further physical impairments, functional limitations, and disability.[2] The information that needs to be processed can be daunting. However, the monitoring equipment provides immediate data regarding the patient's physiologic responses to therapeutic interventions, and appropriate measures can be undertaken to avoid untoward occurrences. In addition, the other health professionals who work in the ICU environment are skilled in providing emergency services in the unlikely event that your patient does not tolerate the therapy session. The physical therapist plays a pivotal role in providing and guiding care throughout the entire acute care continuum with the introduction of patient care often taking place in the ICU. The physical therapist's responsibility is to integrate the patient's pathophysiologic status; the surgical, medical, and pharmacologic interventions; and the technology associated with physiologic monitors and support equipment.

The goal of this chapter is to provide the physical therapist/physical therapist assistant with a working knowledge of the diverse equipment present within the critical care environment and to provide guidelines that will enable the practitioner to provide safe and effective care.

PULMONARY ARTERY CATHETER (SWAN GANZ CATHETER)

The pulmonary artery catheter (PAC) was first introduced by Swan and colleagues in 1970 and has become a widely used tool to measure hemodynamics and modify therapy in the critically ill.[3] Although controversy exists regarding the use of these devices and patient outcomes, their use in the ICU remains the standard of care for concurrent hemodynamic monitoring.[4] The PAC is a flexible, balloon-tipped, flow-directed catheter that is inserted in a large peripheral vein and guided through the right side of the heart into the pulmonary artery (Figure 3–1).[5,6] The PAC catheter is typically inserted into the subclavian or internal jugular veins. The catheter's balloon is inflated upon insertion and rapidly migrates distally into the pulmonary vasculature, carried by the force of pulmonary blood flow against the inflated balloon until it impacts upon a medium-sized pulmonary artery whose internal diameter is the same or less than that of the balloon.[5] The PAC is commonly a triple lumen catheter with a proximal port for measuring right atrial pressure (RAP), a distal port for measuring pulmonary artery pressure (PAP), and a thermistor that allows calculation of the cardiac output (CO) by thermodilution.[7] An estimate of left ventricular preload is obtained with the PAC, utilizing the pulmonary capillary wedge or arterial wedge or occlusion pressure (PCWP/PAWP/PAOP). The PCWP is measured with the balloon inflated, preventing continued flow of blood in the occluded pulmonary artery, creating a static column of fluid. The static column of fluid transmits pressures from the left atrium providing a measure of left atrial pressure (LAP) and, therefore, the left ventricular end diastolic pressure (LVEDP), which is the estimate of preload.[4,5,7] Segmental lung infarction may occur if the catheter balloon is left inflated for long periods. Therefore, PCWP is only measured intermittently. PCWP should be determined at end expiration because respiratory variation of the waveform occurs due to changes in intrathoracic pressures.[8] Other hemodynamic variables can be derived from these basic measures as outlined in Table 3–1.

HEMODYNAMIC PRESSURES AND RESISTANCES

As the therapist begins to review the data that are generated from the PAC, one must remember that there are many assumptions that must be met for the values present to be valid. In addition, the therapist must remember that pressure may not directly reflect volume due to the impact of vascular and cardiac chamber compliance (intrinsic distensibility) and the relative state of vasodilation and relaxation which can impact on pressure, volume, and blood flow creating erroneous interpretations of the data.

Right arterial pressure (RAP)/CVP is recorded from the proximal port of the PA catheter situated in the superior vena cava or right atrium, and is equal to the pressure in the right atrium. The RAP should be equivalent to right ventricular end diastolic pressure (RVEDP) when there is no obstruction and/or valve abnormality between the right atrium and ventricle and typically reflects the blood volume that is returned to the right heart which creates the "filling pressure" or **preload**. The left heart's filling pressure is provided by the PCWP/PAWP/PAOP and is reflective of the volume of blood traversing the pulmonary circulation to the left atria. PAWP/PCWP is measured when there is no flow between the catheter tip and the left atrium (because the balloon on the PA catheter tip is inflated), the PCWP should be the same as the LAP. The LAP should also be

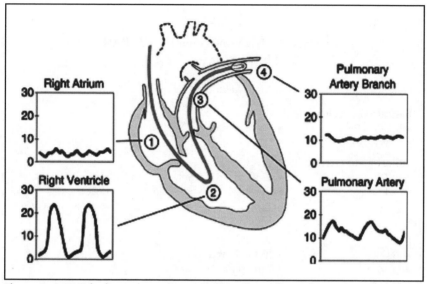

Figure 3–1. PAC for hemodynamic monitoring. The catheter passes through the right atrium and ventricle into the pulmonary artery. (Reprinted with permission from Marino PL. *The ICU Book*. Baltimore, Md: Williams & Wilkins; 1998.)

equivalent to the LVEDP when there is no obstruction and/or valve abnormality between the left atrium and ventricle (PCWP = LAP = LVEDP).[7–9]

The thermodilution (indicator washout) technique involves the calculation of blood flow following a central venous injection of an indicator solution. This method is based on the premise that when an indicator substance is added to circulating blood, the rate of blood flow is inversely proportional to the change in concentration of the indicator over time (washout). The indicator substance can be a dye (dye-dilution method) or a fluid with a different temperature than blood (thermodilution method) and is typically injected proximal to the right heart and sampled in the pulmonary artery.[4,8,10] The change in the indicator concentration measured at the point downstream of the injection site allows calculation of the CO. Delayed washout is indicative of poor blood flow or decreased CO, while rapid blood flow and adequate CO is associated with quick washout of the indicator solution. This technique provides a good estimate of the CO as long as there is no shunting of blood (eg, ventricular septal defect) and the tricuspid valve is normal.[4,7,10] Continuous measures of **CO** is a derivation of the thermodilution method using a catheter equipped with a thermal filament. The filament generates low-energy heat pulses that are transmitted to the surrounding blood. The resulting change in blood temperature is then used to generate a thermodilution curve for determining CO.[8] CO is corrected to body size by indexing the values to the body surface area (BSA) and is expressed as the **cardiac index (CI)**.

Mixed venous oxygen saturation (S_VO_2) is the saturation of hemoglobin in the pulmonary artery. Blood is sampled and analyzed via one of the ports of the PAC. S_VO_2 reflects the balance between oxygen delivery and the amount

Table 3–1

COMMON MEASURED AND CALCULATED HEMODYNAMIC VALUES

Parameter	Normal Value (Mean)	Equation
Indicator of preload		
• RAP/CVP	• 2 to 8 mmHg	
• PAWP/LVEDP	• 8 to 15 mmHg	
Indicators of afterload		
• PVR	• <250 dynes–s/cm^5	PVR = (mean PAP-
• SVR	• 800 to 1200 dynes–s/cm^5	PAWP/CO) x 80
		SVR = (mean BP-CVP/ CO) x 80
PAP		
• Systolic	• 20 to 30 mmHg	
• Diastolic	• 5 to 10 mmHg	
• Mean	• 10 to 20 mmHg	
CO	• 5.2 to 7.4 (L/min) (6)	CO = HR x SV
CI	• 2.6 to 4.2 (L/min-m^2) (3.2)	**Thermodilution:** CO = amount of indicator injected/area under curve
		Fick equation: CO = $VO_2/(CaO_2 - CvO_2)$ CI = CO/BSA
Arterial blood pressure (see Table 6-3)	• <130/85	
Mean Arterial Pressure (MAP)	• 70 to 110 mmHg	DBP + 1/3 PP $\frac{SBP + (2 \times DBP)}{3}$

Pressure (mmHg) = pressure (cm H_2O) x 1.36

Adapted from:

Tibby SM, Murdoch IA. Monitoring cardiac function in intensive care. *Arch Dis Child.* 2003;88:46-52.

Hillegass EA, Sadowsky HS. *Essentials of Cardiopulmonary Physical Therapy.* 2nd ed. Philadelphia, Pa: WB Saunders; 2001.

consumed. Values of 60% to 80% are normal.[9] A low S_VO_2 is associated with a decrease in the CO, anemia, or may indicate pulmonary dysfunction resulting from gas exchanging abnormalities and a low blood oxygen content.[7] If the S_VO_2 changes ±10% from the prior value, confirm that the change reflects a change in the patient's condition and alert the medical team.[9]

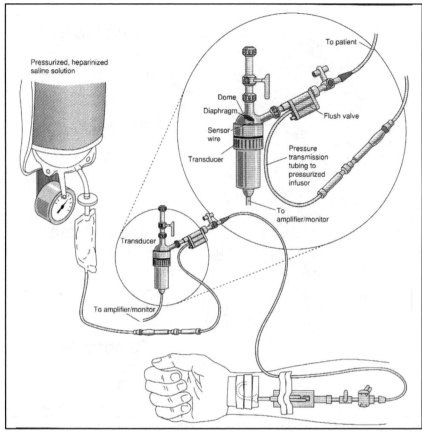

Figure 3–2. Arterial line. (Reprinted from Hillegass E, Sadowsky S. *Essentials of Cardiopulmonary Physical Therapy.* 2nd ed. Philadelphia, Pa: WB Saunders Co; 2001, with permission from Elsevier.)

ARTERIAL BLOOD PRESSURE

Arterial blood pressure (BP) monitoring is accomplished via the use of an indwelling peripheral catheter, which is inserted into a peripheral artery and connected to a transducer and a pressurized flush device (Figure 3–2). The transducer is set at a reference point, usually the level of the left atrium (mid axillary line in supine), and the transducer is "zeroed" to atmospheric pressure. BP is represented by the height of a column of blood that would rise above the zero point.

The systolic BP can increase as much as 20 mmHg from the proximal aorta to the radial or femoral arteries due to the reflection of the pressure waves back from the periphery (Figure 3-3). This increase in peak systolic pressure is offset by the narrowing of the systolic pressure wave, so that the **mean arterial pressure (MAP)** remains unchanged. Therefore, the MAP is a more accurate

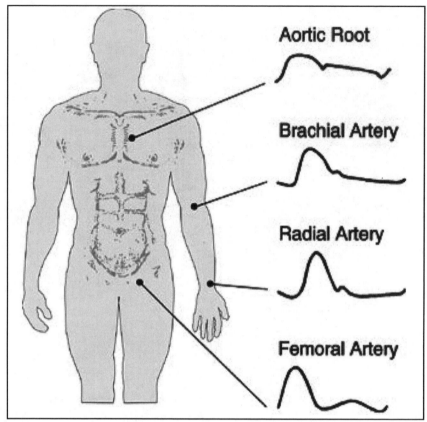

Figure 3–3. Arterial waveforms. (Reprinted with permission from Marino PL. *The ICU Book*. Baltimore, Md: Williams & Wilkins; 1998.)

measure of central aortic pressure and reflects the tissue perfusion pressure.[4,8,11] MAP is the true driving pressure for peripheral blood flow. The electronic measurement of MAP is preferred to the estimated mean pressure, which is derived as the diastolic pressure plus one-third of the pulse pressure. This formula is based on the assumption that diastole represents two-thirds of the cardiac cycle, which corresponds to a heart rate (HR) of 60 beats per minute (bpm). Therefore, heart rates faster than 60 bpm, which are common in critically ill patients, lead to errors in the estimated MAP.[8]

CENTRAL VENOUS AND PULMONARY ARTERY CATHETER MONITORING

For patients who present with a central indwelling catheter, the most common complication is a transient dysrhythmia as the catheter passes through the tricuspid and pulmonary valves during insertion. Dysrhythmias may occur in approximately 50% of insertions, are usually self-limiting, and cause no harm.[7] Other complications include infection of insertion site, line-related sepsis, thrombus, and, rarely, pulmonary infarction, pulmonary artery rupture, and death.[7]

Interpretation of the data obtained via a PAC is complicated, and the ultimate aim is to determine the cardiovascular performance of the individual. This requires an extensive understanding of cardiovascular and pulmonary physio/pathophysiology that is beyond the focus of this text. However, the absolute values of the measured variables are often difficult to decipher, and it is the trend in response to treatment that is most relevant.[7] The physical therapy practitioner must determine the hemodynamic, respiratory, and electrophysiologic stability of the patient prior to initiating therapeutic intervention. Patients with a PAC and other central indwelling catheters can participate in all physical therapy including positioning, airway clearance, and mobilization providing that the patient is stable.[11,12]

ARTERIAL BLOOD PRESSURE MONITORING

Arterial BP monitoring using indwelling catheters inserted into a peripheral artery is a common method of monitoring arterial BP. In addition to continuous BP measurements, these catheters are also used to monitor arterial blood gases and acid/base status (eg, respiratory insufficiency/mechanical ventilation [MV]/weaning, metabolic disorders—kidney failure/diabetes mellitus). Common sites for insertion include the radial artery, femoral artery, and dorsalis pedis artery. Weightbearing and joint movement/range of motion (ROM) near the sites of insertion is typically limited and may be contraindicated depending on institution guidelines and patient presentation. The physical therapist should note the position of the transducer and the arterial pressure waveform to determine the accuracy of the numerical readings prior to initiation of an examination or therapeutic interventions.[10,12] The arterial pressure waveform consists of three distinct components that the physical therapist should recognize as outlined in Figure 3–3:

1. Peak systolic pressure

2. The dicrotic notch indicating retrograde blood flow and closure of the aortic valve

3. The diastolic pressure point

As the case with PAC and other central indwelling catheters, patients can participate in all physical therapy including positioning, airway clearance, and mobilization, providing that the patient is hemodynamically stable and the arterial line is secure.[11,12] The physical therapist should always monitor the waveform to determine if any interventions result in damping of the arterial waveform. Repeated motion should be limited at the joint(s) of catheter insertion to prevent possible arterial damage or dislodgment. If the catheter becomes dislodged, immediately apply direct pressure and call for assistance. While mobilizing the patient, the transducer must be aligned with the heart to maintain an accurate reading. If the transducer height is below the heart, the displayed BP will be falsely high, while a higher transducer height will result in erroneously low BP readings.

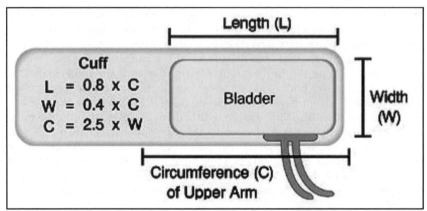

Figure 3–4. BP cuff dimensions for accurate measurements. (Reprinted with permission from Marino PL. *The ICU Book.* Baltimore, Md: Williams & Wilkins; 1998.)

A second and more common approach to BP measurement is the indirect measurement of BP using a sphygmomanometer. The practitioner should remember that cuff size is important. Proper size of the cuff includes the width of the bladder, approximately 40% of the circumference of the limb, and the length of the bladder within the cuff must completely encircle the extremity without overlapping (Figure 3–4). An oversized cuff will provide a falsely low readings and an undersized cuff will result in a falsely high reading (see Table 6–8).[13,14] Brachial arterial pressure can be accurately performed in the obese using the forearm provided that the forearm is cylindrical and not conical in shape and an appropriately sized cuff allows even distribution of pressure.[13] BP should be taken in both arms because the systolic pressure tends to be somewhat higher in the right upper extremity (RUE) (as much as 15 mmHg in adults).[13] Lower extremity (LE) BP tends to be higher than upper extremity (UE) measurements due to the reflection of the pressure wave and the influence of gravity.

CHEST DRAINS

Injury, disease, or surgical procedures that result in the accumulation of air or fluid in the pleural cavity will result in loss of lung volume due to compression with resultant impaired ventilation. The accumulation of fluid within the mediastinum or pericardium can result in cardiac tamponade. A chest drain is a large catheter placed within the pleural space, mediastinum, or pericardium to evacuate fluid and/or air (Figure 3–5). Mediastinal/pericardial tubes are often placed after open-heart surgery. Common indications requiring intrapleural drainage include pneumothorax, hemothorax, pleural effusion, and empyema.[15,16] Chest drainage systems consist of three chambers:

1. Collection chamber
2. Underwater seal chamber
3. Suction chamber

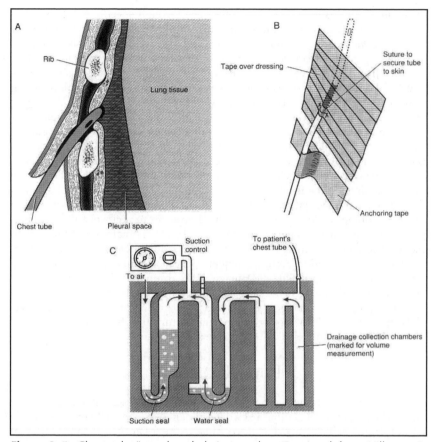

Figure 3–5. Chest tube/intrapleural drainage tube. (Reprinted from Hillegass E, Sadowsky S. *Essentials of Cardiopulmonary Physical Therapy.* 2nd ed. Philadelphia, Pa: WB Saunders Co; 2001, with permission from Elsevier.)

The collection chamber allows measurement, observation of color, and sampling of evacuated fluid for analysis. The underwater seal chamber acts as a one-way valve, allowing escape of fluid and air from the body while preventing retrograde flow into the pleural or mediastinal space. The suction chamber allows the application of negative pressure through the drainage system, promoting the evacuation of fluid/air. Typical goals of drainage systems include the removal of intrapleural and mediastinal collections, promote lung re-expansion and pleural healing, and attempt recurrence prevention.[16–18]

Drain insertion sites may vary depending on the indications for placement. In general, access to the thoracic cavity is through an intercostal space, typically fourth or fifth, in the mid or anterior axillary line with the site of entry posterior to the lateral border of the pectoralis major muscle. If the intention is to drain a pneumothorax, the drain is directed to the apex of the lung, or if it is to drain a fluid collection, the drain is placed lower toward the base or dependent portion of the lung. Drainage of loculated collections through specific points of entry determined by radiologic or ultrasound guidance may also be performed.[16]

The patient's vital signs should be monitored with special emphasis on respiratory status (eg, RR, breathing pattern, breath sounds, and oxygen saturation [see Table 7-7]) and pain level with mobility and coughing. The therapist should note any "bubbling" within the water seal chamber indicating air removal. Bubbling is typically more pronounced during expiration and coughing. If bubbling is noted continuously, either the patient has significant parenchymal damage or there is a leak in the drainage system. If this is a new occurrence, the medical/surgical team should be notified. "Swinging" refers to the usual 5- to 10-cm fluctuation in the underwater seal chamber associated with the pressure fluctuations of the respiratory cycle. If swinging is not identified, check to determine that the drainage tube is not blocked or kinked and alert the medical/surgical team. Obviously, the patient should avoid positions that kink or obstruct the drainage tubing. Patients are frequently allowed to participate fully in therapeutic interventions as long as the drainage system is maintained lower than the insertion site and the prescribed level of suction is continued. The patient should be encouraged to perform frequent position changes and perform deep breathing exercises to facilitate drainage. If the drainage tube becomes disconnected or falls out, an occlusive dressing should be placed at the insertion site or the remaining tube should be clamped to prevent air entry into the pleural space. If the collection bottle falls over, immediately return the chambers to upright to re-establish underwater seal, and alert the medical/surgical team.[11,12,15]

PULSE OXIMETRY

Pulse oximetry provides a noninvasive, continuous assessment of pulse rate and oxyhemoglobin saturation, a key determinant of oxygen delivery to systemic tissues (Figure 3–6).[16] The principles of pulse oximetry are based on the different light-absorbing characteristics of oxyhemoglobin and deoxyhemoglobin and the pulsatile nature of arterial blood flow.[19] The pulse oximeter consists of a probe that emits two wavelengths of light and a photodetector that measures the differences between light absorbances during (systole) and between (diastole) arterial pulsations, providing an estimate of arterial oxygen saturation of available hemoglobin (%SaO_2).[16,19] Pulse oximetry is an accurate assessment of %SaO_2 with values >90%. Values below 90% should trigger additional investigations to confirm the accuracy of the reading.[16] Common sources of error include poor peripheral perfusion (low CO or vasoconstriction), anemia, skin pigmentation and nail polish, presence of carboxyhemoglobin (smokers) or methehemoglobin, hypoxemia, and motion artifact. Accuracy of readings is enhanced if the therapist pays careful attention to signal strength.

To interpret the results of pulse oximetry, the therapist must be familiar with the oxyhemoglobin dissociation curve (see Figure 3–6). The flat portion of the curve illustrates the "loading" of oxygen onto hemoglobin. This portion of the curve demonstrates that with large increases in PaO_2, there is little change in oxygen content or %SaO_2. However, the steep portion of the curve illustrates the "unloading" of oxygen. This portion of the curve demonstrates that large changes in %SaO_2 and oxygen content are associated with small changes in

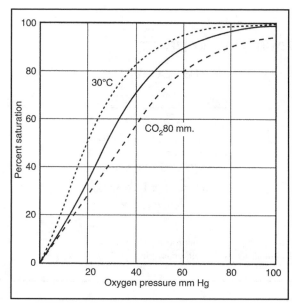

Figure 3–6. Oxyhemoglobin dissociation curve. (Reprinted with permission from Sheldon LK. *Oxygenation.* Sudbury, Mass: Jones and Bartlett; 2001. Available at: www.jbpub.com.)

PaO_2. During this portion of the curve, $\%SaO_2$ <90%, the patient is becoming increasingly hypoxemic and tissue damage may result. Supplemental oxygen is often provided to boost the PaO_2 and increase the oxygen content to limit hypoxemia-induced tissue damage. The therapist must also consider the common factors that shift the oxygemoglobin dissociation curve. A rightward shift results in reduced $\%SaO_2$ and oxygen content for a given PaO_2 due to a reduced affinity of hemoglobin for oxygen. This may result in hypoxemia. A leftward shift results in enhanced binding, a greater affinity, and reduced unloading of oxygen at low PaO_2 values that may limit oxygen delivery to the peripheral tissues.

OXYGEN DELIVERY DEVICES

Oxygen is a medication that is prescribed in specific dosages and delivery modes. Oxygen is administered to raise the PaO_2 to reverse or diminish hypoxemia.[4] Once the hemoglobin is saturated with oxygen, additional oxygen administration will not raise the oxygen content of the blood (ie, flat portion of the oxyhemoglobin dissociation curve) and may result in toxicity. The physical therapist requires a physician prescription to modify either the mode or dose of oxygen provided to the patient. Common delivery devices include low flow and high flow devices as listed in Table 3–2 and Figures 3–7 and 3–8. Low flow refers to a delivery system that does not meet the entire inspiratory flow demands of the patient resulting in the entrainment of ambient air. This results in variable F_iO_2 delivery depending on the patient's respiratory drive and breathing pattern.[4] **Nasal prongs** or **nasal cannula** are inserted into the patient's nose and oxygen can deliver from 0.5 to 5 or 6 lpm. Typically flow rates >6 lpm do not further increase tracheal F_iO_2. High flow systems attempt to minimize the

Table 3–2
OXYGEN DELIVERY DEVICES

Low Flow Devices

Dose	F_iO_2
Nasal cannula:	
1 L/min	0.24
2 L/min	0.28
3 L/min	0.32
4 L/min	0.36
5 L/min	0.40
6 L/min	0.44

High Flow Devices

Dose	F_iO_2
Venturi mask:	
4 L/min	0.24 to 0.28
6 to 8 L/min	0.32 to 0.36
10 to 12 L/min	0.40 to 0.50
Nonrebreather face mask:	
10 to 15 L/min	1.0

Adapted from:
Sheldon LS. Oxygenation. Thorofare, NJ: SLACK Incorporated; 2001.
Hillegass EA, Sadowsky HS. Essentials in Cardiopulmonary Physical Therapy. 2nd ed.
Philadelphia, Pa: WB Saunders; 2001.

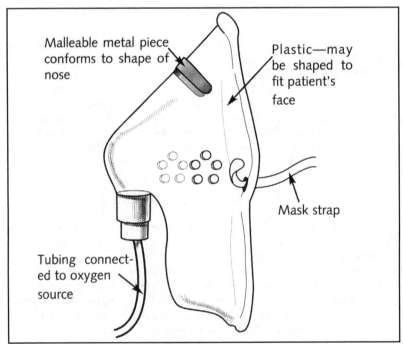

Malleable metal piece conforms to shape of nose

Plastic—may be shaped to fit patient's face

Mask strap

Tubing connected to oxygen source

Figure 3–7. Example of oxygen delivery devices: simple face mask. Oxygen flow rates are 5 to 8 L/minute providing an oxygen concentration between 40% and 60%. The F_iO_2 will be diluted by room air and expired air and will vary depending on the fit of the mask and the patient's RR and breathing pattern. (Reprinted with permission from Sheldon LK. *Oxygenation.* Sudbury, Mass: Jones and Bartlett; 2001:124. Available at: www.jbpub.com.)

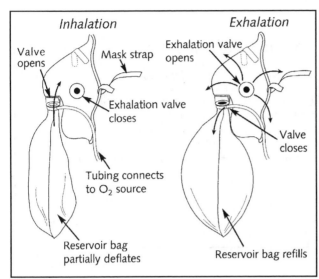

Inhalation

Valve opens

Mask strap

Exhalation valve closes

Tubing connects to O_2 source

Reservoir bag partially deflates

Exhalation

Exhalation valve opens

Valve closes

Reservoir bag refills

Figure 3–8. Example of oxygen delivery devices: nonrebreather face mask. Note oxygen flowing into a reservoir bag and one way valves limiting the rebreathing of expired air. This type of face mask will deliver the highest oxygen concentration. (Reprinted with permission from Sheldon LK. *Oxygenation.* Sudbury, Mass: Jones and Bartlett; 2001:125. Available at: www.jbpub.com.)

variability in F_iO_2 and usually consist of **face masks** that deliver oxygen at any F_iO_2 up to 1.00. The exact F_iO_2 provided to the patient will depend upon the fit of the mask, oxygen flow rate, and the patient's breathing pattern (inspiratory flow rate).[20] **Nonrebreather masks** have one-way valves that prevent the rebreathing of exhaled gas and the inspiration of ambient air. **"Venturi" masks** rely on air entrainment around a jet of oxygen to deliver a precise F_iO_2. The oxygen flow rate and the jet orifice diameter determine the precise F_iO_2.[4,20] A **transtracheal catheter** is another method of providing oxygen directly into the trachea. This delivery device requires a small incision ("mini-trach") for the percutaneous placement of the catheter directly into the trachea. This device provides higher oxygen flows and must be cleaned daily to prevent mucus plugging of the catheter tip.[20]

Oxygen therapy is well tolerated with few complications. Complications include mucosal membrane dryness, potential oxygen toxicity and elevations in $PaCO_2$. Patients with severe lung disease may demonstrate an increase in the $PaCO_2$ due to failure of the hypoxic drive or due to changes in the ventilation/perfusion (V/Q) relationship. V/Q mismatch may result from correction of hypoxemia, which reduces hypoxic pulmonary vasoconstriction. This can increase the perfusion to poorly ventilated alveoli resulting in the V/Q abnormality. Complications are avoided by administering oxygen at the lowest flow rate that provides an acceptable arterial oxygen level.[16,20] Humidification and careful monitoring of the patient's vital signs, breathing pattern, and arterial blood gasses will prevent untoward events. Criteria for the prescription of supplemental oxygen include $PaO_2 \leq 55$ mmHg or $SaO_2 \leq 88\%$ and/or in presence of cor pulmonale, a PaO_2 55 to 59 mmHg or $SaO_2 \geq 89\%$. Therapists should consider these values in relationship to sleep, resting posture, and with ambulation and activities of daily living (ADL) performance. If abnormal readings are noted, the

Table 3–3

MECHANICAL VENTILATION

Indications	Goals (Measure)
• Inadequate alveolar ventilation • Inadequate lung expansion • Inadequate respiratory muscle strength • Excessive work of breathing • Insufficient or unstable respiratory drive • Severe hypoxemia	• Improve alveolar ventilation ($pH/PaCO_2$) • Improve oxygenation (PaO_2/SaO_2) • Decrease work of rebreathing

Adapted from Albert RK, Spiro SG, Jett JR. *Comprehensive Respiratory Medicine.* Philadelphia, Pa: Mosby; 1999.

therapist must confer with the medical team, and provide recommendations if appropriate, regarding oxygen prescription.

MECHANICAL VENTILATION

Mechanical ventilation (MV) is one of the cornerstones of intensive respiratory medicine and is life saving in acute respiratory failure, severe hypoxemia, and worsening respiratory acidosis.[16,20,21] MV is primarily indicated to decrease the work of breathing and improve alveolar gas exchange. Although there are multiple indications and modes of MV, there are common objectives as listed in Table 3–3. MV has historically been accomplished by the application of negative pressure to the thorax (eg, "iron lung") or through the application of positive pressure to the airways and lungs. There are two primary types of ventilators used for adults in the ICU: volume ventilators and pressure ventilators. Virtually all mechanical ventilators used in ICUs today are positive pressure ventilators. Volume ventilators provide a stable minute ventilation (mVe = RR x V_T) with known tidal volumes. However, the tidal volume is maintained at the expense of peak airway pressure. Pressure ventilators prevent sudden changes in inspiratory pressures as lung and chest wall compliance change. However, tidal volume may be variable. For example, if compliance falls due to increased stiffness of the lung, the patient will quickly reach the predetermined peak airway pressure and the MV will stop the inspiration, resulting in an inadequate tidal volume. All ventilators used in the ICU setting provide three basic modes of ventilation:

1. Assist/control mode
2. Pressure support (PS) mode/pressure control (PC) mode
3. Synchronized intermittent mandatory ventilatory (SIMV) mode

Current mechanical ventilator technology allows these modes to be used in isolation or hybrid modes that combine features of volume and pressure targeted

<table>
<tr><td colspan="3" align="center">Table 3-4
MECHANICAL VENTILATION</td></tr>
</table>

Type	Mode	Description
• Conventional positive pressure ventilation: tidal volume (V_T) preset	• Controlled mechanical ventilation (CMV)	• All machine breaths delivered at a fixed respiratory rate (RR), V_T and minute ventilation (mVe) • Variables cannot be changed by patient
	• Assist/control	• All breaths machine delivered at fixed V_T • Patient can increase RR
	• SIMV	• Fixed rate and V_T for machine delivered breaths • Breaths are delivered after patient exhales • Patient can breath spontaneously between machine delivered breaths
• Conventional positive pressure ventilation; peak pressure preset	• Pressure support ventilation (PSV)	• Patient breaths spontaneously and determines rate • V_T is determined by inflation pressure and patient's lung and chest wall compliance • Minute ventilation may vary
	• PC ventilation	• Inflation pressure/inspiratory time and RR are fixed • V_T and mVe are determined by patient's lung and chest wall compliance

Adapted from Albert RK, Spiro SG, Jett JR. *Comprehensive Respiratory Medicine.* Philadelphia, Pa: Mosby; 1999.

ventilation.[4,16,20] A description of the common modes of positive pressure ventilation are provided in Table 3-4.

In addition to the specific mode of ventilation, there are numerous variables that can be manipulated to achieve "optimal" MV settings in a critically ill patient. These variables include the trigger, limit, and cycle variables. The trigger variable determines what initiates inspiration—a preset pressure (pressure triggering), a preset volume, a designated flow, or an elapsed time. The limit variable is the pressure, volume, or flow that cannot be exceeded during inspiration. The cycle variable refers to the factor—pressure, volume, flow, or time—that terminates the inspiration. Typically, the physician and respiratory therapist will determine the appropriate setting for the MV.

Others modes of ventilation include high frequency ventilation ("jet" ventilation), inverse ratio ventilation, proportional assist ventilation, airway-pressure release ventilation, and extra-corporeal carbon dioxide removal. To date, there is no firm evidence that these new methods of ventilatory support have improved adult patient outcomes.[21] However, the therapist may encounter these modes depending on physician experience, physician preference and clinical situations. The dangers of ventilator-induced lung injury have led to many changes in the prescription and monitoring of ventilator settings. Patients are often placed on lung protective ventilation strategies consisting of low tidal volume ventilation to avoid high inflation pressures and alveolar distension.[22] As a result of this protocol, patients may present with acceptable abnormal blood gasses including permissive hypercapnea (reduced pH; elevated $PaCO_2$) and/or mild hypoxemia.[22,23]

Positive end expiratory pressure (PEEP) is a mechanical means of increasing the end-expiratory volume of the lungs, the functional residual capacity (FRC). Pressure is deliberately raised above atmospheric pressure and all inspiratory and expiratory breaths begin and end above ambient. PEEP attempts to improve oxygenation by reinflating completely atelectatic alveoli and expanding alveoli that are partially atelectatic or closed. The result is an enhanced lung volume which attempts to increase the relationship between ventilated and perfused alveoli (V/Q ratio), reduce right to left (intrapulmonary) shunt, and ultimately improve oxygenation.[4,16,20,21] Because lung volume and pressures are increased due to PEEP, this can diminish venous return and increase pulmonary vascular resistance due to vascular compression. The result is decreased CO and possible reduced oxygen delivery to the tissues.[8,16] **Continuous positive airway pressure (CPAP)** is analogous to PEEP during spontaneous breathing. Inspiration and expiration are pressurized, and airway pressure never returns to zero.

WEANING FROM MECHANICAL VENTILATION

Weaning is an individualized process involving a change in the interaction between the patient and the ventilator. The intent of the weaning process is to decrease the level of support provided by the ventilator, requiring the patient to assume a greater proportion of the workload, thereby "liberating" the patient and allowing him or her to breath on his or her own.[4,24] Common parameters that hope to predict a successful weaning trial or may lead the clinician to suspecting a failed extubation are listed in Table 3–5.

Weaning may be accomplished in multiple ways: a modification of the ventilatory settings including a reduction in the PS (PS wean) and/or machine-assisted breaths (SIMV) or the rapid placement onto a "T" piece for a spontaneous breathing trial. A wean may also include a progression of time spent with less ventilatory support coordinated with periods of rest or rapid extubation and observation. The physical therapist needs to understand the physiologic demands placed on the patient during a weaning trial due to the impact that therapy may incur. Routine daily ICU activities including bathing, ROM, and chest physical therapy can significantly alter metabolic rate. Daily ICU

Table 3–5

PREDICTORS OF READINESS TO WEAN
FROM MECHANICAL VENTILATION

- PaO_2 >80 mmHg on F_IO_2 <0.40 (PaO_2/F_IO_2 >200)
- Vital capacity >10 mL/kg
- Minute ventilation (mVe) <10 to 12 L/min to maintain normal $PaCO_2$
- Maximum inspiratory pressure (MIP)/negative inspiratory force (NIF) >20 cm H_2O
- Rapid shallow breathing index (ratio of spontaneous RR to spontaneous V_T) <100

Adapted from Albert RK, Spiro SG, Jett JR. *Comprehensive Respiratory Medicine.* Philadelphia, Pa: Mosby; 1999.

activities can increase HR, BP, and oxygen consumption by 20% to 35% greater than resting.[25,26] In addition, the patient with lung disease may be utilizing upwards of 25% of his or her oxygen consumption simply to breathe at rest due to increases in the work of breathing. Therapists should coordinate with the medical team to determine appropriate times to institute the therapeutic regimen. Coordination of the provision of medications and airway clearance in addition to mobilization activities helps to ensure a positive response. At times it is necessary to initiate therapy during the weaning trial or during the rest period. For patients who are undergoing a prolonged wean, personal experience has prompted scheduling the therapy session during the rest period or the placement of the patient on the "rest settings" during therapy with a return to the "weaning setting" post therapy. Signs and symptoms of weaning intolerance are provided in Table 3–6 and may help guide the therapist in determining the proper timing and intensity of therapeutic interventions. Finally, therapists must also be familiar with common alarms that may sound on the mechanical ventilator as noted in Table 3–6. The therapist should not silence these alarms unless a rationale is determined for the alarm trigger. If the therapist feels confident that he or she can explain the alarm in combination with the patient presentation, the alarm should be terminated.

ARTIFICIAL AIRWAYS

Artificial airways are primarily indicated whenever disease or dysfunction compromises airway protection or the gas-exchanging function of the lungs.[16,20] Airways can be divided into those that occupy the nose or mouth, those that traverse the larynx, and those that are placed directly into the trachea (Figure 3–9). The common advantages and disadvantages of artificial airways are listed in Table 3–7.

An **oropharyngeal airway** prevents obstruction of the upper airway by moving the tongue anteriorly. In addition, these airways attempt to limit biting and compression of the tongue and endotracheal tube. The **nasopharyngeal airway**

<u>Table 3–6</u>

POTENTIAL SIGNS AND SYMPTOMS OF WEANING INTOLERANCE

- Increased RR (>35 bpm)
- Decreased V_T
- Change in HR/rhythm/BP
- Altered level of consciousness (LOC)
- Altered breathing pattern
  - ➢ Rapid, shallow pattern
  - ➢ Paradoxical pattern (abdominal paradox)
- Arterial blood gas (ABG) analysis
  - ➢ Hypercarbia/hypoxemia

Common Alarms and Mechanical Ventilation

Ventilator alarms
High/low pressure: Indicates the need for elevated/decreased pressure to deliver the desired volume of air
- High pressure: Mucus plug/bronchospasm
- Low pressure: Disconnection/tube leak

High/low RR: Patient's RR has exceeded/declined below a preset limit
- High RR: Pain/discomfort/agitation/exercise/fatigue
- Low RR: Fatigue/sedation

---

provides a direct connection between the nose and the upper airway. This airway is often used to facilitate nasotracheal suctioning for those patients with retained secretions, a poor cough, and without an endotracheal tube. An **endotracheal tube (ETT)** or a **tracheostomy tube** are indicated to prevent/relieve upper airway obstruction, to protect the airway from aspiration, to facilitate tracheal suctioning and airway clearance, and to provide a sealed, closed system for MV.[20] The ETT is generally a shorter duration artificial airway as compared to the tracheostomy tube. Tracheostomy tubes are usually inserted between the second or third cartilaginous ring, inferior to the vocal cords, and fixated initially with a stitch and later by knotted string ties or Velcro strapping. The typical tracheostomy tube consists of an outer cannula or flange allowing fixation and stabilization at the neck and a removable inner cannula allowing airway hygiene.[12] Both ETT and tracheostomy tubes terminate above the carina to allow airflow to both lungs. Tracheostomy tubes allow improved communication and potential for oral feeding. A **fenestrated tracheostomy** tube has an opening in the superior aspect of the outer cannula, which allows airflow to enter the upper airway when the inner cannula of the tracheostomy tube is removed.

Tracheostomy buttons are cannulas that extend from the anterior surface of the trachea to the periphery. These airways maintain an open stoma and allow direct tracheal suctioning.

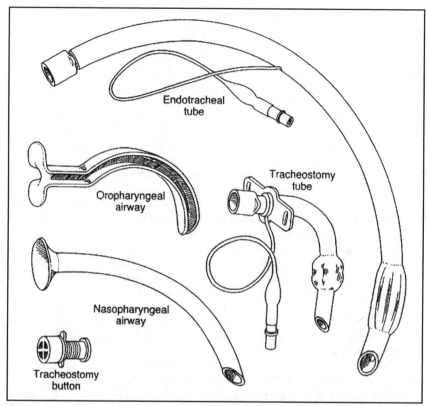

Figure 3–9. Common airways. Reprinted from Luce JM, Pierson DJ, Tyler ML. *Intensive Respiratory Care.* 2nd ed. Philadelphia, Pa: WB Saunders Co; 1993:16, with permission from Elsevier.

Table 3–7

ARTIFICIAL AIRWAYS

Indications	*Disadvantages*
• To prevent/relieve upper airway obstruction	• Decreased cough effectiveness
• To protect the airway from aspiration	• Reduced ciliary motion
• To facilitate tracheal suctioning/airway clearance	• Interference with communication and nutrition
• To provide a sealed, closed system for mechanical ventilation	• Bypasses respiratory defense mechanisms
	• Increased risk of infection
	• Loss of dignity
	• Tracheal stenosis

Speaking valves or caps may be placed over the tracheostomy tube to promote use of the upper airway, assess the patient's ability to clear secretions, allow phonation, and improve communication. Remember that the cuff needs to be deflated to allow these devices to work and that the patient must be able to adequately clear his or her own airway or obstruction and asphyxiation may occur.

Patients with artificial airways can participate in all aspects of therapeutic interventions and usually require special emphasis on airway clearance and mobilization. The insertion of an artificial airway results in loss of the normal upper airway functions of humidification, warming, and filtration of inspired air. As a result, these patients are at risk for impaired mucociliary transport and limited host defense resulting in retained secretions and an increase risk of infections and pneumonia. The physical therapist must determine the stability of the airway prior to initiating therapy. Breath sounds should be assessed to determine the degree of aeration and presence/absence of adventitious sounds throughout the lung fields. ETT should be monitored by checking the position of the tube in relationship to the lip, teeth, or gum line. ETT are usually marked in standard increments along the length of the tube allowing the therapist to check the relative position before, during, and after the therapy session. Excessive movements of all airways, but especially ETT and tracheostomy tubes, should be avoided due to possible tracheal irritation, extubation, or accidental intubation of a single mainstem bronchi. Patients may produce grunting noises due to airleaks around the cuff/balloon of the ETT or tracheostomy tube. Airleaks are common during mobility exercises and are typically a harmless nuisance. An airleak may be hazardous if sufficient volume of air escapes through the upper airway limiting alveolar ventilation. The respiratory therapist should be notified to check the airway stability and cuff inflation pressure (usually <30 cm H_2O).

The removal of an airway or the cessation of mechanical ventilatory support, **extubation**, is considered when the patient demonstrates adequate ventilatory drive, respiratory muscle strength and gas exchange, a satisfactory breathing pattern, a patent airway with intact protective reflexes, improving pulmonary function, and is hemodynamically stable.[27] The therapist should note that a patient who has been extubated or liberated from MV is vulnerable and may require reintubation due to bronchosplasm, laryngospasm, aspiration, inadequate airway patency, impaired ventilatory drive, and/or mucus plugging.[27] The physical therapist needs to adequately examine the patient: assessing vital signs to determine hemodynamic stability, assessing breath sounds and breathing pattern, and using pulse oximetry, which may provide an indication of the patient's respiratory status.

SUCTIONING

The aim of suctioning is to maintain a clear airway, normalize breath sounds and breathing pattern, reduce dyspnea, and limit airway trauma and hypoxemia.[28] However, suctioning is extremely unpleasant, and multiple negative responses may result including bronchial epithelial damage, transient hypoxemia, and bronchospasm. This may increase mucus hypersection and potentiates hemodynamic instability due to vasovagal stimulation (bradycardia and hypotension).[29] Due to the risks and potential complications, suctioning should be reserved and used judiciously. Other noninvasive techniques, such as optimization of positioning, application of assisted coughing and chest wall exercises, splinting of incisions, and instruction in directed coughing or huffing, should be instituted prior to suctioning.[11,29] Proper suction technique is provided in Table 3–8.

INTRA-AORTIC BALLOON PUMP/INTRA-AORTIC BALLOON COUNTERPULSATION

Intra-aortic balloon pump (IABP) is used for patients with cardiac pump dysfunction associated with myocardial infarction and refractory cardiogenic shock due to its ability to reduce afterload, reduce myocardial oxygen consumption, improve coronary blood flow, and improve tissue perfusion.[4,30] The device consists of a balloon mounted on a catheter that is attached to a console (Figure 3–10). The catheter is frequently inserted into the femoral artery and advanced to the descending thoracic aorta. The balloon inflates with the onset of diastole, which increases diastolic pressure promoting increased coronary artery perfusion pressure. Balloon deflation occurs prior to systole, which reduces afterload pressures in the aorta promoting enhanced CO and reduced myocardial oxygen demand. If therapy is indicated, the physical therapist must ensure hemodynamic stability, review HR and BP (myocardial oxygen demand) limits, and maintain patency of the insertion catheter at all times (eg, hip flexion <30 degrees).

EXTRACORPOREAL MEMBRANOUS OXYGENATION AND EXTRACORPOREAL CARBON DIOXIDE REMOVAL

Extracorporeal membranous oxygenation (ECMO) and extracorporeal carbon dioxide removal (ECCO$_2$ R) are methods of replacing the gas exchange functions of the lung via a modified heart-lung bypass machine. Blood is removed from the venous system, and oxygen is added and CO$_2$ removed by a membrane oxygenator outside the body and returned via the arterial or venous pathway.[9] These highly technical methods are reserved for the critically ill and provide a means of limiting lung damage resulting from MV.[31] These methods require the administration of paralytic agents, anticoagulation as well as analgesia and sedation. Physical therapy is typically contraindicated, but if necessary (eg, airway clearance, positioning, ROM), utmost concern to avoid cannula dislodgement or tubing separation must be maintained due to the risk of immediate hemorrhage. Tubing and cannula must be secured, and visible and diligent continuous hemodynamic monitoring is required.[9]

NUTRITION SUPPORT/FEEDING TUBES

Nutrition support plays a vital role in the management of acutely ill patients. Delivery is accomplished through the parenteral route, via central venous access,

Table 3–8

ENDOTRACHEAL SUCTIONING (VIA ARTIFICIAL AIRWAY)

Evaluate patient for ineffective cough/ inability to clear secretions (auscultate lung fields)

1. Explain rationale and procedure to patient.
2. Prepare sterile work area for suctioning. Gloves, catheter, and saline (if used). Size of catheter, length of catheter should be determined by the size of endotracheal tube, size of patient, and amount/ thickness of secretions.
3. Preoxygenate using 100% F_1O_2 prior to, during, and following airway suctioning.
4. Visually measure length of catheter for depth of insertion not to exceed carina (use Angle of Louis as visual landmark or second rib).
5. Insert sterile catheter until resistance and withdraw 1 cm and apply suction no longer then 8 to 10 seconds at a pressure of 80 to 100 mmHg as catheter is withdrawn from airway. (Recommend therapist hold breath to simulate patient's breath hold during suctioning.)
6. Repeat cycle depending on volume of secretions, patient's hemodynamic and respiratory responses, and note time to recovery to baseline status.
7. Document procedure, secretion color/viscosity/amount, patient hemodynamic response, any adverse reactions, and recommendations for follow-up sessions.

Considerations and precautions

- Sterile instilled (2 to 3 ccs) saline may be beneficial for cough stimulation. Some evidence relates that instilled saline may lead to increased pulmonary infections. Use instilled saline cautiously.
- Universal precautions (goggles/ gloves/gown if indicated)

Observe for

- Frank, red blood (hemoptysis)
- Prolonged bronchospasm or wheeze
- Dysrhythmias associated with decreased oxygen
- Vasovagal response with insertion of catheter (bradycardia; hypotension)
- Elevated BP
- Transient or prolonged decline in oxygenation

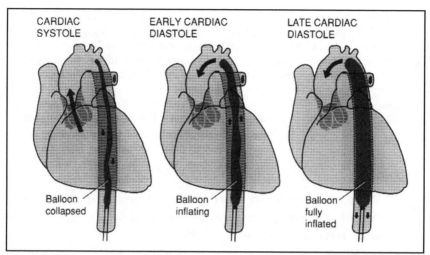

| CARDIAC SYSTOLE | EARLY CARDIAC DIASTOLE | LATE CARDIAC DIASTOLE |

Balloon collapsed | Balloon inflating | Balloon fully inflated

Figure 3–10. Intra-aortic balloon pump. Note deflation of balloon during cardiac diastole and inflation during cardiac systole. Reprinted from Hillegass E, Sadowsky S. *Essentials of Cardiopulmonary Physical Therapy.* 2nd ed. Philadelphia, Pa: WB Saunders Co; 2001, with permission from Elsevier.

or the enteral route, use of the alimentary canal. Enteral nutrition is preferred due to the ease of administration, decreased cost, decreased prevalence of infection, no need for central venous access, and improved gastrointestinal (GI) function. **Total parenteral nutrition (TPN)** is reserved for those patients who cannot use their GI tract due to dysmotility, ischemia, or obstruction or for those who demonstrate an intolerance to tube feedings and cannot meet their nutritional requirements.[4,32] The patient's clinical status will determine the specific contents (carbohydrates, proteins, fats, electrolytes, vitamins, trace elements) of the formula. Special formulations include pulmonary formulas that are designed to be high in fat and low in carbohydrates to reduce CO_2 production, thereby reducing ventilatory demand. Hepatic formulas contain large amounts of branch chain amino acids (BCAA) to improve the nitrogen balance and limit encephalopathy. Renal formulas are usually calorically dense, low in protein, and contain variable amounts of BCAA.[33]

The **nasogastric tube (NG tube)** is a tube inserted through a nostril and terminates in the stomach. This route of administration is usually short term, and well tolerated, but complications may include gastroesophageal reflux, rhinitis, pharyngitis, esophagitis and stricture, upper GI bleeding, and pneumothorax. **Nasoduodenal** and **nasojejunal** feeding may reduce the risk for aspiration. **Percutaneous endoscopic gastrostomy (PEG)** and **percutaneous endoscopic jejunostomy (PEJ)** tubes are surgically inserted directly into the GI tract through the abdominal wall and are usually a longer term solution for nutrition support. PEG and PEJ tubes eliminate nasal and esophageal irritation and reduce potential aspiration. Complications include skin breakdown and wound dehiscence associated with gastric content leak through the incision site and GI bleeding.[34–36]

Patients receiving nutrition support can participate in all aspects of physical therapy. Risk of aspiration should be minimized by maintaining the head in a upright position and limiting Trendelenburg or other head-down positions. If appropriate, place the nutrition support on hold during the session (consider bolus versus continuous feeds, insulin dosing, etc). The physical therapist needs to ensure that the feeding tube is properly secured to prevent problems with leakage and tube migration. Changes in bowel habits or other GI complaints may provide evidence of poor tolerance to the nutritional support, and this information should be passed on to the medical team (see Tables 11-18 and 11–19).

CHAPTER REVIEW QUESTIONS

1. Describe how pulmonary artery wedge pressure is measured.
2. What clinical findings are associated with a low S_VO_2?
3. What does the MAP reflect or represent?
4. What is the most common complication with central venous and pulmonary artery monitoring?
5. What are some common sources of error when interpreting oxygen saturation?

REFERENCES

1. Stiller K. Physiotherapy in intensive care: towards an evidence-based practice. *Crit Care Review.* 2000;118:1801–1813.
2. Sciaky AJ. Mobilizing the intensive care unit patient: pathophysiology and treatment. *Phys Ther Pract.* 1994;3:69–80.
3. Swan HJ, Ganz W, Forrester J, et al. Catheterization of the heart in man with the use of a flow-directed balloon tipped catheter. *N Engl J Med.* 1970;283:447–551.
4. Lanken P. *The Intensive Care Unit Manual.* Philadelphia, Pa: WB Saunders Co; 2001.
5. Pinsky MR. Pulmonary artery occlusion pressure. *Intens Care Med.* 2003;29:19–22.
6. Dulak SB. A PA catheter refresher course. *RN.* 2003;66:28–35.
7. Manikon M, Grounds M, Rhodes A. The pulmonary artery catheter. *Clin Med.* 2002;2:101–104.
8. Marino PL. *The ICU Book.* Baltimore, Md: Williams & Wilkins; 1998.
9. Nettina SM. *The Lippincott Manual of Nursing Practice.* Philadelphia, Pa: Lippincott Williams & Wilkins; 2001.
10. Tibby SM, Murdoch IS. Monitoring cardiac function in intensive care. *Arch Dis Child.* 2003;88:46–62.
11. Hillegass E, Sadowsky S. *Essentials of Cardiopulmonary Physical Therapy.* 2nd ed. Philadelphia, Pa: WB Saunders Co; 2001.
12. Ciesla ND, Murdock KR. Lines, tubes, catheters, and physiologic monitoring in the ICU. *Cardiopulmonary Phys Ther.* 2000;11:10–25.
13. Perloff JK. *Physical Examination of the Heart and Circulation.* Philadelphia, Pa: WB Saunders Co; 2000.

14. Manning DM, Kuchira C, Kaminski J. Miscuffing: inappropriate blood pressure cuff application. *Circulation.* 1983;86:73.
15. Allibone L. Nursing management of chest drains. *Nursing Standard.* 2003;17:45–56.
16. Albert RK, Spiro SG, Jett JR. *Comprehensive Respiratory Medicine.* Philadelphia, Pa: Mosby; 1999.
17. Baumann MH, Strange C, Heffner JE, et al. Management of spontaneous pneumothorax: an American College of Chest Physicians Delphi consensus statement. *Chest.* 2001;119:590–602.
18. Baumann MH, Strange C. Treatment of spontaneous pneumothorax: a more aggressive approach? *Chest.* 1997;112:789–804.
19. Mengelkock LJ, Martin D, Lawler J. A review of the priniciples of pulse oximetry and accuracy of pulse oximeter estimates during exercise. *Physical Therapy.* 1994;74:40–49.
20. Luce JM, Pierson DJ, Tyler ML. *Intensive Respiratory Care.* 2nd ed. Philadelphia, Pa: WB Saunders Co; 1993.
21. Tobin MJ. Current concepts: mechanical ventilation. *N Engl J Med.* 1994; 330:1056–1061.
22. Acute Respiratory Distress Network. Ventilation with lower tidal volumes as compared with traditional tidal volumes for acute lung injury and the acute respiratory distress syndrome. *N Engl J Med.* 2000;342:1301–1308.
23. Tobin MJ. Medical progress: advances in mechanical ventilation. *N Engl J Med.* 2001;344:1986–1996.
24. Hess D. Ventilatory modes used in weaning. *Chest.* 2001;120:474S–476S.
25. Weissman C, Kemper M, Damask MC, et al. Effect of routine intensive care interactions on metabolic rate. *Chest.* 1984;86:815–818.
26. Verderber A, Gallagher KF. Effects of bathing, passive range of motion exercises, and turning on oxygen consumption in healthy men and women. *Am J Crit Care.* 1994;3:374–381.
27. Miller KA, Harkin CP, Bailey PL. Postoperative tracheal extubation. *Anesthesia & Analgesia.* 1995;80:149–172.
28. Griggs A. Tracheostomy: suctioning and humidification. *Nurs Stand.* 1998;13:49–53, 55–56.
29. Bach JR. *Pulmonary Rehabilitation: The Obstructive and Paralytic Conditions.* Philadelphia, Pa: Hanley E. Belfus; 1996.
30. Bavin TK, Self MA. Weaning from intra-aortic balloon pump support. *Am J Nurs.* 1991;10:54–59.
31. Miller RD. *Anesthesia.* 5th ed. Philadelphia, Pa: Churchill Livingstone, Inc; 2000.
32 Smith HG, Orlando R. Enteral nutrition: should we feed the stomach? *Crit Care Med.* 1999;27:1652–1653.
33. Chan S, McGowen KC, Blackburn GL. Nutrition management in the ICU. *Chest.* 1999;115:145S–148S.
34. Barrera R, Schattner M, Nygard S, et al. Outcome of direct percutaneous endoscopic jejunostomy tube placement for nutritional support in critically ill, mechanically ventilated patients. *J Crit Care.* 2001;16:178–181.
35. Kennedy JF. Enteral feeding for the critically ill patient. *Nurs Stand.* 1997;11:39–43.
36. Marik PE, Zaloga GP. Early enteral nutrition in acutely ill patients: a systematic review. *Crit Care Med.* 2001;29:2264–2270.

BED REST, DECONDITIONING, AND HOSPITAL-ACQUIRED NEUROMUSCULAR DISORDERS

Daniel J. Malone, MPT, CCS

"Teach us to live that we may dread unnecessary time in bed. Get people up and we may save our patients from an early grave."[1]

The profound impact of immobility and detraining is well documented, and confinement to bed is, unfortunately, a common treatment for patients with acute and chronic disease and injury. Functional status and maintenance of activity levels in hospitalized patients are often overshadowed by patient care requirements for comfort and pain management, fluid and electrolyte maintenance, medication administration, hemodynamic monitoring, nutrition, wound care, and emotional and psychological support.[2] Patients are often confined to bed due to the severity of their illness, simply feeling poor, multiple lines and tubes, interaction of multiple medications including use of sedatives, depression or other psychological issues, or simply a lack of personnel to assist with mobility. Hospitalization is a major risk for older persons and is often followed by an irreversible decline in functional status and a change in quality and style of life.[3,4] How immobility and detraining directly relates to hospitalized patients has not been adequately addressed in the literature. The spectrum of disuse ranges from a minimal reduction of usual activity levels to the extreme immobilization of spinal cord injury (SCI).[5] This chapter will use information derived from imposed and simulated bed rest, as well as research using microgravity, to draw many correlations of bed rest in hospitalized patients. This chapter will illustrate the sequelae of immobility and bed rest and provide evidence that many of these untoward complications can be attenuated through the provision of physical therapy services.

OVERVIEW

Detraining is defined as the loss of physiologic and performance adaptations and occurs rapidly when a person terminates participation in regular activities of daily living (ADLs) and exercise. Only 1 to 2 weeks of detraining significantly reduces both metabolic and exercise capacity, with many training improvements totally lost within several months.[6]

The resultant physiological adaptations associated with immobilization include reductions in physical work capacity associated with impairment of cardiovascular, pulmonary, hematologic, musculoskeletal, metabolic, thermoregulatory, immune, neuroendocrine, and psychologic functions as noted in Table 4–1.[7–11]

CARDIOVASCULAR

The ability of an individual to perform short-duration, "all-out" tasks requires skill, motivation, and the ability to generate mechanical power. Mechanical power is related to muscular strength and the ability to produce energy via anaerobic metabolic pathways. Many tasks that make up ADLs (eg, toileting, grooming) may challenge the anaerobic power of bed bound patients. Activities of longer duration, such as walking household distances, challenge the aerobic pathways of energy production. Additionally, many ADLs may include both aerobic and anaerobic components, challenging both metabolic pathways. Most ADLs are submaximal in relation to total possible energy production for the community-dwelling individual. However, many hospitalized patients, especially those involved with prolonged hospitalization, may be functioning near their peak aerobic and anaerobic levels during routine ADL performance. It is this challenge to the physical therapy practitioner that prolonged bed rest and immobility creates.

Cardiovascular Adaptations

A common manifestation of prolonged bed rest is a reduction in aerobic power. This reduced maximal oxygen uptake ($VO_{2\,max}$) and the magnitude of this reduction is dependent on the duration of bed rest confinement.[12–14] The longer the duration, the greater the reduction is in aerobic power. Additionally, elevated submaximal heart rates (HRs) as well as reduced maximal cardiac output (CO) are observed due to bed rest and immobility. The elevated HR at rest, with submaximal workloads and maximal workloads, is a compensation to maintain the CO during exercise and stressful situations. However, CO and $VO_{2\,max}$ are primarily reduced due to limitations in stroke volume (SV) resulting from reduced blood volume, limiting ventricular filling or end-diastolic volume.[14,15] The reduction in circulating plasma volume (hypovolemia) and central venous pressures occur most rapidly during the first few days of bed rest due to renal excretion of sodium (natriuresis) and diuresis.[16] Venous compliance also increases, allowing enhanced venous pooling which may be exacerbated with the return to an upright posture. Venous pooling will limit venous return and cardiac filling contributing to orthostatic intolerance.[14,17] Additional contributors to resting tachycardia include reduced cardiac vagal tone, greater plasma norepinephrine, and/or enhanced beta-adrenergic receptor sensitivity.[14,18,19]

Orthostatic hypotension is common manifestation of prolonged bed rest. Bed rest reduces a person's habitual exposure to the upright posture, which deprives the cardiovascular system of stimulation to maintain adequate blood pressure

Table 4–1
CONSEQUENCES OF BED REST AND IMMOBILITY

Cardiovascular

- ↓ Exercise tolerance/ ↓ VO$_2$ $_{max}$
- ↓ CO
- ↑ Resting HR
- ↓ Resting and maximum SV
- ↑ Venous compliance
- ↓ Orthostatic tolerance
- Venous pooling

Hematologic

- ↓ Blood volume
- ↓ Red blood cells (RBCs)
- ↑ Deep venous thrombosis (DVT) risk

Musculoskeletal

- Muscle atrophy (disuse atrophy)
- ↓ Mitochondria density/ ↓ aerobic enzymes
- Bone demineralization/osteopenia/osteoporosis

Pulmonary

- ↓ Lung volumes and capacities
- ↓ Respiratory muscle strength
- ↑ Risk for pneumonia/pulmonary emboli (PE)

Metabolic/Endocrine/Electrolytes

- ↑ Insulin resistance
- Hypercalcemia/renal stone formation
- ↑ Urinary excretion of sodium, potassium, calcium, and phosphorus

Psychiatric

- ↑ Anxiety
- ↑ Agitation
- ↑ Delirium
- ↑ Depression

Nutrition

- Cachexia/malnutrition
- Obesity

(BP) regulation.[16] Initially, orthostasis is related to hypovolemia and resultant decrease in cardiac filling and SV. However, past 1 week, the contribution of autonomic reflex function, impaired carotid-cardiac baroreflex responses, and impaired vascular vasoconstrictive reserve contribute to the inability to tolerate upright.[16,20]

HEMATOLOGIC

Bed rest reduces RBC mass by 5% to 25% resulting in a diminished oxygen carrying capacity that may limit oxygen delivery to exercising muscle. The reduced RBCs combined with the contracted plasma volume may by represented by a normal or slightly elevated hematocrit (HCT). An elevated HCT increases the resistance to blood flow that may overly stress a compromised cardiovascular system as well as increase the risk of DVT. Further exacerbating limited blood flow is a reduction in capillarization of peripheral muscle beds, which impairs blood flow to exercising muscle during exercise and stress.

MUSCULOSKELETAL

Muscle and bone, once considered fixed entities, are in reality, dynamic structures with an extraordinary adaptive potential. Muscle damage can occur during the prolonged immobility of hospitalization and from external sources such as mechanical injury (trauma/surgery) or from the administration of necrotizing or harmful chemical (anesthesia).[21] Multiple interactive factors influence skeletal muscle phenotype or structure including genetics, neural activation, mechanical conditions, and metabolic and hormonal factors.[22] Key elements of bed rest contributing to changes in the musculoskeletal system are as follows:
- The lack of usual weightbearing forces acting on bones of the lower limb in the vertical position
- The decrease in number and/or magnitude of muscle contractions, especially in the postural musculature[5]

Muscle and bone tissue start adapting to the decreased loading of bed rest within a matter of days. The predominant adaptive response to decreased use is skeletal muscle atrophy.[23] Atrophy is the process whereby muscle size is reduced, almost exclusively because of reduction in the contractile proteins actin and myosin.[23] This increased protein degradation results in a negative nitrogen balance and is a diagnostic marker for muscle atrophy.[5] The amount of muscle atrophy a patient will experience depends on the usage prior to bed rest and the function of the muscle.

The pattern of muscular weakness tends to favor decrements in muscle force of the antigravity musculature. For example, antigravity muscles such as the quadriceps will have greater atrophy than the antagonist muscles, the hamstrings.[21] The lower extremity (LE) knee extensors are weaker compared to the knee flexors and plantar flexors greater than the dorsiflexors.[5,21,24] Strength loss in the upper extremity (UE) muscle groups is somewhat spared in relation to LE disuse.[9] The magnitude of loss of muscle mass and strength as well as the decrement in bone mineral density (BMD) is roughly proportional to the duration of the immobilization period.[25] Atrophy accounts for most but not all of the decrease in force production, suggesting that the ability to activate muscle via neuromuscular transmission and electrical contraction coupling is also compromised by the unloading stimulus.[23,26]

Muscle fibers decrease in size with immobilization and detraining impacting type IIB (fast twitch fibers) to a greater extent than type I (slow twitch fibers) and type IIA (intermediate fibers).[23,27,28] Additionally, unloading and immobilization of skeletal muscle result in a fiber type modifications resulting in a slow to fast transition with type IIA transitioning to type IIX and type IIB.[28] Fiber type transition can lead to further exacerbation of endurance impairments.

Positioning may alter the disuse atrophy associated with bed rest. Numerous studies have provided evidence that immobilization in shortened positions enhances atrophy while immobilization in lengthened and stretched positions may attenuate the loss of muscle fiber proteins.[29] This has important clinical considerations for those patients who are diagnosed with an orthopedic or neuromuscular condition limiting active movements of the extremities, who are medically immobilized/paralyzed, or who require excessive sedation.

Muscle metabolism is greatly effected by disuse and bed rest. Decrements are noted in enzymes associated with aerobic metabolism included enzymes of the Krebs cycle and beta-oxidation pathway (fatty acid metabolism). Enzymes associated with anaerobic metabolic pathways, glycolysis, appear to be spared. These changes, loss of aerobic capability and sparing of glycolytic pathways, contribute to the early fatigue observed after disuse and immobility.[25] Fiber atrophy results in lower total mitochondria content resulting in absolute reduction in muscle endurance capacity. However, the mitochondria to fiber ratio may not change significantly, but due to fiber atrophy and mitochondria loss, the remaining muscle and contractile proteins must work against greater absolute workloads. Long-term unloading, as seen in SCI, is associated with fewer mitochondria per muscle fiber.[23]

Skeletal Adaptations

Disuse atrophy of muscle contributes to the loss of bone mass termed disuse osteopenia. This loss of bone mass is delayed compared to the loss of muscle strength. However, the reduced BMD associated with bed rest increases a patient's risk of bone fracture with even minor falls. Normal homeostasis of the skeletal system involves a balance among bone formation, osteoblastic function, and bone resorption via the osteoclasts. Balance is a function of normal mechanical forces acting on bones and the interaction of several endocrine hormones. Parathyroid hormone (PTH) promotes enhanced bone resorption, calcitonin promotes bone formation, and 1, 25 dihydroxyvitamin D promotes absorption of calcium via the intestine (see Chapter 10). Hallmarks of osteopenia include the increased excretion of calcium in the urine and feces that may be observed within 1 week of the onset of bed rest, reflecting an evolving negative calcium balance.[5] Increased blood calcium concentrations and the increase in urinary excretion is associated with PTH while excretion of calcium in the feces indicates reduced calcium absorption via the intestines and the impact of 1, 25 dihydroxy vitamin D/calcitriol. The negative calcium balance associated with bed rest leads to enhanced bone resorption via the osteoclasts with resultant mobilization of calcium and a decrease in the bone mass.

Bony sites in weightbearing lower limbs appear to be the most susceptible to bone loss secondary to disuse. Loss of BMD at the calcaneus is greatest followed by the femoral neck and spine with minimal changes in the UEs.[25] Interestingly, the BMD of the spine of SCI patients is maintained within normal limits possibly reflecting the ongoing mechanical loads associated with wheelchair mobility and transfers.[25] This provides further evidence for the common use of closed chain exercise and the facilitation of weightbearing upright activities for all hospitalized patients.

RESPIRATORY FUNCTION

Pulmonary complications are a leading cause of hospital morbidity resulting in prolonged hospitalization and admission into the intensive care unit (ICU).[30] Pulmonary function is impaired in patients who have undergone prolonged bed rest. Common abnormalities include reductions in lung volumes and capacities, airflow rates, respiratory muscle strength, and potential alterations in gas exchange. Supine positioning and prolonged bed rest result in a diminished vital capacity, the maximal amount of air that can be exhaled after a maximal inspiration, and a reduced expiratory reserve volume. In addition, pulmonary compliance is reduced resulting in increased stiffness of the lung and chest wall.[31] Additional impairments associated with supine positioning and bed rest include a decreased tidal volume, FEV_1 (forced expiratory volume in 1 second), mid-expiratory flow rates (FEF_{25-75}), and respiratory muscle weakness.[32,33]

Reduced lung volumes, decreased pulmonary compliance, and respiratory muscle weakness enhance the patient risk for pneumonia, atelectasis, and other pulmonary complications. This increased risk is potentially exacerbated by thoracic and abdominal surgery as well as advancing age.[3,30] Abnormalities in respiratory muscle strength and limited tidal volume may impair the cough mechanism further increasing the risk for pulmonary complications during a prolonged hospitalization. Finally, the alterations in lung function may lead to immobility due to increased work of breathing and complaints of dyspnea on exertion.

METABOLIC ALTERATIONS

Insulin resistance increases as a result of bed rest, and physical inactivity has been implicated in type 2 diabetes, obesity, and the metabolic syndrome. Glucose transport into skeletal muscle is primarily a function of the glucose transporter protein 4 (Glut4). In the absence of insulin, Glut4 resides predominantly in intracellular vesicles resulting in minimal diffusion of blood glucose into the cell. During insulin stimulation, the Glut4 protein translocates to the cell surface membrane leading to an increase in the uptake of blood glucose.[34] Muscle activity is of paramount importance for the expression of Glut4 proteins in muscle. Detraining and immobilization have been shown to decrease the expression of Glut4 in skeletal muscle, and glucose intolerance due to decreases in insulin receptor sensitivity has been demonstrated after only 3 days of bed rest.[34,35]

Bed rest can also elicit marked changes in plasma and urinary electrolyte concentrations. Enforced bed rest of 7 days results in enhanced urinary excretion of sodium, potassium, calcium, and phosphorus[36] (see Chapter 2). This increased calcium excretion enhances stone formation in the kidney and urinary systems.

Bed rest can also lead to alterations in endocrine function leading to changes in hormone production and subsequent effects. For example, decreased erythropoietin concentrations have been noted, which may partially explain the reduced RBC number associated with prolonged bed rest.[37]

THERMOREGULATORY CHANGES

Thermoregulatory responses are altered secondary to bed rest and physical inactivity. The primary source of heat gain is internal heat generated by energy metabolism. Patients in the hospital may have elevated basal metabolic rates due to infections, fever, or stress reactions, leading to elevations in body temperature. The primary responses to elevated body temperatures is to increase HR to promote elevations in CO, vasodilate cutaneous blood vessels to promote convective and radiative heat loss, and to initiate sweating to promote evaporative heat exchange with the environment.[25] Deconditioning and bed rest alters thermoregulatory abilities resulting in increases in internal core temperatures with exercise stimuli. The threshold for cutaneous vasodilation and sweating to promote heat dissipation is shifted to a higher core temperature.[38] Impaired regulation of body heat limits exercise performance resulting in increased complaints of fatigue, and can increase the risk of heat-related abnormalities including cramping in fatigued muscles and in extreme circumstances syncope and heat stroke.[25]

PSYCHIATRIC

Alterations in mood often accompany a prolonged hospitalization, and alterations in psychological functioning promote functional decline leading to enhanced morbidity and mortality of hospitalized adults.[39] Anxiety, agitation, delirium, and depression are common findings in the acute care setting affecting greater than 50% of all patients young and old.[40,41] Alterations in sleep patterns, presence of noxious stimuli, noise, and loss of circadian light patterns can lead to intellectual and perceptual deficits limiting patient mobility and safety and prolonging hospital lengths of stay and elevating costs.[3] The physical therapist needs to recognize these untoward psychiatric events; alert the medical/surgical teams so appropriate interventions can be initiated.

Delirium may be characterized by disturbances in consciousness, orientation, memory, thought, perception, and behavior. Delirium is typically abrupt in onset and fluctuating in its course and may be delineated into hyperactive, hypoactive, and mixed forms. Hyperactive delirium is characterized by agitation, diaphoresis, tachycardia, and tremor. Patients with hypoactive delirium are often passive and at risk for dehydration, pressure sores, and nutrition abnormalities.[40] Anxiety is a condition characterized by apprehension and increased motor activity, with autonomic arousal.[42] The features include physiologic hyperreactivity, tremor, shaking, and avoidance behaviors. Agitation is typified by excessive motor activity leading to inappropriate verbal behavior and physical aggression. Agitation is driven by internal factors such as disease, pain, anxiety, and delirium. Consequences can be deleterious and include removal of catheters and indwelling vascular access, self-extubation, and increased oxygen consumption leading to myocardial or cerebral ischemia and respiratory abnormalities including hypoxemia, hypercarbia, and ventilator dysynchrony.[41] Depression is the persistence of a low mood or loss of interest in most activities for at least 2 weeks. It is associated with weight change, altered sleep patterns, lack of energy, agitation, poor self-esteem, and suicidal ideations.[39,43] Patients with symptoms of depression are more likely to be dependent and require assistance with basic ADLs or instrumental ADLs (IADLs) independent of comorbidities or illness severity.[39]

NUTRITION ISSUES

Cachexia and malnutrition are prominent in prolonged hospitalization, and impaired nutrition status is associated with poor outcomes. Critical illness results in a well-orchestrated set of metabolic consequences encompassed by hypermetabolism and hypercatabolism.[44] These terms refer to an increase in energy expenditure and increased destruction of existing tissues. The sum of these effects is a rapid depletion of body tissue stores and critical protein elements leading to reduced protein synthesis, enhanced protein breakdown, and malnutrition.[44,45] Nutrition dysfunction can lead to muscle wasting, reduced respiratory and peripheral muscle strength and endurance, increased rates of infection, increased mortality, and reduced pulmonary function. Cachexia is associated with a broad spectrum of clinical diseases including HIV/AIDS, cancers, rheumatologic diseases, chronic heart failure, chronic obstructive pulmonary disease (COPD), end-stage renal disease, inflammatory bowel disease, and hepatitis and the elderly.[45] Nutritional issues will impact the rehabilitation program of the patient in the acute care setting (see Chapter 11).

ACQUIRED NEUROMUSCULAR DISORDERS OF ACUTE CARE

Severe weakness with respiratory failure is a common complication of critically ill patients. Neuromuscular disorders are recognized as common causes of weakness occurring in critically ill patients with an incidence approaching 70% to 80% of patients hospitalized with sepsis or multiorgan failure.[46,47] The most common acquired neuromuscular disorders include **acute myopathy syndrome (AMS)** and **critical illness polyneuropathy (CIP)**. Afflicted patients develop acute, diffuse, flaccid weakness often first identified due to the failure to wean from mechanical ventilation.[48] AMS, also known as critical care myopathy or acute necrotizing myopathy, is associated with neuromuscular blocking agents, intravenous corticosteroids, or both, and aminoglycosides.[48–50] Other predisposing conditions include liver and lung transplantation, hepatic failure, and acidosis.[50] AMS is associated with preferential derangement of the type II (myosin heavy chain) muscle fibers resulting in profound weakness and atrophy. Sensory function is typically spared. CIP is defined as an axonal neuropathy associated with intense inflammatory responses associated with sepsis and multiorgan failure. Features of CIP include flaccid tetraplegia, hyporeflexia, muscle atrophy, and distal sensory disturbances.[51] Both of these acquired neuromuscular syndromes can result in profound paralysis requiring months of recovery and rehabilitation.

Transient causes of acute muscle weakness include endocrine disorders and electrolyte disturbances, particularly hypophosphatemia or hypokalemia[52,53] (see Chapter 2).

Steroid-induced myopathy can occur acutely or may be associated with chronic glucocorticoid maintenance therapy. The risk of developing myopathy is dose dependent, and risk is increased for the elderly, those who are inactive, those with cancer, and patients who are nutritionally depleted.[54] Steroids alter muscle lipids, carbohydrates, and protein metabolism; however, the main effect of glucocorticoids is to induce muscle protein catabolism and myocyte apoptosis leading to the preferential atrophy of the type 2 muscle fiber.[54,55] Particular concern for the hospitalized patient is that fasting and inactivity worsen the course of steroid-induced myopathy. The additive effects of inactivity and glucocorticoid treatment on muscle function may partially explain why patients who receive neuromuscular blocking agents may develop steroid myopathy quickly. Weakness is primarily proximal, with the legs more severely involved than the arms; cranial nerve-innervated muscles and sphincters are spared. Myalgias and electrolyte abnormalities occur frequently.[54,55] Weakness typically improves with reduction of the steroid dose, but full recovery may require extensive rehabilitation and prolonged periods of time.

Rhabdomyolysis is a syndrome characterized by muscle necrosis and the release of cellular contents into the circulation due to disruption of the sarcolemma and influx of extracellular calcium. The elevated intracellular calcium causes a pathologic interaction of actin and myosin resulting in muscle destruction and fiber necrosis.[56,57] This syndrome is often associated with:

- Trauma and crush injuries
- Prolonged muscle compression and ischemia, static positioning due to excessive alcohol ingestion, operative positioning, or coma/paralysis
- Seizures and agitation
- Heat stress and extreme exertion
- Electrolyte disturbances including hypokalemia, hypophosphatemia, hypocalcemia, hypernatremia, and hyponatremia

Patient presentation may include acute muscle necrosis resulting in myalgias, pigmenturia due to renal filtration of myoglobin, elevated serum creatine kinase (CK) levels, and acute renal failure. Muscle weakness is often associated with the severity of muscle damage.

INFLAMMATORY MYOPATHIES

The inflammatory myopathies include **dermatomyositis** (DM), **polymyositis** (PM), and **inclusion body myositis** (IBM). These disorders are often associated with connective tissue diseases (scleroderma, mixed connective-tissue disease), cancers (gastrointestinal [GI], lung, breast, ovarian, non-Hodgkin's lymphoma), and autoimmune diseases (systemic lupus erythematosus [SLE], rheumatoid arthritis [RA], Sjörgren's syndrome, sarcoidosis, primary biliary cirrhosis). Common to these disorders are moderate to severe weakness and muscle inflammation. Symptoms typically develop over weeks to months, but acute cases have been noted.[58] Symmetric proximal muscle weakness is common to DM and PM including trunk muscle weakness, but IBM may be asymmetric and present with distal to proximal weakness. DM patients present with characteristic rashes on the extremities and trunk, while all inflammatory myopathies demonstrate elevations in serum creatine phosphokinase (CK). Diagnosis is confirmed by muscle biopsy. Facial muscles and cranial nerves are typically spared, and myalgias are noted early in disease course.[58,59] Patients typically complain of difficulty with stair climbing, out of bed (OOB) transfers, arising from supine, and may have experienced frequent falls or loss of balance.

THERAPEUTIC INTERVENTIONS/INTERVENTIONS FOR BED REST

Examination of neuromuscular status is important in all patients, but is especially important for those who have maintained bed rest for a prolonged period of time. Initial signs of neuromuscular dysfunction may not be evident until the patient attempts to move. The physical therapist is often the first to attempt to mobilize the patient and abnormalities become evident. Movement patterns may provide a quick insight into the neurologic integrity of the patient. Tone, motor control, and sensation should be noted to further evaluate the patient's condition and may trigger the need for a further work-up if neurologic abnormalities are encountered. Patient presentation is important for those who have been on bed rest for prolonged periods of time. These patients will present with LE > UE weakness with noted decrements in the antigravity muscle groups. Orthostatic hypotension should be expected if OOB and upright activities have been performed minimally. Treatment interventions are diverse and specific programs cannot be recommended. Maintenance of aerobic work capacity, strength, and endurance during prolonged bed rest may be attained best by exercise regimens requiring development of maximal muscular tension intermittently rather than performance of longer duration submaximal exercise continuously as reported in ambulatory subjects.[60] Many studies address the use of various exercise programs including isometric, isokinetic, and isotonic exercise as countermeasures to alleviate or prevent the untoward effects of bed rest. Few studies, however, directly address hospitalized patients with multiple co-morbid medical conditions; the majority of these studies use normal men and women as subjects, and the typical exercise workloads are >50% the one repetition maximum for resistive exercise prescriptions or >50% of $VO_{2\ max}$ for aerobic work. These factors limit generalizations to the acute care setting, however, the premise that bed rest deconditioning can be partly explained independent of disease underscores the importance of physical activity, resistive exercise, and early intermittent ambulation.[11] Reductions in bone mass after a period of bed rest are associated with decrements in muscle strength and possible alterations in balance and gait significantly increase the risk of bone fracture with even minor falls.[5] Although passive range of motion (PROM) is routinely used to prevent pressure ulcers and contractures and to stimulate circulation, PROM can not prevent atrophy of affected muscles.[21] Muscle contraction of certain minimal force and frequency are necessary to maintain strength. Additionally, the continued performance of ADLs supports the cardiovascular system and improves muscle strength alleviating many of the hazards of bed rest and inactivity.[11,21] Overall, exercise can diminish and potentially alleviate the muscle atrophy in an exercise-specific manner. This specificity of training is demonstrated in studies addressing LE strengthening. For example, leg press type exercises promote definitive improvements in quadriceps and hamstring force production with minimal changes in plantar and dorsiflexion strength,[61-63] whereas specific programs aimed at the plantar flexor muscle group can attenuate the deconditioning of this muscle group associated with bed rest.[64] Specificity of training is important considering that bed rest promotes the greatest loss of strength in the postural and LEs. Specificity issues also relate to orthostatic intolerance. Attenuation of carotid vagal baroreflex after inactivity was found to be dependent on posture occurring only in supine rest. Numerous studies note that supine exercise does not correct orthostatic intolerance even with correction of plasma volumes (euvolemia).[60,65] This provides further evidence of the importance of facilitating OOB activities and maximizing upright positioning including sitting.

Additional benefits of exercise training during prolonged bed rest include increased fluid intake and maintenance of a positive fluid balance and attenuation in the loss of RBC volume.[60,62,63] There are decreased incidences of DVT, PE, pneumonia, and urinary tract infections with programs emphasizing standard mobility and activity guidelines which attempt to promote reductions in unnecessary bed rest.[2] Exercise tends to maintain quality of sleep and concentration and leads to improvements in depression symptoms.[60,62,63] Finally, exercise may lead to maintenance or improvements in proprioception, further reducing fall and fracture risk.[60]

Positioning in functional or lengthened/stretched positions and frequent range of motion (ROM) needs to be considered for those who are unable to move, are pharmacologically sedated, or paralyzed. Static positioning in shortened positions should be avoided and active assisted and active muscular activity and upright positioning should be promoted as much as possible.

Finally, it has been shown that physical therapy including deep breathing exercises, huffing, coughing and early mobilization can improve oxygen saturation and reduce the incidence of postoperative pulmonary complications.[66,67] All hospitalized patients should be involved in an airway clearance and mobility regimens.

CASE STUDY

Mrs. Morton is a 60-year-old female transferred from a local community hospital to the academic teaching center per the family's request for further treatment of a severe exacerbation of COPD and possible evaluation for lung transplantation. She was transferred to the medical intensive care unit (MICU), intubated and sedated. Physical therapy is consulted for evaluation and treatment as part of the "mechanical ventilation challenge to wean" protocol.

Patient/Client History

General Demographics/Social History/ Living Environment

Her husband states that they live in a split-level with four steps to enter from the outside, two from the garage, and that there is a bathroom on each of the levels of the house. On clarification, the bathrooms are either up or down six steps in the house. Mrs. Morton is a retired pharmacist, but still manages a chain of pharmacies.

General Health Status/Family History

Mrs. Morton's father died of a heart attack at age 55, and she had lost a brother to a heart attack last year.

Medical/Surgical History

Chart review reveals that Mrs. Morton had been a 100 pack/year smoker, had quit smoking 5 years ago, but was dependent on 15 mg of prednisone for the past 6 months. She has a past medical history (PMH) that includes HTN (hypertension) that has been well controlled with medication and diet. Her weight on admission to the outside hospital was 205 pounds at a height of 70 inches. Her surgical history is significant for an anterior cruciate ligament (ACL) repair on the right 20 years ago while skiing.

Current Conditions/Chief Complaints

Mrs. Morton was admitted to the community hospital 3 weeks ago for an exacerbation of her COPD. She has not responded to intravenous (IV) antibiotics and corticosteroids, bronchodilators, supplemental oxygen therapy, non-invasive mechanical ventilation, and airway clearance. She is on synchronized intermittent mandatory ventilation (SIMV),[12] pressure support (PS),[15] F_iO_2 40%, positive end expiratory pressure (PEEP).[10] She is not awake or responsive, most likely due to sedation to lessen her "fighting" the ventilator. The chest x-ray demonstrates hyperinflation, flattened diaphragms, and some patchy haziness at the right base. The medical staff has noticed minimal active muscle activity during examination. Reflexes are diminished.

Functional Status and Activity Level

Mrs. Morton was independent with all ADLs, enjoyed getting together with her children and grandchildren, and played golf with friends at least twice a week prior to hospital admission.

Other Clinical Tests

Laboratory results of the complete blood cell count (CBC) revealed white blood cell (WBC) elevation, hemoglobin of 9.4 g/dL, and HCT 33%. The electrolyte panel results were sodium 131 mEq/L, creatinine 1.7 mg/dL, albumin

2.8 g/dL. Arterial blood gas (ABG) values were pH 7.34/PCO_2 48/PO_2 70/HCO_3^- 26.

Systems Review

Cardiovascular/Pulmonary

Patient is minimally responsive and has resting vital signs (VS) of HR 94 sinus, respiratory rate (RR) 12, BP 130/90, and SpO_2 93% on SIMV 12, PS 15, F_iO_2 40%, and PEEP of 10. Manual muscle test (MMT), ROM, and bed mobility were evaluated with a vital sign response of HR 128, RR 20, BP 166/96, and SpO_2 89%. Anemia is noted on the CBC. Seven minutes was required for VS to return to baseline. Her breath sounds on the ventilator are coarse anteriorly and laterally, but diminished posteriorly at the lung bases. A weak cough was elicited with moving side to side while assessing bed mobility.

Integumentary

Mrs. Morton has a radial arterial line in her right forearm with a supportive board, an IV line in her left antecubital space, and a central line in the right subclavian. She also has a Foley catheter in place. Her skin appears dry and fragile with purplish marks on the forearms. Her legs have pneumatic boots on, but upon removal the skin is also very dry and fragile, but there are no pressure sores on elbows, heels, or buttocks region. Slight pitting edema (+2) noted in the buttock area and distal extremities.

Musculoskeletal

MMT reveals 2-/5 UE elbow flexion and grasp, and 1 to 2-/5 quadriceps, hip flexion and extension, and dorsiflexion bilaterally, trace shoulder flexion and abduction right > left. ROM is limited to <100 degrees at bilateral shoulders, hip flexion is limited to <50 degrees bilaterally, knee extension is within normal limits (WNL), but flexion is limited to 40 degrees, and dorsiflexion is minus 10 bilaterally. Bed mobility is dependent.

Neuromuscular

Mrs. Morton will squeeze her eyelids for yes/no questions. Gross sensation appeared intact for light touch and sharp/dull. Reflexes are diminished (1+). Proprioception was not evaluated. Further mobility testing was postponed at this time due to fatigue as demonstrated by subjective complaints and vital sign changes with minimal exertion.

Communication, Affect, Cognition, Language, and Learning Style

Mrs. Morton speaks primarily English per her husband. She did follow simple direction as demonstrated by attempts to squeeze eyelids with one-step direction. Presently she is intubated and did not attempt to mouth words. She is somnolent and easily aroused.

Tests and Measures

Aerobic Capacity and Endurance

Poor endurance as demonstrated by supine evaluation of MMT, ROM, and bed mobility. Mrs. Morton had a significant change in HR, BP, RR, and a drop in SpO_2 with a minimal intensity challenge. Laboratory results are indicative of hypoxemia along with borderline nutritional, pulmonary, and kidney function. PT/PTT should also be monitored because she is anticoagulated due to her risk for deep vein thrombosis.

Assistive and Adaptive Devices

Recommend resting ankle/foot orthosis to prevent breakdown and prevent worsening of distal LE ROM deficits. Recommend elevation of distal UE/LE in supine position and placing patient on a pressure relief mattress for wound prevention.

Gait, Locomotion, and Balance

During bed mobility the patient demonstrated no adjustments in the neck and trunk area.

Pain

Unable to quantify but patient confirmed pain by squeezing her eyelids with end ROM at the ankles, knees, hips, and shoulders.

Evaluation

Mrs. Morton presents with profound motor weakness with intact sensation. The therapist cannot distinguish between disuse atrophy or myopathic process, but an acquired neuromuscular disorder would be consistent with the history and subsequent hospital course. Additionally, the cardiopulmonary reserve is diminished as evidenced by the VS responses during bed mobility activities.

Diagnosis

Mrs. Morton demonstrates a severe quadriparesis, potentially myopathy, related to deconditioning, bedrest, and complicated by chronic corticosteroid use. Recommend treatment pattern 5G: impaired motor function and sensory integrity associated with acute or chronic polyneuropathies.[68]

Prognosis

Mrs. Morton will need daily physical therapy services for progression of functional level and to assist with weaning from mechanical ventilation. She will need prolonged rehabilitation services that will span acute care through inpatient rehabilitation.

Intervention

Mrs. Morton will receive daily physical therapy consisting of airway clearance, therapeutic exercise, proprioceptive neuromuscular facilitation techniques, and mobility training. She will also benefit from occupational and speech therapy as well as a nutrition consult for weight loss of >25 pounds and decreased albumin since outside hospital admission. The nursing assistants and the patient's family are instructed in ROM exercises to be performed daily.

Reexamination

Mrs. Morton was transferred to the intermediate medical care unit (IMCU) and underwent a tracheostomy and gastric tube insertion for supplemental feeding 5 days post admission to this facility. Her arterial line was removed, but the Foley catheter was continued. Mrs. Morton is OOB in a pneumatic lift chair 1 hour twice a day. She is able to sit at a 45-degree angle in the chair. Her ventilator settings have been decreased to SIMV 8, PS 10, PEEP 10, F_iO_2 40%. Her quadriceps, hip flexors, dorsiflexors are 2 to 3-/5, shoulder shrugs 2/5 bilaterally, and elbow flexion and grasp 3/5. She is able to roll side to side in bed with the head of the bed flat with maximum assistance of one, transfer to dangling with maximum assist of one, and tolerate dangle sitting for 60 seconds times 2. Her VS take <5 minutes to return to baseline compared to 7 minutes on initial evaluation.

Outcomes

Mrs. Morton needs to continue with the present therapy services and will remain in the acute care setting for another 2 weeks. Her functional limitations continue to be inability to perform bed mobility, transfers, or ADLs without maximal assistance. She is being evaluated for discharge to a skilled nursing unit. Her insurance does not cover inpatient acute level rehabilitation.

CHAPTER REVIEW QUESTIONS

1. How does prolonged bed rest affect aerobic capacity of the patient, and what are the physiological mechanisms of detraining?

2. How does an elevated HCT increase the risk for deep vein thrombosis?

3. Describe the predominant adaptive response to reduced muscle use and how muscle metabolism is affected.

4. Which skeletal sites are most susceptible to bone loss secondary to disuse?

5. Do PROM exercises maintain the strength of a patient confined to bed rest? Why or why not?

REFERENCES

1. Asher RA. The dangers of going to bed. *Br Med J.* 1947;4:967–968.
2. Markey DW, Brown RJ. An interdisciplinary approach to addressing patient activity and mobility in the medical-surgical patient. *J Nurs Care Qual.* 2002;16:1–12.
3. Creditor MC. Hazards of hospitalization of the elderly. *Annals of Intern Med.* 1993;18:219–223.

4. Lamont CT, Sampson S, Matthias R, Kane R. The outcome of hospitalization for acute illness in the elderly. *J Am Geriatr Soc.* 1983;31:282–288.
5. Bloomfield S. Changes in musculoskeletal structure and function with prolonged bed rest. *Med Sci Sports Exerc.* 1997;29:197–206.
6. McArdle WD, Katch FI, Katch VL. *Exercise Physiology: Energy, Nutrition and Human Performance.* Philadelphia, Pa: Lippincott Williams & Wilkins; 2001.
7. Bassey E, Bennett T, Birmingham AT, et al. Effects of surgical operation and bed rest on cardiovascular responses to exercise in hospital patients. *Cardiovasc Res.* 1973;7:588–592.
8. Convertino V. Effects of exercise and inactivity on intravascular volume and cardiovascular control mechanisms. *Acta Astronautica.* 1992;27:123–129.
9. Gogia P, Schneider V, LeBlanc AD, et al. Bed rest effect on extremity muscle torque in healthy men. *Arch Phys Med Rehab.* 1988;69:1030–1032.
10. Crandall C, Johnson V, Convertino VA, et al. Altered thermoregulatory responses after 15-days of head-down tilt. *J Appl Phys.* 1994;77:1863–1867.
11. Convertino V, Bloomfield S, Greenleaf J. An overview of the issues: physiological effects of bed rest and restricted physical activity. *Med Sci Sports Exerc.* 1997;29:187–190.
12. Convertino V. Effects of orthostatic stress on exercise performance after bed rest: relation to in hospital rehabilitation. *J Cardiac Rehabil.* 1983;3:660–663.
13. Greenleaf J, Bernauer A, Ertl AC, et al. Work capacity during 30-days of bed rest with isotonic and isokinetic exercise training. *J Appl Phys.* 1989;67:1820–1826.
14. Convertino V. Cardiovascular consequences of bed rest: effect on maximal oxygen uptake. *Medicine and Science in Sports and Exercise.* 1997;29:191–196.
15. Saltin B, Bloomqv, Mitchell JH, et al. Response to exercise after bed rest and after training. *Circulation.* 1968;38:1–78.
16. Convertino VA. Value of orthostatic stress in maintaining functional status soon after myocardial infarction or cardiac artery bypass grafting. *J Cardiovasc Nurs.* 2003;18:124–130.
17. Convertino V, Doerr DF, Mathes KL, et al. Changes in size and compliance of the calf following 30 days of exposure to simulated microgravity. *Aviat Space Environ Med.* 1989;60:653–658.
18. Englelke J, Convertino V. Catecholamine response to maximal exercise following 16 days of simulated microgravity. *Aviat Space Environ Med.* 1996;67:243–247.
19. Crandall C, Englelke J, Pawelczyk JA, et al. Power spectral and time based analysis of heart rate variability following 15 days head-down bed rest.. *Aviat Space Environ Med.* 1994;65:1105–1109.
20. Convertino VA, Doerr DF, Eckberg DL, et al. Head-down bed rest impairs vagal baroreflex responses and provokes orthostatic hypotension. *J Appl Phys.* 1990;68:1458–1464.
21. Kasper CE, Talbot LA, Gaines JM. Skeletal muscle damage and recovery. *AACN Clin Issues.* 2002;13:237–247.
22. Edgerton VR, Roy RR, Allen DL, Monti RJ. Adaptations in skeletal muscle disuse or decreased-use atrophy. *Am J Phys Med Rehab.* 2002;81:S127–S147.
23. *ACSM's Resource Manual for Guidelines for Exercise Testing and Prescription.* 4th ed. Philadelphia, Pa: Lippincott Williams & Wilkins; 2001.
24. LeBlanc A, Gogia V, Schneider V, et al. Calf muscle area and strength changes after five weeks of horizontal bed rest. *Am J Sports Med.* 1988;16:624–629.
25. *ACSM Resource Manual for Guidelines for Exercise Testing and Prescription.* Philadelphia, Pa: Lea & Febiger; 1993.

26. Kawakami Y, Akima H, Kubo K, et al. Changes in muscle size, architecture, and neural activation after 20 days of bed rest with and without resistance exercise. *Eur J Appl Physiol.* 2001;84:7–12.

27. Hikida RS, Gollnick, Dudley GA, et al. Structural and metabolic characteristics of human skeletal muscle following 30 days of simulated microgravity. *Aviat Space Environ Med.* 1989;60:664–670.

28. Pette D, Staron RS. Transitions of muscle fiber phenotypic profiles. *Histochem Cell Biol.* 2001;115:359–372.

29. Goldspink G. Changes in muscle mass and phenotype and the expression of autocrine and systemic growth factors by muscle in response to stretch and overload. *J Anat.* 1998;194:323–334.

30. Lawrence VA, Hilsenbeck SG, Mulrow DC. Incidence and hospital stay for cardiac and pulmonary complications after abdominal surgery. *J Gen Intern Med.* 1995;10:671–678.

31. Venturoli D, Semino P, Negrini D, et al. Respiratory mechanics after 180 days space mission. *Acta Astronaut.* 1998;42:185–204.

32. Montmerle S, Spaak J, Linnarsson, D. Lung function during and after prolonged head-down bed rest. *J Appl Physiol.* 2002;92:75–83.

33. Vitacca M, Clini E, Spassini W, et al. Does the supine position worsen respiratory function in elderly subjects? *Gerontology.* 1996;42:46–53.

34. Daugaard JR, Richter EA. Relationship between muscle fibre composition, glucose transporter protein 4 and exercise training: possible consequences in non-insulin-dependent diabetes mellitus. *Acta Physiol Scand.* 2001;171:267–276.

35. Greenleaf JE. Physiologic consequences of reduced physical activity during bed rest. *Exerc Sports Sci Reviews.* 1982;10:84.

36. Zorbas YG, Kakurin VJ, Afonin VB, et al. Electrolyte changes in plasma and urine of athletes during acute and rigorous bed rest and ambulatory conditions. *Biol Trace Elem Res.* 2001;79:49–65.

37. Tipton CM, Greenleaf JE, Jackson CG. Neuroendocrine and immune system responses with spaceflights. *Med Sci Sports Exerc.* 1996;28:988–998.

38. Shibasaki M, Wilson TE, Cui J, et al. Exercise throughout 6-degree head-down tilt bed rest preserves thermoregulatory responses. *J Appl Physiol.* 2003;95:1817–1823.

39. Covinsky KE, Fortinsky RH, Palmer RM, et al. Relation between symptoms of depression and health status outcomes in acutely ill hospitalized older persons. *Ann Intern Med.* 1997;126:417–425.

40. Cole MG. Delirium in elderly patients. *Am J Geriatr Psychiatry.* 2004;12:7–21.

41. Siegel MD. Management of agitation in the intensive care unit. *Clin Chest Med.* 2003;24:713–725.

42. Szokol JW, Vender JS. Anxiety, delirium, and pain in the intensive care unit. *Crit Care Clin.* 2001;17:821–842.

43. Davies SJ, Jackson PR, Protokar J, Nutt DJ. Treatment of anxiety and depressive disorders in patients with cardiovascular disease. *BMJ.* 2004;17:939–943.

44. Lanken P. *The Intensive Care Unit Manual.* Philadelphia, Pa: WB Saunders Co; 2001.

45. Kotler DP. Cachexia. *Annals of Internal Med.* 2000;17:622–634.

46. Berek K, Margreiter J, Willeit J, et al. Polyneuropathies in critically patients: a prospective evaluation. *Int Care Med.* 1996;22:849–855.

47. Hund E. Mypoathy in critically ill patients. *Crit Care Med.* 1999;27:2544–2547.

48. Lacomis D, Giuliani MJ, Van Cott A, et al. Acute myopathy of intensive care: clinical, electromyographic, and pathologic aspects. *Ann Neurol.* 1996;40:645–654.

49. Partridge BL, Abroms JH, Bazemore C, et al. Prolonged neuromuscular block-ade after long-term infusion of vecuronium bromide in the intensive care unit. *Crit Care Med.* 1990;18:1177–1179.
50. Gutmann L. Critical Illness neuropathy and myopathy. *Archiv Neurol.* 1999;56:527–528.
51. Leijten FS, Harinck-de Weerd JE, Poortvliet DC, et al. The role of polyneuropathy in motor convalescence after prolonged mechanical ventilation. *JAMA.* 1995;274:1221–1225.
52. Polkey MI, Lyall RA, Moxham J, et al. Respiratory aspects of neurologic disease. *J Neurol Neurosurg Psychiatry.* 1999;66:5–15.
53. Huether SE, McCance KL. *Understanding Pathophysiology.* St. Louis, Mo: Mosby-Year Book Inc; 1996.
54. Alshekhlee A, Kaminski HJ, Ruff RL. Neuromuscular manifestations of endocrine disorders. *Neurologic Clinics.* 2002;20:35–58.
55. Anagnos A, Ruff RL, Kaminski HJ. Endocrine neuromyopathies. *Neurol Clin.* 1997;15:673–696.
56. Malinoski DJ, Slater MS, Mullins RJ. Crush injury and rhabdomyolysis. *Crit Care Clin.* 2004;20:171–192.
57. Warren JD, Blumbergs PC, Thompson PD. Rhabdomyolysis: a review. *Muscle Nerve.* 2002;25:332–347.
58. Dalakas, MC, Hohlfeld R. Polymyositis and dermatomyositis. *Lancet.* 2003;362:971–982.
59. Yazici Y, Kagen LJ. Clinical presentation of the idiopathic inflammatory myopathies. *Rheum Dis Clin North Am.* 2002;28:823–832.
60. Greenleaf JE. Intensive exercise training during bed rest attenuates deconditioning. *Med Sci Sports Exerc.* 1997;29:207–215.
61. Kawakami Y, Muraoka Y, Kubo K, et al. Changes in muscle size and architecture following 20 days of bed rest. *J Gravit Physiol.* 2000;7:53-59.
62. Bamman MM, Clarke MS, Feeback DI, et al. Impact of resistance exercise during bed rest on skeletal muscle sarcopenia and myosin isoform distribution. *J Appl Physiol.* 1998;84:157–163.
63. Akima H, Kubo K, Kanehisa H, et al. Leg-press resistance training during 20 days of 6 degrees head-down-tilt bed rest prevents muscle deconditioning. *Eur J Appl Physiol.* 2000;82:30–38.
64. Bamman MM, Hunter GR, Stevens BR, et al. Resistance exercise prevents plantar flexor deconditioning during bed rest. *Med Sci Sports Exerc.* 1997;29:1462–1468.
65. Haruna Y, Suzuki Y, Kawakubo K, et al. Baroreflex during exercise in different postures before and after 20-days bed rest. *J Gravit Physiol.* 1997;4:S53–S57.
66. Oslen MF, Hahn I, Nordgren S, et al. Randomized controlled trial of prophylactic chest physiotherapy in major abdominal surgery. *Br J Surg.* 1997;84:1535–1538.
67. Thomas JA, McIntosh JM. Are incentive spirometry, intermittent positive pressure breathing, and deep breathing exercises effective in the prevention of postoperative pulmonary complications after upper abdominal surgery? A systematic overview and meta-analysis. *Phys Ther.* 1994;74:3–10.
68. Guide to Physical Therapist Practice. 2nd ed. *Phys Ther.* January 2001;81(1).

The Immune System and Infectious Diseases and Disorders

Zoher F. Kapasi, PT, PhD

The primary function of the immune system is to defend the body against infectious microbes—bacteria, viruses, fungi, protozoa, and multicellular parasites. These microbes can cause disease, and if they multiply unchecked they will eventually kill their host. The immune system is effective in curtailing most infections in normal individuals such that infectious disease is short lived and leaves little permanent damage. In addition to infectious microbes, even noninfectious foreign substances can elicit immune responses. Finally, the immune system also reacts against many tumors. Note that not all immune system responses are helpful, as in the case of organ or tissue transplant rejection (see Chapter 14). Additionally, excessive or inappropriate activity of the immune system can result in different hypersensitivity states, immune complex disease, or autoimmune disease. This chapter will focus and briefly review the immune responses useful in combating infections including general clinical manifestations common to most infectious diseases. While discussion of specific infectious diseases is beyond the scope of this chapter, the physical therapist will be provided with guidelines to follow that apply in treating patients with an infectious disease. These guidelines will include the impact of exercise, a therapeutic intervention, on the immune system and infection.

IMMUNE RESPONSE TO INFECTION

The microbes that infect our body come in many different forms, and hence, a wide variety of immune responses are required to deal with each type of infection. However, any immune response involves recognition of the pathogen (disease-causing microbe) or other foreign material, and then a reaction to eliminate it. The different types of immune responses fall into two categories: innate, or nonadaptive, immune responses and adaptive immune responses (Table 5-1). **Innate** immunity, also called natural or native immunity, is constitutional and

Table 5–1

THE IMMUNE RESPONSE

Innate Immunity	Adaptive Immunity	
	Humoral	**Cell-Mediated**
Nonspecific interaction with different antigens, lacks immunologic memory	Specific interaction with different antigens, immunologic memory present	Specific interaction with different antigens, immunologic memory present
Exterior defenses: skin, mucosa, secretions, nasal hair, ear wax	Mediated by antibodies, present as serum globulins	Mediated by T lymphocytes
Soluble mediators: complement, acute phase proteins and interferons (IFNs)	Antibodies are produced by plasma cells (differentiated form of B lymphocytes)	Production of helper T cells (CD4+) and cytotoxic T cells (CD8+)
Phagocytes (leukocytes): neutrophils (PMNs) monocytes/macrophages eosinophils basophils	Globulins having antibody activity are called immunoglobulins (Ig)	Secretion of lymphokines
Mast cells and platelets (inflammation)	Primary and secondary (memory) antibody response	Primary and secondary (memory) T cell response
Natural killer (NK) cells or large granular lymphocytes		

does not improve on repeated contact with the same infectious agent. Innate immunity is the body's first line of defense to prevent the entry of pathogens. Through mutation, the microbes can evolve strategies to evade innate defenses. Therefore, our body is equipped with **adaptive immunity**. The two features of adaptive immunity, also called **acquired** or **specific immunity**, are specificity and memory. An adaptive immune response is highly specific for a particular pathogen and improves with each successive encounter with the same pathogen. In other words, the adaptive immune system "remembers" the infectious agent and can prevent it from causing disease later due to an improved immune response. There are two types of adaptive immune responses, called humoral and cell-mediated immunity, which are mediated by different components of the immune system and function to eliminate different types of microbes.

INNATE IMMUNITY

The components of innate immunity include exterior defenses like skin; soluble mediators like complement, acute-phase proteins and IFNs; cells that are involved in phagocytosis and inflammation (neutrophils, macrophages, eosinophils, basophils, mast cells), and NK cells.

Exterior Defenses

Infection can be avoided by preventing the microbes from gaining access to the body. When intact, the skin is impermeable to most infectious agents. Infection becomes a major problem when there is skin loss as in burns. In areas where there are openings in the body (mouth, nostrils, ears, eyes, etc), unique protection is provided. For example, saliva and stomach acid destroy organisms ingested through the mouth. Nasal hair and secretions protect against microbes entering the nostrils. A waxy secretion prevents microbes from advancing inside the ear canal. The washing action and presence of lysozyme in tears can kill bacteria in the eye. Finally, protective low pH of vaginal secretions and acidic urine protect the genitourinary (GU) openings. When microbes enter the body by penetrating the skin or the epithelial surface of the respiratory, gastrointestinal (GI), or GU tract, two main defensive operations come into play: the destructive effect of soluble mediators and the mechanism of phagocytosis carried out by the phagocytes.

Soluble Mediators

The complement system is a group of about 20 serum proteins produced by the liver that have an intrinsic ability to recognize microbial components and antibodies (produced by B cells during the humoral immune response) bound to the microbe. The complement system of proteins can lyse the cell membranes of many bacterial species. Complement products released in this reaction attract phagocytes to the site of the reaction (**chemotaxis**). Furthermore, complement components can coat the bacterial surface (**opsonization**) allowing the phagocytes to recognize the bacteria and engulf them. A number of serum proteins increase rapidly during infection and tissue injury and are, therefore, collectively called acute phase proteins (C-reactive and mannose binding proteins). The acute phase proteins bind to microbes and promote their uptake by phagocytes (opsonization). IFNs are important in limiting the spread of certain viral infections. IFNα and IFNβ are produced by cells that have become virally infected, and IFNγ is released by certain activated T cells. IFNs induce a state of antiviral resistance in surrounding uninfected tissue cells. The IFNs are produced very early in infection and are the first line of resistance to several viral infections.

Neutrophils

The function of ingesting and destroying microbes is mediated by phagocytes, which include **neutrophils** early in the innate immune response and macrophages later in the response. Because of their multi-lobed nucleus, neutrophils are also called **polymorphonuclear cells (PMNs)** and are the most abundant leukocytes (white blood cells [WBCs]). Neutrophils are short lived (2 to 3 days) relative to monocytes/macrophages, which may live for months or years. The importance of these cells is evident in individuals with reduced white cell numbers such as following chemotherapy or radiotherapy in cancer or with rare genetic defects which prevent PMN emigration in tissues in response to chemotactic stimuli. Both defects markedly increase susceptibility to infection.

Macrophages

Macrophages are "big eaters." Macrophages develop from blood monocytes after monocytes enter into tissues. Macrophages are particularly concentrated in the lung (alveolar macrophages), liver (Kupffer cells), and lining of spleen sinusoids and lymph node medullary sinuses where they are strategically placed to filter foreign material including microbes. Macrophages persist much longer at sites of inflammation, and are the dominant effector cells of the later stages of the innate immune response, 1 or 2 days after infection.

Neutrophils and macrophages both have receptors for complement and antibodies (opsonins) so coating of microbes with opsonins enhances phagocytosis.

Eosinophils

Eosinophils are derived from bone marrow like other WBCs and are involved in destroying large parasites that cannot physically be phagocytosed. Eosinophils secrete chemicals that damage the parasite's membrane leading to organism destruction.

Basophils, Mast Cells, and Platelets

These play a role in immunity against microbes by releasing mediators that enhance inflammation. In particular, mediators such as histamine, released by basophils and mast cells, propagate inflammatory reactions controlling parasitic infections.

Natural Killer Cells

NK cells are large granular lymphocytes that are neither T or B lymphocytes. The function of NK cells is to kill viruses, other intracellular microbe infected cells, and tumor cells. NK cells account for 15% of blood lymphocytes.

ADAPTIVE IMMUNITY

While innate immunity provides early defense against pathogenic microbes, adaptive immunity is the later reaction. Adaptive immunity enhances the protective mechanisms of innate immunity and directs these mechanisms to sites of infection. Adaptive immune responses to microbes induce effector cells that eliminate the microbes and activate memory cells that protect the individual from subsequent infections, so-called protective immunity. There are two types of adaptive immune responses: humoral and cell-mediated immunity.

Humoral Immunity

Humoral immunity is the mechanism of defense against extracellular microbes (including viruses before they enter a cell) and their toxins. It is mediated by antibodies present in different secretions (humors) such as saliva, blood, or vaginal secretions. Humoral immunity is mediated by B lymphocytes or B cells (called as such because they originate and mature in Bone marrow, a primary lymphoid organ). Each B cell can recognize a specific antigen and then proliferate and differentiate into antibody-producing plasma cells or B memory cells. The plasma cells produce antibodies of different isotypes, like IgG, IgA, IgM, IgD, and IgE (serum globulins having antibody activity are called immunoglobulins [Ig]). Antibodies combat infections by numerous mechanisms. High-affinity antibodies bind to and neutralize microbes and their toxins. Antibodies of different isotypes perform different effector functions. Some IgG antibodies opsonize microbes and are recognized by phagocytes with subsequent ingestion and degradation of the microbes. IgM and some IgG antibodies bound to microbes activate the complement system and promote phagocytosis and lysis of the microbes. IgA antibodies are secreted through mucosal epithelia and neutralize microbes in the lumens of mucosal organs such as the GI tract. In pregnant females, some IgG antibodies are transported through the placenta and later IgA antibodies are transported via the breastmilk to provide passive immunity to the newborn while the immune system is developing. Memory B cells circulate throughout the body and are responsible for the more rapid and stronger immune response that occurs with repeated exposure to the same antigen.

Cell-Mediated Immunity

Cell-mediated immunity is the mechanism of defense against intracellular microbes that are either ingested by and survive in phagocytes or infect non-phagocytic cells. Since antibodies cannot reach inside the cell, cell-mediated immunity is necessary to destroy the microbes inside a cell. T lymphocytes or T cells (called as such because their precursors arise in bone marrow and mature in Thymus, primary lymphoid organs) mediate this form of immunity. T cells are classified as CD4 T cells or CD8 T cells (based on distinctive molecules called cluster designation [CD] present on their cell surface). CD4 T cells are generally referred to as helper T cells and CD8 T cells are also called cytotoxic T lymphocytes (CTLs). CD4 T cells secrete cytokines (protein molecules that encompass molecules such as interleukins, lymphokines, monokines, and IFN) that activate macrophages to destroy microbes and also help B cells augment antibody production. CTLs recognize peptide antigens of microbes, such as viruses, that infect and survive or replicate in the cytoplasm of any nucleated host cell. Once the CTLs recognize the cell in which the microbe is hiding, they secrete granule proteins and express surface molecules that kill the infected cells and, thereby, eliminate a reservoir of infection.

The complexity of the cellular interactions that occur during adaptive immune responses requires specialized microenvironments in which relevant cells can collaborate efficiently. These microenvironments are provided in secondary lymphoid organs. Secondary lymphoid organs include lymph nodes that filter lymph, the spleen which filters blood, and mucosal-associated lymphoid tissues (MALTs) such as tonsils, adenoids, and Peyer's patches in the small intestine that handle microbes that enter thorough the nasal and oral cavity. Because only a few lymphocytes are specific for any given antigen, T cells and B cells need to migrate throughout the body in blood and secondary lymphoid organs to increase the probability that they will encounter that particular antigen.

INFECTIOUS DISEASE

Infectious disease occurs when pathogens cause signs and symptoms of illness. The interactions between a host, such as a human, and the microbes that reside on or in the host are not always detrimental and in certain situations may benefit both organisms. Harmless inhabitation of the skin and mucous membranes by these microbes is called **colonization**. Normal flora that reside in the host can become opportunistic pathogens, capable of producing an infectious disease when the immunity of the host is compromised.

Factors Affecting Immunity

Immunity of the host is weakened by several factors. For example, skin and mucous membrane that act as important mechanical and biochemical barriers are compromised in patients with incisions, intravenous or urinary catheters, endotracheal tubes, chest tubes, and other invasive monitoring catheters. Adequate nutrition is necessary to maintain a healthy immune system. Malnutrition (protein-energy malnutrition, vitamin and trace element deficiencies) is a risk factor for development of infections. Chronic illnesses such as diabetes, cancer, heart disease, and renal failure are associated with an increased risk of infection. Diabetes alters the host's ability to resist infection. Phagocytosis is impaired with hyperglycemia, and detection of pain from infection may be delayed because of neuropathies. The virulence of some microbes is increased when exposed to hyperglycemic conditions. Circulatory problems associated with cardiac failure or peripheral vascular disease are risk factors for infection since the cellular components of the immune system and antimicrobial agents are dependent on the circulatory system for delivery to the site of infection. Many pathogens thrive in areas with poor tissue perfusion. Age of the host is an important variable in the ability to resist infections. Infants are at an increased risk for infection because of an immature immune system. The elderly are more susceptible to infection because immune function declines with aging leading to greater morbidity and mortality. The lungs and the urinary tract are the most common sites of infection in the elderly. Infection in the elderly may also be manifested atypically, with absence of fever and sudden onset of confusion. Finally, a host may be immunocompromised due to defects in one or more components of the immune system as in the acquired immunodeficiency syndrome (AIDS) wherein the human immunodeficiency virus (HIV) destroys the CD4 T cells. Agents such as antimetabolites, corticosteroids, cyclosporine, and antibiotics can cause immunosuppression. Surgery and anesthesia can also suppress both T and B cell function for up to 1 month postoperatively. Stress has been implicated in predisposing individuals to an infectious process by causing release of stress hormones that are known to depress immune function.

Transmission of Infection

For infection to be transmitted, the microbe must be transported from an infected source to a susceptible host. The five main routes of transmission are as follows:

1. Contact
2. Airborne
3. Droplet
4. Vehicle
5. Vectorborne

Contact transmission occurs directly or indirectly. Direct contact is the transfer of microbes that come into physical contact either by skin-to-skin or mucous membrane-to-mucous membrane (eg, sexual contact, biting, touching, and kissing). Indirect contact involves transfer of microbes from a source to a host by passive transfer from an inanimate, intermediate object, called a fomite. Inanimate objects include assistive devices, goniometer, cuff weights, sphygmomanometer, bedside rail, tray tables, or any item that comes in direct contact with the infected person.

Airborne transmission occurs when microbes are so small (<5 µm) that they float on air currents within a room and remain suspended for several hours. They are often propelled from the respiratory tract through coughing or sneezing. A host then inhales the particles directly into the respiratory tract (eg, tuberculosis, chickenpox).

Droplet transmission is different from airborne transmission because droplets are larger particles (>5 µm) and therefore do not remain suspended in air and fall within 3 feet of the source. Droplets are produced when a person coughs or sneezes and transmission occurs when droplets containing the microorganisms are propelled a short distance through air and are deposited on another person's conjunctiva, nasal mucosa, or mouth. An example of droplet transmission of a microbe is the influenza virus. People in closest proximity to the infected source have the highest risk for infection through droplet transmission.

Vehicle transmission occurs when infectious organisms (eg, Salmonella) are transmitted through a common source (eg, contaminated food, water, and intravenous fluid) to susceptible hosts. **Vectorborne transmission** of infectious organisms involves insects and/or animals that act as intermediaries between two or more hosts. Lyme disease, Rocky Mountain spotted fever, and Creutzfeldt-Jakob disease are examples of vectorborne diseases.

An infection acquired during hospitalization of a patient is referred to as **nosocomial infection**. Nosocomial infections result in prolongation of hospital stays, increases in cost of care, significant morbidity, and can result in death. The most common infections are urinary tract infections (usually associated with Foley catheters or urologic procedures) or bloodstream infections. Prevention is of critical importance in controlling nosocomial infections.

Clinical Presentation and Management of Infectious Disease

Clinical presentation of infectious disease depends on the type of infecting microbe (eg, bacteria, virus) and the body system affected (eg, GU, GI, nervous system, cardiopulmonary system). The symptoms of an infectious disease may be specific and reflect the site of infection. For example, painful urination (dysuria) can result from a urinary tract infection, a skin rash and red streaks can represent a manifestation of a skin infection, and diarrhea can result from a GI infection. Conversely, systemic symptoms such as fever, chills, sweating, malaise, and myalgia are shared by a number of diverse infectious diseases. Elderly persons may experience a change in mentation (eg, confusion, memory loss, difficulty concentrating).

Infections can cause a hypermetabolic state which presents clinically as an increase in heart rate (HR), respiratory rate (RR), and blood pressure (BP). However, BP can decrease secondary to vasodilation from inflammatory responses in the body. Inflammatory response to infection can also lead to an increase in erythrocyte sedimentation rate (ESR) and leukocyte or WBC count. A differential WBC count (granulocytes—neutrophils, basophils, and eosinophils; lymphocytes and monocytes) can assist in identification of the type of infection. For example, a bacterial infection leads to an increase in neutrophils, whereas a parasitic infection leads to increased eosinophils in blood.

In addition to clinical presentation, diagnosis of infectious disease requires the recovery of a probable pathogen or evidence of its presence from the infected sites of a disease host. In the laboratory, the diagnosis of an infectious agent is accomplished using three basic techniques:

1. Culture

2. Serology

3. Direct antigen detection

Culture refers to the propagation of a microbe outside the body using an artificial growth media such as agar plates or broth. The specimen (eg, urine, feces, sputum, cerebrospinal fluid, pleural fluid, synovial fluid) from the diseased host is inoculated into broth or placed on the surface of an agar plate, and the culture is placed in an incubator until the growth of the microbe becomes detectable. In the case of bacteria, identification is based on microscopic appearance and Gram's stain reaction (positive or negative), shape, texture, and color (ie, morphology) of the colonies. **Serology**, the study of serum, is an indirect means of identifying infectious agents by measuring serum antibodies in the diseased host. **Direct antigen detection** relies on purified antibodies to detect antigens of infectious agents in specimens obtained from a diseased host. Identification of microbes is also done through detection of sequences of deoxyribonucleic acids (DNA) or ribonucleic acids (RNA) unique to that microbe using techniques like DNA probe hybridization and polymerase chain reaction (PCR). Each technique has a different degree of sensitivity regarding the number of microbes that need to be present in a specimen for detection. Most infectious diseases of humans are self-limiting and require little or no medical therapy for a complete cure. However, when therapeutic intervention is essential the choice of treatment may be use of the following:

- Antimicrobial agents (see Pharmacological Information)
- Immunologic therapies with antibody preparations, vaccine, or substances that stimulate and improve the host's immune function
- Surgery to remove infected tissues

PHYSICAL THERAPY IMPLICATIONS

Physical therapists and physical therapy assistants need to be aware of two-tier precautions that have to be followed in an acute-care hospital setting—standard precautions and transmission-based precautions—related to infection control.

Standard precautions are designed for the care of all patients in hospitals regardless of their diagnosis or presumed infection status. Implementation of standard precautions is the primary strategy for successfully controlling nosocomial infections. Standard precautions are designed to reduce the risk of transmission of blood-borne pathogens and reduce the risk of transmission of pathogens from moist body substances. Standard precautions apply to:

- Blood
- All body fluids, secretions, and excretions, except sweat, regardless of whether or not they contain visible blood
- Nonintact skin
- Mucous membranes

Standard precautions are designed to reduce the risk of transmission of microbes from both recognized and unrecognized sources of infection in hospitals. Use **personal protective equipment (PPE)** to implement barrier precautions:

- All health care workers should routinely use appropriate barrier precautions to prevent skin and mucous membrane exposure when contact with blood or body fluids or generation of droplets is anticipated. For whirlpool or pulsatile lavage with suction consider hair coverings, masks face shields, and protective eyewear to protect mucus membranes of the eyes, nose, and mouth. Shoulder length gloves should be available for those working with whirlpools, but may fill with contaminated water, limiting effectiveness.
- Gloves should be worn for touching blood and body fluids, mucous membranes, and nonintact skin of all persons.
- Gloves should be changed and hands washed after contact with each client.
- Hand cream should be applied after glove removal to prevent skin chapping, which is a potential risk factor for employees. Petroleum-based hand creams or lotions should not be used, which can damage latex gloves.
- Fluid-resistant gowns or aprons should be worn during procedures that are likely to generate splashes of blood or other body fluids.
- Hand hygiene (ie, hand washing or use of alcohol-based hand rubs) should be practiced before and after client contact and after removing PPE.
- Hands and other skin surfaces should be washed immediately and thoroughly if contaminated with blood or other body fluids. If hands are

visibly soiled, they should be washed with soap and water immediately after gloves are removed. However, if hands are not visibly soiled, an alcohol-based hand hygiene product is the preferred method of hand cleansing.

- Sharp instruments, such as scissors or scalpels, should be handled with great care and disposed of in puncture-resistant containers. Needles should never be manipulated, bent, broken, or recapped.

- Pocket masks or mechanical ventilation devices should be available in areas in which cardiopulmonary resuscitation procedures are likely.

- Health care workers who have exudative lesions or weeping dermatitis should refrain from all direct client care and from handling equipment belonging to the client until the condition resolves.

- Eating, drinking, applying lip balm or lipstick, and handling contact lenses is prohibited in any area where clients or their body fluids are present.

Note that hand hygiene has been cited as the easiest and most effective means of preventing nosocomial infection and must be done routinely even when gloves are used. Before beginning handwashing with soap and water, prepare to have access to a paper towel. This will ensure that once the hands are cleansed, the health care worker does not contaminate his or her hands by touching the paper towel dispenser. Moisten hands before applying soap to ensure that the soap starts lathering as soon as it touches the hands. Avoid using hot water, because repeated exposure to hot water may increase the risk of dermatitis. Effective handwashing technique involves scrubbing for at least 15 seconds (as long as it takes to sing "Happy Birthday" or "Twinkle, Twinkle Little Star" twice). Both sides of both hands must be scrubbed along with wrists, web space between the fingers, and under the nails. Use a paper towel to turn off the faucet and if leaving the room use the paper towel to open the door before discarding the towel. When dealing with antimicrobial-resistant gram-positive cocci (eg, methicillin resistant staphylococcus aureus [MRSA] and vancomycin resistant enterococci [VRE]), an antimicrobial soap is recommended. When using an alcohol-based hand rub, apply product to palm of one hand and rub hands together, covering all surfaces of hands and fingers, until hands are dry. Note that the volume needed to reduce the number of bacteria on hands varies by product. Alcohol-based handrubs significantly reduce the number of microbes on skin, are fast acting, cause less skin irritation, and take less time to use than traditional hand washing. Health care personnel should avoid wearing artificial nails and keep natural nails less than one quarter of an inch long if they care for patients at high risk of acquiring infections. Hand hygiene must be practiced after taking gloves off and before touching anything and before and after each and every client (before to protect the client and after to protect yourself and others). Do not touch a chart with gloved hands. Apart from hand hygiene, every health care worker should be adequately immunized against hepatitis B, influenza (every year), measles, mumps, rubella, polio, tetanus, diphtheria, and varicella to control nosocomial infections. Since urinary tract infection associated with Foley catheter is a common nosocomial infection, a physical therapist should take certain precautions (over and above the standard precautions) when handling the drainage bag while working with the client. Before turning, moving, or transferring a catheterized person, locate the proximal end of the tubing and either clamp it to the person's gown or hold it to allow necessary slack during movement. This will help prevent the catheter from accidentally and traumatically being pulled out. Avoid raising the drainage bag above the level of the person's bladder to prevent backflow of the urine from the tube toward the bladder. If it becomes necessary to raise the bag during transfers, clamp the tubing to prevent backflow as you move the bag and then release the clamp. Avoid allowing large loops of tubing to dangle from the bedside, wheelchair, or walker. Drain all the urine from tubing into the bag before the person exercises or ambulates.

Transmission-based precautions are designed for patients documented or suspected to be infected or colonized with highly transmissible or epidemiologically important pathogens for which additional precautions beyond standard precautions are needed to interrupt transmission in hospitals. There are three types of **transmission-based precautions**:

1. Airborne precautions

2. Droplet precautions

3. Contact precautions

They may be combined for diseases that have multiple routes of transmission. When used either singularly or in combination, they are to be used in addition to standard precautions. Make sure to identify each client's individual transmission precautions and procedures. When in doubt, ask the nursing staff regarding the status of the person in question. Some transmission-based precautions include:

- Private, negative pressure room (airborne transmission isolation room) with doors kept closed (note that airborne transmission isolation room is not required for droplet or contact transmission-based precautions).

- Wear a mask when entering the room (for airborne and droplet transmission-based precautions).

- Limit transport of client from room. Place surgical mask on client when transported.

- Remove gown and gloves before leaving client environment, wash hands immediately with antimicrobial soap, and then do not touch potentially contaminated materials or surfaces as you leave the room (for contact transmission-based precautions).

- Dedicate use of non-critical client care items to only this person (eg, leave the stethoscope, gait belt, cuff weights, goniometer, and assistive devices in the client's room) (for contact transmission-based precautions).

- Disinfect equipment with approved disinfectant prior to use with other people (for contact transmission-based precautions).

Optimizing the client's mobility and endurance are frequently the goals of physical therapy in an acute care setting, and, consequently, the physical therapist should be aware of the effects of physical exercise on immune function. A detailed review[1] of these effects is beyond the scope of this chapter, however, the physical therapist should be aware that intense exercise (exercising at

>80% of maximum oxygen consumption [$VO_{2\,max}$]) is known to suppress immune function, particularly in young individuals. The immune system takes 6 to 24 hours to recover from the acute effects of intense exercise. Each individual client must be evaluated after exercise to determine the perceived intensity of the exercise or intervention session. For example, in the deconditioned older adult with compromised cardiopulmonary function, reduced oxygen transport, and impaired mobility, ambulating from the bed to the bathroom may be perceived by his or her body as intense exercise. However, in a recent study, intense exercise was shown not to have a detrimental effect on immune function and incidence of infections in the elderly.[2] While the suppressive effects of exercise on immune function may differ between young and elderly persons, intense exercise during an infectious episode should be avoided in both the young and elderly clients. For anyone (especially competitive athletes) wondering whether or not to exercise in the presence of acute bacterial or viral infection (eg, when manifesting constitutional symptoms), do a "neck check." If the symptoms are located above the neck, such as stuffy or runny nose, sneezing, or a scratchy throat, exercise should be performed cautiously through the scheduled workout at half the usual intensity and duration. If, after 10 minutes, the symptoms are alleviated, the workout can be completed using the usual exercise prescription (frequency/intensity/duration). If, instead, the symptoms are worse and the head is pounding or throbbing with every footstep, the exercise program should be stopped and the person should rest. If there is fever or there are symptoms below the neck, such as aching muscles, a hacking cough, diarrhea, or vomiting, exercise should not be initiated. Finally, because of vasodilation occurring from inflammation associated with infection, patients may experience orthostatic hypotension and hypotension with functional activities. Consequently, frequent BP monitoring and gradual changes in positions, particularly from recumbent to upright positions, are important to promote tolerance to functional activities.

SUMMARY

The immune system protects the body against pathogens by means of innate and adaptive immunity. Infectious disease occurs when the pathogen overwhelms the immune system resulting in signs and symptoms of the disease. Immune function is compromised by several factors, including malnutrition, loss of skin integrity, coexisting chronic illnesses like diabetes, stress, drugs like steroids, and the age of the patient (elderly and children), and may predispose a person to infection. The physical therapist and physical therapist assistants should follow standard and transmission-based precautions to ensure infection control. Moreover, the therapist should understand the impact of exercise on the immune response and tailor their mobility and endurance exercise programs to the clinical presentation of the infectious disease their client is manifesting.

CASE STUDY

A 66-year-old male, Mr. O'Baxter, diagnosed with type 2 diabetes mellitus, is admitted with fever, inflammation of the dorsum right foot, and a large ulcer on the plantar surface of the right foot. In the past 2 days, the amount of drainage from the ulcer has increased. Physical therapy is consulted for wound management.

Patient/Client History

General Demographics/Social History/Living Environment

Mr. O'Baxter lives with his wife and children on the third floor of a walk-up apartment building. He is formally employed as a manager of a construction company. He presently works part-time helping in his wife's dry cleaning business.

General Health Status/Family History

Mr. O'Baxter quit smoking 2 years ago after smoking for 25 years. He states he enjoys a beer a couple times a week.

Medical/Surgical History

Past medical history includes a positive annual PPD tuberculin skin tests with negative chest x-rays since returning from Vietnam several years ago. Patient completed 6 months of INH (isoniazid) chemotherapy after his positive PPD.

Current Conditions/Chief Complaints

Mr. O'Baxter is complaining of right foot discomfort, fever, and a noticeable increase in drainage in his right sock and shoe. On physical examination, the patient has a fever of 101.8°F with decreased breath sounds in left apical lung fields and a frequent dry cough. The chest x-ray shows a suspicious 2.5-cm diameter area of consolidation in left apical lobe. The dorsal surface of right foot is red with induration from mid-foot distally. There is a large callous with an ulcer draining large amounts of malodorous purulent material on the plantar surface of the right foot. The wound is covered with fibrous yellow and black necrotic debris and wound depth is unable to be determined. The patient is on full respiratory precautions until cleared by infection control and sputum cultures.

Functional Status and Activity Level

Mr. O'Baxter was functionally independent prior to the foot infection.

Other Clinical Tests

Laboratory findings reveals the following data: Hgb A_1c 9.9%, WBC 11,560/mm^3, creatinine 1.5 mg/dL, iron 60 μg/dL, and ABGs pH 7.34/PCO_2 38/PO_2 88/HCO_3^- 26, and ABI 0.8.

Systems Review

Cardiovascular/Pulmonary

Resting VS in bed (head of bed raised >45 degrees) are oxygen saturation (SpO_2) 94% on 0.35 F_iO_2 (35%) via face mask, HR 108, pulse regular, RR 28 with accessory muscle use, BP 108/76, and pain 2/10 with right foot elevated in bed. Breath sounds are decreased in left apical lung fields and a frequent dry cough. Patient is on respiratory precautions. Following transfers and evaluation, his VS were 95% SpO_2, HR 114, RR 30, BP 110/76, and pain 4/10.

Integumentary

The dorsal surface of right foot is red with induration from mid-foot distally. There is a large callous with an ulcer draining large amounts of malodorous purulent material on the plantar surface of the right foot. The wound is covered with fibrous yellow and black necrotic debris. The wound measures 5 cm across and 3 cm in width. No depth was measured at this time.

Musculoskeletal

Manual muscle test (MMT), range of motion (ROM), of bilateral upper extremities (BUE) and left lower extremity (LLE) within normal limits (WNL). Right lower extremity (RLE) hip/knee MMT and ROM WFL. Ankle motion appears intact, but due to pain on movement did not fully assess. Bed mobility and non-weightbearing sit-to-stand transfers to wheelchair require only contact guard and verbal cues.

Neuromuscular

BUE sensation intact, sharp/dull diminished below bilateral knees.

Communication, Affect, Cognition, Language, and Learning Style

Mr. O'Baxter is awake, alert, and oriented times 4. He does complain of chills and discomfort. His primary language is English.

Tests and Measures

Aerobic Capacity and Endurance

Mr. O'Baxter demonstrated elevated resting HR, RR and apparent respiratory distress with accessory muscle usage. His vital signs (VS) responses during functional examination were appropriate. He appears short of breath and uses his accessory muscles for minimal activity. Laboratory findings support poor diabetes management, probable infection, renal insufficiency, and large vessel disease most likely from complications of diabetes. Await sputum results for tuberculosis/AFB screen.

Assistive and Adaptive Devices

Recommend a standard walker for the patient's room to assist with non-weightbearing transfers and eventual ambulation.

Gait, Locomotion, and Balance

At this time, transfers only were attempted. Patient's static and dynamic balance were fair and required only contact guard assistance.

Pain

Mr. O'Baxter had increased pain with non-weightbearing transfers. This may change with further wound evaluation and treatment. Pain management should be optimized prior to and during therapy sessions.

Evaluation

Mr. O'Baxter's functional limitations are related to his non-weightbearing status and limited pulmonary reserve. The provision of physical therapy services is challenged by his isolation status. Appropriate wound care and medical management should enable this elderly man to return to his home.

Diagnosis

Mr. O'Baxter presents with a respiratory impairment as well as a non-healing wound in his RLE. He needs to remain on full respiratory precautions until his cultures return and rule out TB. He will have to be treated bedside for wound care. Recommend treatment pattern 7C: impaired integumentary integrity associated with partial-thickness skin involvement and scar formation.[3] This pattern may change once the wound is fully visible.

Prognosis

Diabetes impairs immune function, and chronic illnesses like diabetes are associated with increased infection risk. Furthermore, immune function declines with aging and infection in the elderly is associated with greater morbidity and mortality. Although there is a history of a positive skin test for exposure to tuberculosis, the patient completed preventive drug therapy. However, since the patient's immune system is depressed, there is a possibility for reactivation of the infection. The patient's cough and the small area of consolidation on the chest x-ray made it necessary to put the patient on respiratory precautions. These precautions include housing the patient in a private room with doors closed and monitored negative airflow. Finally, because the patient has a fever, he should be advised to balance rest with activities that are not exhausting. He is restricted to bathroom privileges and ambulation within his room.

Intervention

Recommend aggressive wound care as well as deep breathing and AROM exercises to prevent possible pneumonia from limited activity. Gait, transfer, and wheelchair training are performed maintaining NWB until independent with use of walker.

Reexamination

Mr. O'Baxter remains on full respiratory precautions, is independent with mobility within the confines of his room, and bedside wound care continues.

Outcomes

Recommend continued outpatient wound care once cleared to leave hospital by infectious disease specialist.

CHAPTER REVIEW QUESTIONS

1. Define the primary function of the immune system.
2. Contrast the two types of immunity.
3. What are the clinical presentation features of an infectious disease?
4. Describe standard and transmission-based precautions for infection control.
5. Discuss the impact of exercise on immune function and infectious disease.

DISEASE INFORMATION: COMMON INFECTIOUS DISEASES WORLDWIDE

The following is a list of the most common infectious diseases throughout the world today. Accurate caseload numbers are difficult to determine, especially because so many of these diseases are endemic to developing countries, where many people do not have access to modern medical care. Approximately half of all deaths caused by infectious diseases each year can be attributed to just three diseases: tuberculosis, malaria, and AIDS. Together, these diseases cause more than 300 million illnesses and more than 5 million deaths each year.

The list does not include diseases that have received a significant amount of media attention in recent years—such as Ebola hemorrhagic fever or West Nile virus—but which in fact have infected a relatively small number of people.

African Trypanosomiasis ("Sleeping Sickness")

African trypanosomiasis is spread by the tsetse fly, which is common to many African countries. The World Health Organization (WHO) estimates that nearly 450,000 cases occur each year. Symptoms of the disease include fever, headaches, joint pains, and itching in the early stage and confusion, sensory disturbances, poor coordination, and disrupted sleep cycles in the second stage. If the disease goes untreated in its first stage, it causes irreparable neurological damage; if it goes untreated in its second stage, it is fatal.

Cholera

Cholera is a disease spread mostly through contaminated drinking water and unsanitary conditions. It is endemic in the Indian subcontinent, Russia, and sub-Saharan Africa. It is an acute infection of the intestines with the bacterium *Vibrio cholerae*. Its main symptom is copious diarrhea. Between 5% and 10% of those infected with the disease will develop severe symptoms, which also include vomiting and leg cramps. In its severe form, cholera can cause death by dehydration. An estimated 200,000 cases are reported to WHO annually.

Cryptosporidiosis

Cryptosporidiosis has become one of the most common causes of waterborne disease in the United States and in recent years; it is also found throughout the rest of the world. It is caused by a parasite that spreads when a water source is contaminated, usually with the feces of infected animals or humans. Symptoms include diarrhea, stomach cramps, an upset stomach, and slight fever. Some people do not exhibit any symptoms.

Dengue

WHO estimates that 50 million cases of dengue fever appear each year. The spread of dengue fever is through the bite of the *Aedes aegypti* mosquito. Recent years have seen dengue outbreaks all over Asia and Africa. Dengue fever can be mild to moderate, and occasionally severe, though it is rarely fatal. Mild cases, which usually affect infants and young children, involve a nonspecific febrile illness, while moderate cases, seen in older children and adults, display high fever, severe headaches, muscle and joint pains, and rash. Severe cases develop into dengue hemorrhagic fever, which involves high fever, hemorrhaging, and sometimes circulatory failure.

Hepatitis A

Hepatitis A is a highly contagious liver disease caused by the hepatitis A virus. Spread primarily by the fecal-oral route or by ingestion of contaminated water or food, the number of annual infections worldwide is estimated at 1.4 million. Symptoms include fever, fatigue, jaundice, and dark urine. Although those exposed usually develop life-long immunity, the best protection against hepatitis A is vaccination.

Hepatitis B

Approximately 2 billion people are infected with the hepatitis B virus (HBV), making it the most common infectious disease in the world today. More than 350 million of those infected never rid themselves of the infection. Hepatitis is an inflammation of the liver that causes symptoms such as jaundice, extreme fatigue, nausea, vomiting, and stomach pain; hepatitis B is the most serious form of the disease. Chronic infections can cause cirrhosis of the liver or liver cancer in later years.

Hepatitis C

Hepatitis C is a less common, and less severe, form of hepatitis. An estimated 170 million people worldwide are infected with hepatitis C virus (HCV); 3 to 4 million more are infected every year. The majority of HCV cases are asymptomatic, even in people who develop chronic infection.

HIV/AIDS

Acquired immune deficiency syndrome, or AIDS, was first reported in mid-1981 in the United States and is believed to have originated in sub-Saharan Africa. The HIV that causes AIDS was identified in 1983, and by 1985 tests to detect the virus were available. The clinical consequences of HIV infection are due to the ability of this retrovirus to target crucial cells of the immune system, the lymphocyte, that expresses the cell surface marker CD4, which serves as a receptor that binds the envelope protein of the virus. Two major types of HIV have been recognized, HIV-1 and HIV-2. HIV-1 is the dominant type worldwide. HIV-2 is found principally in West Africa but cases have been reported in East Africa, Europe, Asia, and Latin America. There are at least 10 different genetic subtypes of HIV-1, but their biological and epidemiological significance is unclear at present. Both HIV-1 and HIV-2 are transmitted in the same ways. Although the first reported cases involved homosexual men in Los Angeles who were infected through sexual contact, the principal mode of transmission throughout the world is through the exchange of bodily fluids during heterosexual intercourse. HIV is transmitted by sexual contact, intravenous drug users sharing infected hypodermic needles, through transfused blood or its components, and it may also be transmitted from infected mother to infant before, during, or shortly after birth.

HIV infection is characterized by the progressive loss of CD4+ lymphocytes, and immunodeficiency results not only from a lack of effective immunity against HIV itself, but also because the virus damages CD4 cell subsets that are crucial for containing other pathogens. AIDS is the fatal and incurable disease caused by HIV. AIDS attacks and destroys the immune system, gradually leaving the individual defenseless against illnesses that lead to death. These illnesses are referred to as "opportunistic" infections or diseases; in AIDS patients the most common are Pneumocystis carinii pneumonia (PCP), a parasitic infection of the lungs, and a type of cancer known as Kaposi's sarcoma (KS). Other opportunistic infections include unusually severe infections with yeast, cytomegalovirus, herpes virus, and parasites such as Toxoplasma or Cryptosporidia. Milder infections with these organisms do not suggest immune deficiencies. Symptoms of full-blown AIDS include a persistent cough, fever, and difficulty in breathing. Multiple purplish blotches and bumps on the skin may indicate Kaposi's sarcoma. The virus can also cause brain damage. People infected with the virus can have a wide range of symptoms—from none to mild to severe. At least one fourth to one half of those infected with HIV will develop AIDS within 4 to 10 years.

The introduction of highly active antiretroviral (ARV) therapy in 1996 was a turning point for those with access to sophisticated health care systems. Although they cannot cure HIV/AIDS, ARVs and their use in combination, "cocktails," have dramatically reduced mortality and morbidity and prolonged and improved the lives of sufferers. With no cure at present, prudence could save thousands of people who have yet to be exposed to the virus. Use of condoms lessens the possibility of transmission, as does the elimination of sharing hypodermic needles. The fate of many will depend less on science than on the ability of large numbers of human beings to change their behavior in the face of growing danger.

Influenza

Several influenza epidemics in the 20th century caused millions of deaths worldwide, including the worst epidemic in American history, the Spanish influenza outbreak that killed more than 500,000 in 1918. Today influenza is less of a public health threat, though it continues to be a serious disease that affects many people. Approximately 20,000 people die of the flu in the United States every year. The influenza virus attacks the human respiratory tract, causing symptoms such as fever, headaches, fatigue, coughing, sore throat, nasal congestion, and body aches.

Japanese Encephalitis

Japanese encephalitis is a mosquito-borne disease endemic in Asia. Around 50,000 cases occur each year; 25% to 30% of all cases are fatal.

Leishmaniasis

Leishmaniasis is a disease spread by the bite of the sandfly. It is found mostly in tropical countries. There are several types of leishmaniasis, and they vary in symptoms and severity. Visceral leishmaniasis (VL, or *kala azar*) is the most severe; left untreated, it is always fatal. Symptoms include fever, weight loss, anemia, and a swelling of the spleen and liver. Mucocutaneous leishmaniasis (MCL, or *espundia*) produces lesions that affect the nose, mouth, and throat and can destroy their mucous membranes. Cutaneous leishmaniasis (CL) produces skin ulcers, sometimes as many as 200, that cause disability and extensive scarring. Diffuse cutaneous leishmaniasis (DCL) is similar to CL, and infected people are prone to relapses. Approximately 12 million cases of leishmaniasis exist today.

Malaria

Malaria is a mosquito-borne disease that affects 300 to 500 million people annually, causing nearly 3 million deaths. Most common in tropical and subtropical climates, malaria is found in more than 100 countries, including many parts of Central and South America, Africa, Southeast Asia and the Indian subcontinent, and the Middle East. Symptoms include several stages of illness. The first stage consists of shaking and chills, the next stage involves high fever and severe headache, and in the final stage the infected person's temperature drops and he or she sweats profusely. Infected people also often suffer from anemia, weakness, and a swelling of the spleen. Malaria was almost eradicated 30 years ago; now it is on the rise again.

Measles

Measles is a disease that has seen a drastic reduction in countries where a vaccine is readily available, but it is still prevalent in developing countries, where most of the 777,000 deaths (out of 30 million cases) it caused in 2001 occurred. Symptoms include high fever, coughing, and a maculopapular rash; common complications include diarrhea, pneumonia, and ear infections.

Meningitis

Meningitis, often known as spinal meningitis, is an infection of the spinal cord and usually the result of a viral or bacterial infection. Bacterial meningitis is more severe than viral meningitis and may cause brain damage, hearing loss, and learning disabilities. An estimated 1.2 million cases of bacterial meningitis occur every year, over a tenth of which are fatal. Symptoms include severe headache, fever, nausea, vomiting, lethargy, delirium, photophobia, and a stiff neck.

Onchocerciasis ("River Blindness")

Onchocerciasis is caused by the larvae of *Onchocerca volvulus*, a parasitic worm that lives in the human body for years. It is endemic in Africa, where nearly all of the 18 million people infected with the disease live. Of those infected, over 6.5 million have developed dermatitis and 270,000 have gone blind. Symptoms include visual impairment, rashes, lesions, intense itching, skin depigmentation, and lymphadenitis.

Pneumonia

Pneumonia has many possible causes, but it is usually an infection of the streptococcus or mycoplasma bacteria. These bacteria can live in the human body without causing infection for years, and only surface when another illness has lowered the person's immunity to disease. *Streptococcus pneumoniae* causes streptococcal pneumonia, the most common kind, which is more severe than mycoplasmal pneumonia. *S. pneumoniae* is responsible for more than 100,000 hospitalizations for pneumonia annually, as well as 6 million cases of otitis media and over 60,000 cases of invasive diseases such as meningitis.

Rotavirus

Rotavirus is the most common cause of viral gastroenteritis worldwide. It kills more than 600,000 children each year, mostly in developing countries. Symptoms include vomiting, watery diarrhea, fever, and abdominal pain.

Schistosomiasis

Schistosomiasis is a parasitic disease that is endemic in many developing countries. Roughly 200 million people worldwide are infected with the flukeworm, whose eggs cause the symptoms of the disease. Some 120 million of those infected are symptomatic, and 20 million suffer severely from the infection. Symptoms include rash and itchiness soon after becoming infected, followed by fever, chills, coughing, and muscle aches.

Shigellosis

Shigella infection causes an estimated 600,000 deaths worldwide every year. It is most common in developing countries with poor sanitation. Shigella bacteria cause bacillary dysentery, or shigellosis. Symptoms include diarrhea with bloody stool, vomiting, and abdominal cramps.

Strep Throat

Strep throat is caused by the streptococcus bacteria. Several million cases of strep throat occur every year. Symptoms include a sore throat, fever, headache, fatigue, and nausea.

Tuberculosis

Tuberculosis causes nearly 2 million deaths every year, and WHO estimates that nearly 1 billion people will be infected between 2000 and 2020 if more effective preventive procedures are not adopted. The TB bacteria are most often found in the lungs, where they can cause chest pain and a bad cough that brings up bloody phlegm. Other symptoms include fatigue, weight loss, appetite loss, chills, fever, and night sweats.

Typhoid

Typhoid fever causes an estimated 600,000 deaths annually, out of 12 to 17 million cases. It is usually the spread through infected food or water. Symptoms include a sudden and sustained fever, severe headache, nausea, severe appetite loss, constipation, and sometimes diarrhea.

Yellow Fever

Yellow fever causes an estimated 30,000 deaths each year, out of 200,000 cases. The disease has two phases. In the acute phase, symptoms include fever, muscle pain, headache, shivers, appetite loss, nausea, and vomiting. This lasts for 3 to 4 days, after which most patients recover. But 15% will enter the toxic phase, in which fever reappears, along with other symptoms, including jaundice; abdominal pain; vomiting; bleeding from the mouth, nose, eyes, and stomach; and deterioration of kidney function (sometimes complete kidney failure). Half of all patients in the toxic phase die within 2 weeks; the other half recover.

Pharmacological Information: Infectious Diseases and Pharmacology

Antifungals

Action
Antifungal agents can kill susceptible fungi, fungicidal, or stop growth, fungistatic. Antifungals bind and disrupt the cell membrane of the fungi or alter protein or lipid synthesis within the fungi leading to the therapeutic effects.

Side Effects
Central nervous system (CNS): Headache, dizziness
Cardiovascular (CV): Hypotension, dysrhythmias
GI: Vomiting, abdominal pain
Misc: Arthralgias, myalgias, peripheral neuropathy, skin exfoliation

Common Medications
Systemic: Amphotericin, Fluconazole (Diflucan), Itraconazole
Local/Topical: Ciclopirox, clotrimazole (Lotrimin), keoconazole (Nizoral), miconazole (Micatin/Desenex), nystatin

Anti-Infectives

Aminoglycosides

Action
Aminoglycosides are used for the treatment or prophylaxis of gram-negative bacterial infections including Pseudomonas Aeruginosa, Klebsiella pneumonia, Escherichia coli, Serratia, Acinetobacter, Staphylococcus aureus. Aminoglycosides are bacteriocidal through inhibition of ribosomal protein synthesis.

Side Effects
GU: Nephrotoxicity
Misc: Ototoxicity, hypersensitivity reactions

Common Medications
Gentamicin, Neomycin, Streptomycin, Tobramycin

Carbapenem

Action
Carbapenems bind to bacterial cell walls resulting in cell death. These are broad spectrum antibiotics that are active against most gram-positive infectious agents including Streptococcus pneumonia, enterococcus, staphylococcus aureus, and gram-negative infections including Pseudomonas Aeruginosa, Klebsiella, Escherichia coli. Imipenem may be combined with cilastatin to decrease renal inactivation of drug.

Side Effects
CNS: Seizures, dizziness
CV: Hypotension
GI: Diarrhea, nausea, vomiting, colitis
Misc: Anaphylaxis

Common Medications
Imipenem/cilastatin (Primaxin)

Cephalosporins

Action
Cephalosporins are bacteriocidal to gram-positive cocci including Streptococcus pneumonia, staphylococci, streptococci. Second- and third-generation cephalosporins have greater gram-negative bacteriocidal activity.

Side Effects
CNS: Seizures, dizziness
CV: Hypotension
GI: Diarrhea, nausea, vomiting, colitis
Misc: Anaphylaxis, pain/phlebitis at administration site

Common Medications
First generation: Cefazolin (Ancef), Cephalexin (Biocef, Keflex)
Second generation: Cefmetazole (Monocid), cefprozil (Cefzil), cefuroxime (Ceftin, Kefurox, Zinacef)
Third generation: Cefepime, ceftazidime (Ceftaz)

Penicillins

Action
Penicillins are bacteriocidal by preventing bacterial cell wall synthesis. They are commonly prescribed for respiratory and GU infections, sepsis, endocarditis, peptic ulcer disease, sexually transmitted diseases (chlamydia, syphillis, gonorrhea), lymes disease. Penicillins are effective against streptococcal, pneumococcal, gonococcal, and meningococcal infections.

Side Effects
CNS: Seizures
GI: Diarrhea, nausea, vomiting, colitis
Misc: Allergic reactions (rash, bronchospasm), anaphylaxis

Common Medications
Penicillins: Benzylpenicillin (Penicillin G), Phenoxymethylpenicillin (Penicillin V)
Extended-Spectrum Penicillins: Ampicillin, Amoxicillin, Piperacillin
Penicillinase-Resistant Penicillins: Methicillin, Nafcillin, Oxacillin, Cloxacillin, Dicloxacillin

Fluoroquinolones

Action

Fluoroquinolones are bacteriostatic by inhibiting DNA synthesis. These broad spectrum agents are prescribed for the prophylaxis and treatment of many gram-positive pathogens including methicillin-resistant staphylococcus aureus (MRSA) and streptococcus pneumonia; gram-negative activity against Escherichia coli (E. coli), Pseudomonal aeruginosa, Acinetobacter. Common in respiratory, GU and GI tract infections, meningitis, and septicemia.

Side Effects

CNS: Seizures, dizziness, drowsiness, fatigue, headache
CV: Dysrhythmias
GI: Diarrhea, nausea, vomiting, colitis, hepatotoxicity
Misc: Hyper/hypoglycemia, tendinitis/tendon rupture, anaphylaxis, skin exfoliation (Stevens-Johnson Syndrome)

Common Medications

Ciprofloxacin (Cipro), Levofloxacin (Levaquin)

Macrolides

Action

Macrolides are bacteriostatic by binding to bacterial ribosomes inhibiting protein synthesis. Macrolides are frequently prescribed for gram-positive and gram-negative pathogens. Commonly used in cellulitis, respiratory infections, and chronic bronchitis.

Side Effects

CNS: Dizziness, drowsiness, fatigue, headache
CV: Chest pain, palpitations
GI: Diarrhea, nausea, vomiting, abdominal cramps
Misc: Angioedema, pain/phlebitis at administration site

Common Medications

Erhythromycin, Clarithromycin (Biaxin), Azithromycin (Zithromax)

Tetracyclines

Action

Tetracyclines are bacteriostatic by binding to bacterial ribosomes inhibiting protein synthesis of gram-positive and gram-negative pathogens. They are frequently prescribed for atypical pneumonias and chronic bronchitis, acne, periodontitis.

Side Effects

CNS: Dizziness/fatigue
Derm: Light sensitivity, rash

GI: Diarrhea, nausea, colitis
Misc: Ataxia, discoloration of teeth
Common Medications
Tetracycline, doxycycline (Doxy), minocycline (Minocin)

Sulfonamides

Action
Sulfonamides inhibit the bacterial synthesis of folic acid that is essential for growth. These broad-spectrum antibiotics are prescribed for multiple gram-positive and gram-negative pathogens. Most notably, these agents are used for urinary tract infections, meningitis, intestinal and lower respiratory tract infections.

Side Effects
CNS: Fatigue, hallucinations, headache
GI: Diarrhea, vomiting, nausea
Misc: Hypersensitivity, skin rash, thrombocytopenia, fever

Common Medications
Trimethoprim/Sulfamethoxazole (Bactrim)

Antiretrovirals

Action
Antiretrovirals are used in the management of HIV to improve the CD4 cell counts and decrease viral load. These medications include nucleoside and non-nucleoside reverse transciptase inhibitors and protease inhibitors. Viruses use the infected cell to replicate new viral particles through the process of reverse transcription. Reverse transciptase inhibitors limit viral reproduction. Protease inhibitors limit the cleavage and activation of HIV proteins that are necessary for viral replication leading to reductions in viral levels in the blood.

Side Effects
CNS: Dizziness, drowsiness, fatigue, headache, weakness
CV: Orthostatic hypotension
GI: Abdominal pain, diarrhea, vomiting, nausea
Misc: Hypersensitivity/anaphylaxis (Stevens-Johnson Syndrome), musculoskeletal pain, fat redistribution, peripheral neuropathy

Common Medications
Nonnucleoside Reverse Transcriptase Inhibitors: Delavirdine (rescriptor), Efavirenz (Sustiva), Nevirapine (Viramune)
Nucleoside Reverse Transcriptase Inhibitors: Abacavir (Ziagen), Didanosine (ddI, Videx), Zalcitabine (ddC), Zidovudine (AZT, Retrovir)
Protease Inhibitors: Amprenavir (Agenerase), Indinavir (Crixivan)

Antituberculars

Action

Antituberculars are medications used in the treatment and prevention of tuberculosis. These medications inhibit RNA synthesis by blocking RNA transcription or disrupt formation of the bacterial cell wall.

Side Effects

CNS: Ataxia, confusion, drowsiness, fatigue, weakness, headache

GI: Abdominal pain, diarrhea, vomiting, nausea, hepatitis

Misc: Arthralgias, myalgias, peripheral neuropathy

Common Medications

Ethambutol, Isoniazid (INH), Pyrazinamide, Rifampin (Rifadin), rifapentine (Priftin)

Antivirals

Action

Antiviral agents limit replication and spread of viruses through multiple mechanisms. Common viral infections treated by antiviral medications include herpes simplex, herpes zoster ("shingles"), varicella ("chicken pox"), influenza, and CMV.

Side Effects

CNS: Seizures, dizziness, headache, drowsiness

CV: Dysrhythmias, hypo/hypertension

GI: GI bleeding, diarrhea, vomiting, nausea

Misc: Arthralgias, tremor, ataxia, peripheral neuropathy

Common Medications

Acyclovir (Avirax, Zovirax), ganciclovir (Vitrasert), oseltamivir (Tamiflu), valacyclovir (Valtrex), zanamivir (Relenza)

References

1. Goodman CC, Kapasi ZF. The effect of exercise on the immune system. *Rehabilitation Oncology.* 2002;20(1):13–15.
2. Kapasi ZF, Ouslander JG, Schnelle JF, Kutner M, Fahey JL. Effects of an exercise intervention on immunologic parameters in frail elderly nursing home residents. *J Gerontol Series A—Biol Sci Med Sci.* 2003;58:636–643.
3. Guide to Physical Therapist Practice. 2nd ed. *Physical Therapy.* 2001;81(1).

Bibliography

Abbas AK, Lichtman AH, Pober JS. *Cellular and Molecular Immunology.* 4th ed. Philadelphia, Pa: WB Saunders; 2000.

Copstead LC, Banasik JL. *Pathophysiology: Biological and Behavioral Perspectives.* 2nd ed. Philadelphia, Pa: WB Saunders; 2000.

Craig CR, Stitzel RE. *Modern Pharmacology with Clinical Applications.* New York, NY: Little, Brown, and Co; 1997.

Deglin JH, Vallerand AH. *Davis's Drug Guide for Nurses.* 8th ed. Philadelphia, Pa: FA Davis Co; 2003.

Goodman CC, Boissonnault WG, Fuller KS. *Pathology: Implications for the Physical Therapist.* 2nd ed. Philadelphia, Pa: WB Saunders; 2003.

Guideline for hand hygiene in health-care settings. *MMWR.* 51(RR16):1–44.

Inforplease. Common Infectious Disease Worldwide. Pearson Education, publishing as Infoplease. Available at: http://www.infoplease.com/ipa/A0903696.html. Accessed on September 13, 2005.

Karch AM. *Lippincott's Nursing Drug Guide.* Springhouse, Pa: Lippincott Williams & Wilkins; 2004.

Porth CM. *Pathophysiology: Concepts of Altered Health States.* 6th ed. Philadelphia, Pa: Lippincott Williams & Wilkins; 2002.

Ritter JM, Lewis LD, Mant TG. *Textbook of Clinical Pharmacology.* London, England: Edward Arnold Co; 1995.

Roitt I, Brostoff J, Male D. *Immunology.* 6th ed. London, UK: Mosby; 2001.

Chapter

6

CARDIOVASCULAR DISEASES AND DISORDERS

Daniel J. Malone, MPT, CCS

Cardiovascular disease is the leading cause of morbidity and mortality in the United States, responsible for almost 50% of all deaths. More than 13.5 million Americans have a history of having myocardial infarction (MI) or experience chest pain. Heart failure is associated with over 20% of all hospital admissions for those over 65 years old, and the rate of hospital admission has increased over 159% over the past decade. Heart failure is the most common discharge diagnosis for hospitalized Medicare patients, and the fourth most common discharge diagnosis for all patients hospitalized in the United States.[1–3] Cardiovascular disease is more than coronary artery disease (CAD) and heart failure, but also includes hypertension (HTN), cerebrovascular disease, congenital heart diseases, and valve dysfunction. Clearly rehabilitation professionals will interact with patients who have primary or secondary cardiovascular disease in their practice every day. This chapter will review basic anatomy and physiology of the cardiovascular system and describe the most common pathologies encountered in the acute care setting. Physical therapy implications of cardiovascular disease will be presented in the context of cardiac rehabilitation. Monitoring information will expand on electrophysiology, the electrocardiogram (ECG), pacemakers, and defibrillators.

ANATOMY AND PHYSIOLOGY

The cardiovascular system's primary purpose is to deliver adequate amounts of oxygen and remove wastes from the body.[4,5] The heart's pumping action provides the motive force to open the heart's valves and push blood throughout the body. The blood vessels provide the conduit for the distribution and return of blood and waste products to their appropriate destinations. In order to perform its functions, the cardiovascular system works together with the respiratory, neurologic, urinary, digestive, endocrine, and integumentary systems in maintaining homeostasis.[6–8]

Figure 6–1. Relationship of the heart and the principle valves to the overlying rib cage. A = aortic valve, M = mitral valve, P = pulmonary valve, T = tricuspid valve. (Reprinted from Hillegass EA, Sadowsky HS. *Essentials of Cardiopulmonary Physical Therapy.* 2nd ed. Philadelphia, Pa: WB Saunders Co; 2001: 30 with permission from Elsevier.)

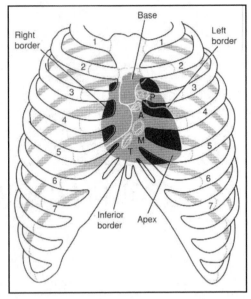

Anatomically, the cardiovascular system includes the heart, the pericardium, and all the blood vessels including the arteries, veins, and lymphatics. Physiologically, you must consider the anatomic structures and the presence of disease, but in addition, you must consider the nervous supply, the fluid volume, and metabolic state of the body to assess proper function.

The heart is located within the **mediastinum** of the thorax. By definition the mediastinum is the space superior to the diaphragm, inferior to the cranium, and medial to the lungs. It contains the heart encased in its protective layer, the **pericardium**, the great vessels including the aorta, the SVC and IVC, the pulmonary arteries and veins, as well as the esophagus, the phrenic nerves, and the sympathetic chain ganglia.

Normally, the heart is conical in shape and is roughly the size of an individual's fist. It is located anteriorly in the mediastinum behind the sternum with approximately two-thirds of the heart left of midline. The surface marking of the heart can be identified over the anterior chest wall. The heart extends from the second to fifth intercostal spaces, and extends from the sternum to the left midclavicular line[1,7,9,10] (Figure 6–1).

The **base** of the heart faces posteriorly and is made up largely of the left atrium (LA) and a portion of the right atrium. The base is the superior portion of the heart and is related to the second intercostal space parasternally. The **apex** points downward, toward the left and forward. The apex projects into the fifth intercostal space in the midclavicular line. The apex is the inferior portion of the heart and is comprised primarily of the left ventricle (LV).[1,9,11] The **point of maximal impulse (PMI)** refers to the apex of the heart and may be palpated to determine the relative position of the LV.[9]

Table 6–1

IMPACT OF COMMON VASOACTIVE ELEMENTS ON ARTERIES AND VEINS

Vasodilation

- Vaso-vagal syncope
- Deep pain (eg, joint disruption, crush injury), visceral pain/distension
- Autonomic dysfunction (eg, Parkinson's disease/DM) inflammatory mediators/sepsis/septic shock
- Fever/hyperthermia
- Pain medications/narcotic analgesics (eg, opiods)
- Anxiolytics/sedatives

Cardiovascular Medications:
- Nitric oxide/nitrates
- Calcium channel blockers
- Beta blockers
- Vasodilators

Vasoconstriction

- Superficial pain
- Endothelin
- Angiotensin II/Aldosterone
- Beta agonists (eg, norepinephrine, epinephrine, isoproteronol)
- Vasopressin/antidiuretic hormone (ADH)
- Cold temperature/hypothermia

Sympathetic nervous system-activation/catecholamines:
- Norepinephrine

Pulmonary Vessels (ie, hypoxic vasocontriction):
- Hypoxemia/acidosis

Blood Vessels

The blood vessels form a tubular network that allows blood to flow from the heart to all cells of the body. This network consists of vessels of progressively smaller diameters and increased total surface area called arteries, arterioles, and capillaries. The capillaries are microscopic vessels that join the arterial flow to the venous flow. Blood returns to the heart from the capillaries passing through vessels of progressively larger diameters called venules and veins.[4] The blood vessels actively control the flow and distribution of blood throughout the body by smooth muscle vasoconstriction or dilatation which results from the influences of vasosoactive substances, hormones, and neurologic input (Table 6–1).

All vessels larger than the capillaries consist of three distinct layers—the intima tunica, the media, and the adventitia (Figure 6–2). The anatomic distribution of these three distinct layers provides the functional differences among the arteries, arterioles, venules, and veins. The innermost layer, the intima tunica, consists of a smooth layer of endothelial cells, supporting connective tissue, and isolated smooth muscle cells. The **endothelium** allows smooth laminar blood flow and is selectively permeable to many different molecules (eg, low density lipoprotein [LDL] cholesterol). The endothelium secretes and responds to a variety of vasoactive substances that determine the diameter of the vessel lumen (see Table 6–1). The middle layer, the media, consists of multiple layers of smooth muscle cells and elastic tissue. The media is the site of vasoconstriction/

Figure 6–2. Arteries and veins. (Reprinted with permission from Sheldon LK. *Oxygenation.* Sudbury, Mass: Jones and Bartlett Publishers; 2001. Available at: www.jbpub.com.)

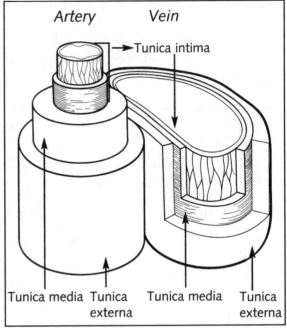

dilation through chemical, mechanical, and neurologic stimuli. The outer layer, the adventitia, consists of collagenous fibers and loose connective tissues. The adventitia provides the basic support structure for the vessels, binds the vessel loosely to the connective tissue in which they run, and contains nerves and small blood vessels, the vaso vasorum, that supply the walls of the vessels.[9,11–13]

The Heart

The heart is a four-chambered muscular pump divided into to right and left halves with each half containing an **atria** and a **ventricle**. The atria receive blood returning to the heart from the veins (inferior vena cava [IVC]/superior vena cava [SVC]/pulmonary veins), while the ventricles receive blood from the atria and eject into the main arteries (pulmonary artery/aorta/coronary arteries). A muscular wall, the **interventricular septum**, prevents the mixing of blood from the two sides of the heart and contributes to the contractile function of the heart. The right heart pumps to the lungs and is referred to as the pulmonary circuit while the left heart is the systemic circuit pumping to the remainder of the body (Figure 6–3).

The walls of the heart are made up of three layers: an inner layer (endocardium), an outer protective layer (epicardium), and muscular middle layer (myocardium).[12] The innermost layer, the **endocardium**, is a thin layer of endothelial cells supported by underlying connective tissue. This layer repeatedly folds on itself to form the valves of the heart and is continuous with the innermost layer of the large blood vessels (intima). The middle layer, the **myocardium**, is the contractile layer of the heart and is composed primarily of cardiac muscle fibers.

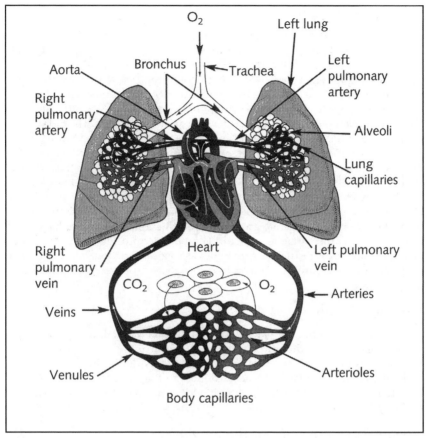

Figure 6–3. The vascular circuits: pulmonic and systemic. (Reprinted with permission from Sheldon LK. *Oxygenation*. Sudbury, Mass: Jones and Bartlett Publishers; 2001. Available at: www.jbpub.com.)

The outer layer, the **epicardium**, is a thin membrane that encases the myocardium and is the root of the great vessels. The epicardium turns back on itself to form a sac which surrounds the heart, the **pericardium**. Between the layers of the pericardium is a thin layer of pericardial fluid.[11,12]

The **pericardium** is the fibrous sac encompassing the heart and the root of the great vessels as they enter or leave the heart. This sac consists of the inner serous pericardium, made up of the inner visceral and outer parietal layers separated by a virtual space containing the pericardial fluid, and the external fibrous pericardium. Primary functions of the pericardium include lubricating the moving surfaces of the heart to limit friction, maintaining the position and limiting distension of the heart within the thoracic cavity, protecting the heart from external trauma and infection, and distributing contractile forces via mechanical coupling of the heart's chambers.[14,15]

Pulmonary Circuit

The right atrium (RA) receives deoxygenated blood returning from the body via the **SVC and IVC.** The SVC drains blood from the head and upper extremities (UEs), and the IVC drains blood from the lower extremities (LEs) and abdomen. Dividing the right atria (RA) from the right ventricle (RV) is the **tricuspid valve (TV).** The RV receives the blood from the RA and pumps blood through the pulmonary valve (PV) into the main pulmonary artery, which bifurcates into the right and left pulmonary arteries for transport to the lungs. The pulmonary circuit is a low pressure, high capacitance system that receives the entire cardiac output (CO) while maintaining pressures that are usually one fourth to one-fifth of the systemic circulation. The RV has a thicker myocardium than the atria, but is approximately one third the thickness of the LV. This thinner myocardium is related to the lower pulmonary vascular resistance within the pulmonary circuit compared to the vascular resistance of the systemic circuit. Normally, the RV is not required to generate great pressures due to the high compliance and low resistance of the pulmonary circuit. This becomes problematic during states of high pulmonary resistance (eg, **hypoxic vasoconstriction**/left ventricular dysfunction and failure) which can lead to right ventricular hypertrophy and failure.

Systemic Circuit

Blood returns to the LA via the four pulmonary veins draining the lungs. Blood passes through the **mitral valve (MV)** (bicuspid valve) en route to the LV. The LV is roughly three times thicker than the RV due to the large total systemic/peripheral vascular resistance that it must pump against. Blood leaves the LV through the **aortic valve (AoV)** entering the **aorta** for distribution throughout the body.

Atrioventricular and Semilunar Valves

There are two atrioventricular valves, the **TV** and **MV,** and two semilunar valves, the **PV** and **AoV.** The primary functions of the valves are to direct the one-way flow of blood through the pulmonary and systemic circuits. Within the interior of the ventricles are the papillary muscles that attach to the atrioventricular valves, the MV and TV, via the chordae tendinae. The papillary muscle-chordae tendinae apparatus contract and provides an inward directed force during ejection that prevents the eversion of the valves into the atria.

Conduction System and Electrocardiography

Myocardial cells have the potential for spontaneous electrical activity that can lead to a variety of abnormal heart rhythms. However, in the normal heart, spontaneous electrical activity is limited to a small region located in the superior aspect of the RA, the **sinoatrial node (SA node).** The SA node is the usual pacemaker of the heart secondary to the rapidity of its inherent depolarizations. Generally, the region of the heart with the most rapid rate of depolarization will take over pacemaker function. Once the SA node fires, this depolarization wave is transmitted throughout the entire heart over the conduction system as outlined in Figure 6–4. From the SA node, the impulses travel over

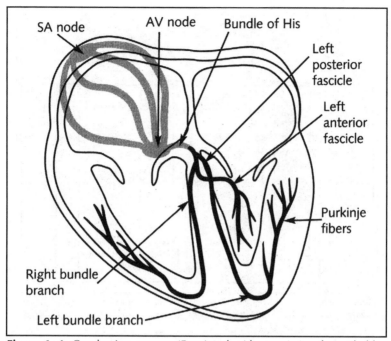

Figure 6–4. Conduction system. (Reprinted with permission from Sheldon LK. *Oxygenation.* Sudbury, Mass: Jones and Bartlett Publishers; 2001. Available at: www.jbpub.com.)

Bachman's Bundle to the LA and down the internodal fasciculi through the RA to the ventricles. A connective tissue sheath preventing the transmission of the impulse into the ventricles separates the atria and ventricles. A group of specialized myocardial cells, the **atrioventricular node (AV node)**, the **atrioventricular bundle (Bundle of His)**, and **purkinje fibers**, complete the conduction of impulses throughout the ventricles. The impulse is delayed at the AV node allowing the atria to fully contract prior to ventricular systole. This time delay and coordination between the atria and ventricles allows maximal filling during diastole (filling) in order to maximize ventricular systole (ejection) and stroke volume (SV). Abnormalities in the conduction system can lead to a change in the heart's rhythm impacting on the diastolic and systolic functions of the heart. These "dysrhythmias" can impair filling (eg, atrial fibrillation) or ejection (eg, ventricular fibrillation [VF]) to such an extent that SV and CO do not meet the demands of the body (see Figure 6–15).

The Cardiac Cycle

The cardiac cycle (Figure 6–5) defines the combined electrical and mechanical forces acting within the heart to complete one heartbeat. This cycle consists of a phase of contraction, **systole**, and a phase of relaxation/filling, **diastole**. Systole begins with the contraction of the ventricle resulting from electrical stimulation by the pacemaker of the heart transmitted through the conduction system. This

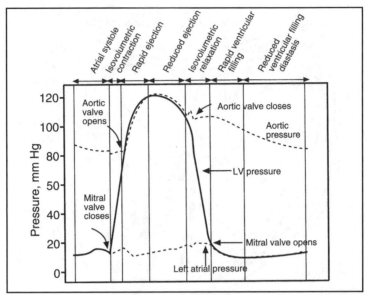

Figure 6–5. The car-diac cycle. (Reprinted with permission from Sheldon LK. *Oxygenation*. Sudbury, Mass: Jones and Bartlett Publishers; 2001. Available at: www.jbpub.com.)

electrical stimulation (QRS complex on ECG) initiates ventricular contraction thus generating the pressure required to force open the aortic/pulmonic valves and propel blood into the major arteries. Initially, as the ventricle contracts, there is no movement of blood (**isovolumic contraction**). However, as contraction continues, the intraventricular pressure becomes greater than the pressure within the great arteries, and the aortic/pulmonic valves open and blood is ejected into the aorta and pulmonary arteries. As the ventricles continue to contract and sarcomeres shorten, the pressure generated falls below the pressures within the major arteries resulting in closure of the aortic/pulmonic valves (**S2 heart sound**). With closure of the valves, ejection ends, the ventricles begin to relax, and diastole begins. Diastole begins with all valves closed. As the ventricle continues to relax, the myocardium lengthens, increasing the intraventricular volume and resultant reductions in the intraventricular pressure (**isovolumic relaxation**). Pressure within the ventricles falls below that of the atria and major veins allowing the MV/TV to open and blood to flow passively into the ventricles. Passive filling accounts for approximately 80% of the ventricular preload. The atria depolarize (P wave on ECG) and contract providing the active contribution of ventricular filling. As blood fills the ventricles, pressure increases. Filling will continue until ventricular pressure equals atrial pressure. With the initiation of ventricular contraction (QRS complex), pressure increases dramatically closing the MV/TV (**S1 heart sound**). This signals the end of diastole and the beginning of systole.

The amount of blood ejected from the heart with each ventricular contraction, ventricular systole, is **SV.** If we consider that the heart can only eject what enters it during diastole, it is evident that the SV is highly dependent upon the amount of blood filling the heart prior to ejection, the **preload or end-diastolic volume (EDV)**.

The amount of blood ejected from the ventricles per minute defines the **CO**. Mathematically, CO is the product of heart rate (HR) times SV (CO = HR x SV).

One heartbeat typically lasts approximately 0.8 seconds with two-thirds of that time spent in diastole. Increases in HR will reduce the filling time of the heart resulting from shortening of the diastolic time during the cardiac cycle. This may partially explain SV and CO limitation associated with tachyarrhythmias.

PATHOPHYSIOLOGY

Electrocardiogram/Dysrhythmias

The acute care practitioner should be aware of the major dysrhythmias and the impact of these rhythm disturbances on cardiovascular physiology and subsequent therapeutic interventions and monitoring. As outlined in Monitoring Information, most dysrhythmias impact on the normal filling or ejection of the ventricles leading to abnormalities in SV and CO. The clinician must also consider the impact on myocardial oxygen supply and demand in relation to the patient's underlying condition to determine the appropriate interventions or noninterventions for the episode of care. Cardiac dysrhythmia interpretation is not limited to critical care and is often necessary in a variety of medical and surgical environments.

Coronary Artery Disease/Angina/Myocardial Infarction Revascularization Procedures

Atherosclerosis is a multifactorial disease process affecting the large and medium-sized arteries throughout the body. When it occurs in the vessels of the heart, it is known as CAD. When atherosclerosis occurs in the extremities, aorta, or iliac arteries, it is called peripheral arterial disease (PAD) or peripheral arterial occlusive disease (PAOD) and is a common manifestation of systemic atherosclerosis. CAD and cerebrovascular disease are present in a large portion of individuals with PAD, and PAD itself confers sharply increased risks for cardiac and cerebral atherothrombotic events.[16] Athersclerosis is associated with known risk factors that are amenable to rehabilitation input (Table 6–2). Atherosclerosis involves the formation of fibromuscular plaques within the walls of the arteries that limit the flow of blood to the tissues. Plaque formation begins with the leaking of blood lipids (LDL cholesterol) and inflammatory cells into the subendothelial layer of the vessel forming a fatty streak. Damage to the intima and the endothelial cells associated with smoking, shear stress related to HTN, age, diabetes, and other risk factors increase the permeability of the inner lining of the vasculature. Smooth muscle cells migrate from the media to this region of damage. This cellular material, known as a fibromuscular plaque, begins to decrease the lumen diameter of the blood vessel.[13,17] The result is reduced blood flow, leading to ischemia, and eventually to cell necrosis. **Angina,** the result of ischemia, is the complaint of chest pain or pressure commonly behind the

Table 6–2

RISK FACTORS AND CORONARY ARTERY DISEASE

Modifiable Risk Factors and CAD	Non-Modifiable
• Smoking	• Age
• HTN	• Sex
• Hypercholesterolemia	• Genetics/family history
• Sedentary lifestyle	
• Diabetes mellitus (DM)	
• Obesity/diet/stress/personality	

sternum, jaw, and left shoulder of individuals with CAD. **MI** implies permanent damage and death of heart cells. Peripheral vasculature is also impacted by atherosclerosis. PAD is a leading cause of LE discomfort associated with walking, **intermittent claudication**, as well as wounds, limb loss, and amputation.

Angina, ischemia, intermittent claudication, and MI typically result from oxygen supply-demand inequalities. Decreases in myocardial oxygen supply are primarily related to coronary stenosis associated with atherosclerosis. Other factors that reduce myocardial blood flow include coronary vasospasm, coronary thrombosis, or platelet thrombi. The process of atherosclerosis damages the endothelium leading to abnormalities in vasomotor tone and blood coagulation exacerbating the already reduced coronary blood flow.

The main determinants of oxygen demand are HR, myocardial contractility, and ventricular wall stress[6,8,14] (Figure 6–6). The ventricular wall stress is related to the ventricular volume and systemic blood pressure (BP). Increases in myocardial oxygen demand are associated with physical work and exercise and mental stress. Most studies indicate that increased oxygen demand is the most frequent cause of myocardial ischemia during daily life in patients with CAD. The treatments of these conditions are to increase oxygen supply or reduce oxygen demand through various pharmacological and/or surgical procedures, risk factors, and behavior modifications through cardiac rehabilitation.[1,13,18]

Medical Management/Nonsurgical Intervention

The rehabilitation professional is an integral member of the health care team involved in the medical management of atherosclerosis. Pharmacological intervention involves the use of medications to reduce oxygen demand (beta blockers/calcium channel blockers/ace inhibitors/diuretics) and improve or maintain oxygen supply (antiplatelet/anticoagulants/calcium channel blockers).

Surgical Intervention/Revascularization Procedures

Percutaneous transluminal coronary angioplasty (PTCA) involves the insertion of a balloon-tipped catheter through a peripheral artery (usually femoral or brachial artery) which is guided through the peripheral circulation to the heart and coronary vessels. Once inside the offending coronary vessel, the catheter is placed so that it straddles the stenotic lesion. The balloon is inflated to

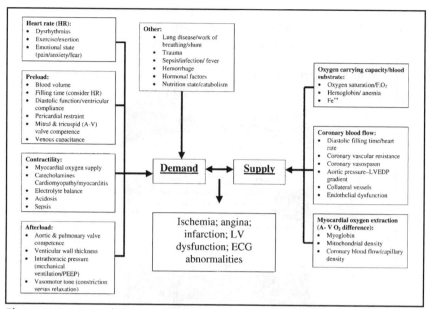

Figure 6–6. Myocardial oxygen supply-demand relationship. (Adapted from Tibby SM, Murdoch IA. Monitoring cardiac function in intensive care. *Arch Dis Child.* 2003;88:46–52.)

a specific compressive pressure and the plaque is literally crushed between the vessel wall and the balloon.[13] An **endoluminal stent** may be placed at the site of the atherosclerotic lesion to maintain the patency of the coronary artery lumen after the angioplasty procedure (Figure 6–7). The most significant complications associated with PTCA include vascular trauma, perioperative MI and restenosis. Restenosis typically occurs within the first 3 to 6 months after the procedure. Endoluminal stents and antiplatelet medications have decreased the incidence of restenosis to <10% to 30%. The rehabilitation team rarely is consulted on an inpatient basis for someone who has undergone PTCA. The procedure is often performed as outpatient and prolonged hospitalization would occur only if complications have arisen.

Coronary artery bypass grafting (CABG) involves segments of arteries and/or veins to bypass around a complete occlusion, multiple plaques not amenable to PTCA, or severe CAD. The vascular sections connect the aorta and a coronary artery distal to the obstruction (Figure 6–8). The vascular segments are often taken from the LEs (saphenous veins), anterior chest wall (internal mammary artery), or forearms (radial artery). The surgical approach is usually a median sternotomy where the sternum is transected from the sternal notch extending below the xiphoid process. The sternum is generally closed with stainless steel sutures either through or around the sternum to provide stability. Primary complications include postoperative dysrhythmias, HTN, wound infection, cerebral vascular accident (CVA), and MI.[19] The patient will often present with a mediastinal chest tube, external pacemaker, and multiple intravascular catheters impacting on the rehabilitation team. Postoperative

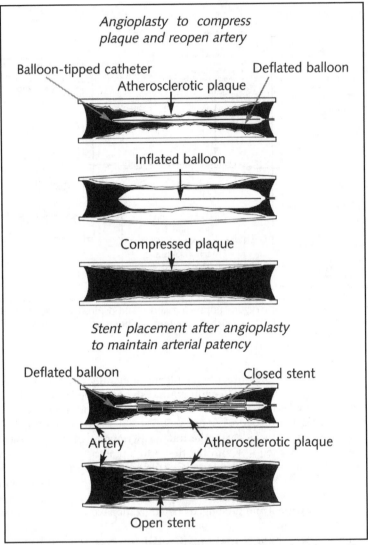

Figure 6–7. Angioplasty and stent placement. (Adapted with permission from Sheldon LK. *Oxygenation*. Sudbury, Mass: Jones and Bartlett Publishers; 2001. Available at: www.jbpub.com.)

HTN, abnormal laboratory values, incision pain, and dysrhythmias warrant special consideration by the rehabilitation team. The new onsets of brady- or tachyarrhythmias are most frequent during the first postoperative week, and the most frequent abnormal rhythm is rapid atrial arrhythmias.[19,20]

Transmyocardial revascularization (TMR) uses a surgical laser to create a channel in ischemic myocardium. This channel facilitates microcirculatory blood flow and possible new vessel formation (neovascularization/angiogenesis)

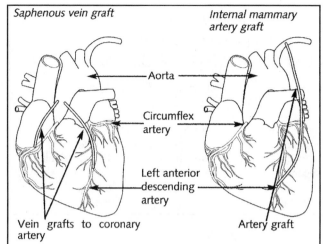

Figure 6–8. CABG. (Reprinted with permission from Sheldon LK. *Oxygenation.* Sudbury, Mass: Jones and Bartlett Publishers; 2001. Available at: www.jbpub.com.)

Saphenous vein graft

Internal mammary artery graft

Aorta

Circumflex artery

Left anterior descending artery

Vein grafts to coronary artery

Artery graft

Table 6–3

CLASSIFICATION OF BLOOD PRESSURE FOR ADULTS

Category	Systolic (mmHg)	Diastolic (mmHg)
• Optimal	• <120	• <80
• Normal	• <130	• <85
• Pre-HTN	• 120 to 139	• 80 to 90
• HTN		
• Stage 1	• 140 to 159	• 90 to 99
• Stage 2	• 160 to 179	• 100 to 109
• Stage 3	• ≥180	• ≥110

leading to reduced anginal symptoms. This procedure is performed for patients with CAD and chronic angina that is not amenable to CABG or PTCA.[21,22]

Hypertension

HTN is classified as an elevated BP greater than 140/90 (Table 6–3).[23] HTN affects nearly 50 million or over 24% of the US population and is an important modifiable cardiovascular risk factor.[24] The relationship between elevated BP and cardiovascular risk (stroke or TIA, CAD, heart failure) has long been recognized. BP is the product of CO times the total peripheral resistance (TPR) (BP=CO x TPR). Therefore, factors impacting on CO and/or TPR will influence the BP. HTN is generally considered an abnormality of TPR regulation. Primary, idiopathic, or essential HTN accounts for 90% of the cases and its causes are unknown even though there are known risk factors. Secondary HTN is most often associated with renal disease (glomerulonephritis, nephritis, diabetic nephropathy), endocrine disorders (acromegaly, hyperthyroidism, adrenal disorders—Cushings

Table 6–4
CARDIOMYOPATHY
(AS DEFINED BY THE WORLD HEALTH ORGANIZATION)

Specific (Secondary to External Processes)	*Intrinsic to Myocardium*
• Hypertensive cardiomyopathy • Valvular cardiomyopathy • Ischemic cardiomyopathy • Cardiomyopathy secondary to systemic disease • Ischemic cardiomyopathy	• Dilated cardiomyopathy • Hypertrophic cardiomyopathy • Arrhythmogenic right ventricular dysplasia • Obliterative cardiomyopathy

syndrome/aldosteronism, pheochromocytoma) sleep disorders, pregnancy, and acute stress (postoperative, hypoglycemia, alcohol withdrawal).[17]

Cardiomyopathy

The cardiomyopathies are a diverse group of disorders involving the myocardium that can be classified in multiple ways. Table 6–4 provides a classification system related to etiological causes.[25] Table 6–5 defines cardiomyopathy by morphologic expression:

- Dilated
- Hypertrophic
- Restrictive[25,26]

The cardiomyopathies have distinct anatomic variants, and the late presentations of the disorders are typically one of systolic or diastolic heart failure as outlined in Table 6–5.[17,25,26]

Valve Disease

Valvular heart disease (VHD) in the adult is attributed to rheumatic fever in childhood, congenital disorders, or degenerative changes. Degenerative changes occur with aging and are often associated with calcification and infections.[26–28] Valve dysfunction can occur in all valves of the heart but principally impact on the aortic and MVs. Valve dysfunction is generally described as stenotic lesions or insufficiency resulting in regurgitation (Table 6–6).

Aortic Stenosis

Aortic stenosis (AS) results in obstruction to flow from the LV into the ascending aorta resulting from narrowing of the aortic outflow tract.[27,28] It may be associated with rheumatic fever, but is more commonly associated with age and a congenital bicuspid valve. Etiological factors contributing to AS are progressive calcification, hypercholesterolemia, and inflammation. AS occurs in men more than women, is generally asymptomatic until middle age or older, and is the most common cardiac valve lesion in the United States.[29] Ventricular

Table 6–5

SIGNS AND SYMPTOMS OF CARDIOMYOPATHY

Dilated	*Hypertrophic*	*Restrictive*
• CHF • ECG: Ventricular dysrhythmias, non-specific repolarization abnormalities (ST-T changes) • LV dilation/dysfunction • High diastolic pressure/low CO	• Dyspnea, chest pain, syncope • ECG: LVH, exaggerated Q waves • LVH, hypercontractile function • Diastolic dysfunction	• Dyspnea, fatigue, right-sided CHF • ECG: Nonspecific repolarization abnormalities (ST-T changes) • Small LV, normal or mildly reduced LV function • High diastolic pressures

Adapted from:
Berkow R. *The Merck Manual of Diagnosis and Therapy*. Rahway, NJ: Merck Sharp & Dome Research Laboratories; 1987.
Carabello BS. Aortic stenosis. *N Engl J Med*. 2002;346:677–682.
Carabello BS, Crawford FA. Medical progress: valvular heart disease. *N Engl J Med*. 1997;337:32–41.
Tierney LM, McPhee SJ, Papadakis MA. *Current Medical Diagnosis and Treatment*. Norwalk, Conn: Appleton & Lange; 1994.
Way LW. *Current Surgical Diagnosis and Treatment*. 9th ed. Norwalk, Conn: Appleton & Lange; 1991.

strain and excessive demand result in a pressure overload as the heart attempts to eject against a narrowed opening. Ventricular hypertrophy maintains SV and CO during a prolonged latency period, but chronic obstruction and pressure overload lead to angina, syncope, and the terminal manifestations of the disease, systolic heart failure.[26–29] Typical signs and symptoms are listed in Table 6–6.

Aortic Insufficiency/Regurgitation

Aortic regurgitation results in retrograde blood flow from the aorta into the LV through incompetent aortic cusps. Aortic incompetence leading to regurgitation may develop gradually (chronic regurgitation) or rapidly (acute regurgitation) and most are associated with rheumatic heart disease, congenital bicuspid AoV, infective endocarditis, HTN, and aortic root diseases (eg, Marfan's syndrome/aortic dissection and aneurysms).[13,26] Initially, left ventricular hypertrophy due to dilation allows maintenance of SV and forward CO. However, progressive regurgitation results in diastolic run-off leading to volume overload and left ventricular failure.

Mitral Stenosis

Mitral stenosis (MS) may be defined as an obstruction of flow from the LA to LV because of a narrowed mitral orifice.[17,26] MS is most commonly associated

---

Table 6–6
SIGNS AND SYMPTOMS OF VALVE DYSFUNCTION

Aortic Stenosis

- Harsh, systolic murmur, often radiating to the neck
- ECG: Left ventricular hypertrophy
- Dampened peripheral pulses
- Angina on exertion, syncope, dyspnea/orthopnea/PND

Aortic Insufficiency/Regurgitation

- Wide pulse pressure
- Chest pain
- ECG: Left ventricular hypertrophy
- Diastolic murmur along left sternal border
- PMI in left axilla

Mitral Stenosis

- ECG: Atrial fibrillation (common), left atrial enlargement
- Prominent S1 heart sound
- Right ventricular heave
- Dyspnea/orthopnea/PND

Mitral Insufficiency/Regurgitation

- ECG: Left atrial enlargement
- Pulmonary congestion (crackles)
- Systolic murmur
- Palpitations/fatigue/dyspnea/ wheezing/orthopnea/ND

---

with rheumatic heart disease resulting in fibrotic thickening and fusion of the valve leaflets. MS limits LA outflow reducing LV filling during diastole, thereby limiting CO. Pulmonary vascular pressures rise resulting in elevated RV afterload and RV function is compromised as it strains to propel blood through the pulmonary circuit. Patients present with symptoms of LV failure due to reduced CO, but LV ejection fraction (EF) is often maintained.[17,30]

Mitral Insufficiency/Mitral Regurgitation

Mitral regurgitation is the retrograde flow of blood from the LV into the LA through an incompetent MV. Common causes of this disorder include rheumatic heart damage, rupture of papillary muscle or chordae tendinae, infective endocarditis, collagen vascular disease, myxomatous degeneration, and cardiomyopathy-related annular distension.[30,31] MR results in elevated filling volumes of the LV due to the retrograde blood flow during systole flowing back into the LV during the next diastole. The increased preload allows a forceful systolic contraction and emptying of the LV (recall the Starling Law of the Heart). LV hypertrophy progresses over time and eventual contractile dysfunction leads to symptoms of LV failure.[30,31]

Medical and Surgical Management of Valvular Heart Disease

Repair Versus Replacement

The decision to manage valve dysfunction medically or to proceed with repair or replacement of a damaged valve is based on the hemodynamic burden and subsequent muscle dysfunction of the RV or LV (EF/end systolic dimension), repairability of the lesion, presence of comorbid conditions (ischemic heart disease), and age.[32] Goals of maintaining the valve apparatus are to allow sustained ventricular function, reduce operative mortality, promote better late outcomes, restrict anticoagulation therapy, reduce endocarditis, and avoid possible failure of prosthetic valves.[30] As a result, valve repair surgeries, when feasible, are viewed as superior to replacement procedures. The surgical approach for valve surgery is variable. Minimally invasive techniques that attempt to limit blood loss, pain, and hospital stay are becoming increasingly common. Valve surgery may employ median sternotomy, partial sternotomy, transverse sternotomy, and/or limited lateral thoracotomy as the surgical approach. Robotically maneuvered instruments or computer-assisted surgery have been introduced in association with small incisions and minimally invasive procedures.[33,34] Common procedures include the following.

Stenosis: Valvulotomies are procedures to enlarge a narrowed opening of a heart valve. These procedures can be performed by cutting through the commissures with a knife or by a finger thrust, also termed **commissurotomy**, or may be performed through the insertion of a balloon catheter across the stenotic valve, **balloon valvotomy.**[34–36] These techniques may be performed in closed fashion through the insertion of a catheter through a large peripheral vein or in an open fashion associated with cardiopulmonary bypass.[17,34]

Regurgitation: Annuloplasty involves the placement of a prosthetic ring to recreate the normal annular geometry and improve leaflet coaptation or closure. Annuloplasty is performed with regurgitant or prolapsed valves. Other repair procedures include **chordal transfer or shortening, artificial chordae tendinae** via sutures, **cusp plication or cusp extension,** or replacement using autologous pericardium. These procedures attempt to normalize the valvular apparatus by promoting complete closure of the valves thereby preventing regurgitation.[34,35]

Valve replacement surgeries use either mechanical valves or biologic/bioprosthetic valves. Common mechanical valves include the caged-ball type, Starr-Edwards, bileaflet-tilting-disc, St. Jude Medical, or the single-tilting-disk, Bjork-Shiley. The bioprosthetic valves are termed heterografts, composed of either porcine or bovine tissue, or homografts, which are preserved human valves.[17,37] Prosthetic valves differ from one another with regard to several characteristics, including durability (longevity), thrombogenicity, and hemodynamic profile. Mechanical valves are thrombogenic and, therefore, require that the patient receive long-term anticoagulant therapy.[37]

Complications after valve surgery include valve thrombosis and embolism, which is often attributable to inadequate anticoagulation, atrial fibrillation, age greater than 70 years, and depressed LV function.[37] Early endocarditis may occur in 3% to 6% of patients, who acquire perioperative bacteremia arising from skin, wound, or contaminated intravascular devices. Valve failure or regurgitation occurs minimally, but may be a complication of prosthetic-valve endocarditis.[37] Close anatomic relationship between the valves, especially the AoV, and the conduction tissue may lead to conduction defects are and are frequently encountered in the early postoperative period.[38]

Aneurysm

An aneurysm is a localized abnormal dilation of a blood vessel, usually an artery. Thrombus generation, progressive expansion, and eventual rupture characterize the natural history of aneurysms. Most aneurysms are associated

Figure 6–9. The DeBakey classification system for aortic dissection. Type I originates in the ascending aorta and may propagate beyond the aortic arch. Type II is confined to the ascending aorta, and Type III originates in the descending aorta and extends distally. Proximal dissection includes DeBakey Types I and II, while distal dissection are DeBakey III. (Reprinted with permission from Braunwald E. *Heart Disease: A Textbook of Cardiovascular Medicine.* 6th ed. 2001. with permission from Elsevier.)

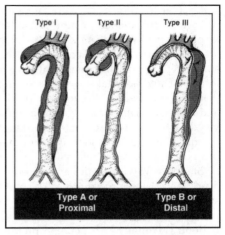

with atherosclerosis, HTN, male gender, cigarette smoking, chronic obstructive pulmonary disease (COPD), and the incidence increases over the age of 70 years.[39] Aneurysms may be classified as saccular, a local outpouching, or more commonly as fusiform, an enlargement of the entire vessel lumen.[28] Clinically, aortic aneurysms are classified according to anatomic features as shown in Figure 6–9. Aneurysms are often asymptomatic making diagnosis difficult. Dissection involves intimal rupture followed by intraluminal splitting and separation of the medial layers of the vessel by a column of blood.[40] Classic signs and symptoms of aortic aneurysm dissection are related to the size and location of the defect, but typically include severe "tearing" anterior chest, back, and abdominal pain; pulse and BP differentials between extremities; signs of altered cerebral hypoperfusion (stroke, syncope, altered MS); or less frequently spinal cord ischemia.[28,40]

Medical Management

Medical therapy is directed to decrease the risk of rupture and slow the advancement of dissection by reducing the force of LV contractions and lowering arterial BP without compromising vital organ perfusion.[40] Common agents employed include beta-blockers, nitrates, and vasodilators.

Surgical Management

Surgical repair is performed to prevent rupture at a time that the risk of rupture is greater than the risk of death from the operation.[41] Surgical techniques for aneurysms may be endovascular or a traditional open approach via a thoracotomy for thoracic aortic aneurysm (TAA) or transperitoneal, midline, or left retroperitoneal exposures for abdominal aortic aneurysms (AAA) depending on the anatomical characteristics of the lesion. The aim of open surgical treatment is to excise and replace the aortic segment containing the origin of the dissection, and not to replace the entire dissected aorta. Open repairs involves the use of synthetic grafts of woven or knitted Dacron.[40] Endovascular-stent grafting is minimally invasive and utilizes stents to bridge or buttress the aneurysm.

Complications are typically reduced via the endovascular approach versus the open techniques. However, AAA and TAA repairs are risky surgeries, and complications are not infrequent. Complications include MI, hemorrhage, pulmonary insufficiency, renal failure, impaired bowel function including paralytic ileus and colonic ischemia, graft infection, and spinal cord injury.[39,42]

Endocarditis/Myocarditis

Endocarditis is a microbial infection of the endocardium resulting in fever, valvular vegetations and dysfunction, systemic emboli, and heart murmurs. It is most common in those with underlying heart disease, intravenous (IV) drug users, hospital-acquired infections, diabetes mellitus (DM), hemodialysis, and those with poor dental hygiene.[26,27,43] Common symptoms are nonspecific and include fever, fatigue, dyspnea, arthralgias, weight loss, night sweats, heart murmur, and petechiae on the skin.[26,43] Diagnosis is via blood cultures that guide antimicrobial therapy. Complications include embolic CVA, abscess formation, valve dysfunction resulting in regurgitation, and conduction disturbances.

Myocarditis is a focal or diffuse inflammation of the myocardium due primarily to viral, bacterial, or fungal infections and secondarily to drugs and immunologic reactions. Myocarditis is most common following a respiratory infection and patient presentation may include chest pain, tachycardia, and symptoms of heart failure (dyspnea, orthopnea, fatigue).

Pericardial Disease

Pericarditis is an inflammatory process involving the visceral and parietal layers of the pericardium and the epicardial surface. This process is common after an acute MI, open heart surgery, uremia (kidney failure), and viral and bacterial infections. Patients will frequently complain of chest pain, fever, and present with a pericardial friction rub via auscultation. Complications include tamponade physiology and heart failure.

Cardiac tamponade results from the rapid development of a **pericardial effusion**, fluid within the pericardial sac, interfering with diastolic filling and coronary artery blood flow. Patients will present with elevated right atrial pressure (RAP)/jugular venous distention (JVD), diminished heart sounds, falling BP, and tachyarrhythmias. Cardiac tamponade results in poor venous return which compromises SV and CO. Although uncommon, tamponade may be a complication following removal of epicardial pacemaker wires.

Heart Failure

Heart failure may be defined as the inability of the heart to pump sufficient amounts of blood to meet the physiologic demands of the body.[17,44] Nearly 5 million Americans are affected with an incidence approaching 10 per 1000 persons and is the admitting diagnosis for over 20% of persons older than 65.[2,3] Heart failure is the final pathway for virtually all forms of heart disease including CAD/ischemic heart disease, HTN, cardiomyopathies, valve disorders, arrhythmogenic diseases, congenital heart disease, as well as other causes (Figure 6–10).[17] Clinically, heart failure may be categorized in multiple ways, including high output/low output, right sided/left sided, but the most frequent description is **systolic heart failure**—failure of the

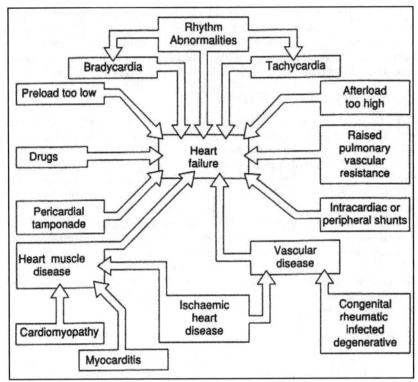

Figure 6–10. Causes of heart failure.

ventricular pump—or **diastolic heart failure**—inability to fill properly thereby limiting output. The common denominator for all descriptions of heart failure is that the clinical manifestations of the disease result from an inadequate CO. The pathogenesis of heart failure is multifactorial resulting from a complex blend of structural, functional, and biological alterations including altered loading conditions, altered energy metabolism, altered neurohumoral activation and signal transduction, abnormal expression and function of contractile proteins, abnormal excitation-contraction coupling, and an altered cytoskeleton (Table 6–7).[3,45] Multiple compensatory mechanisms attempt to increase blood volume and raise cardiac filling pressure to maintain the CO, raise BP, and redistribute blood flow as shown in Figure 6–10. However, as heart failure proceeds, the heart's ability to contract and relax declines progressively and the failure worsens.[17,44] Common symptoms of heart failure are listed in Table 6–8.

Medical and Surgical Management of Heart Failure

The goals of therapy in patients with heart failure are to improve quality and quantity of life and to prevent progression of the syndrome. This is accomplished through three principal components:

1. Removal or amelioration of the underlying cause (eg, AVR secondary to AS)

Table 6–7

POTENTIAL PATHOPHYSIOLOGIC MECHANISM IMPORTANT IN THE SYNDROME OF HEART FAILURE

Structural	*Functional*	*Biological*
• Hypertrophy • Fibrosis/extracellular matrix changes • Myocyte apoptosis • LV remodeling Dilation/increased spherical shape Wall thinning/aneurysm formation • Coronary artery obstruction/ inflammation • Expression of fetal contractile proteins	• Valve disease/ dysfunction • Ischemic/hibernating myocardium • Atrial/ventricular arrhythmias • Altered ventricular interaction	• Activation of renin-angiotensin-aldoste-rone system • Activation of sympa-thetic nervous system • Increased expression of cytokines • Impaired calcium handling

Adapted from Jessup M, Brozena S. Medical progress: heart failure. *N Engl J Med.* 2003;348:2007–2018.

Table 6–8

SIGNS AND SYMPTOMS OF HEART FAILURE

Respiratory Distress

- DOE/SOB
- Orthopnea
- Paroxysmal nocturnal dyspnea
- Cough/pink, frothy sputum
- ↑ respiratory rate

Reduced Exercise Capacity

- Fatigue/weakness
- Limited ability to perform ADLs (6 MWT)

Physical Exam:

- Pulmonary crackles
- S3 heart sound
- Jugular venous distension/ ↑ central venous pressure (CVP)/right atrial pressure (RAP)

2. Removal of precipitating cause (eg, dysrhythmia identification and treatment antibiotics for endocarditis)

3. Control of the heart failure state

Pharmacologic control of the heart failure state is accomplished through the prescription of ACE inhibitors, diuretic therapy, beta-blockers, inotropic agents, and vasodilators (see Monitoring Information).[3,17,46] These drugs attempt to limit the pathophysiologic consequences related to activation of the renin-angiotensin-aldosterone system and sympathetic nervous system. Medications reduce afterload, correct fluid balance, and augment ventricular contractility to enhance the SV and CO. Other medications encountered include anti-arrhythmia drugs.

Surgical interventions include heart transplantation (see Chapter 14), high risk CABG and valve repairs/replacement surgeries, TMR, partial left ventriculostomy, and implantation of pacemakers and defibrillators and mechanical assist devices (intra-aortic balloon counterpulsation [IABP]/left ventricular assist devices [LVAD], total artificial heart).[17,22]

IABP provides support to a patient's failing myocardium and is indicated for patients in cardiogenic shock following cardiac surgery or an acute MI. The device consists of a balloon-tipped flexible catheter attached to a console. The catheter is inserted through the femoral artery and guided to the descending thoracic aorta. The patient's ECG and pressure waveforms are monitored and the balloon is triggered to inflate during ventricular diastole and deflate during systole. Recalling that left ventricular myocardial blood flow primarily occurs during diastole, the inflation of the balloon displaces blood and increases diastolic pressure in the arch of the aorta (behind balloon) augmenting blood flow through the coronary vessels. Additionally, the deflation enhances CO by reducing aortic pressures (afterload) prior to ejection.[17,47] Patients are critically ill and physical therapy is not typically indicated. However, patients may be referred for bed mobility, range of motion (ROM) exercises, and airway clearance. Precautions for IABP include maintaining hip flexion <70 degrees of the involved limb and careful monitoring of device patency and patient's hemodynamics.[7] Complications include LE ischemia, line infections, and vascular injuries (aortic dissection/laceration, lymphocele).[17]

Ventricular assist devices (VAD) are designed to unload the right **(RVAD)** or left **(LVAD)** ventricle and completely support the pulmonary or systemic circulation by restoring normal hemodynamics and end-organ blood flow (Figure 6–11).[17,48] VAD support was previously viewed as rescue therapy as a bridge to transplantation. Now, the VAD can be considered terminal or destination therapy as well as a bridge to heart transplant.[49,50] The implanted LVAD has an outflow line connected to the left ventricular apex, where blood is diverted through a pump and returned to the circulation via an aortic inflow line. The RVAD withdraws blood from the right atrium and returns to the main pulmonary artery. Two blood pumps can be used for biventricular support.[17,22,48] VAD support has led to reverse remodeling or improvements in ventricular size, shape, and contractile function leading to device removal in select patients. VADs are connected to a central console that allows monitoring and recording of device data (eg, device stroke rate, SV, output flows [CO]). Physical therapy will be consulted to initiate exercise conditioning with these patients. Therapeutic

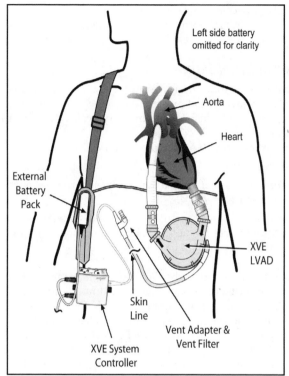

Left side battery
omitted for clarity

Aorta

Heart

External
Battery
Pack

XVE
LVAD

Skin
Line

Vent Adapter &
Vent Filter

XVE System
Controller

Figure 6–11. Heart Mate XVE LVAS (left ventricular assist system). (Reprinted with permission from Thoratec Corp.)

interventions include treadmill walking and progressive resistive exercises as patients participate in phase I–II cardiac rehab programs with improvements in quality of life and exercise capacity.[51,52] VADs can operate on batteries to allow greater mobility, and the therapist must be familiar with emergency procedures in case of battery failure. The physical therapist/physical therapist assistant must maintain the patency of the drive lines with external pumps to ensure adequate flows and monitor the patient's and the device's hemodynamic information (rates/BP/outputs). Complications of VADs include thrombus formation associated with blood stasis within the pump or inadequate anticoagulation, CVA, hemorrhage, line infections, and renal or hepatic insufficiency.[17]

Left ventricular and **biventricular pacing** has proven effective to improve the electrical and mechanical activation sequence or "synchrony" for patients with congestive heart failure, intraventricular conduction delay, or left bundle branch block. Synchrony refers to the normal coordinated, electrically induced contraction of the RV and LV. CHF and LBBB lead to RV and LV contraction abnormalities. Biventricular pacing synchronizes the RV/LV contractions leading to enhanced EF, augmented SV, CO, and cardiac index.[53] **Automatic implantable cardiac defibrillators (AICD/ICD)** are devices used for the prevention of sudden cardiac death due to life-threatening ventricular dysrhythmias (ventricular tachycardia (VT), VF).[54]

Patients who have received a pacemaker or ICD can participate in therapy. The therapist should review the ECG information and standard precautions provided for pacemakers/ICDs.

Differential Diagnosis of Chest Pain

Angina pectoris, or chest pain, results from myocardial ischemia, which is caused by an imbalance between myocardial oxygen requirements and oxygen supply and delivery (see Figure 6–6).[17] Unstable angina is typically defined as having three possible presentations:

1. Symptoms of angina at rest or with minimal exertion

2. New onset of exertional angina

3. Recent acceleration or crescendo of angina symptoms superimposed on a preexisting pattern of angina[13,55]

Unstable angina may be a symptom of the onset of an acute coronary syndrome leading to eventual MI. Physical therapy is usually contraindicated for patients with unstable angina until the patient has been medically or surgically stabilized.

Chest pain occurs frequently and is usually benign. Despite this, myocardial ischemia remains important, because of the impact on patient morbidity and is potentially fatal.[56] Certainly, the patient's complaint of chest pain will influence the physical therapy practitioner and the rapid recognition of chest pain that is cardiac or noncardiac in origin will impact on intervention decision making. Table 6–9 provides a general schema to determine the origins of chest pain. Patient complaints of chest pain should be forwarded to the nursing and medical team for continued triage. The evaluation of acute chest pain should begin with a clinical history that focuses on the characteristics of pain, the time of onset, and the duration of symptoms and an examination that emphasizes vital signs and cardiovascular status.[57] Secondary questions should include an assessment of cardiac risk factors and for gastric or pulmonary disease, as well as psychological disorders.[57] About 50% of all patients with chest pain and normal coronary anatomy have esophageal reflux or motility disorders, approximately 60% have evidence of breathing disorders, and 60%, psychological abnormalities.[58]

REHABILITATION OVERVIEW

Phase I Cardiac Rehabilitation

The rehabilitation professional must be aware of the principles of cardiac rehabilitation in the treatment of patients with cardiovascular disease. Cardiac rehabilitation may be defined as a program of education and exercise established to assist individuals with heart disease in achieving optimal physical, psychosocial, and functional status within the limits of their disease. Additionally, comprehensive risk factor intervention can extend overall survival, improve quality of life, decrease need for interventional procedures such as angioplasty and bypass grafting, and reduces the incidence of subsequent MI.[1] Exercise training improves exercise tolerance, reduces the severity of anginal symptoms, and improves both physical and psychological functioning.[59]

Table 6–9
DIFFERENTIAL DIAGNOSIS OF CHEST PAIN

Descriptor (questions to ask)	Angina	Other Cardiac (eg, pericarditis)	Musculoskeletal (eg, subacromial bursitis)	Gastrointestinal
Symptoms	Nonfocal, dull, vague	Sharp, cutting; difficulty swallowing	Intense, constant, dull, sometimes throbbing, vague onset	Vague onset; symptoms ↑ related to food consumption
Location	Anything above the waist (classic: substernal/LUE/jaw)	Substernal, and may radiate to neck, upper back, upper traps, left arm	Anterolateral shoulder region	
CV exercise	↑ symptoms	↓ symptoms or no effect	↑ symptoms with motions of involved UE, especially overhead movements	May exacerbate symptoms (eg, peptic ulcers), but often no effect
Rest	↓ symptoms; may awaken from sleep	No effect	↓ symptoms; sleep delayed	No effect; may awaken from sleep
Body position/ROM	No effect	Symptoms ↓ by quadruped, leaning forward, sitting upright. Symptoms ↑ by trunk rotation/sidebending	Symptoms ↑ with lying on involved side	Symptoms with head down positioning (eg, GERD)
Deep breath/cough	No effect	↑ symptoms with any activity that causes chest wall to move	No effect	No effect
Palpation	No effect	Painful over left, anterior/lower chest wall	Painful over bursa; area may be warm/swollen	No effect

(continued)

Table 6–9   (continued)

DIFFERENTIAL DIAGNOSIS OF CHEST PAIN

Descriptor (questions to ask)	Angina	Other Cardiac (eg, pericarditis)	Musculoskeletal (eg, subacrominial bursitis)	Gastrointestinal
Nitroglycerine	↓ symptoms	No effect	No effect	No effect
Other		H/o of fever/chills, recent MI, c/o weakness	Relief with heat, non-steroidal anti-inflammatory agents	Relief with antacids

Adapted from:
Heibert J, Coffman S. Presentation: Chest Pain—Now What? Recognition and Management of Angina. Combined Sections Meeting, San Antionio, Tex 2001.
Seidel HM, Ball JW, Benedict GW, et al. *Mosby's Guide to Physical Examination.* St. Louis, Mo: Mosby, Inc; 2003.

Table 6–10

CARDIAC REHABILITATION ASSESSMENT PARAMETERS

Patient is considered **stable**:
No new/recurrent episode of chest pain in 8 hours.

No new signs of uncompensated heart failure including:
• Dyspnea at rest
• Bilateral crackles >0.5 of lung
• Hypotension

No new significant, abnormal rhythm or ECG changes in past 8 hours.
• If atrial fibrillation: Ventricular rate <110 bpm at rest

Able to speak comfortably with a RR <30 breaths/ minute

Cardiac index (CO/body mass) >2 $L/min/m^2$
CVP <12 mmHg

Adapted from AACVPR. *Guidelines for Cardiac Rehabilitation and Secondary Prevention Programs.* Champaign, Ill: Human Kinetics; 1999.

Phase I cardiac rehabilitation occurs in the acute care, transitional care units (skilled nursing facilities/subacute rehabilitation/acute rehabilitation), and home health settings. Rehabilitation should begin once a referral is made and the patient is determined to be "stable" (Table 6–10). Following the interview/ history and review of systems, a physical examination is performed which should include assessment of gross musculoskeletal strength, flexibility and coordination, palpation of pulses, determination of heart/pulse rate, BP, review of cardiovascular symptoms, and auscultation of the heart and lungs as noted in Tables 1–2, 6–11, and 7–7.[7] Progression of rehabilitation depends on the initial examination as well as daily assessments. Progression may vary from a more rapid increase in activity tolerance in the low risk patient to a slower progression in higher risk or more debilitated patients.[7] A framework to determine relative risk of untoward cardiovascular events at rest and with exercise is presented in Table 6–12. Contraindications and relative contraindications for exercise training are provided in Table 6–13. This framework may help guide the physical therapy practitioner to determine an appropriate exercise prescription for the rehabilitation sessions. The general goal of phase I rehabilitation is to enable the patient to tolerate activities of daily living (ADLs), including self-care activities, stair climbing, toileting, and walking functional distances (1 to 4 METS of activity), with minimal to no cardiovascular symptoms and appropriate vital sign responses (Tables 6–14 and 6–15). During phase I cardiac rehabilitation, education is of paramount importance, and this is a time to initiate intensive risk factor and behavior modification. It is well established that risk factor modification and living a more "heart healthy" lifestyle can reduce secondary complications and future coronary events.

Additional Considerations

Rehabilitation of the hospitalized patient who has undergone open-heart surgery follows a phase I cardiac rehabilitation philosophy. Special considerations would include review of **ECG**, laboratory values, determination of hemodynamic stability through review of vital signs over the past 12 to 24 hours, and wound/incision assessment. ECG monitoring often reveals postoperative changes. The most common postoperative ECG changes include atrial fibrillation/flutter and ventricular beats. In atrial fibrillation/flutter and ventricular ectopy, the heart does not fill correctly. Recall that the atria typically contribute 20% to the active filling of the ventricles during diastole. These abnormal heart rhythms may result in impaired filling and reduced preload. With inadequate filling, there is a reduced SV and limited CO, which can cause hypotension/dizziness/orthostasis. Generally, rehabilitation is held if the patient is experiencing atrial fibrillation/flutter with a rapid ventricular response (HR >110).

Laboratory values are important to monitor because the electrolyte and blood cells counts will impact on the intensity and appropriateness of therapy for that day. Special consideration is given to potassium and calcium levels as well as white blood cell (WBC) and hemoglobin concentrations (see Chapter 2). Potassium and calcium are molecules, which determine the normal myocardial cell depolarization. When these values are abnormal, dysrhythmias can develop that compromise CO or can be life threatening. The complete blood cell count (CBC) will provide the practitioner with knowledge of oxygen carrying capacity (hemoglobin/red blood cells (RBCs)/hematocrit), presence of infection (WBCs are often elevated post surgery), and blood coagulation (platelets). The physical therapist/physical therapist assistant should be familiar with the coagulation profile of the patient. The **PT/PTT/INR** will provide information regarding the ability the blood to clot. If the PT/PTT/INR are elevated, the patient is at an increased risk of bleeding secondary to a prolonged time to form a blood clot. After valve replacement, MI, PTCA, the coagulation profile indices are often maintained in

Table 6–11

CARDIOVASCULAR SYSTEM EXAMINATION

Examination Technique	Description of Technique	Examination Findings in Common Diseases/ Disorders
Observation and palpation of chest wall and extremities	• See Table 1–4 regarding grading edema. • See Table 7–7 regarding chest wall and extremity observation and configuration. • See Table 15–1 regarding wound examination and skin inspection.	↑ **accessory muscle hypertrophy:** Chronic respiratory disease, heart failure. **Unilateral edema:** Suspect occlusion of major vein. **Bilateral edema:** Suspect CHF, liver dysfunction, malnutrition, etc.
BP	• Warm and clean diaphragm of stethoscope before placement on patient skin. • Review the patient's history to determine if there is a contraindication/relative contraindication for BP measurements on a particular extremity (eg, PICC line, recent mastectomy or lymph drainage impairment, arterial-venous fistula for hemodialysis, arterial line, recent fracture, etc). • Palpate the brachial pulse (medial to biceps tendon)—this is where the diaphragm of the stethoscope will be placed. • Place the appropriate-sized cuff around the upper arm at least two fingers (2 to 3 cm) width above the elbow crease. The cuff measurements will vary depending on the size of the upper arm. The length of the bladder should be twice the width (~ 80% of the limb circumference).	**BP differences:** It is not uncommon for BP to differ by 10 mmHg between the right and left extremities. The RUE BP is typically higher. Record the higher BP. **False BP reading:** • A cuff too large will underestimate BP. • A cuff too small will overestimate BP. • **Auscultatory gap:** The period of silence when the Korotkoff sound disappears and reappears 10 to 15 mmHg lower. Note the first sound as SBP. Auscultatory gap may lead to an underestimate of BP. **High BP/HTN** is typically diagnosed over time. Select reading on a single day may not be conclusive.

(continued)

Table 6–11 (continued)

CARDIOVASCULAR SYSTEM EXAMINATION

Examination Technique	*Description of Technique*	*Examination Findings in Common Diseases/ Disorders*
	• Raise the UE to heart level and pump the cuff up to >180 mmHg or until the brachial pulse is absent. • Lower the cuff pressure by 2 to 3 mmHg per second. • Note the first "clear" Korotkoff sound (systolic BP [SBP]) and when this sound disappears (diastolic BP [DBP]). • LE BP measurement: Make sure the cuff fits the LE correctly; in most cases at least a large to extra large adult cuff is needed. LE BP is typically greater than UE BP (note Ankle Brachial Index) (see Table 15-2).	**Classification of BP:** Table 6–3. **Hypotension or blunted BP rise with activity:** Suspect LV pump dysfunction/heart failure, dehydration, medication side effect, etc.
Pulse or HR	**Arterial pulses:** A bounding wave of blood that diminishes with increasing distance from the heart. • Palpate a radial pulse using 2 to 3 fingers (not your thumb) on the underside of the forearm. • Follow the patient's thumb from the thenar eminence to just proximal of the wrist crease. • Gently press until a beating sensation is palpated. • Count for a minimum of 15 seconds and then multiply by 4. If there is an irregularity or the pulse feels extremely slow, weak, or fast, count for 30 to 60 seconds and multiply accordingly.	**Pulse rhythm:** • An irregular pulse may accompany or signify a dysrhythmia (eg, atrial fibrillation = irregularly irregular pulse; ventricular bigeminy, sinus arrhythmia = regularly irregular pulse) • The heart rhythm cannot be inferred from the pulse quality; an ECG is required to confirm the presence of a dysrhythmia **Bradycardia:** Pulse rate <60 (eg, cardiac conduction abnormality, hypothyroidism, hypothermia, drug intoxication, athlete)

(continued)

Table 6–11 (continued)

CARDIOVASCULAR SYSTEM EXAMINATION

Examination Technique	Description of Technique	Examination Findings in Common Diseases/Disorders
	• LE pulses (eg, femoral, popliteal, dorsalis pedis) can be palpated if UE pulses are unidentified. • Carotid pulses can be palpated, but only one at a time. Carotid pulses should be avoided during exercise due to risk for vasovagal response (eg, bradycardia and hypotension). • Apical pulse can be auscultated when peripheral palpation is difficult. • Determine the point of maximal impulse (PMI)—left fifth intercostal space, midclavicular region. • Listen and count the number of cardiac cycles and multiply accordingly (each cardiac cycle is one S1 and one S2—see heart sounds below). Document the • Calculated pulse rate • Rhythm of the pulse (eg, regular, regularly irregular, or irregularly irregular) • Quality of pulse (see Table 1–7) 4+: Bounding 3+: Full, strong 2+: Normal 1+: Weak, thready 0: Absent	**Tachycardia:** Pulse rate >100 (eg, heart disease, lung disease, fever, hyperthyroidism, anemia, shock, anxiety, exercise) **Pulses alternans:** Amplitude of pulse varies between weak and strong beats (eg, heart failure/left ventricular failure) **Pulses paradoxus:** Pulse strength falls with inspiration (eg, restrictive pericarditis, pericardial effusion, COPD) **Pulses differens:** Unequal pulses between left and right extremities (eg, impaired circulation/unilateral vascular obstruction) **Bounding pulse (+4):** Hyperkinetic or strong pulse (eg, aortic rigidity, atherosclerosis, anxiety, fever, hyperthyroidism, exercise)
Auscultation	**Heart sounds:** Listen to determine the S1, the first heart sound ("lub"), and S2, the second heart sound ("dub"). S1 signifies the onset of systole while S2 marks	**S1:** Best heard toward the apex of the heart (PMI/mitral region) **S2:** Best heard at the base of the heart (aortic region)

(continued)

Table 6–11 (continued)

CARDIOVASCULAR SYSTEM EXAMINATION

Examination Technique	*Description of Technique*	*Examination Findings in Common Diseases/ Disorders*
	the end of systole/beginning of diastole. Abnormal heart sounds include S3, S4, pericardial friction rub, and heart murmurs (see Table 6-6). • **Apical pulse and mitral region:** fifth intercostal space, midclavicular region • **Aortic area:** second intercostal space just to the right of sternum • **Pulmonic area:** second intercostal space just to the left of the sternum • **Tricuspid area:** fourth or fifth intercostals space border of left sternal area	**S3 ("ventricular gallop"):** An abnormal heart sound occurring early in diastole (passive filling phase) (eg, CHF). Sounds like "lub-dub-*dub*" **S4 ("atrial gallop"):** An abnormal heart sound occurring late in ventricular diastole (atrial systole). (eg, HTN, MI) Sounds like "*la*-lub-dub" **Pericardial friction rub:** Pericardial inflammation/ pericarditis **Systolic murmurs:** Heard between S1 and S2. Sounds like "lub-*swoosh*-dub" (eg, aortic and pulmonic stenosis, mitral and tricuspid regurgitation) **Diastolic murmurs:** Heard post S2 preceding S1. Sounds like "lub-dub-*swoosh*" (eg, mitral and tricuspid stenosis, aortic regurgitation)
	Arterial bruits: A murmur in an artery indicative of turbulent blood flow Sites to auscultate include the temporal, carotid, subclavian abdominal aortal, renal, iliac and femoral arteries	**Arterial bruits:** May reflect the transmitting of murmurs resulting from aortic or MV disorders (eg, stentosis and/or regurgitation; may indicate obstructive arterial disease (eg, artherosclerosis, arteritis)
Electrocardiogram review	See Monitoring Information	

(continued)

Table 6–11 (continued)

CARDIOVASCULAR SYSTEM EXAMINATION

Examination Technique	Description of Technique	Examination Findings in Common Diseases/Disorders	
Chest pain	See Table 6-9	Causes of Chest Pain:	
		Cardiac:	**Pulmonary:**
		Angina/MI/peri-	Pleurisy/pneumo-
		carditis/MV pro-	thorax/mediasti-
		lapse	nal emphysema
		Musculoskeletal:	**Gastrointestinal:**
		Cervical radicu-	Hiatus hernia/
		lopathy/shoulder	reflex esophagi-
		arthritis/rotator	tis, esophageal
		cuff injury/costo-	spasm/peptic
		chondral disorder	ulcer/pancreatitis

Adapted from:
Frownfelter D, Dean E. *Principles and Practice of Cardiopulmonary Physical Therapy.* St. Louis, Mo: Mosby-Year Book, Inc; 1996.
Hillegass EA, Sadowsky HS. *Essentials of Cardiopulmonary Physical Therapy.* 2nd ed. Philadelphia, Pa: WB Saunders Co; 2001.
Irwin S, Tecklin JS. *Cardiopulmonary Physical Therapy: A Guide to Practice.* 4th ed. St. Louis, Mo: Mosby Inc; 2004.
Perloff JK. *Physical Examination of the Heart and Circulation.* 3rd ed. Philadelphia, Pa: WB Saunders Co; 2000.
Reid WD, Chung F. *Clinical Management Notes and Case Histories in Cardiopulmonary Physical Therapy.* Thorofare, NJ: SLACK Incorporated; 2004.
Seidel HM, Ball JW, Benedict GW, et al. *Mosby's Guide to Physical Examination.* St. Louis, Mo: Mosby, Inc; 2003.
Watchie J. *Cardiopulmonary Physical Therapy: A Clinical Manual.* Philadelphia, Pa: WB Saunders Co; 1995.

a slightly elevated range to prevent blood clot formation and maintain smooth laminar blood flow. Review institutional guidelines or communicate with the physician and nursing personnel to determine optimal ranges for each patient.

Wound assessment should include assessing for the presence of infection, inadequate healing, and determine the stability of wound closure. Wound infection is suspected if there is excessive, foul-smelling, and/or discolored drainage. Some serosanguinous drainage may be present. Determining the presence of a sternal "click" quickly assesses sternal stability. To determine stability, the practitioner should place two fingers on either side of the incision or place a stethoscope over top of the incision. You then ask the patient to take a deep breath or cough gently. With a stable sternum, you should feel both sides of the wound rise and fall together and no click/rubbing noise should be auscultated via the stethoscope. If there is asymmetry via palpation or if a loud "click" is heard, the wound is considered unstable and caution should be exercised with

Table 6–12

RISK STRATIFICATION IN CARDIAC REHABILITATION

Lowest Risk	*Moderate Risk*	*Highest Risk*
• No significant LV dysfunction (EF >50%) • No resting/exercise complex dysrhythmias • Uncomplicated MI/CABG/angioplasty • Normal hemodynamics with exercise/recovery • Asymptomatic/absence of angina • Absence of clinical depression	• Moderate LV dysfunction (EF = 40% to 49%) • Signs/symptoms at moderate levels of exercise (5 to 7 METs) • **Moderate risk is assumed for patients who do not meet the low or high risk criteria**	• Decreased LV function (EF <40%) • Survivor of cardiac arrest or sudden death • Complex ventricular dysrhythmia at rest/exercise • Complicated MI or CABG: • Perioperative ischemia/MI • CHF/shock • MI: Pericarditis • Abnormal hemodynamics with exercise • Flat/decreasing SBP • Chronotropic incompetence w/ ↑ workload • Clinically significant depression

Adapted from:
AACVPR. *Guidelines for Cardiac Rehabilitation and Secondary Prevention Programs.* Champaign, IL: Human Kinetics; 1999.
ACSM Guidelines for Exercise Testing and Prescription. 6th ed. Philadelphia, Pa: Lippincott Williams & Wilkins; 2000.

UE activities. Patients are often instructed in sternal precautions to limit unnecessary stress on the healing surgical approach (Table 6–16).

Postoperative lung injury is a complication of all major surgeries due to general anesthesia induced atelectasis and surfactant abnormalities resulting in decreased pulmonary compliance and potentially limited ventilation. Abnormalities are noted after cardiac surgery involving cardiopulmonary bypass. Bypass is associated with increased inflammatory cytokines and pulmonary vascular permeability leading to leakage of plasma proteins creating increased extravascular water and pulmonary edema. Additionally, the surgical approach and patient complaints of chest wall pain will limit chest expansion. Lung compliance is reduced postsurgery due to altered surfactant, increased vascular permeability and pulmonary edema. The sum of these factors leads to impairments in gas exchange and musculoskeletal pump performance. All cardiovascular patients should be involved in an airway clearance and mobility regimen to reduce the incidence of postoperative pulmonary complication.

Table 6-13

CONTRAINDICATIONS/RELATIVE CONTRAINDICATIONS TO EXERCISE TRAINING

Contraindications:

- Unstable angina
- Moderate to severe angina
- Uncompensated heart failure
- Acute aortic dissection
- Severe/symptomatic valve dysfunction
- Uncontrolled dysrhythmias:
  - ➢ Sustained VT
  - ➢ Second/third degree heart block
  - ➢ New onset SVT (atrial fibrillation/flutter/PAT)
  - ➢ New onset brady/tachy arrhythmias with hemodynamic compromise
- Drop in SBP >10 mmHg
- Resting SBP >210; DBP >110
- Inability to monitor pulse or BP
- Signs or symptoms of exercise intolerance or poor perfusion including
  - ➢ Angina
  - ➢ Marked dyspnea
  - ➢ Palor
  - ➢ Cyanosis

Relative Containdications:

- Acute myocarditis/pericarditis
- Electrolyte abnormalities
- Severe HTN (stage 2/3)
- New onset brady/tachy arrhythmias without hemodynamic compromise
- Symptomatic valve dysfunction
- Inability to monitor ECG
- Subjective complaints of fatigue/SOB/wheezing/leg cramps
- SBP >210; DBP >110
- Rating of perceived exertion >15
- Peak HR >40 beats/min above resting or 75% of predicted HR maximum

Adapted from AACVPR. *Guidelines for Cardiac Rehabilitation and Secondary Prevention Programs.* Champaign, Ill: Human Kinetics; 1999.

CASE STUDY

Mrs. Hayes is a 74 year old (y/o) female with a history of (h/o) coronary atherosclerotic heart disease. She had a heart catheterization 1 month ago showing diffuse disease. Her medical management has included beta-blockers, statins, and aspirin. The patient was admitted to the hospital with worsening dyspnea on exertion. She experienced an episode of supraventricular tachycardia (SVT) and atrial fibrillation that was rate controlled with metoprolol and IV procainamide. An echocardiogram revealed an EF of 40%. She was cardioverted to sinus rhythm. On auscultation she had bilateral crackles 1/3 bilaterally, no S3 or JVD, and 1+ pitting edema. Her current ECG revealed atrial fibrillation at a rate of 121. She underwent another catheterization that revealed a complex LAD/bifurcation stenosis, left circumflex stenosis, and diagonal involvement. On the third

Table 6–14

SAMPLE PHASE I CARDIAC REHABILITATION PROGRAM/ ACTIVITY PRESCRIPTION

	MET Level	Activity
Day 1: Critical care unit	• 1 to 2	• Bedrest until stable • OOB in chair • Toileting • Airway clearance techniques (ACT): Deep breathing/cough/incentive spirometry
Day 2: Transfer to step down unit	• 2 to 3	• Sitting UE/LE AROM exercise/ calisthenics • Continued airway clearance • Walking in room
Days 3 to 5:	• 2 to 3	• OOB as tolerated • Standing warm ups • Walking 5 to 10 minutes in hall up to BID/TID • Continue ACT
	• 3 to 4	• Shower with seat • Standing warm ups • Walking 5 to 10 minutes in hall up to BID/TID • Initiate stair climbing

Adapted from AACVPR. *Guidelines for Cardiac Rehabilitation and Secondary Prevention Programs.* Champaign, Ill: Human Kinetics; 1999.

hospital day she underwent a CABG using the left internal mammary artery (LIMA) and the saphenous vein from the left LE (LLE). Physical therapy was consulted on postoperative day 2.

Patient/Client History

General Demographics/Social History/ Living Environment

Mrs. Hayes has been married for 50 years and lives in a ranch style home with four steps to enter and no handrail. She has one son that lives with her with two grandchildren (ages 5 and 7). She is a retired postal worker.

General Health Status/Family History

Mrs. Hayes states she smoked for 40 years and quit 10 years ago when she got short of breath at a work picnic. She enjoys a beer or glass of wine at night when her son gets home from work.

Table 6–15

ACTIVITIES OF DAILY LIVING AND METABOLIC EQUIVALENTS

Activity	Method	METs	Average HR Response
• Toileting	• Bed pan • Commode • Urinal (in bed) • Urinal (standing)	• 1 to 2	• 5 to 15 bpm ↑ from resting heart rate (RHR)
• Bathing	• Bed bath • Tub bath • Shower	• 2 to 3	• 10 to 20 bpm ↑ from RHR
• Walking	Flat surface • 2 mph • 2.5 mph • 3 mph	• 2 to 2.5 • 2.5 to 2.9 • 3 to 3.3	• 5 to 15 bpm ↑ from RHR
• Stair climbing	1 flight=12 steps • Down 1 FOS • Up 1-2 FOS	• 2.5 • 4.0	• 10 bpm ↑ from RHR • 10 to 25 bpm ↑ from RHR
• Upper body exercise	While standing • UE • Trunk	• 2.6 to 3.1 • 2 to 2.2	• 10 to 20 bpm ↑ from RHR
• Leg calisthenics		• 2.5 to 4.5	• 15 to 25 bpm ↑ from RHR

Adapted from AACVPR. *Guidelines for Cardiac Rehabilitation and Secondary Prevention Programs.* Champaign, Ill: Human Kinetics; 1999.

Table 6–16

STERNAL PRECAUTIONS

- Limit bilateral upper extremity (BUE) overhead movements
- Limit UE horizontal adduction across midline and horizontal abduction past the coronal plane
- UE weight lifting is limited to 5 to 10 pounds
- No driving

*Restrictions are typically maintained for 6 weeks or until cleared by cardiovascular surgeon or cardiologist. Check with institutional guidelines.

Medical/Surgical History

Mrs. Hayes is a 74 y/o female who has a long history of CAD and is 2 days status post (s/p) CABG. Her medical history includes stable angina >2 years, HTN, Type 2 DM for >10 years, and she is moderately overweight. She is s/p transmetarsal amputation of the LLE 4 years ago for complications of a foot ulcer.

Current Condition/Chief Complaint

Mrs. Hayes is lethargic and complaining of being uncomfortable. She has a face mask delivering 35% F_iO_2 (fraction of inspired oxygen), a right radial arterial line with arm board, pneumatic boots on both LE, and a Foley catheter in place. The chest tube and central lines have been removed. She remains monitored for oxygen saturation and ECG examination.

Functional Status and Activity Level

Mrs. Hayes used a straight cane to ambulate on all surfaces prior to admission. She does not have an orthopedic shoe for the LLE. Her husband drives because she has been having difficulty with her vision lately. They enjoy playing bridge with their church group, but no longer travel outside their hometown.

Other Clinical Tests

Laboratory results revealed hyperkalemia of 5.2, CPK of 500 ng/mL, glucose 200, Hgb A_{1c} 9.0%, +ketones in urine, and elevated WBCs at 14,000.

Systems Review

Cardiovascular/Pulmonary

Resting vital signs in bed (head of bed raised >30 degrees) are oxygen saturation (SpO_2) 92% on 35% F_iO_2, HR 90 and pulse irregularly irregular, RR 24 with accessory muscle use, BP 100/88, and pain 6/10. ROM, MMT, bed mobility, and transfer to dangling revealed a vital sign response of SpO_2 95%, HR 96 to 115, RR 26 with continued accessory muscle use, BP 88/86, and pain 6/10. She complained of dizziness and was transferred back to sidelying. She was able to tolerate 30 seconds of dangling. Her cough is weak and nonproductive. Her breath sounds are diminished throughout with the right posterior lower lobe being absent. "E" to "A" changes were auscultated in the same area. There is decreased chest wall movement comparing the right lateral chest wall to the left. Mediate percussion reveals a "dull" sound in the right posterior lobe. The chest x-ray demonstrates pneumonia in the right lower lobe and slight flattening of the diaphragms bilaterally. The nursing staff was informed of her vital sign response and levels of discomfort during the evaluation.

Integumentary

Mrs. Hayes has a Foley catheter, an arterial line, and a surgical bandage in the center of her thorax with epicardial pacing wires exiting. There appears to be some brownish, dried drainage around the edges of the dressing. The transmetarsal incision is well healed. The LLE has a surgical dressing extending from below the knee to just below the groin area. There is also some brownish, dried drainage on this dressing. She has some pitting edema in her left > right ankle area (+2).

Musculoskeletal

Her MMT revealed 2–3/5 for bilateral lower extremity (BLE), with 3/5 for BUE. Her ROM is >90 degrees in bilateral shoulder area; the radial board limits wrist movements on the right side, otherwise UEs are within functional limits (WFL). There is a decreased ROM in bilateral ankles due to edema, but appears to be functional. Bed mobility is moderate assistance of one with rolling side to side even using the bedrail. She transferred to dangling with moderate assistance of one. Due to drop in BP with transfer and complaints of dizziness, a standing transfer was not attempted at this time.

Neuromuscular

Mrs. Hayes had decreased sharp sensation below the knees bilaterally, and prioprioception is intact BUE/LE.

Communication, Affect, Cognition, Language, and Learning Style

Mrs. Hayes was awake, but lethargic. She was able to recognize where she was, but did not know the current president or the month. Her primary language is English. She was also able to perform one-and two-step directions without cues.

Tests and Measures

Aerobic Capacity and Endurance

Mrs. Hayes demonstrated orthostatic hypotension with transfer from sidelying to dangling at the edge of the bed. She is tachycardic and tachypnic at rest and has a poor ventilation pattern as well as a poor cough. Laboratory results are suspicious for poorly controlled diabetes which will impact healing, elevated potassium which could result in dysrhythmias, and elevated WBC which may correspond with clinical pulmonary findings, possible infection, and/or a common postoperative finding. An elevated CPK is expected following trauma or surgery. If there is suspicion of perioperative MI, cardiac troponins or other cardiac enzymes should be reviewed (see Chapter 12).

Assistive and Adaptive Devices

Recommend Mrs. Hayes have a rolling walker when she is ready for out of bed activities.

Gait, Locomotion, and Balance

Unable to evaluate gait at this time and she required assistance with her sitting static/dynamic balance.

Pain

Mrs. Hayes had increased pain with activity; recommend coordinating therapy with pain management.

Diagnosis

Mrs. Hayes presents with deconditioning from inactivity prior to surgery and complications related to atrial fibrillation. She has a pneumonia that needs aggressive treatment to prevent possible reintubation and prolonged hospital stay. Recommend treatment pattern 6D: impaired aerobic capacity/endurance associated with cardiovascular pump dysfunction.[60]

Prognosis

Mrs. Hayes should progress functionally with therapy in conjunction with aggressive airway clearance and pain management.

Intervention

Recommend frequent incentive spirometry and splinted coughing (10x/hour while awake), and mobilization three to four times per day once hemodynamically stable. Recommend out of bed with nurses a minimum of 45 minutes twice a day (eg, meals). Elevate LE and monitor skin integrity closely. Educate patient and family members on precautions due to decrease sensation, sternal precautions, importance of airway clearance and OOB activities, and cardiac risk factor reduction.

Reexamination

Following 4 days: Foley catheter and arterial line removed. Bulky surgical dressings removed revealing adhesive strips in areas of incisions. MMT grossly 4–/5 BUE/LE, pain 3/10 with activity and 0/10 at rest. Cough when splinted is effective following gentle percussion/vibration and incentive spirometry. Chest x-ray is clearing. Gait with rolling walker moderate assistance of one, 50 feet x 2 trials on 3 liters nasal cannula.

Outcomes

Recommend transfer to inpatient rehabilitation unit for continued progress in functional level.

CHAPTER REVIEW QUESTIONS

1. What are four factors that determine myocardial oxygen demand, and how does exercise impact these factors?

2. Describe the clinical presentation of a patient with LLE PAD.

3. What are the standard precautions for a patient who has a temporary pacemaker? A permanent pacemaker/ICD?

4. What are five modifiable risk factors for coronary heart disease?

5. How does general anesthesia promote lung injury as a complication of all major surgeries?

MONITORING INFORMATION: THE ELECTROCARDIOGRAM, INTERPRETATION, AND ANTIARRHYTHMIC DEVICES

Daniel Malone, MPT, CCS

Monitoring of the ECG and interacting with patients who require pacemakers or defibrillators is common practice in the acute care setting. This section will provide an overview of electrophysiology and electrocardiography, provide the definitions and examples of common dysrhythmias, and discuss devices used to manage electrophysiologic abnormalities.

The Electrocardiogram

The electrical events within the heart initiate the cardiac cycle resulting in myocardial contraction and pressure generation, the opening and closing of the valves, and the ejection of blood. The action potential (AP) of the cardiac myocyte is divided into depolarization, or the change of the membrane potential from negative to positive, and repolarization, or the return to the resting negative steady state. The AP consists of four phases as noted in Figure 6–12. These phases result from changes in the permeability of the cell membrane associated with the opening and closing of ion channels. These channels allow the diffusion of sodium, potassium, and calcium ions across the cell membrane leading to the alterations in the membrane potential and ultimately cardiac contraction.

Cardiac myocytes are characterized by unique properties termed automaticity and conductivity. Automaticity refers to the ability of a cardiac myocyte to discharge an electrical current without stimulation from the nervous system. The pacemaker cells of the SA node, AV node, and purkinje system highlight this property (Table 6–17), but other regions of the myocardium can initiate electrical impulses and take over pacemaker function. **Conductivity** defines the ability of the myocytes to transmit impulses rapidly to successive cells. Cardiac myocytes are connected via intercalated discs that couple the cells both mechanically and electrically allowing the heart to contract as a unit.

A **dysrhythmia** results from a disturbance in the discharge of cardiac impulses or transmission of the impulse through the conduction system. Dysrhythmias may result from:

- Disturbance in automaticity: This may involve a speeding up or slowing down of the sinus node (sinus bradycardia/tachycardia), the formation of premature beats (often called premature complexes or depolarizations) from the atria, the atrioventricular (AV) junction or the ventricles (PAC/PJC/PVCs).

- Disturbance in conductivity: Conduction may be too rapid (eg, Wolf-Parkinson-White syndrome) or too slow (as in AV block).

- Combinations of altered automaticity and conductivity.

The **ECG** is a recording of the electrical forces produced by the heart and inscribed on graph paper. The ECG paper is divided into five small squares

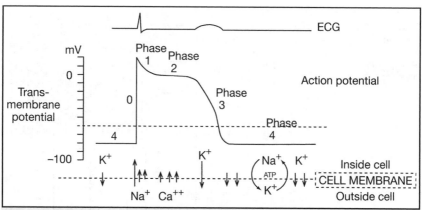

Figure 6–12. Phases of AP. (Reprinted with permission from the American Heart Association.)

Table 6–17
PACEMAKERS OF THE HEART

Pacemaker	Intrinsic Rate
Primary Pacemaker:	60 to 100
• SA node	
Latent or Secondary Pacemakers:	40 to 60
• AV node	20 to 40
• Ventricles/purkinje system	

comprising one large square and advances at 25 mm/sec. Each small square corresponds to 0.04 sec and each large square is 0.20 sec (0.04 sec x 5 small boxes) as noted in Figure 6–13. Electrodes, placed on the skin of the patient, record the electrical activity that precedes the mechanical contraction and relaxation of the myocardium. Changing the location of the recording electrodes provides different perspectives a nd different waveforms, enabling the observer to gain a more complete picture of the electrical forces within the heart. The selection of a particular lead configuration is based upon which lead provides the clearest picture or allows the observer to focus on particular regions of the heart. The standard 12-lead ECG consists of tracings from six limb leads (I, II, III, aVR, aVL, aVF) and six chest leads (V1, V2, V3, V4, V5, V6) (Figure 6–14). The physical therapist should be familiar with a single lead tracing termed a rhythm strip and be able to interpret the HR, rhythm, and presence (or absence) of dysrhythmias. Once the rhythm strip has been interpreted, it is imperative that the therapist understands the impact of these electrical events on the hemodynamic profile of the patient (Figure 6–15).

Figure 6–13. The ECG paper displays time on the horizontal axis and voltage on the vertical axis. (Reprinted from Hillegass EA, Sadowsky HS. *Essentials of Cardiopulmonary Physical Therapy*, page 387, with permission from Elsevier.)

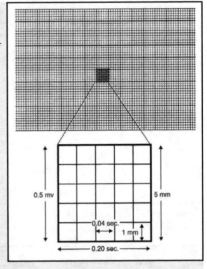

Figure 6–14. The ECG tracing from the chest leads (V1 to V6) showing the changes in the QRS configuration. (Reprinted from Hillegass EA, Sadowsky HS. *Essentials of Cardiopulmonary Physical Therapy*, page 387, with permission from Elsevier.)

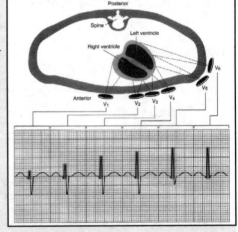

Electrocardiogram Interpretation

ECG interpretation begins with identification of the electrical waveforms and intervals as noted in Figure 6–16 including:

- **P wave:** Atrial depolarization.

- **QRS complex:** Ventricular depolarization.

- **T wave:** Ventricular repolarization.

- **U wave:** Possible repolarization of the Purkinje system (minimal significance).

- **PR interval:** Extends from the beginning of the P wave to the onset of the QRS complex. This interval represents conduction through the atria to the

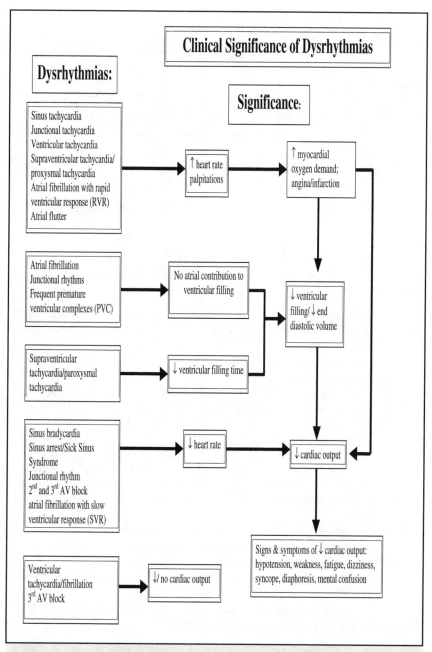

Figure 6–15. Impact of various dysrhythmias on hemodynamic responses and patient complaints. (Adapted from Watchie J. *Cardiopulmonary Physical Therapy: A Clinical Manual.* Philadelphia, Pa: WB Saunders Co; 1995. With permission from Elsevier.)

Figure 6–16. Electrical waveforms and intervals of an ECG. (Reprinted from Hillegass EA, Sadowsky HS. *Essentials of Cardiopulmonary Physical Therapy*, page 468, with permission from Elsevier.)

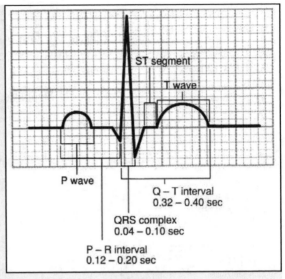

AV node and the Bundle of His. PRI is measured from the onset of the P wave to the onset of the QRS complex, and its normal duration is **0.12 to 0.20 sec.**

- **QRS interval:** Extends from the end of the PR interval (noted by change in the waveform deflection) and ends with the return to baseline. The QRS interval represents the time it takes for the ventricles to depolarize or conduction from the AV node, through the Bundle of His, the Bundle Branches, and the Purkinje System. The normal QRS duration is **0.04 to 0.11 sec.**

- **ST segment:** Interval measured from the end of the QRS complex and the beginning of the T wave. It represents the time during which the ventricles have completed depolarization and repolarization begins. ST segment elevation and depression are observed as an early ECG sign of infarction.

- **Q-T interval:** Extends from the beginning of the QRS complex until the end of the T wave and represents the time interval for ventricular depolarization and repolarization. The normal Q-T interval is **0.32 to 0.40 sec** and prolongation is associated with drug toxicity and increased risk of dysrhythmias.

ECG interpretation should be performed in an organized and systematic fashion. Table 6–18 provides a step-wise approach.

Common Rhythms/Dysrhythmias

Normal Sinus Rhythm
Rate: 60 to 100.
Rhythm: Regular.

Table 6–18

SYSTEMATIC APPROACH TO DYSRHYTHMIA INTERPRETATION

1. Regularity (Also Called Rhythm):
- Is it regular?
- Is it irregular? } √ R-R' interval
- Are there any patterns to the irregularity?
- Are there any ectopic beats; if so, are they early or late?

2. Rate:
- What is the exact rate?
- Is the atrial rate the same as the ventricular rate?

3. P Waves:
- Are the P waves regular?
- Is there one P wave for every QRS?
- Is the P wave in front of the QRS or behind it?
- Is the P wave normal or upright in Lead II?
- Are there more P waves than QRS complexes?
- Do all the P waves look alike?
- Are the irregular P waves associated with ectopic beats?

4. PR Interval:
- Are all the PRIs constant?
- Is the PRI measurement within the normal range?
- If the PRI varies, is there a pattern to the changing measurements?

5. QRS Complex:
- Are all the QRS complexes of equal duration?
- What is the measurement of the QRS complex?
- Is the QRS measurement within normal limits?
- Do all the QRS complexes look alike?
- Are the unusual QRS complexes associated with ectopic beats?

Adapted from:
Dysrhythmia Review Manual. Nursing Staff Development. University of Pennsylvania Health System. Hospital of the University of Pennsylvania.
Hillegass EA. Electrocardiography. In: Hillegass EA, Sadowsky HS, eds. Essentials of Cardiopulmonary Physical Therapy. 2nd ed. Philadelphia, PA: WB Saunders; 2001.
Mammen BA, Irwin S, Tecklin JS. Common cardiac and pulmonary clinical measures. In: Irwin S, Tecklin JS. Cardiopulmonary Physical Therapy: A Guide to Practice. 4th ed. St. Louis, Mo: Mosby Inc: 2004.

P wave: Sinus, P followed by QRS.
PRI: 0.12 to 0.20 sec.
QRS: 0.06 to 0.11 sec.

Sinus Bradycardia (Figure 6–17)
Rate: <60.

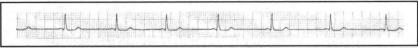

Figure 6–17. Sinus bradycardia.

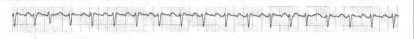

Figure 6–18. Sinus tachycardia.

Rhythm: Regular.
P wave: Sinus, P f/b QRS.
PRI: 0.12 to 0.20 sec.
QRS: 0.06 to 0.11 sec.
Common causes:

- Normal in well-trained athlete secondary to enhanced SV and influence of the parasympathetic nervous system.

- Beta-blocking medications.

- Decrease in automaticity of the SA node (eg, sick sinus syndrome).

- Increased vagal stimulation/enhanced parasympathetic nervous system stimulation (eg, vasovagal stimulus—suctioning, vomiting).

- Increased intracranial pressure (eg, traumatic brain injury).

- Bradycardia may be present with second or third-degree heart block.

Treatment:

- No treatment necessary if asymptomatic.

- If symptomatic (eg, dizziness/hypotension), increase HR via drugs (eg, atropine) or pacemaker.

Sinus Tachycardia (Figure 6–18)
Rate: >100.
Rhythm: Regular.
P wave: Sinus, P followed by QRS.
PRI: 0.12 to 0.20 sec.
QRS: 0.06 to 0.11 sec.
Common causes:

- Increased SA node automaticity (eg, increased sympathetic nervous system stimulation).

- Pain, fear, exertion/exercise, artificial stimulants (eg, caffeine, nicotine, atropine, amphetamines).

- Conditions that increase oxygen demand (eg, fever, CHF, infection, anemia, hemorrhage, myocardial injury, hyperthyroidism, pulmonary disease).

Treatment:

- Elimination of the underlying cause or initiation of beta blockers.

Sinus Arrhythmia

Definition: An irregularity in rhythm in which the impulse is initiated by the SA node but with phasic quickening and slowing of the impulse formation.

Rate: 40 to 100.

Rhythm: Irregular. Impulse is originated in the SA node but with phasic quickening and slowing of the impulse formation. The irregularity is usually caused by an alternation in vagal stimulation (eg, inspiration—increases rate; expiration—decreases rate).

P wave: Sinus, P followed by QRS.

PRI: 0.12 to 0.20 sec.

QRS: 0.06 to 0.12 sec.

Common causes:

- Most common type is associated with the respiratory cycle and is usually observed in the young and the elderly. Sinus arrhythmia often disappears with activity.

- Nonrespiratory sinus arrhythmia may occur in conditions of infection, fever, and medication administration (particularly toxicity with digoxin or morphine).

Treatment:

- The respiratory type is benign and does not require treatment.

- The nonrespiratory type should be evaluated for the underlying cause and then managed.

Sinus Pause or Block

Definition: Occurs when the SA node fails to initiate an impulse, usually only for one cycle.

Rate: Usually 60 to 100.

Rhythm: Underlying rhythm is regular, but occasional pauses are noted

P wave: Sinus, P followed by QRS.

PRI: 0.12 to 0.20 sec.

QRS: 0.06 to 0.12 sec.

Common causes:

- Sudden increases in parasympathetic activity.

- Organic disease of the SA node (eg, sick sinus syndrome).

- Other causes may include: infection, rheumatic disease, severe ischemia, or infarction to the SA node and/or digoxin toxicity.

Treatment:

- Required only if symptomatic. Remove or correct causative agent.

Atrial Dysrhythmias

Premature Atrial Complexes (PAC)

Definition: An ectopic, or abnormal, focus in either atria that initiates an impulse before the next impulse is initiated by the SA node. Conduction through the ventricles is normal.

Significance:

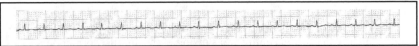

Figure 6–19. Paroxysmal atrial tachycardia/atrial tacyardia.

- PACs reflect the irritability of atrial muscle. May reflect a predisposition to other atrial dysrhythmias.

Rate: Underlying rhythm usually sinus. Therefore rate is 60 to 100.

Rhythm: Irregular. The premature ectopic beat will interrupt the regularity of the underlying rhythm. Note the irregular P-P and R-R intervals if you include the ectopic beat.

P waves: A P' wave, differing in morphology from that of the sinus node, occurring before the next expected sinus beat, hence the P-P' interval is shorter than the normal P-P interval. PACs originating from the same focus will have similar P' waves. A noncompensatory pause is usually present.

PRI: Normal or prolonged. The PRI of the ectopic will probably be different from the PRI of the other complexes.

QRS: Normal or aberrant.

Assessment findings:
1. Pulse: Irregular.
2. Identification: By ECG.

Common causes:
- Stimulants, infectious disorders, MI.
- Stress, exertion, anxiety drug toxicity.
- Metabolic disorders, cor pulmonale.

Treatment:
- Treat the underlying cause.
- Antiarrhythmic drugs (eg, procainamide, verapamil).

Paroxysmal Atrial Tachycardia/Atrial Tachycardia (Figure 6–19)

PAT: A distinct clinical syndrome characterized by repeated episodes (ie, paroxysms) of AT with abrupt onset lasting from a few seconds to many hours.

Significance:
- May result in a decrease in SV and CO and eventually BP.
- Predispose to heart failure.
- Increases myocardial oxygen consumption which can lead to angina or infarction in ischemic heart disease (ie, CAD).

Rate: Atrial rate is usually 150 to 250 beats/min.

Rhythm: Atrial rhythm is usually regular. The ventricular rhythm is often regular with 1:1 AV conduction when the atrial rate is <200. With atrial rate >200, 2:1 AV block (or higher) is common.

P waves: May be difficult to identify because the P wave may be buried within preceding T wave. The P waves will differ morphologically from sinus P waves.

PRI: Normal or prolonged.

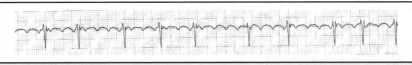

Figure 6–20. Atrial flutter.

QRS: Normal.
Assessment:
1. Pulse and HR are rapid.
2. CO and BP may be lower due to reduced ventricular filling time and limited SV.
3. May c/o dizziness, anxiety, generalized weakness, palpitations, chest thumping.

Common causes:
- Emotional factors.
- Overexertion, hyperventilation.
- Potassium depletion.
- Caffeine, nicotine, or aspirin sensitivity, digitalis toxicity.
- Rheumatic heart disease, MV dysfunction (ie, MV prolapse).
- Pulmonary embolism.
- Thyroid disease.

Treatment:
- Identify underlying cause.
- Discontinuation of medications.
- Performance of autonomic stimulation/vagal maneuvers (ie, valsalva maneuvers, breath holding, coughing).
- If episodes are prolonged, medications may be indicated (eg, beta blockers, verapamil).

Atrial Flutter (Figure 6–20)
Definition: An ectopic atrial focus depolarizes at a rate of 250 to 350 beats/min exciting nearby areas repeatedly forming a reentry pathway. If only one ectopic focus is firing repetitively, the P waves look identical and have a characteristic "sawtooth" pattern.
Significance:
- Decrease CO.
- Increased myocardial oxygen demand.
- Predisposition to LV failure.

Rate: Atrial rate=250 to 350 beats/min. Ventricular rate may vary depending on conductance to the ventricles. Commonly there is a physiologic block at the AV node because of the refractory period resulting in a 2:1 conduction.

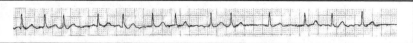

Figure 6–21. Atrial fibrillation.

Rhythm: Atrial rhythm usually regular. Ventricular rhythm will be regular if a constant degree of AV block or may be irregular if variable block is present.
P waves: Flutter waves ("sawtooth").
PRI: Normal or may vary. Often it is impossible to identify a PRI because of the unusual configuration of the P waves (Flutter waves).
QRS: Normal or aberrant.
Assessment findings:

1. Pulse: Regular if conduction is constant. Irregular if conduction ratio varies.

2. If CO is decreased, BP is diminished. Patients frequently c/o angina, palpitations, and/or dizziness.

3. Identification via ECG.

Common causes:

•   Multiple pathologic conditions including: rheumatic heart disease, cardiomyopathy, MV disease, CAD, MI, stress, drugs, renal failure, hypoxemia, and pericarditis.

Treatment:

•   With increased ventricular rate, CO may become compromised.

•   Medications: Antiarrhythmic: verapamil, procainamide. Drugs to reduce AV conduction: Digitalis, beta blockers (propranolol).

•   Cardioversion or pacemaker.

Atrial Fibrillation (Figure 6–21)
Definition: An erratic quivering or twitching of the atrial muscle caused by multiple ectopic foci in the atria or multiple reentry pathways. There is a loss of atrial contraction and potential thrombi formation. The AV node attempts to control the entry of impulses that initiate QRS complexes; therefore a totally irregular rhythm is present.
Rate: Atrial rate is 400 to 700 beats/min (usually cannot be counted). Ventricular rate may be normal, slow, or rapid.
Rhythm: Irregularly irregular ventricular rhythm. Atrial rhythm is unmeasurable because atrial activity is chaotic.
P waves: None of the ectopic foci fully depolarize the atria, so no true P waves are present. There is no organized atrial activity and fibrillatory waves are present.
PRI: Not identified.
QRS: Normal or aberrant.
Assessment findings:

1. Pulse: Irregularly, irregular.
2. Sign/symptoms of decreased CO.

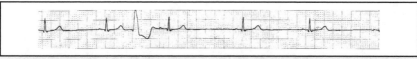

Figure 6–22. Premature ventricular contractions.

Common causes:
- Multiple factors including: age, CHF, ischemia, infarction, cardiomyopathy, digoxin toxicity, drug use, stress or pain, renal failure, or rheumatic heart disease.

Treatment:
- If loss of atrial activity ("atrial kick"), CO may be compromised (up to a 20% to 30% decrease). With ventricular response rates <100, the decrease in CO is usually not problematic. With ventricular rates >100, CO may be diminished and signs and symptoms of hemodynamic compromise may occur (eg, decreased BP/hypotension, c/o dizziness, palpitations, SOB).

- Increased potential to develop mural thrombi. Therefore, patients are prescribed anticoagulant therapy.

- Medications: Verapamil, digoxin.

- Cardioversion.

Ventricular Dysrhythmias

Premature Ventricular Complexes (PVCs) (Figure 6–22)
Definition: A depolarization that arises in either ventricle prior to the next expected sinus beat. Since the impulse originates outside of the normal conduction system, conduction is slowed resulting in a bizarre and widened QRS complex without a P wave and followed by a complete compensatory pause. PVCs may be identical (**unifocal**—originating from the same foci) or look different (**multifocal**—originating from different foci).
Significance:
May indicate a predisposition to developing other lethal dysrhythmias especially if PVCs existing in the following forms:
1. Frequent: >5 per min.

2. Multifocal: Configuration varies (indicates a varying focus).

3. Bigeminy (1:1), trigeminy (2:1), quadrageminy (3:1), etc.

4. R on T pattern.

5. Sequential salvos: Short runs of two or three beats.

Rhythm: Irregular; underlying rhythm usually sinus.
P waves: Sinus P waves are usually obscured by the QRS, ST segment, or the T wave of the PVC. The presence of a sinus P wave can be inferred by the presence of a fully compensatory pause.
PRI: Depends upon underlying rhythm. Cannot determine PRI of PVC.
QRS: >0.12 sec.; wide and distorted.

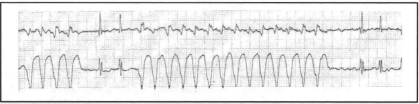

Figure 6–23. Ventricular tachycardia.

Assessment:
1. Conscious sensation: Palpitations, skipping a beat, thumping.
2. Pulse: Irregular.
3. BP may be lower than usual.
4. Decreased CO: Patient may c/o dizziness, angina, weakness.

Common causes:
- Caffeine or nicotine sensitivity.
- Electrolyte imbalances (particularly hypokalemia or hyperkalemia).
- Cardiac ischemia, cardiomyopathy, MI, CHF.
- Chronic lung disease and/or hypoxemia.

Treatment:
- Depends on the underlying cause, frequency and severity of the PVCs and the associated symptoms. PVCs may indicate increased irritability of the ventricle and may progress to lethal VT or VF.

Ventricular Tachycardia (Figure 6–23)
Definition: A series of three or more PVCs in a row.
- Occurs because of rapid firing by a single ventricular focus with increased automaticity.

Significance:
- Indicates extensive myocardial ischemia and irritability.
- Decreased CO and BP.
- Unreliable pacemaker.
- Predisposing to VF and ventricular standstill.

Rate: Ventricular rate 100 to 250 beats/min.
Rhythm: Usually regular.
P waves: Absent (buried in QRS complex).
PRI: Absent.
QRS: >0.12 sec.; wide and bizarre in appearance.
Assessment:
1. Signs and symptoms of decreased CO.
- Angina.
- Dizziness.

- Low BP to no BP.
- Syncope.
- Weak, thready pulse.

2. If conscious, may c/o anxiety, confusion, disorientation, thumping, racing heartbeat.
3. Patient may be unconscious.

Common causes:
- Ischemia, acute infarction, CAD.
- Respiratory failure (hypoxia), massive PE.
- Electric shock.
- Cardiac pacing.
- Heart block (advanced).

Treatment:
- Emergency situation secondary to compromised CO and BP.
- Initiate CPR/ACLS (advanced cardiac life support).
- Cardioversion/defibrillation.
- Immediate pharmacological injection (eg, lidocaine, bretylium, procainamide, epinephrine).

Ventricular Fibrillation
Definition: Erratic quivering of the ventricular muscle resulting in no CO. As in AF, multiple ectopic foci fire creating asynchrony.
Significance:
- No CO.
- Death is inevitable unless the situation is reversed immediately.

Rate: Chaotic.
Rhythm: Absent.
P waves: Absent.
QRS: Widened and bizarre, fibrillatory waves present.
Assessment:
1. Pulse: None.
2. Heart sounds: None.
3. BP: None.
4. Unconsciousness.
5. Cyanosis.
6. Convulsions, pupils dilated.

Common causes:
Same as VT.
Treatment:
- Defibrillation followed by CPR, supplemental oxygen, and medication injection.

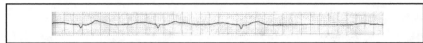

Figure 6–24. Idioventricular rhythm. Asystole.

Idioventricular Rhythm (Figure 6–24)
Definition: In the absence of a higher pacemaker, the ventricles will function as the dominant pacemaker and initiate a regular impulse at their inherent rate of 20 to 40 beats per minute (bpm).
Significance:
- Indicates extensive myocardial ischemia and irritability.
- Decreased CO.
- Unreliable pacemaker.
- Predisposing to VF and ventricular standstill.

Rate: Ventricular rate usually 20 to 40 bpm. (Accelerated idioventricular rhythm 40 to 100 bpm.)
Rhythm: Regular.
P waves: Absent.
PRI: Absent
QRS: >0.12 sec.; wide and distorted.
Assessment:
1. Signs and symptoms of decreased CO.
   - Angina.
   - Dizziness.
   - Low BP to no BP.
   - Syncope.
   - Weak, thready pulse.
2. If conscious, may c/o anxiety, confusion, disorientation, thumping in chest.
3. Patient may be unconscious.

Common causes:
- Ischemia, acute infarction, CAD.
- Respiratory failure (hypoxia, massive PE).
- Electric shock.
- Cardiac pacing malfunction.
- Heart block (advanced).

Treatment:
- Attempt to increase sinus rate for capture, atropine.
- Antiarrhythmic drugs.
- Treat underlying cause.

Asystole (Figure 6–24)

Definition: There is no electrical pacemaker to initiate measurable electrical flow.

Significance:

- Cardiovascular collapse/ventricular standstill.

- Death is imminent.

Rate: None.
Rhythm: None.
P waves: None.
PRI: None.
QRS: None.

Heart Blocks

Definition: Heart blocks are due to delayed, erratic, or absent conduction through the AV node.

First-Degree Heart Block

Rate: Depend on underlying rhythm.
Rhythm: Regular.
P waves: Sinus, P followed by QRS.
PRI: PR-interval is lengthened >0.20 sec. The interval is usually constant, but may vary.
QRS: 0.06 to 0.11 sec.
Assessment:
Patients are typically asymptomatic.
Common causes:

- CAD/MI.

- Rheumatic heart disease.

- Digoxin or beta blockers.

Treatment: None, unless due to medication reaction.

Type I Second-Degree Heart Block (Mobitz Type I; Wenckebach)

Definition: This type of block usually occurs at the AV node and is highlighted by the prolongation of the PR interval.
Rate: Depends on underlying rhythm; atrial rate will be greater than ventricular rate.
Rhythm: Irregular. The R-R interval will vary
P waves: P followed by QRS until "dropped" beat (QRS).
PRI: PR-interval progressively lengthens until one P wave is not followed by a QRS ("dropped" beat).
QRS: 0.06 to 0.11 sec.
Assessment:

- Patients are typically asymptomatic.

- Pulse is irregular. If the block is cyclic, the pulse will be regularly irregular.

Common causes:

- CAD/MI.

- Excessive beta blockade.
- Increased vagal/parasympathetic tone (eg, athlete).

Treatment:
- None is usually necessary, unless the patient exhibits signs and symptoms of hemodynamic compromise (eg, hypotension, dizziness, shortness of breath).

Type II Second-Degree (Mobitz Type II; Classic Heart Block)

Definition: This type of block occurs typically along the bundle branches or less commonly the Bundle of His. This block is associated with a poorer prognosis and may lead to complete heart block.

Rate: Depends on underlying rhythm; atrial rate will be greater than ventricular rate.

Rhythm: Irregular. The R-R interval will vary depending on the constancy of blocked beats.

P waves: All P waves are not followed by QRS. There will be more P waves than QRS complexes.

PRI: The PRI on conducted beats are constant and may be normal (<0.20 sec) or prolonged (>0.20 sec).

QRS: May be normal (0.06 to 0.11 sec), but is often wide (>0.12 sec).

Assessment:
- If the block is constant, the pulse will be regular.
- If the ventricular rate is low, patients may present with hypotension and c/o dizziness.

Common causes:
- MI.
- Lesion of conducting pathways.

Treatment:
- Pacemaker placement (temporary pacing [eg, transcutaneous or transvenous] until a permanent pacemaker can be inserted).

Third-Degree Heart Block (Complete Heart Block)

Definition: Third-degree heart block indicates that all impulses originating from the atria are blocked at the AV node, the Bundle of His, or the bundle branches. There is an absence of conduction between the atria and ventricles. This is an unstable rhythm.

Rate: The atrial may be equal to or greater than the ventricular rate.

Rhythm: The atria and ventricles are firing independently, and at regular intervals. The P-P interval and the R-R interval are regular.

P waves: The P waves are uniform and usually outnumber the QRS complexes.

PRI: There is no conduction between the atria and ventricles. Therefore, there is no PRI.

QRS: If the ventricles are being stimulated from a junctional foci, the QRS will be normal (<0.12 sec), but if the focus is ventricular, the QRS will be wide (>0.12 sec).

Assessment:
- Signs and symptoms of decreased CO (see above).

Common causes:
- MI.
- Digoxin toxicity.

Treatment:
- Pacemaker placement (temporary pacing [eg, transcutaneous or transvenous] until a permanent pacemaker can be inserted).

AV Junctional Dysrhythmias (Nodal Dysrhythmias)

Definition: Conduction tissue near the AV node can take over pacemaker function if higher pacemaker sites fail. These rhythms are highlighted by slow HRs and retrograde P waves (eg, upside down in Lead II, III, and aVF).

Premature Junctional Complexes (PJCs)
Rate: Depends on underlying rhythm.
Rhythm: Irregular due to PJC. The R-R interval will vary.
P waves: The P wave of the ectopic beat can come before, during, or after the QRS complex and will be inverted in lead II, III, and aVF.
PRI: If the P wave is before the QRS, the PRI will be less than 0.12 sec. If the P wave falls with or after the QRS, there is no PRI.
QRS: Normal (<0.12 sec).

Junctional Escape Rhythm
Rate: Usually between 40 and 60.
Rhythm: Regular.
P waves: The P waves can come before, during, or after the QRS complex and will be inverted in lead II, III, and aVF.
PRI: If the P wave is before the QRS, the PRI will be less than 0.12 sec. If the P wave falls with or after the QRS, there is no PRI.
QRS: normal (<0.12 sec).

Accelerated Junctional Rhythm/Junctional Tachycardia
Rate: Usually between 100 to 180.
Rhythm: Regular.
P waves: The P waves can come before, during, or after the QRS complex and will be inverted in lead II, III, and aVF.
PRI: If the P wave is before the QRS, the PRI will be less than 0.12 sec. If the P wave falls with or after the QRS, there is no PRI.
QRS: Normal (<0.12 sec).
Assessment:
- CO and BP can be reduced with slow rates or decreased due to limited filling times with tachycardia.
- Pulses may be weak, thready, and irregular or regular.
- Patients may c/o dizziness/palpitations/fatigue.

Common causes:
- MI, CAD.
- S/p heart surgery.
- Myocarditis.
- Digitalis intoxication.
- Hyperventilation.

Treatment:
- Identify and treat the underlying cause.
- If rate is slow and patient symptomatic, medications (eg, atropine) or pacemaker are indicated.
- Often treatment is not necessary.

Pacemakers, Defibrillators, and Cardioversion

Pacemakers are mechanical devices used prophylactically (eg, post open heart surgery) to initiate myocardial contractions when intrinsic electrical impulses are insufficient (eg, bradycardia associated with MI), the native impulses are not being conducted (eg, second or third heart block), the HR is too slow to maintain an adequate CO (eg, sinus node dysfunction and syncope) or overdriving tachydysrhythmias (eg, atrial flutter). Left **ventricular** and **biventricular** pacing, also known as cardiac resynchronization, is becoming more common in severe CHF, left bundle branch block, and intraventricular conduction delay. Biventricular pacing attempts to coordinate the electrical and mechanical ventricular activation sequence leading to a more efficient ventricular contraction. These devices can be inserted on a temporary or permanent basis. **Temporary pacemaker** implantation is most commonly achieved by transvenous, transcutaneous, or direct placement of electrodes on the epicardial surface of the heart. **Transvenous** cardiac pacing is achieved by threading an electrode through a central vein (eg, subclavian, internal or external jugular or femoral veins) to the endocardial surface of the RV or less commonly the right atrium. **Transcutaneous** or external pacing is indicated for emergent situations such as asystole and severe bradycardias and involves placement of anterior and posterior electrode pads on the chest wall. **Epicardial** pacing is common following open-heart procedures such as CABG, valve repair, or replacement and transplant surgery. The electrodes connecting the pulse generator to the heart are embedded or lightly sutured to the epicardium, the outer surface of the heart, externalized prior to closing the thorax, and secured to the chest wall. **Permanent pacemakers (PPM)** are usually placed along the left anterior chest wall in an infraclavicular pocket and endocardial leads are affixed to the heart via the cephalic vein as noted in Figure 6–25.

A pacemaker's function is typically described by a coding system outlined in Table 6–19 that defines the chambers paced and sensed and the pacemaker responses. Sensing is the identification of intrinsic cardiac electrical activity while capture or pacing describes the pacemaker's stimulus resulting in electrical activity leading to myocardial contraction. For example, a VVI

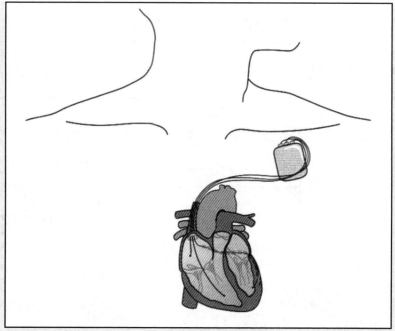

Figure 6–25. Permanent pacemakers (PPM) are usually placed along the left anterior chest wall in an infraclavicular pocket and endocardial leads are affixed to the heart via the cephalic vein. Example of permanent pacemaker with three leads. (Reprinted from Hillegass EA, Sadowsky HS. *Essentials of Cardiopulmonary Physical Therapy*, page 468, with permission from Elsevier.)

Table 6–19
NBG PACEMAKER CODES

Pacing Location	Sensing Location	Response to Pacing	Modulation	Antiarrhythmia Function
A = atrium	A = atrium	O = no response	O = none	O = none
V=ventricle	V=ventricle	I=inhibited	R = rate modulation	P = pacing
D = dual (A & V)	D = dual (A & V)	T = triggered	M = multi-program	S = shock
D = dual (T & I)	C = commu-nicating	D = dual (P & S)		

Adapted from Bernstein AD, Camm AJ, Flecher RD, et al. The NASPE/BPEG generic pacemaker code for antibradyarrhythmias and adaptive-rate pacing and antitachyarrhythmia devices. *PACE.* 1987;10:794.

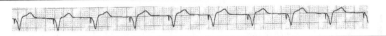

Figure 6–26. Example of ventricular paced rhythm. Note pacemaker spike preceding wide QRS complex.

Table 6–20

PHYSICAL THERAPY CONSIDERATIONS FOR PACEMAKERS AND ICDs

Temporary Pacemakers:

- Determine that the epicardial wires are taped securely to the skin to prevent accidental dislodgement.
- After epicardial wires are removed, patients should be monitored closely for signs of cardiac tamponade (eg, tachycardia/hypotension). Patients are frequently maintained on 1 to 2 hours bed rest post removal.

Permanent Pacemakers and ICDs:

- Limit weightbearing and heavy lifting (>10 pounds) of the involved UE x 6 to 8 weeks after placement.
- Shoulder elevation of the involved UE is limited to <90 x 6 to 8 weeks after placement.
- No driving until cleared by physician.
- Check incision daily: Redness/ swelling; drainage.
- Monitor for fever (temperature >100.5 degrees or develops chills).

---

pacemaker will sense and stimulate ventricular activity and is inhibited if sufficient intrinsic ventricular depolarizations are sensed. If native ventricular activity is not sensed, the pacemaker will provide electrical stimulation to the ventricle initiating depolarization. Figure 6–26 provides an example of a ventricle paced rhythm.

Automatic Implantable Cardiovertor-Defibrillators (AICD/ICD) are devices that detect life-threatening dysrhythmias including VF and VT. The ICD provides an electrical shock to temporarily depolarize an irregularly beating heart allowing normal electrical and coordinated contractile activity to resume. ICDs are implanted just as a permanent pacemaker and are generally indicated for those who have survived cardiac arrest due to VT or VF, those with recurrent tachydysrhythmias with CAD/MI or LV dysfunction, and those with inducible VT or VF. **Cardioversion** is similar to defibrillation in concept, but the energy requirements and emergent nature are reduced. Cardioversion can be accomplished through medications (eg, adenosine) or through the application of transcutaneous electrical current. Cardioversion is often performed to terminate dysrhythmias including atrial fibrillation, atrial flutter, and VT.

Common physical therapy precautions associated with pacemakers and ICDs are provided in Table 6–20.

PHARMACOLOGICAL INFORMATION: CARDIOVASCULAR DISEASES AND DISORDERS PHARMACOLOGY

Nitrates

Action

Produces vasodilatation (venous > arterial) through the production of nitric oxide. The vasodilatation of coronary arteries increases blood supply to ischemic regions. The vasodilatation of peripheral vessels increases venous capacitance resulting in decreased venous return and end-diastolic volume. The net result is improved oxygen supply and reduced oxygen consumption (starling mechanism). Nitrates are commonly prescribed for patients with ischemic heart disease, angina, CHF, HTN, and pulmonary edema.

Side Effects
CNS: Dizziness, headache, weakness
CV: Hypotension, syncope, reflex tachycardia
GI: Nausea, vomiting, abdominal pain
Misc: Flushing

Common Medications
Isosorbide dinitrate (Isordil, Isorbid), Isosorbide mononitrate (Imdur), Nitroglycerine (Nitrostat, Nitro-Dur, Nitrocot)

Calcium Channel Blockers

Action

CCB inhibit the transport of calcium into myocardial and vascular smooth muscle cells. The result is inhibited excitation-contraction coupling leading to muscular relaxation and vasodilatation. CCB are indicated for patients with ischemic heart disease, coronary vasospasm (Prinzmetal angina), s/p MI, HTN, and SVTs.

Side Effects
CNS: Headache, dizziness, fatigue
CV: Bradycardia, tachycardia, palpitations, hypotension, peripheral edema, angina
GI: Nausea, constipation, diarrhea
Misc: Flushing, sexual dysfunction

Common Medications
Amlodipine (Norvasc), Diltiazam (Cardizem), Nifedipine (Procardia, Adalat), Verapamil (Calan), Bepridil (Vascor)

Beta Blockers

Action
Beta blockers inhibit the stimulation of the beta$_1$ (myocardial) and/or beta$_2$ (pulmonary, vascular) adrenergic receptors. Nonselective agents block both beta$_{1\&2}$; selective agents block only beta$_1$. Beta blockers decrease HR and BP and are frequently prescribed for those with ischemic heart disease, s/p MI, HTN, anxiety, and to decrease progression of CHF.

Side Effects
CNS: Dizziness, fatigue, weakness, anxiety/nervousness
CV: Bradycardia, orthostatic hypotension
GI: Diarrhea, constipation, nausea
Misc: Arthralgias, back pain, muscle cramp
Pulm: Bronchospasm (nonselective agents)

Common Medications
Non-Selective: Carvedilol (Coreg), Labetalol (Normodyne, Trandate), Timolol
Selective: Atenolol (Tenormin), Metoprolol (Lopressor, Toprol)

Angiotensive-Converting Enzyme Inhibitors

Action
ACE inhibitors block the conversion of Angiotensin I to the vasoconstrictor Angiotensin II and reduce the production of aldosterone. ACE inhibitors are indicated for heart failure, HTN, MI and diabetic nephropathy.

Side Effects
CNS: Dizziness, fatigue, headache, weakness, insomnia
CV: Hypotension, tachycardia, angina
GI: Diarrhea, nausea
Misc: Angioedema, fever
Pulm: Cough

Common Medications
Benazapril, captopril (Capoten), enalapril (Vasotec), Fosinopril (Monopril), Lisinopril (Zestril), Quiapril (Accupril), Ramipril (Altace).

Angiotensin II Receptor Antagonists/Angiotensin II Receptor Blockers

Action
Angiotensin II receptor antagonists are used in the treatment of HTN. They block the receptor for the vasoconstrictor angiotensin II leading to vasodilatation. Additionally, these medications decrease the production of aldosterone.

Side Effects
CNS: Dizziness, fatigue, headache

CV: Hypotension
GI: Diarrhea, hepatitis
GU: Renal failure
Misc: Hyperkalemia

Common Medications
Candesartan (Atacand), Eprosartan (Teveten), Losartan (Cozaar)

Centrally Acting Adrenergic Agonists

Action
Centrally acting adrenergic agonists stimulates the alpha-adrenergic receptors within the CNS, which inhibits peripheral sympathetic outflow. The result is reduced BP, and inhibited HR acceleration. Additionally these medications provide pain relief.

Side Effects
CNS: Sedation/drowsiness, depression, dizziness
CV: Bradycardia, hypotension, palpitations
GI: Dry mouth, constipation, nausea, vomiting
Misc: Weight gain, rash, impotence

Common Medications
Clonidine (Catapres), methyldopa (Aldomet), Reserpine

Diuretics

Action
Diuretics increase tubular secretion or inhibit reabsorption of electrolytes (Na^+, K^+, Cl^-) within the loop of henle or distal tubule leading to enhanced renal excretion of electrolytes and water. Diuretics are prescribed for HTN, pulmonary edema and effusions, and hypervolemia states.

Side Effects
CNS: Dizziness, headache
CV: Hypotension (hypovolemia)
GI: Dry mouth, constipation, dyspepsia
Misc: Electrolyte abnormalities including hyper/hypokalemia, hyponatremia, hypochloremia, hypomagnesemia; metabolic alkalosis; muscle cramping

Common Medications
Loop Diuretics: Bumetanide (Bumex), Furosemide (Lasix), Toresemide (Demadex)
Osmotic Diuretics: Mannitol
Potassium-Sparing Diuretics: Amiloride (Midamor), Spironolactone (Aldactone)
Thiazide Diuretics: Hydrochlorothiazide

Alpha-Adrenergic Blockers

Action
These medications block the postsynaptic alpha-adrenergic receptors leading to vascular smooth muscle relaxation.

Side Effects
CNS: Dizziness, headache, fatigue, weakness
CV: Orthostatic hypotension, tachycardia
GI: Dry mouth, constipation, nausea, vomiting
Misc: Fluid retention/edema, arthritis/gout, sexual dysfunction

Common Medications
Prazosin (Minipress), Doxazosin (Cardura)

Vasodilators

Action
Vasodilators relax the smooth muscle of arteries and veins through varied mechanisms. For example, nitroprusside liberates nitric oxide, a potent vasodilator

Side Effects
CNS: Dizziness, headache, blurred vision
CV: Hypotension, dyspnea
GI: Nausea, vomiting, GI pain

Common Medications
Nitroprusside (Nitropress), Hydralazine (Apresoline), minoxidil (Loniten)

Anticoagulants

Action
Anticoagulants inhibit the clotting mechanism at various points in the clotting cascade (eg, oral anticoagulants interfere with the hepatic synthesis of vitamin K—dependent clotting factors (factors II, prothrombin, VII, IX, and X). Parenteral anticoagulants interfere with the conversion of prothrombin to thrombin). Patients will have the INR or APTT monitored to adjust dosage (see Chapter 2).

Side Effects
CNS: Dizziness, headache, bleeding
CV: Edema
GI/GU: Bleeding (GIB; hematuria), nausea, vomiting, anorexia, abdominal cramping, diarrhea
Misc: Fever

Common Medications
Oral: Coumarin (Warfarin)

Parenteral: Heparin; low-molecular weight heparins (dalteparin [Fragmin], danaparoid [Orgaran], enoxaparin [Lovenox])

Antiplatelet Agents

Action
Antiplatelet agents disrupt the activation, aggregation or adhesion of platelets. Aspirin inhibits the formation of thromboxane A2, glycoprotein IIb/IIIa inhibitors block fibrinogen receptors on platelets: Clopidogrel block ADP receptors on platelets.

Side Effects
CNS: Dizziness, tinnitus, difficulty hearing
CV/Pulm: Hypotension, bronchospasm
GI: Bleeding, nausea, dyspepsia, heartburn, abdominal discomfort, hepatotoxicity
GU: Hematuria

Common Medications
Aspirin (acetylsalicylic acid, Bayer, Ecotrin), Tirofiban (Aggrastat), Eptifibatide (Integrilin), Clopidogrel (Plavix)

Thrombolytics

Action
Thrombolytic agents convert plasminogen to plasmin, which degrades fibrin clots and lyse thrombi and emboli. These agents are used in acute coronary events (eg, MI), embolic CVA, DVT and clearing of blockage in catheters/cannulae.

Side Effects
CNS: Bleeding/intracranial hemorrhage
CV/Pulm: Reperfusion dysrhythmias, hypotension; bronchospasm
GI: Bleeding
Pulm: Bronchospasm, hemoptysis
Misc: Allergic reaction, fever

Common Medications
Alteplase (Tissue plasminogen activator (t-PA), Streptokinase, Urokinase

Antiarrhythmics

Action
Antiarrhythmics interfere with myocardial excitability and automaticity modifying the AP of the myocytes. These drugs alter the duration of the AP, slow conduction or prolong the refractory periods and are beneficial for reentry and tachyarrhythmias. These drugs are divided into four classifications and most may cause new or worsened arrhythmias (proarrhythmic effect).
Class IA: Inhibits the fast sodium channels depressing phase 0 of the AP.

Additionally, they prolong the duration of the AP (similar to Class III).

Common Medications

Quinidine, disopyramide, procainamide

Class IB: Inhibits the fast sodium channels and shortens the AP selectively in diseased heart tissue.

Common Medications

Lidocaine, phenytoin (Dilantin)

Class IC: Inhibits the fast sodium channels depressing phase 0 and have an affinity to slow conduction and shorten AP duration of HIS/pukinje fibers.

Common Medications

Flecainide (Tambocor), Propafenone (Rythmol), Moricizine (Ethmozine)

Class II: Inhibits phase 4 spontaneous depolarization of nodal tissue and indirectly close calcium channels leading to reduced nodal automaticity and slower conduction.

Common Medications

Beta blockers: Propranolol, esmolol, acebutolol

Class III: Block outward potassium channels thereby prolonging the AP duration and refractoriness.

Common Medications

Amiodarone (Cordarone), Sotalol (Betapace), bretylium

Class IV: Calcium channel blockers (CCBs) slow conduction and increase the duration of the refractory period of the AV node by inhibiting the inward calcium channel.

Common Medications

Verapamil (Calan), diltiazem (Cardiazem)

Miscellaneous:

Atropine: Inhibits the action of postsynaptic acetylcholine diminishing the influence of the parasympathetic nervous system leading to increased HR.

Adenosine: Inhibits both the sinus and AV nodes by opening potassium channels and indirectly inhibiting the calcium channels.

Digoxin: Augments parasympathetic tone on the atria and AV node and is prescribed for the treatment of atrial fibrillation.

Lipid Lowering Agents (HMG CoA Inhibitors—Statins)

Action

"Statins" inhibit an enzyme (HMG CoA) that is essential for hepatic cholesterol synthesis resulting in reduced LDL and potentially a slight increase in HDL cholesterols.

Side Effects
CNS: Headache, blurred vision, dizziness, insomnia, fatigue
GI: Flatulence, abdominal pain/cramps, constipation, nausea, vomiting, heartburn, elevated liver enzymes
Misc: Rhabdomyolysis with possible renal failure; arthralgias, rash, muscle cramps

Common Medications
Atorvastatin (Lipitor), fluvastatin (Lescol), lovastatin (Mevacor), pravastatin (Pravachol), simvastatin (Zocor)

Inotropes

Action
Inotropic medications increase the intracellular myocyte concentrations of calcium leading to enhanced myocardial contractility, prolongation of the refractory period of the AV node and slower conduction velocities through the SA and AV nodes. These agents are indicated for CHF, atrial fibrillation, SVT

Side Effects
CNS: Fatigue, headache, weakness
CV: Dysrhythmias (bradycardia/SVT/Ventricular dysrhythmias), hypotension, chest pain
GI: Nausea, vomiting
Misc: thrombocytopenia

Common Medications
Digitalis, Digoxin (Lanoxin), Dopamine, Dobutamine, Milrinone (Primacor)

REFERENCES

1. Wenger NK, Froelicher ES, Smith LK, et al. *Cardiac Rehabilitation as Secondary Prevention:* Clinical Practice Guidelines. Department of Health and Human Services, Public Heatlth Service, Agency for Health Care Policy and Research and National Heart, Lung and Blood Institute. AHCPR Pub. No. 96–0673. October 1995.
2. *2001 Heart and Stroke Statistical Update.* Dallas, Tex: American Heart Association; 2000.
3. Jessup M, Brozena S. Medical progress: heart failure. *N Engl J Med.* 2003;348:2007–2018.
4. Peel G. The cardiopulmonary system and movement dysfunction. *Physical Therapy.* 1996;76:448–455.
5. Foss ML, Keteyian SJ. *Fox's Physiologic Basis for Exercise and Sport.* 6th ed. Boston, Mass: McGraw-Hill; 1998.
6. Rhoades, RA, Tanner GA. *Medical Physiology.* Baltimore, Md: Lippincott Williams & Wilkins; 1995.
7. Hillegass EA, Sadowsky HS. *Essentials of Cardiopulmonary Physical Therapy.* 2nd ed. Philadelphia, Pa: WB Saunders Co; 2001.
8. Guyton AC, Hall JE. *Textbook of Medical Physiology.* Philadelphia, Pa: WB Saunders Co; 2000.
9. Perloff JK. *Physical Examination of the Heart and Circulation.* 3rd ed. Philadelphia, Pa: WB Saunders Co; 2000.
10. Frownfelter D, Dean E. *Principles and Practice of Cardiopulmonary Physical Therapy.* St. Louis, Mo: Mosby-Year Book, Inc; 1996.
11. AACVPR. *Guidelines for Cardiac Rehabilitation and Secondary Prevention Programs.* Champaign, Ill: Human Kinetics; 1999.
12. Powers SK, Howley ET. *Exercise Physiology: Theory and Application to Fitness and Performance.* Dubuque, Iowa: Brown & Benchmark Publishers; 1997.
13. Cheng JW. Recognition, pathophysiology, and management of acute myocardial infarction. *Am J Health Syst Pharm.* 2001;58:1709–1721.
14. Berne RM, Levy MN. *Cardiovascular Physiology.* 8th ed. St. Louis, Mo: Mosby, Inc; 2001.
15. Hollinshead WH, Rosse C. *Textbook Anatomy.* 4th ed. Philadelphia, Pa: Harper & Row, Publishers Inc; 1985.
16. Criqui MH, Langer RD, Fronek A, et al. Mortality over a period of 10 years in patients with peripheral arterial disease. *N Engl J Med.* 1992;326:381–386.
17. Braunwald E. *Heart Disease: A Textbook of Cardiovascular Medicine.* Philadelphia, Pa: WB Saunders Co; 1997.
18. Ades P. Medical progress: cardiac rehabilitation and secondary prevention of coronary heart disease. *N Engl J Med.* 2001;345:892–902.
19. Matthew JP, Parks R, Savino JS, et al. Atrial fibrillation following coronary artery bypass graft surgery: predictors, outcomes and resource utilization. *JAMA.* 1996;276:300–306.
20. Atlee JL. Perioperative cardiac dysrhythmias: diagnosis and management. *Anesthesiology.* 1997;76:1397–1424.
21. Kantor B, McKenna CJ, Caccitolo JA, et al. Transmyocardial and percutaneous myocardial revascularization: current and future role in the treatment of coronary artery disease. *Mayo Clinic Proc.* 1999;74:585–592.
22. Humphrey R, Arena R. Surgical innovations for chronic heart failure in the context of cardiopulmonary rehabilitation. *Physical Therapy.* 2000;80:61–69.

23. Canzanello VJ, Sheps SG. The sixth report of the Joint National Committee on Prevention, Detection, Evaluation, and Treatment of High Blood Pressure. *Cardio Rev.* 1998;5(6):272-277.
24. Wolz M, Cutler J, Roccella EJ, et al. Statement from the National High Blood Pressure Education Program: prevalence of hypertension. *Am J Hypertens.* 2000;13:103–104.
25. Davies MJ. The cardiomyopathies: an overview. *Heart.* 2000;83:469–474.
26. Tierney LM, McPhee SJ, Papadakis MA. *Current Medical Diagnosis and Treatment.* Norwalk, Conn: Appleton & Lange; 1994.
27. Berkow R. *The Merck Manual of Diagnosis and Therapy.* Rahway, NJ: Merck Sharp & Dome Research Laboratories; 1987.
28. Way LW. *Current Surgical Diagnosis and Treatment.* 9th ed. Norwalk, Conn: Appleton & Lange; 1991.
29. Carabello BS. Aortic stenosis. *N Engl J Med.* 2002;346:677–682.
30. Carabello BS, Crawford FA. Medical progress: valvular heart disease. *N Engl J Med.* 1997;337:32–41.
31. Otto CM. Evaluation and management of chronic mitral regurgitation. *N Engl J Med.* 2001;345:740–746.
32. Enriquez-Sarano M. Timing of mitral valve surgery. *Heart.* 2002;87:79–85.
33. Diodato MD, Damiano RJ. Robotic cardiac surgery: overview. *Surg Clin North Am.* 2003;83:1351–1367.
34. Aazami M, Schafers HJ. Advances in heart valve surgery. *J Interventional Cardiol.* 2003;16:535–541.
35. Dreyfus G, Milaiheanu S. Mitral valve repair in cardiomyopathy. *J Heart Lung Transplant.* 2000;19(Suppl): S73–S76.
36. Vahanian A. Balloon valvuloplasty. *Heart.* 2001;85:223–228.
37. Vongpatanasin W, Hillis DL, Lange RA. Medical progress: prosthetic heart valves. *N Engl J Med.* 1996;335:407–416.
38. Groves P. Surgery of valve disease: late results and late complications. *Heart.* 2001;86:715–721.
39. Shames ML, Thompson RW. Abdominal aortic aneurysms: surgical treatment. *Cardiol Clin.* 2002;20:563–578.
40. Khan I, Nair C. Clinical, diagnostic, and management perspective of aortic dissection. *Chest.* 2002;122:311–328.
41. Dimick JB, Upchurch GR. The quality of care for patients with abdominal aortic aneurysms. *Cardiovascular Surg.* 2003;5:331–336.
42. Bick C. Abdominal aortic aneurysm repair. *Nursing Standard.* 2000;15:47–52,54–56.
43. Mylonakis E, Calderwood SB. Medical progress: infective endocarditis in adults. *N Engl J Med.* 2001;345:1318–1330.
44. Report of the Task Force on Research in Heart Failure. National Heart, Lung and Blood Institute. 1994.
45. Braunwald E, Bristow MR. Congestive heart failure: fifty years of progress. *Circulation.* 2000;102:IV–14–IV–23.
46. Opie LH, Gersh BJ. *Drugs for the Heart.* 5th ed. Philadelphia, Pa: WB Saunders Co; 2001.
47. Bavin TK, Self MA. Weaning from intra-aortic balloon pump support. *AJN.* 1991;Oct:54–59.
48. Goldstein DJ, Oz MC, Rose EA. Implantable left ventricular assist devices. *N Engl J Med.* 1998;339:1522–1533.
49. Rose EA, Gelijins AC, Moskowitz AJ, et al. Long-term mechanical left ventricular assistance for end-stage heart failure. *N Engl J Med.* 2001;345:2285–2296.

50. Jessup M, Brozena S. Epilogue: support devices for end stage heart failure. *Cardiol Clin.* 2003;21:135–139.
51. Morrone TM, Buck LA, Catanese KA, et al. Early progressive mobilization of patients with left ventricular assist devices is safe and optimizes recovery before heart transplantation. *J Heart Lung Transplant.* 1996;15:423–429.
52. Mancini D, Goldsmith R, Levin H, et al. Comparison of exercise performance in patients with chronic severe heart failure versus left ventricular assist devices. *Circulation.* 1998;98:1178–1183.
53. Gerber TC, Nishimura RA, Holmes DR Jr, et al. Left ventricular and biventricular pacing in congestive heart failure. *Mayo Clinic Proceedings.* 2001;76:803–812.
54. Atlee JL, Bernstein AD. Cardiac rhythm management devices (part 1). *Anesthesiology.* 2001;95:1265–1280.
55. Braunwald E, Jones RH, Mark DB, et al. Diagnosing and managing unstable angina. *Circulation.* 1994;90:613–622.
56. Cooke RA, Smeeton N, Chambers JB. Comparative study of chest pain characteristics in patients with normal and abnormal coronary angiograms. *Heart.* 1997;78:142–146.
57. Lee TH, Goldman L. Primary care: evaluation of the patient with acute chest pain. *Clin Med.* 2000;342:1187–1195.
58. Botoman VA. Noncardiac chest pain. *J Clin Gastroenterol.* 2002;34:6–14.
59. Charlson ME, Isom OW. Care after coronary artery bypass surgery. *N Engl J Med.* 2003;348:456–1463.
60. Guide to Physical Therapist Practice. 2nd ed. *Physical Therapy.* 2001;81(1).

BIBLIOGRAPHY

Barold SS, Zipes DP. Cardiac pacemakers and antiarrhythmic devices. In: Braunwald E, ed. *Heart Disease: A Textbook of Cardiovascular Medicine.* Philadelphia, Pa: WB Saunders Co; 1997.

Berne RM, Levy MN, eds. Electrical activity of the heart. In: *Cardiovascular Physiology.* 8th ed. St. Louis, Mo: Mosby, Inc; 2001.

Bubien RS, Ching EA, Kay GN. Cardiac defibrillation and resynchronization therapies. *AACN Clinical Issues.* 2004;15:340–361.

Craig CR, Stitzel RE. *Modern Pharmacology with Clinical Applications.* New York, NY: Little, Brown, and Co; 1997.

Deglin JH, Vallerand AH. *Davis's Drug Guide for Nurses.* 8th ed. Philadelphia, Pa: FA Davis Co; 2003.

Dysrhythmia Review Manual. Nursing Staff Development. University of Pennsylvania Health System. Hospital of the University of Pennsylvania.

Gerber TC, Nishimura RA, Holmes DR Jr, et al. Left ventricular and biventricular pacing in congestive heart failure. *Mayo Clinic Proceedings.* 2001;76L:803–812.

Hand H. Common cardiac arrhythmias. *Nursing Standard.* 2002;16:43–58.

Hillegass EA. Electrocardiography. In: Hillegass EA, Sadowsky HS, eds. *Essentials of Cardiopulmonary Physical Therapy.* 2nd ed. Philadelphia,Pa: WB Saunders Co; 2001.

Houghton T, Kaye GC. ABC of interventional cardiology: implantable devices for treating tachyarrhythmias. *BMJ.* 2003;327:333–336.

Karch AM. *Lippincott's Nursing Drug Guide.* Springhouse, Pa: Lippincott Williams & Wilkins; 2004.

Mammen BA, Irwin S, Tecklin JS. Common cardiac and pulmonary clinical measures. In: Irwin S, Tecklin JS, eds. *Cardiopulmonary Physical Therapy: A Guide to Practice.* 4th ed. St. Louis, Mo: Mosby Inc; 2004.

Overbay D, Criddle L. Mastering temporary invasive cardiac pacing. *Critical Care Nurse.* 2004;24:25–32.

Ritter JM, Lewis LD, Mant TG. *Textbook of Clinical Pharmacology.* London, England: Edward Arnold Co; 1995

Timothy PR, Rodeman BJ. Temporary pacemakers in critically ill patients. *AACN Clinical Issues.* 2004;15:305–325.

Zipes DP. Genesis of cardiac arrhythmias: electrophysiological considerations. In: Braunwald E, ed. *Heart Disease: A Textbook of Cardiovascular Medicine.* Philadelphia, Pa: WB Saunders Co; 1997.

Zipes DP. Specific arrhythmias: diagnosis and treatment. In: Braunwald E, ed. *Heart Disease: A Textbook of Cardiovascular Medicine.* Philadelphia, Pa: WB Saunders Co; 1997.

Chapter 7

PULMONARY DISEASES AND DISORDERS

Kathy Lee Bishop Lindsay, MS, PT, CCS
Daniel J. Malone, MPT, CCS

INTRODUCTION

Diseases of the respiratory tract are the fourth leading cause of death in the United States and are ranked eighth in primary hospital admission diagnoses.[1,2] Chronic obstructive pulmonary disease (COPD) is symptomatic in approximately 16 million Americans.[3] A decade ago the economic health care impact of COPD alone was 15 billion dollars. Regretfully, COPD is the only major disease in the top 10 list of diseases that is showing an increase in mortality and prevalence. There has been a significant rise in the COPD death rate in women from 1971 to 2000, and current mortality rates are higher for women than men.[4] In 2000, 8 million hospital outpatient and physician office visits were directly related to COPD. Worldwide, COPD is one of the leading causes of mortality and disability.[5] Tobacco remains the number one preventable risk factor for lung disease.[3,6,7]

The goals of this chapter are to review basic anatomy and physiology of the pulmonary system and to define common pathologies. Surgical options, therapeutic interventions, a case study, and chapter review questions are also included.

ANATOMY AND PHYSIOLOGY

A simple way to analyze the pulmonary system is to split the system into the gas-exchanging organ and the musculoskeletal pump.

The Gas-Exchanging Organ

The gas-exchanging organ is composed of the conduits that allow oxygen to travel to the alveoli and the specialized interface between inspired air and the circulation, the alveolar-capillary membrane. The conduits consist of the

Figure 7–1. Interconnecting alveoli through the pore of Kohn. Reprinted with permission from Mackin L, Bullock BL. Normal pulmonary function. In: Bullock BA, Henze RL, eds. *Focus on Pathophysiology.* Philadelphia, Pa: Lippincott Williams & Wilkins; 2000:531.

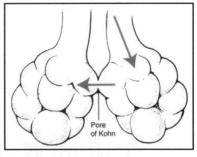

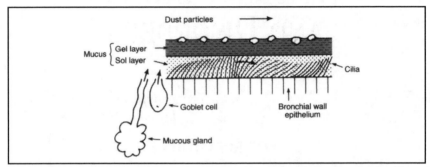

Figure 7–2. Mucociliary escalator. The mucous film consists of a superficial gel layer that traps inhaled particles and a deeper sol layer. It is propelled by cilia. Reprinted with permission from West JB, ed. *Pulmonary Physiology and Pathophysiology: An Integrated, Case-Based Approach.* Philadelphia, Pa: Lippincott Williams & Wilkins; 2001:119.

conducting airway and extend from the oral-nasal pharynx to the seventeenth generation of bronchi and do not contribute to gas exchange. The transitional zone consists of respiratory bronchioles, alveolar ducts, and the alveolar sacs and is the site of gas exchange.[8,9] Three specific conduits allow for collateral ventilation and act as a transit area for cells of the pulmonary immune defenses (Figure 7–1). The pores of Kohn couple adjacent alveoli, Lambert's canals connect the alveoli and the respiratory bronchioles, and the channels of Martin go between the respiratory bronchioles.[9] Airflow can enter neighboring alveoli and bronchioles through these conduits. These are important aspects of anatomy to remember when airway clearance and collateral ventilation is discussed later in the chapter.

The upper respiratory tract, the first line of pulmonary immune defense, warms, humidifies, and filters inspired air.[8,10,11] The mucociliary escalator, the second line of defense, is a specialized transport system consisting of two layers (Figure 7–2). The superficial gel layer is relatively more viscous while the deeper layers contain the motile cilia.[12] Particles imbed within the gel layer and are transported upward by the beating action of the cilia where they are either coughed or swallowed. This protective escalator lines the conducting airways.[10,11] Abnormalities of ciliary function are noted in cystic fibrosis (CF), primary ciliary dyskinesia (Kartagener's syndrome), and bacterial infections

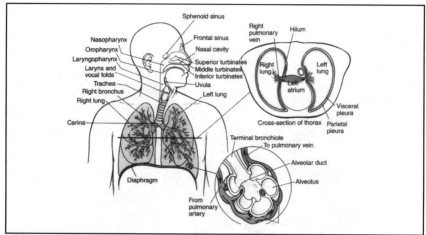

Figure 7–3. The respiratory system. Reprinted with permission from Mackin L, Bullock BL. Normal pulmonary function. In: Bullock BA, Henze RL, eds. *Focus on Pathophysiology*. Philadelphia, Pa: Lippincott Willams & Wilkins; 2000:528.

leading to deficient pulmonary defense.[12,13] Pulmonary defense is completed by immune cells such as macrophages, the most abundant cell in the alveolar space, and neutrophils (see Chapter 5).[10]

The lower respiratory tract divides at the carina into the right and left mainstem bronchi as noted in Figure 7–3. This division corresponds anteriorly with the "angle of Louis," the joint between the manubrium and body of the sternum, and the fourth thoracic vertebrae posteriorly.[14] This anatomic location is important during airway clearance when a suction catheter must be inserted into the trachea (see Table 7-11). The right mainstem bronchus is aligned more vertically than the left promoting more frequent aspiration in the right lung.[14] The right lung divides into three lobes: the middle, upper, and lower lobe. The left lung is divided into two lobes: the upper and lower. Part of the left upper lobe, the lingula, is considered anatomically similar to the right middle lobe (RML).

The pulmonary circulation serves many purposes including filtering of blood, participating in gas exchange at the alveolar-capillary junction, providing nutrients to the lungs, and metabolizing many blood borne chemicals (eg, conversion of angiotensin I to angiotensin II).[8] The pulmonary circulation is a high capacity, low resistance circuit that receives the entire cardiac output. Anatomically, it begins at the main pulmonary artery, branches repeatedly like the airways to the alveolar-capillary interface, and carries oxygenated blood to the left atrium via the pulmonary veins as noted in Figure 7–4.[8] The bronchial circulation arises from the aorta or from intercostal arteries and supplies oxygenated blood to the conducting airways, pulmonary vessels, nerves, interstitium, and pleura.

The capillary system is well developed surrounding the alveoli to promote optimal exchange of oxygen and carbon dioxide. The alveolar-capillary junction plays a critical role in optimizing gas exchange. The thickness of the alveolar-capillary junction (increased with pulmonary edema or pulmonary fibrosis), the anatomic availability and viability (destroyed in emphysema or obstructed by

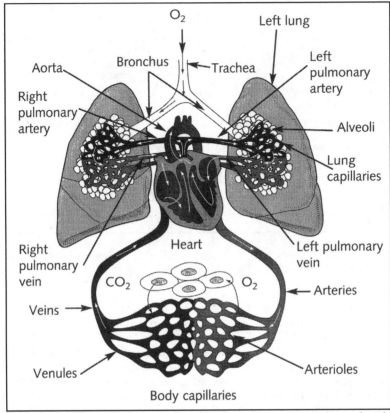

Figure 7–4. The vascular circuits: pulmonic and systemic. (Reprinted with permission from Sheldon LK. *Oxygenation*. Sudbury, Mass: Jones and Bartlett Publishers; 2001. Available at: www.jbpub.com.)

pneumonia), and the oxygen-carrying capacity of hemoglobin may be altered in various diseases leading to shortness of breath (SOB), fatigue, decreased physical function, and hypoxemia. The pulmonary vasculature is sensitive to low oxygen and high carbon dioxide tensions and will adapt by "shunting" blood to better ventilated areas of the lungs for gas exchange, by the process of hypoxic vasoconstriction.[8] This adaptive mechanism attempts to optimize the ventilation (V) and perfusion (Q) (V/Q) relationship but becomes pathologic when there is extensive tissue destruction or alterations of the pulmonary vascular bed leading to increased pulmonary vascular resistance. This can lead to right ventricular hypertrophy, and eventually to right-sided heart failure or "**corpulmonale**." This maladaptive mechanism may be evident in end-stage CF, chronic bronchitis, and emphysema.[15]

The V/Q ratio defines the relationship between airflow and blood flow and describes the gas-exchanging function of the lung. The mismatch between V and Q is the most common cause of hypoxemia in the adult population. Regions of low V/Q, are known as shunt and result in decreased arterial concentration of

Table 7–1
ARTERIAL BLOOD GASES

Components	Normal Values on Room Air
Partial pressure of oxygen (PaO₂)	80 to 100 mmHg
Partial pressure of carbon dioxide (PaCo₂)	35 to 45 mmHg
Bicarbonate (Hco3-)	22 to 28 ,Eq:
Acid/base balance (pH)	7.35 to 7.45

oxygen (PaO_2) and elevated arterial concentrations of carbon dioxide ($PaCO_2$). Regions of high V/Q are termed dead space and result in reduced $PaCO_2$ and insignificant changes in PaO_2. V/Q matching can also be influenced by posture and specific changes in either ventilation or circulation due to disease, abnormal hemodynamic pressures, and abnormal vasoconstriction or bronchoconstriction.[8,14,15] Table 7–1 depicts normal arterial blood gas (ABG) reference values on room air.

The Musculoskeletal Pump

The thoracic rib cage, cervical and thoracic spine, and upper pelvic area comprise the bony components of the musculoskeletal pump (Figure 7–5). These bony structures allow for the origin and insertion of the respiratory muscles and provide protection and support of the lung tissue.[9,11,15] Bony or muscular injury in this region, whether it be a rib or clavicular fracture or a surgical incision, can influence efficiency of the ventilatory pump. Any untoward event impacting the musculoskeletal pump may lead to complaints of pain (eg, thoracic incision, rib fracture) and potential alterations in ventilation. A tibial fracture can be immobilized internally or covered with a cast, but a rib fracture or a surgical incision in the thoracic region is not fixated. As a result, the thoracic rib cage is in constant motion, and patients will complain of difficulty taking deep breaths and soreness with coughing, sneezing, or laughing. Pain and discomfort limit deep breaths following surgery or trauma, increasing the risk for atelectasis and pneumonia. A balance of pain medication, early mobilization, and frequent position change can help to optimize ventilation.

The muscles of respiration alter the configuration of the thoracic cage and produce the pressure fluctuations resulting in inspiration and expiration.[9] These muscles must contract in synchrony on inhalation and relax during a normal exhalation. Expiration is normally a passive process resulting from relaxation of the inspiratory muscles and the elastic recoil of the lungs, airways, and chest wall (Figure 7–6). Exceptions to this are forced expiration (coughing, sneezing, huffing, exercise) and expiration for patients with increased airway resistance (eg, COPD). On forced exhalation the abdominals, the primary expiratory muscles, and the postural back, cervical, and pelvic muscles contribute to force development (Figure 7–7).[9] Postural muscles stabilize the thorax allowing the abdominals to contract, increasing intra-abdominal pressure, forcing the

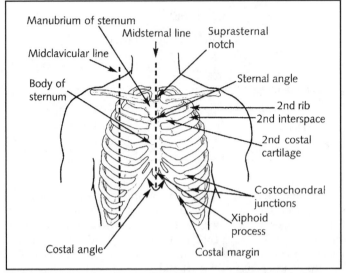

Figure 7–5. Anterior thorax, ribs, and sternum. (Reprinted with permission from Sheldon LK. *Oxygenation*. Sudbury, Mass: Jones and Bartlett Publishers; 2001. Available at: www.jbpub.com.)

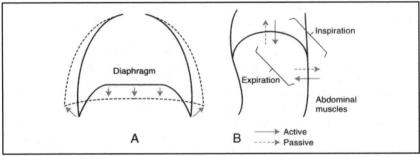

Figure 7–6. A. On inspiration, the dome-shaped diaphragm contracts, the abdominal contents are forced down and forward, and the rib cage is lifted. The volume of the thorax is therefore increased. B. On forced expiration, the abdominal muscles contract and push the diaphragm up. (Reprinted with permission from West JB, ed. *Pulmonary Physiology and Pathophysiology: An Integrated, Case-Based Approach.* Philadelphia, Pa: Lippincott Williams & Wilkins; 2001:3.)

diaphragm cephalad. The pressure gradient between the thorax and abdomen promotes exhalation. Additionally, the respiratory muscles assist with vomiting leading to complaints of abdominal and postural muscle soreness with severe nausea and prolonged episodes of emesis.

The respiratory muscles must develop force to overcome the resistances of the airways, lung tissue, and chest wall.[9] Airway resistance is impacted by the geometry of the airways (bronchodilation versus constriction) and velocity and type of airflow (laminar versus turbulent, slow versus rapid breathing

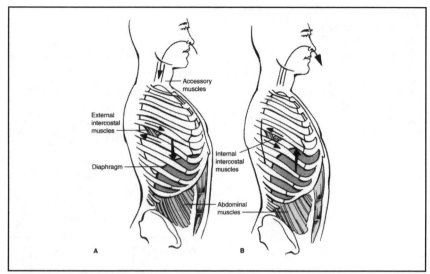

Figure 7–7. Muscles of ventilation. A. Inspiratory muscles. B. Expiratory muscles. (Reprinted with permission from Mackin L, Bullock BL. Normal pulmonary function. In: Bullock BA, Henze RL, eds. *Focus on Pathophysiology.* Philadelphia, Pa: Lippincott Willams & Wilkins; 2000:533.)

frequency). The majority of airway resistance is related to turbulent airflow in the large bronchi extending from the trachea to the fourth or fifth generation (Figure 7–8). Lung tissue and chest wall resistance refers to the compliance, or ease of expansion, which is influenced by the fluid content of pulmonary tissues and the structural make up of the lung parenchyma and musculoskeletal pump.[9,15] Changes in these factors can increase the work of breathing resulting in a greater oxygen consumption for these muscles. Length tension relationships of the muscles, body positioning, organ size (eg, hepatomegaly, ascites), pregnancy, obesity, scoliotic deformities, chest wall deformities (eg, pectus excuvatum), and neurologic disorders (eg, Guillian-Barre, muscular dystrophy, amyotrophic lateral sclerosis) can influence the respiratory muscles and, therefore, the cost of breathing.[9,15]

The primary muscle of inspiration is the diaphragm.[9] This dome-shaped muscle separates the abdomen from the thoracic cavity. The phrenic nerve, originating from cervical nerve roots C_3 to C_5 (remember "3, 4, 5 stay alive"), innervates the diaphragm.[9,15] The diaphragm is divided into two separate domes for the left and the right thoracic cavities. The muscle fans out to originate within the inner surface of the rib cage, termed the costal diaphragm, and inserts into a central tendon that attaches to the lumbar vertebrae, the crural diaphragm.[9] This dome-shaped position correlates with the length tension relationship of a skeletal muscle. There are many influences on the shape and position of the diaphragm including hyperinflation, obesity, and ascites, as previously mentioned. Contraction of the diaphragm pulls the central tendon downward promoting thoracic expansion. The descent of the diaphragm pushes the abdominal organs outward during inspiration. A patient in respiratory distress may reverse this

Figure 7–8. Idealization of the human airways according to Weibel. (Reprinted with permission from West JB, ed. *Pulmonary Physiology and Pathophysiology: An Integrated, Case-Based Approach.* Philadelphia, Pa: Lippincott Williams & Wilkins; 2001:4.)

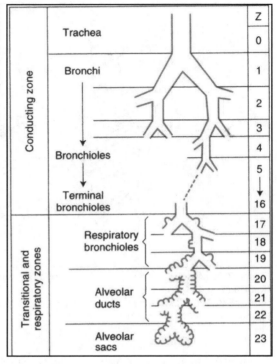

pattern termed respiratory bump, or "paradoxical breathing," where the stomach is "drawn in on inhalation."[16]

The accessory muscle of inspiration, the sternocleidomastoid, erector spinae, trapezius, and scalenus activate during tasks that require increased ventilation (exercise), disorders that increase the resistances of the airways (eg, COPD, asthma), lung tissue (eg, interstitial pulmonary fibrosis [IPF], pneumonia) or chest wall (eg, scoliosis, ankylosing spondylitis), or alter the normal configuration or force production of the diaphragm (eg, COPD, neuromuscular disease).[9,15,16] Accessory muscle usage reflects an increased work of breathing and demands greater oxygen consumption.

Respiratory Control and Innervation

The respiratory control system's primary goal is to maintain adequate oxygen supply and carbon dioxide removal.[8,11,15] Respiratory control is influenced by the autonomic nervous system, chemical and mechanical receptors, and voluntary behaviors. The breathing pattern is usually an automatic function and relies on stimulus from the respiratory centers of the brain stem (medulla, pons) to maintain a normal sequence (breathing pattern, respiratory rate [RR]). The cortex (eg, breath holding, volitional hyperventilation), hypothalamus, and limbic system (eg, emotional states) can influence the breathing pattern.[8]

The central chemoreceptors, located in the medulla, and peripheral chemoreceptors, within the aortic arch and carotid bodies (Figure 7–9), respond to

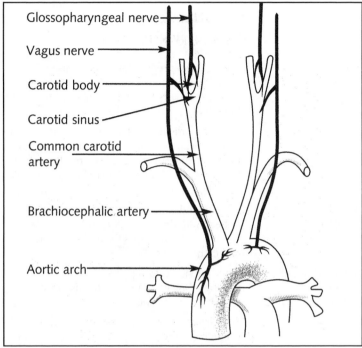

Glossopharyngeal nerve

Vagus nerve

Carotid body

Carotid sinus

Common carotid
artery

Brachiocephalic artery

Aortic arch

Figure 7–9. Location of peripheral chemoreceptors. (Reprinted with permission from Sheldon LK. *Oxygenation*. Sudbury, Mass: Jones and Bartlett Publishers; 2001. Available at: www.jbpub.com.)

chemical stimuli and are sensitive to levels of PaO_2 and $PaCO_2$.[8,14–16] Elevated $PaCO_2$ increases the hydrogen ion concentrations (H^+) (decreasing pH [acidosis]) stimulating the central chemoreceptors, while decreased PaO_2 and increased $PaCO_2$ stimulate the peripheral chemoreceptors resulting in enhanced rates and depth of breathing. Therapists must consider that certain disease states (eg, COPD) lead to impaired sensitivity of the chemoreceptors. For example, a patient who chronically retains CO_2 (elevated $PaCO_2$ via an ABG) and presents with reduced PaO_2 may rely on his or her peripheral chemoreceptors to stimulate the respiratory control center (**hypoxic drive**). The peripheral chemoreceptors are more responsive to lower oxygen concentrations. Providing this patient with supplemental oxygen may elevate the PaO_2 leading to reductions in the rate and depth of breathing, hypoventilation, leading to an elevated $PaCO_2$ and respiratory acidosis. Supplemental oxygen must be titrated carefully in this select patient group.

Additional pulmonary reflexes are outlined in Table 7–2.

PATHOLOGIES

Pulmonary pathologies can primarily be divided into either obstructive or restrictive disease patterns. The therapist should keep in mind that many

Table 7–2
PULMONARY REFLEXES

Deflation reflex	Hering Breuer reflex; "amount of distention of a breath will influence frequency/expiration time." Receptors located in walls of bronchi and bronchioles.
Irritant reflex	Lung compression, deflation, or exposure to noxious gases (mechanical/chemical stimulus) results in cough and bronchoconstriction. Receptors located in subepithelial layer along bronchioles, bronchi, and trachea.
Aortic and carotid sinus baroreceptors	Changes in blood pressure (BP) result in alteration in heart rate (HR) and RR ($\uparrow$ BP = $\downarrow$ HR/RR; $\downarrow$ BP = $\uparrow$ HR/RR). Receptors located near aortic arch and carotid sinus.
Juxtapulmonary-capillary receptors (J receptors)	Stimulation causes rapid, shallow breathing. Receptors located in interstitial tissue between alveoli and capillaries.
Stretch reflex	Stimulation (stretch) of skeletal muscle will $\uparrow$ strength of contraction. Receptors located in muscle spindles.
Joint/muscle receptors	Stimulation enhances ventilation in preparation for activity. Receptors located in peripheral joints/muscles.

end-stage disease processes may cross over to more restrictive patterns. In some cases, there may be a combination of both patterns, but the pathology was put in one category for simplification. History and physical examination and pulmonary diagnostic testing confirm diagnosis. Tables 7–3 and 7–4 and Figure 7–10 provide descriptions of common pulmonary function tests and procedures.

Obstructive

Chronic Obstructive Pulmonary Disease

COPD, also referred to as chronic obstructive lung disease (COLD) or chronic obstructive airway disease (COAD), is a slowly progressive disorder characterized by chronic airflow limitation (Figure 7–11).[4,7] COPD is a combination of emphysema, chronic bronchitis, and in some cases, asthma.[17] Cigarette smoking is the primary preventable cause of COPD, and 10% to 15% of all smokers are expected to develop the disease.[7,18] Age and smoking duration and amount influence the timing of symptoms and diagnosis. The clinical pattern is defined by increased airway resistance, air trapping, termed **hyperinflation**, increased anterior to posterior chest wall diameter, or **barrel chest deformity**, and

Table 7–3
PULMONARY FUNCTION TESTS DEFINITIONS

Type of Test	*Definition*
Forced expiratory volume in 1 second (FEV_1)	Amount of air expired in the first second of forced exhalation, used to assess obstruction in larger airways
Total lung capacity (TLC)	Amount of gas in lungs at end of maximum inhalation
Residual volume (RV)	Amount of air remaining in lungs following maximum expiration
Inspiratory capacity (IC)	Maximal amount of air inspired from resting expiratory levels (V_T + IRV)
Expiratory reserve volume (ERV)	Maximum amount of air expired beyond a normal (quiet) expiration
Inspiratory reserve volume (IRV)	Maximum amount of air inspired above a normal breath
Vital capacity (VC)	Maximum amount inspired and expired with a single breath
Tidal volume (V_T)	Normal amount of air ventilated at rest ("quiet breathing")
Minute ventilation (MV)	Volume of air ventilated in 1 minute (V_T x RR)
Forced expiratory flow % ($FEF_{25\% \text{ to } 75\%}$)	Maximum midexpiratory flow rate (average flow rate during the middle 50% of forced VC), used to assess obstruction in smaller airways
FEV_1/FVC ratio	Used as general indicator of airway obstruction (normal >75%, obstruction <75%)
Peak expiratory flow rate (PEFR)	Maximum expiratory flow rate
Function residual capacity (FRC)	Volume of air in lungs at the resting expiratory level (RV + ERV)
Diffusing capacity of carbon monoxide (DLCO)	Amount of gas that moves across alveolar-capillary membrane, carbon monoxide single breath technique; provides information regarding the gas exchanging function of the lung
Maximal voluntary ventilation (MVV)	Measures maximal breathing capacity (MBC), used as a marker of respiratory muscle endurance
Maximal inspiratory pressure (MIP), or negative inspiratory force (NIF)	Measures maximal pressure developed during inspiration, measures inspiratory muscle strength
Maximal expiratory pressure (MEP)	Measures maximal pressure developed during expiration, measures expiratory muscle strength
Restriction pattern	Reduced lung volumes (V_t, RV) and capacities (FRC, VC), preserved flow rates with reduced FEV_1, FVC due to small lung volumes
Obstruction	Increased FRC/RV, limited V_t, reduced flow rates (FEV_1, FVC)

Table 7–4

TESTS AND PROCEDURES ASSOCIATED WITH THE PULMONARY SYSTEM

Test Name	Clinical Impact for Physical Therapy
Chest x-ray	A radiographic study to determine the size, shape, and location of the heart will determine the presence of extravascular fluid (eg, pulmonary edema/pleural effusion), anatomic integrity of ribs and diaphragm, and attempts to localize lung consolidation, hyperdensities (eg, tumor), or translucency (eg, hyperinflation)
Bronchoscopy	An endoscopic procedure allowing direct visualization of the tracheobronchial tree. Used to localize airway abnormalities: tumors/lesions; bleeding/hemoptysis; airway stenosis; used for biopsy, tissue resection, and secretion removal
ABG	Determines adequacy of ventilation and gas exchange (see Table 7–1)
Pulmonary function test	Will determine restrictive/obstructive patterns and diffusion abnormalities (see Table 7–3 and Figure 7–10)
Thoracentesis	A surgical procedure that drains fluid from pleural space, may be used for biopsy
V/Q scan	A nuclear scan that studies airflow (V) and blood flow (Q) to determine V/Q defects (eg, pulmonary embolism)
Bronchial/alveolar lavage	Fluid is instilled down a patient's airway and removed via gentle suction. This allows access to pulmonary fluids and cells of the lower respiratory tract that are unable to be obtained via coughing

---

lattened diaphragms. The American Thoracic Society has outlined criteria for staging COPD based on pulmonary function criteria:

- Stage I, FEV_1 (forced expiratory volume in 1 second) 50% to 79% predicted
- Stage II, FEV_1 35% to 49% predicted
- Stage III, FEV_1 <5% predicted value[19]

Patients present with higher RRs, wheezing via auscultation, barrel chest deformity, lower oxygen saturations (SpO_2) on room air, accessory muscle usage, dyspnea, and functional limitations depending on disease and symptom severity.

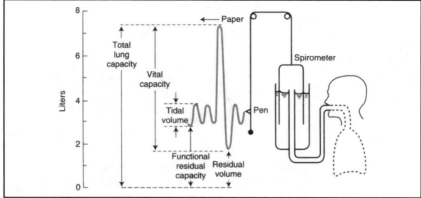

Figure 7–10. Pulmonary function test. Lung volumes. TLC, functional residual capacity, and RV cannot be measured with the spirometer. (Reprinted with permission from West JB, ed. *Pulmonary Physiology and Pathophysiology: An Integrated, Case-Based Approach.* Philadelphia, Pa: Lippincott Williams & Wilkins; 2001:39.)

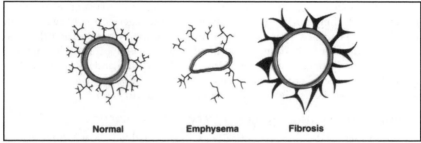

Figure 7–11. Airway caliber in normal lung, emphysema, and interstitial fibrosis. In emphysema, the airways tend to collapse because of the loss of radial traction. By contrast, in fibrosis, radial traction may be excessive, with the result that airway caliber is large when related to lung volume. (Reprinted with permission from West JB, ed. *Pulmonary Physiology and Pathophysiology: An Integrated, Case-Based Approach.* Philadelphia, Pa: Lippincott Williams & Wilkins; 2001:78.)

One of the challenges working with the COPD population is that the levels of dyspnea may not correlate with the disease severity.[19] Recurrent exacerbations result in worsening of symptoms and loss of lung function which may inhibit the individual's functional return.[5] Exacerbation prevention and disease progression are influenced by smoking cessation, long-term oxygen usage, prophylactic vaccinations and airway clearance, limiting exposure to communicable diseases, environmental pollutants and allergens, and remaining physically active or participating in pulmonary rehabilitation programs.

Asthma

Asthma is a reversible or reactive airway disease. The patient has an intrinsic (eg, dust, pollen, pet dander) or extrinsic exposure (eg, medications, infections,

Figure 7–12. Normal bronchiole and bronchiole in asthma. (Reprinted with permission from Sheldon LK. *Oxygenation.* Sudbury, Mass: Jones and Bartlett Publishers; 2001. Available at: www.jbpub.com.)

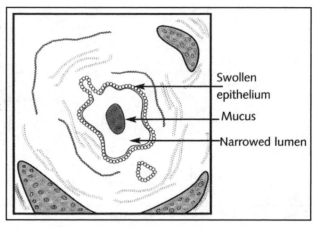

Swollen epithelium

Mucus

Narrowed lumen

exercise, cold air) resulting in airway **bronchoconstriction** and hyperplasia, **inflammation** with resultant swelling, and **hypersecretion** of mucus.[10,16,20] The sum of these factors narrows the airways resulting in obstruction as noted in Figure 7–12. Asthma can be life threatening if not managed properly by eliminating trigger exposures and using preventative medications to stabilize inflammation and reduce bronchopasm. Daily medications include bronchodilators and anti-inflammatory agents via meter dose inhalers (MDI) and intravenous (IV) corticosteroids for severe exacerbations. Patients should be instructed in proper technique for MDIs. See Table 7–5 for recommended directions.

Emphysema and Alpha$_1$ Antitrypsin Deficiency

Emphysema is defined anatomically as an irreversible increase in the size of air spaces distal to the terminal bronchioles with destruction of alveolar septa.[13,21] Patients are described as "pink puffers" due to malnutrition and cachexia, CO_2 retention with flushing and pursed lip breathing (PLB). The disease results from loss of the mechanical tethering or distending function of the lung parenchyma. The loss of lung elasticity results in premature **airway collapse** with expiration producing airtrapping and wheezing.[22] **Hyperinflation** creates flattening of the diaphragms, use of accessory muscles, development of a barrel chest, and functional decline due to chronic symptoms of SOB and fatigue. Alveolar destruction reduces surface area for gas exchange. Although, emphysema's etiology is unknown, theories suggest the disease may be caused by proteases released from inflammatory cells including macrophages and neutrophils.[22] **Alpha$_1$ antitrypsin deficiency (A1AD)** is a genetic form of emphysema. Alpha$_1$ antitrypsin is a glycoprotein that inhibits proteolytic enzymes.[16] Patients who are alpha$_1$ antitrypsin deficient lack this enzyme, the lung architecture will be destroyed, and the clinical symptoms of emphysema will develop at an earlier age. Cigarette smoking accelerates the onset of symptoms.

Chronic Bronchitis

Chronic bronchitis is a clinical diagnosis and is defined by complaint of chronic respiratory symptoms for 2 years in a row for 3 consecutive months.[10,15,16]

Table 7–5

RECOMMENDED USE OF METER DOSE INHALER

1. Shake MDI if prescribed.
2. Practice controlled breathing.
3. Place the opening of the MDI two finger lengths away from the lips.
4. Use a spacer if prescribed by physician or poor technique is demonstrated.
5. Slowly inhale and at the same time compress the MDI.
6. Now hold breath for 8 to 10 seconds.
7. Reshake MDI if prescribed by instructions.
8. Wait 3 to 5 minutes.
9. Repeat steps 3 through 6.
10. Precautions: Watch for signs of medications being deposited in throat and mouth (thrush, continued complaints of shortness of breath, audible wheezing, continued dyspnea, or thickness in mucus if mucolytic).

Adapted from Casaburi R, Petty TL, eds. *Principles and Practice of Pulmonary Rehabilitation.* Philadelphia, Pa: WB Saunders Co; 1993.

Patients are described as "blue bloaters" due to the accompanying hypoxemia, cyanosis, and peripheral edema. The disease is highlighted by airway obstruction due to excessive mucus production secondary to hyperplasia and hypertrophy of mucus-secreting cells of the airways.[13] Factors contributing to the development of chronic bronchitis include cigarette smoking and chronic exposures to dust, fumes, and air pollution.[21]

Bronchiectasis

Bronchiectasis is the permanent dilatation of medium-sized bronchi due to chronic infection and retained mucus.[10,15,16,20] Bronchiectasis can result from abnormal ciliary function (eg, primary ciliary dyskinesia [Kartagener's syndrome], CF), systemic illnesses (eg, CF, HIV), or following prolonged or repeated infectious diseases (eg, tuberculosis (TB), frequent pneumonias).[21] The dilated regions become ideal areas for progressive infections and airway destruction. **Hemoptysis,** or coughing blood, is a complication associated with erosion of the bronchial wall and surrounding pulmonary vessels. Three forms are usually described: cylindrical, fusiform, and saccular dilatation.[16] Secretions tend to be thick and constant and this population benefits from airway clearance programs.

Cystic Fibrosis

CF, an abnormality of chromosome 7, is an inherited autosomal recessive disease affecting the mucus-producing glands in the lungs, sweat glands, digestive tract, and the genitourinary system. To date, over 800 defects have been identified, and CF is the most common inherited disease in Caucasians.[23,24] The genetic defect impairs sodium and chloride transport in the airways resulting in thick, sticky mucus.[25] Patient presentation is variable, but abnormalities may include bronchiectatic lung disease, pancreatic insufficiency with resultant impaired fat absorption, malnutrition, diabetes, potential osteoporosis, and arthropathies. Patients with CF are susceptible to opportunistic lung infections (eg, pseudomonas aeruginosa, burkholdia cepacia). The median age for survival is 33, but unvarying disease progression ends with respiratory failure, pulmonary hypertension (PH), cor pulmonale, and death.[23,25,26] Acute care therapists must be sensitive to infection control and universal precautions. Equipment should not be shared with other CF patients or those who are immunocompromised. All surfaces must be disinfected. Optimizing airway clearance, nutrition, medication delivery, and exercise are mainstays of both outpatient and inpatient programs for patients with CF. Awareness of risks for diabetes, osteopenia, osteoporosis, liver dysfunction, and dehydration should be incorporated into the plan of care.

Bronchiolitis Obliterans

Bronchiolitis obliterans (BO) is a late complication following lung or heart-lung transplant (see Chapter 14) or can also occur independently. **Cryptogenic organizing pneumonia (COP)** and **bronchiolitis obliterans organizing pneumonia (BOOP)** are rare inflammatory disorders characterized by bronchial fibrosis and intraluminal connective tissue plugs extending into the alveoli.[27,28] Men and women in the fifth and sixth decade are affected similarly. Symptoms include progressive dyspnea, new cough, general malaise, weight loss, and fever. Radiographic examination, lung biopsy, and bronchoalveolar lavage are key to accurate diagnosis. The therapist may see elevated RR and HR, decreased SpO_2, and little sputum. Corticosteroids are the mainstay of treatment and prognosis is typically excellent; however, some patients may have permanent fibrotic lung disease.[27–30]

BO, also termed obliterative bronchiolitis (OB), is the aggressive manifestations of chronic rejection following transplantation.[31] Prevalence post lung transplant is upwards of 40% with 25% mortality.[32] Irreversible, progressive airway narrowing by granulation tissue is characteristic of OB.[31] Suspicious clinical findings include dyspnea on exertion (DOE), cough, and reduced pulmonary function studies (decreased FEV_1).[32] Specific risk factors for development of OB post-transplant include primary graft failure, cytomegalovirus infection, airway ischemia, human leukocyte antigen (HLA) mismatching, and recurrent, severe acute rejection episodes (see Chapter 14).[32,33]

Restrictive

Interstitial Lung Disease and Pulmonary Fibrosis

Interstitial lung disease (ILD) is a generic term to describe a diverse group of acute and chronic lung processes. The interstitium refers to the microscopic anatomic space made up of cellular (fibroblasts, neutrophils) and connective tissue (collagen, elastin, proteoglycans) elements between the alveoli and the pulmonary capillaries. ILD pathologies involve the interstitium as well as the endothelial and epithelial linings of the vasculature and alveoli respectively.[13,34] Disease development may be idiopathic (sarcoidosis, collagen vascular diseases, rheumatoid arthritis (RA), systemic lupus erhythematosus (SLE), Sjögren's syndrome, BOOP/OB, lymphangioleiomyomatosis [LAM]), related to chronic infections (eg, TB, Aspergillosis), environmental exposures (eg, asbestosis, silicosis, bird fanciers lung), drug induced (eg, chemotherapeutic agents, methotrexate, amiodorone), or physical agents (eg, radiation exposure, oxygen toxicity).[34] These disorders typically result in mixed pulmonary restriction or obstructive patterns as noted with pulmonary function testing, impaired diffusion (decreased DLCO), and decreased pulmonary compliance. The most common presenting symptoms are SOB and cough. Resting vital signs may be stable, but functional challenges such as ambulation and stair climbing can lead to rapid desaturation and disabling dyspnea. The following section will highlight several ILD disorders.

Idiopathic Pulmonary Fibrosis

Idiopathic pulmonary fibrosis (IPF) is an insidious, progressive restrictive lung disease characterized by interstitial inflammation and fibrosis. Histopathologically, IPF may be described as **usual interstitial pneumonitis (UIP)** or **desquamative interstitial pneumonia (DIP).**[13] Pathogenesis is not clearly defined, but repeated immune and inflammatory responses lead to tissue injury promote widespread fibrotic changes in lung architecture (see Figure 7–11).[13,35] Patients present with progressive DOE, nonproductive paroxysmal cough (often refractory to anti-tussives), crackles via auscultation, fatigue, weight loss, hypoxemia, digital clubbing, and often severely restricted exercise capacity. Five-year mortality is >40% primarily due to respiratory insufficiency. Additional causes of death include cardiac ischemia, PE, infections, and neoplasms.[35,36] Diagnosis is confirmed by lung biopsy, radiologic testing including high-resolution computerized tomography (HRCT), and x-ray. Medical management most commonly includes high-dose corticosteroids, immunosuppressive (azathioprine, cyclosporine) and cytotoxic agents (cytoxan [cyclophsphamide]), inhibitors of collagen synthesis or fibrosis (cholchicine, penicillamine), oxygen therapy, opiates for respiratory distress and dyspnea, and lung transplantation.[35,36]

Sarcoidosis

Sarcoidosis is an idiopathic multisystem disease highlighted by the formation of inflammatory granulomas, masses, or nodules consisting of varied cell types (eg, phagocytes, macrophages, lymphocytes) in the affected organs. Sarcoidosis most commonly affects the lungs and intrathoracic lymph nodes and leads to a progressive restrictive lung disease (reduced lung volumes and flow rates) resulting in SOB, cough, and chest discomfort.[37,38] Therapists need to consider extrapulmonary involvement including cardiac (eg, dysrhythmias, cardiomyopathy, and sudden death), neurologic (eg, Bell's palsy, seizures, polyneuropathy, hydrocephalus), and musculoskeletal systems (eg, myopathy, bone cysts, arthritic-type pain).[37] Bronchoscopy, biopsy, and radiological studies confirm diagnosis. Corticosteroids are the cornerstone of treatment, and additional medications include cytotoxic and immunosuppressive agents.

Lymphangioleiomyomatosis

LAM is a rare, slowly progressive disease characterized by abnormal smooth-muscle cell proliferation affecting women of childbearing age almost exclusively.[39] The smooth-muscle cells are distributed throughout the peribronchial, perivascular, and perilymphatic areas of the lung. Clinically, patients present

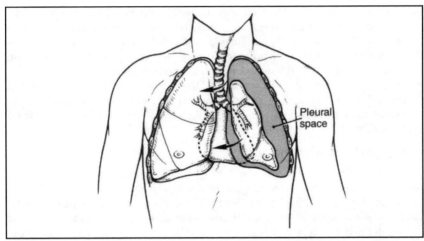

Figure 7–13. Pleural effusion. Shaded area shows fluid collection in the pleural space. Lung tissue is displaced and mediastinal structures are compressed. (Reprinted with permission from Mackin L, Bullock BL. Altered pulmonary function. In: Bullock BA, Henze RL, eds. *Focus on Pathophysiology*. Philadelphia, Pa: Lippincott Willams & Wilkins; 2000:574.)

with a persistent obstructive or mixed pulmonary defect, cough, DOE, recurrent pneumothoraces and less commonly chest pain, and pleural effusions (chylous).[39,40] Figure 7–13 shows an example of a pleural effusion. Hormonal manipulation (oophorectomy, progesterone, leutonizing hormone-releasing hormone analogues) and lung transplantation are the basis of treatment.[40]

Tuberculosis

The incidence of **TB**, an infection with *mycobacterium tuberculosis*, had been declining until 1985. TB is associated with the immunocompromised, poor socioeconomic status, homelessness, alcoholism, and health care workers.[41] TB is the most common infectious disease in adults worldwide due to the development of multiresistant TB and HIV.[42,43] The *mycobacterium tuberculosis* is contained within an airborne droplet; is spread by coughing, talking, or sneezing; and may be held aloft by air currents.[41] The bacilli bypass the pulmonary defenses of the upper respiratory tract and deposit in the alveolus. Bacilli are ingested by alveolar macrophage, where they multiply, destroying the macrophage. Lysis of the marcophage releases the bacilli triggering a greater immune response from the infected host. Monocytes/macrophages and lymphocytes accumulate at the infection site forming a microscopic lesion or granuloma. The immune response may contain the infection within a fibrotic cavity, or tubercle (Gohn Complex), or fail, leading to progression and destruction of surrounding lung structures.[13,41,44] **Reactivation TB** is the most common form and represents exacerbation of latent infection weeks to years after the primary insult. **Miliary TB** results from bacilli invasion and spread by the circulatory system. Patients with active TB will present with cough, fever, malaise, and night sweats and need to be in negative pressure rooms or use designated facemasks to prevent infection spread (see Chapter 5). **Extrapulmonary TB** may affect the musculoskeletal system (particularly the spine and weightbearing joints), pericardium, and meninges.[41]

Respiratory Failure

Respiratory insufficiency and failure can be defined broadly as the impairment of respiratory gas exchange between the ambient air and circulating blood.[20,45] It is generally categorized as either hypercapnic or hypoxemic as defined by specific changes in ABGes and may arise either acutely or chronically. Although the causes of respiratory insufficiency and failure are diverse, generally there are three pathogenic categories of diseases leading to respiratory failure:

1. Progressive airway obstruction (eg, asthma, emphysema, chronic bronchitis, and CF)

2. Altered lung parenchyma (eg, IPF and sarcoidosis)

3. Defects from regulation of ventilation caused either by abnormalities of the musculoskeletal structures of the chest wall (eg, spinal cord injury [SCI], trauma/flail chest and neuromuscular disease) or as a primary dysfunction of the respiratory center (eg, cerebrovascular accident or drug overdose)[46]

Each of these disorders can occur individually or may occur in combination (eg, chronic COPD with superimposed pneumonia).

Acute respiratory failure is sudden and the ABG reveals a pH less than 7.35 with the $PaCO_2$ >50 mmHg (hypercapnea) and PaO_2 is <50 mmHg (hypoxemia).[20] The metabolic system is not able to compensate for the sudden respiratory acidosis. Endotracheal intubation and mechanical ventilation are standard components of treatment for acute respiratory failure.[47] Noninvasive positive-pressure ventilation is being applied as an alternative therapy to minimize invasive procedures and is discussed later in this chapter.

Chronic respiratory failure can be a late manifestation of pulmonary pathologies such as COPD.[20] This regression to failure may take days to weeks to develop. Chronic respiratory failure may follow an acute episode of respiratory failure. The roles of therapists on the team weaning a patient from mechanical ventilation following respiratory failure may range from airway clearance and bedside exercise programs to progressive mobilization and discharge planning.

Acute Lung Injury and Acute Respiratory Distress Syndrome

Acute lung injury (ALI) and acute respiratory distress syndrome (ARDS) are syndromes consisting of acute, severe alterations in lung structure and function characterized by hypoxemia, low compliance, diffuse radiologic infiltrates, and increased pulmonary vascular endothelial and alveolar epithelial permeability leading to pulmonary edema.[48] Pathologically, ARDS/ALI is described as **diffuse alveolar damage (DAD)**. The annual incidence of ARDS and ALI in the United States may be as high as 150,000 cases with mortality rates ranging between 10% and 90%.[49] All ages are potentially susceptible to ARDS and the term *adult respiratory distress syndrome* has been replaced by *ARDS*. Within the continuum of pulmonary insults, ARDS represents the most severe form of ALI.

ARDS may develop after direct lung injury (pneumonia, aspiration, thoracic trauma) or indirect causes (sepsis/systemic inflammatory response syndrome [SIRS]/multiple organ dysfunction [MOD] or failure [MOF], pancreatitis).[50] Regardless of inciting event, intense inflammation is a common pathway leading to pulmonary damage and dysfunction.

ARDS may be divided into three phases of variable duration:

1. Inflammation and exudation (protein rich pulmonary edema)

2. Fibrosis

3. Resolution

The resolution of ARDS is marked by partial or complete return of lung function, or fibrosis and gas-exchanging abnormalities may persist long term. Management is largely supportive and consists of mechanical ventilation (low stretch/reduced V_T protocols, permissive hypercapnea) to alleviate gas-exchanging abnormalities and increased work of breathing, judicious fluid management, anti-inflammatory agents, correction of coagulation disorders, and antibiotics. Physical therapy interventions frequently include positioning and contracture prevention, airway clearance, early mobilization, and patient/family education. Acquired neuromuscular abnormalities are common in this population and often are discovered during physical therapy examination (see Chapter 4).

Pneumonia

The respiratory system is continuously exposed to a myriad of microorganisms that may lead to disease. Pneumonia is an inflammatory process in which fluid or blood cells fill alveoli, interstitial tissue, and bronchioles.[16,20] Individuals who are hospitalized, the very young or old, and immunocompromised patients are at the greatest risk for developing pneumonia. Pneumonia can result from bacterial, viral, fungal, parasitic infection, or even chemical (aspiration) exposure in the lungs where the pulmonary defense mechanisms were overwhelmed. The human body reacts to this infectious exposure through innate and specific immunity and inflammatory responses by recruitment and activation of alveolar macrophages, neutrophils, lymphocytes, complement, immunoglobulins, etc (see Chapter 5).

A full discussion of pneumonic infections is beyond the scope of this chapter, but pneumonia can be classified by the infectious agent (bacterial, viral, fungal, atypical), hospital or community acquired, or aspiration.[16] Risk factors for hospital-acquired **pneumonias (nosocomial)** are admission to the intensive care unit (ICU), endotracheal intubation, thoracoabdominal surgery, nasogastric tubes, inappropriate use of antibiotics, and altered level of consciousness.[20]

Pneumocystis carinii pneumonia (PCP) is considered an opportunistic infection seen in patients with acquired immunodeficiency syndrome (AIDS) or on immunosuppressive therapy.[20] The exact cause is not clearly understood. Exposure may occur in early childhood and an intact immune system is able to respond, but when there is an alteration in the normal T cell immunity, reactivation or susceptibility occurs. The clinical course depends on the host and whether there is immune dysfunction. In the non-HIV-infected patient the symptoms can range from a fever and nonproductive cough to diffuse alveolar infiltrates and respiratory failure.[20] The clinical course is more sinister in the HIV-infected patient. Radiographic changes may be more subtle, combined with a low grade fever, nonproductive cough, and weight loss.

Aspiration pneumonia can occur when a patient cannot protect his or her airway from inhaling fluids or foreign substances. Swallowing dysfunction and altered mental state from medication, drugs, alcohol, anesthesia, cerebral vascular accident (CVA), a loss of consciousness, drowning, or trauma can put the patient at risk. Aspiration can be categorized into inert objects (eg, teeth, food, water), chemicals, and bacteria.[20] Inert objects may become lodged in airways causing a local inflammatory response and wheezing. ALI occurs with a chemical inhalation such as bile and gastric acid leading to airway inflammation, fibrosis, and necrosis.[20] Additionally, over 50% of aspirations result in secondary bacterial infections with the most common source of bacterial substances from the mouth.

Airway clearance, antibiotics, and hydration aid sputum expectoration and improvement in V/Q matching. Therapists may observe elevated RR, HR, accessory muscle use, possible pleuritic chest pain, thick tenacious mucus (bacterial), and decreased SpO_2 depending on the V/Q relationships in patients with pneumonia. Radiographic changes may take a few weeks to completely resolve. In the case of inhalation of an inert substance, bronchoscopy may be needed to identify and remove the foreign substance.

Lung Cancer

The leading cause of death from cancer in this country for both men and women is **lung cancer.**[51] Smoking and secondhand smoke have been linked to lung cancer, specifically small cell and nonsmall cell cancers (Figure 7–14).[20] The three cornerstones of treatment—surgery, radiation, and chemotherapy—can each negatively impact lung function resulting in restrictive lung pathology. Patients are at risk for opportunistic infections due to immunocompromise and universal precautions should be observed at all times. Fatigue, cachexia, poor nutritional state, altered blood cell counts, frequent bouts of nausea and vomiting, and limited pulmonary reserve can lead to functional limitations and impact the physical therapy care plan (see Chapter 13).

Mesothelioma

Mesothelioma is a rare cancer related to asbestos exposure but is the most common cancer of the pleura.[52] Patients are typically in their 60s and exposure may have occurred 30 to 45 years prior to diagnosis.[52] Occupational risk is increased in automotive mechanics, ship builders, and asbestos miners. The tumor originates mainly on the parietal pleura and progressively spreads to encase the lung surfaces, penetrates the chest wall, infiltrates the diaphragm, and invades mediastinal structures.[53] Patients frequently complain of SOB, chest pain, fever, cough, and weakness. Prognosis is poor and physical therapy may be consulted for discharge planning, patient/family education, and prevention of secondary pulmonary complications.

Chest Wall Deformities and Musculoskeletal Disorders

Congenital defects are the primary cause of chest wall abnormalities.[20] **Kyphoscoliosis** (idiopathic or from muscle weakness/denervation), **pectus**

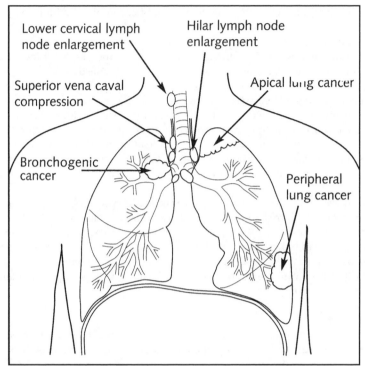

Lower cervical lymph
node enlargement

Hilar lymph node
enlargement

Superior vena caval
compression

Apical lung cancer

Bronchogenic
cancer

Peripheral
lung cancer

Figure 7–14. Clinical features of lung cancer. (Reprinted with permission from Sheldon LK. *Oxygenation*. Sudbury, Mass: Jones and Bartlett Publishers; 2001. Available at: www.jbpub.com.)

excavatum, and **pectus carinatum** result in deformities of the chest wall limiting thoracic expansion (Figure 7–15).[54] TLC, VC, and other volume measurements will be decreased. Some patients do not have difficulty in compensating for the loss of volume and adapt by increasing the rate of respiration. Atelectasis can occur in the areas of lung compression and retained secretions may promote pneumonias.[20] The length tension relationship of the accessory muscles of respiration may be compromised from these chest wall deformities. Instruction in stacking breaths and positions to enhance ventilation can be beneficial.[54] Exercise alone for fixed chest wall deformities remains controversial.

Neuromuscular disorders like Guillain Barre syndrome, SCI, myasthenia gravis, and critical care myopathy/polyneuropathy as well as degenerative diseases like amyotrophic lateral sclerosis, muscular dystrophy, and multiple sclerosis can pose a challenge to the therapist in the acute care setting. The respiratory muscles fail to provide adequate ventilation for gas exchange due to fatigue, weakness, or denervation and respiratory failure ensues. Mechanical ventilation is indicated for acute respiratory failure. However, patients with progressive respiratory insufficiency may benefit from noninvasive ventilation to avoid the complications of intubation.[55] Airway clearance and cough enhancements are vital to progression from the acute care setting to the rehabilitation facility.

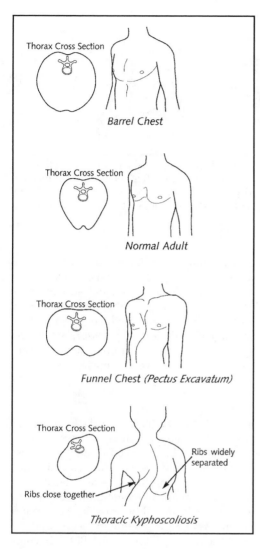

Figure 7–15. Abnor-malities of the chest. (Reprinted with permission from Sheldon LK. *Oxygenation.* Sudbury, Mass: Jones and Bartlett Publishers; 2001. Available at: www.jbpub.com.)

Therapists dealing with spinal cord injured or neuromuscular patients must be familiar with assistive coughing maneuvers. Understanding the hemodynamics (autonomic dysreflexia, vasovagal) and altered state of the pulmonary system (impaired cough and increased production of secretions) of the patient following a cervical level SCI is imperative. Once the patient has been stabilized or fixated (see Chapter 9) and ready for out of bed (OOB) activity, the therapist must be prepared to prevent hypotensive and reflexive type events.

Autonomic dysreflexia is unpredictable and may arise years after the initial injury.[20] Life-threatening conditions like seizures, cerebral hemorrhage, severe hypertension (HTN), and even myocardial infarction may occur in response to the blocked afferent sensory transmission in a patient with a SCI above the sixth

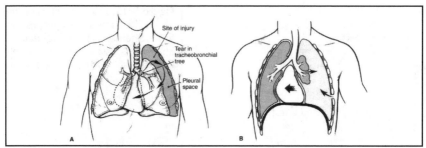

Figure 7–16. Pneumothorax. A. Atmospheric air entering the pleural space through a tracheobronchial tear. B. Tension pneumothorax. (Reprinted with permission from Mackin L, Bullock BL. Altered pulmonary function. In: Bullock BA, Henze RL, eds. *Focus on Pathophysiology*. Philadelphia, Pa: Lippincott Willams & Wilkins; 2000:574.)

or seventh cord segment.[20] Some precipitating factors include bowel or bladder distention, pressure ulcers, and even spasticity or pressure on the penis.

Vasovagal syncope is neurally mediated.[56] This is a common cause of unexplained recurrent syncope. Transient and sudden decline in brain perfusion with vasovagal syncope is related to hypotension by abrupt vasodilation and is often accompanied by a vagally mediated reflex bradycardia.[56] Pressure stockings, tilt tables, abdominal binders, emptying the bladder, and doing airway clearance prior to mobilization may lessen the chance of compromising events (see Chapter 9).

Pneumothorax

A **pneumothorax** literally means "air in the thorax." Air leaks between the visceral and parietal pleura linings of the lungs and chest wall respectively as noted in Figure 7–16. Pneumothoraces are characterized in multiple ways: **primary pneumothorax** typically occurs in 20- to 40-year-old men and is not associated with lung disease; **secondary pneumothorax** is associated with underlying lung disease (eg, COPD); **iatrogenic pneumothorax** can follow a diagnostic or therapeutic procedure (mechanical ventilation, subclavian cannulation, intercostal nerve block), and **traumatic pneumothorax** occurs due to penetrating or nonpenetrating chest trauma (eg, rib fracture, CPR).[57] **Tension pneumothorax**, a life-threatening complication, is the development of high intrapleural pressures leading to lung collapse and hypoxemia and cardiac and vascular compression, resulting in limited venous return, cardiac output, and hypotension. Patients will frequently complain of acute dyspnea and localized pain. Physical examination may reveal absent or diminished breath sounds, hyperresonance on percussion, tachycardia, and potentially tracheal deviation.[58] Radiologic studies (chest x-rays) will confirm diagnosis. Treatments attempt to expand the lung and include needle aspiration, pleural/chest drainage tubes (see Chapter 3), Heimlich flutter valve, pleurodesis, minimally invasive surgery (video-assisted thoracostomy) or open thoracotomy.[57,58] **Pleurodesis** attempts to obliterate the pleural space by producing inflammation and adhesions through physical abrasion or chemical irritants termed sclerosing agents such as talc or tetracylcine. This procedure can be very painful.[58]

Pulmonary Edema

Pulmonary edema is the accumulation of extravascular water in the lungs and classically develops due to increased pulmonary vascular permeability (eg, noncardiogenic [ALI/ARDS]), increased hydrostatic pressures (eg, cardiogenic [CHF], volume overload), or a combination.[59] **Cardiogenic pulmonary edema** results from elevated filling pressures in the left ventricle or atrium. This elevated pressure is reflected into the pulmonary vasculature and promotes the efflux of fluid across the pulmonary capillaries and venules. **Noncardiogenic pulmonary edema** results from alterations in the capillary endothelium, allowing enhanced fluid flux into the lung parenchyma and alveoli (see Chapter 2). Pulmonary edema leads to atelectasis and fluid-filled alveoli causing hypoxemia. Additionally, the work of breathing will be increased due to surfactant dysfunction, reduced lung compliance, and increased airway resistance.

Pulmonary Emboli

Pulmonary emboli (PE) are clots from the systemic venous circulation that obstruct pulmonary arteries/arterioles. Therapists should recognize any sudden complaints of chest pain, dyspnea, and cough. Symptoms include tachypnea, tachycardia, and crackles via auscultation.[60] Risk factors include genetics/family history (eg, venothromboembolic disease, antithrombin III deficiency, increased factor VIII), recent surgery or trauma, bed rest and immobilization (eg, plane travel), pregnancy, and oral contraceptives.[60] Lab values such as PT/PTT or INR can also be reviewed for indicators of risk for PEs (see Chapter 2). Diagnosis is accomplished through V/Q scanning, pulmonary angiography, and spiral computed tomography. V/Q scans do not confirm or exclude PE, but provide an estimate of likelihood.[60] Prevention of deep vein thrombosis and PE are accomplished through prophylactic administration of heparin, pneumatic compression sleeves, and early mobilization.

Rib Fractures and Flail Chest

A **flail chest** is defined as two or three sequential ribs fractured in at least two places resulting in floating of the rib segment during inhalation or exhalation.[61] Flail chest results from blunt chest wall trauma (eg, motor vehicle accident). Complications are multifactorial and depend on the size of the flail segment and the associated damage to the lung parenchyma and other organs.[61] Hemothorax, blood in the pleural space, pneumothorax, and pulmonary contusions will contribute to V/Q mismatching, hypoxemia, and increased work of breathing. Patients complain of tremendous discomfort from rib fractures leading to altered breathing patterns and ineffective coughing with resultant retained secretions, atelectasis, and increased risk for pneumonia and respiratory failure. Physical therapy is consulted for airway clearance (deep breathing/incentive spirometry, effective coughing) and mobilization and must work closely with the medical team and patient for proper pain control (eg, intercostal nerve block, epidural analgesia).

Figure 7–17. Atelectasis due to obstruction. (Reprinted with permission from Sheldon LK. *Oxygenation.* Sudbury, Mass: Jones and Bartlett Publishers; 2001. Available at: www.jbpub. com.)

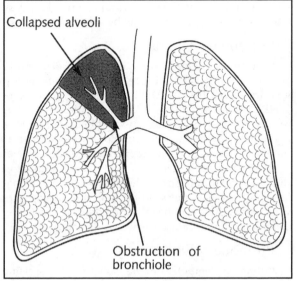

Collapsed alveoli

Obstruction of bronchiole

Atelectasis

Atelectasis is essentially "lung collapse" due to loss of air volume. Three types of atelectasis are described: absorption, compression, and contraction.[20,22] **Absorption atelectasis** occurs when ventilation is limited to a lung region and the air in the alveoli is absorbed and not replenished as described in Figure 7–17. Absorption atelectasis is common postsurgery and in disorders like CF where thick mucus occludes the airway. **Compression atelectasis** occurs when air or fluid occupies the pleural space. Examples include pleural effusion, pneumothorax, hemothorax, or tumor. **Contraction atelectasis** results from decreased pulmonary compliance that limits lung expansion and promotes lung collapse. This is observed in pulmonary fibrosis.[20]

Early mobilization, coughing, and deep breathing are critical to prevent atelectasis.

Pulmonary Hypertension

The pulmonary circulation is described as a high capacitance, low-pressure system and the normal right ventricle is a thin-walled, distensible chamber.[62,63] Pulmonary pressures can increase due to increased pulmonary vascular resistance or augmented flow.[13] Normally, however, pulmonary blood flow can increase three- to five-fold with minimal changes in pulmonary artery pressures because of recruitment and distension of the pulmonary vasculature.[64] **PH** is defined as a mean pulmonary artery pressure >25 mmHg at rest or >30 mmHg with exercise and typically results from increased pulmonary vascular resistance. PH is categorized into five subgroups:

1. Pulmonary arterial HTN (primary PH [PPH], collagen vascular disease, portal HTN, HIV infections, drugs/toxins, anorexic/diet drugs [fenfluramine], and congenital shunts)

2. Pulmonary venous HTN

3. PH associated with hypoxemia (hypoxic vasoconstriction)

4. PH related to chronic embolic/thrombotic disease

5. PH related to disorders impacting the pulmonary vasculature[65]

PH leads to vascular remodeling (medial hypertrophy, intimal proliferation and fibrosis and reduced lumen diameter) and loss of cross sectional area due to occlusion and obstruction of the vasculature.[13,62] These abnormalities increase the pulmonary vascular resistance creating a chronic pressure overload which may progress to RV dysfunction or cor pulmonale. **Cor pulmonale** denotes RV hypertrophy or dilatation due to lung or musculoskeletal pump pathology or impaired respiratory control (sleep apnea/hypoventilation syndrome).[62] Symptoms associated with PH are dyspnea, chest pain, dizziness, or syncope, but PH is generally asymptomatic until significant disease is noted.[62]

PPH is a rare phenomenon with no known cause.[65] The disease has a female predominance and usually manifests between 30 and 36 years old.[62] Prognosis and survival are poor if PPH remains untreated. **Secondary PH** is commonly associated with diseases that destroy the lung parenchyma and result in hypoxemia (eg, CF, COPD, and IPF) or occlude the pulmonary vasculature (eg, thromboembolic disease, PE).[66]

Treatment is aimed at selective vasodilation of the vascular bed (calcium channel blockers [eg, nifedipine, diltiazem], epoprostenol [flolan]), anticoagulation (eg, warfarin, heparin), and transplantation.[63] Patients are instructed to avoid extreme physical exertion, limit air travel (hypoxia at altitude), and use prescribed supplemental oxygen.

Sleep Apnea

Obstructive sleep apnea (OSA) affects thousands of patients each year in the United States and is the most common form of sleep-deprived breathing.[67] Four percent of the population is reported to suffer from this disorder.[68,69] OSA is associated with the development of systemic HTN, PH, congestive heart failure, dysrhythmias, insulin resistance, and CVAs.[67,68] Prevalence of OSA in HTN is approximately 50%, 30% in acute coronary syndromes, and as high as 60% in strokes.[67] Upwards of 25% of patients with heart failure have been reported having OSA.[67,70,71] OSA is characterized by episodes of partial or complete occlusion of the upper airway limiting ventilation, resulting in repetitive drops in oxygen saturation and fragmented sleep.[69] **Central sleep apnea** differs from OSA in that there is a periodic cessation of breathing with no respiratory effort, followed by hyperventilation.[67] The apnea-hypopnea index (AHI) refers to the number of obstructive events per hour and is used as a measure to quantify OSA.[67] An AHI range of five to 15 events per hour defines mild OSA and ≥30 events per hour classifies severe disease.

Recommended treatments include alcohol avoidance, weight loss in obese patients, and continuous positive airway pressure (CPAP) ventilation at night to brace the airways to improve ventilation.[67,68] Oral appliance and postural devices have not proven to be as effective as CPAP. Compliance remains a hurdle with CPAP due to poor fitting masks, skin and eye irritation, and complaints of claustrophobia.[67,72] Therapists should consider including simple questionnaires

Table 7–6
EPWORTH SLEEPINESS SCALE

Scale:	Score:
No chance of dozing	0
Slight	1
Moderate	2
High	3

Situation:
Sitting and reading
Watching TV
Sitting in an inactive place (movie theater)
As a passenger in a car without a break for an hour
Lying down to rest in the afternoon when the circumstances permit
Sitting and talking to someone
Sitting quietly after lunch without alcohol
In a car, while stopped for a few minutes

Total: ≤6 = Less tired than average
              7 to 8 = Average
              ≥9 = Tiredness requiring investigation

to screen for the presence of sleep apnea. The Epworth Sleep Scale is an easily administered standardized measure of tiredness and should be a standard evaluation tools of patients with HTN, obesity, CVA, and heart failure[67] (Table 7–6).

Lung Volume Reduction Surgery

Lung volume reduction surgery (LVRS) was a surgical technique developed in the 1950s for emphysema but abandoned for years because of poor outcomes.[73] The surgery reduces the size of the thorax through excision of diseased lung, enhancing elastic recoil and improving mechanical advantage of the diaphragm and improving pulmonary function (FEV_1, FVC, and PaO_2).[73] Patients report improved quality of life, reduction in dyspnea, and increased 6-minute walk distance. Currently, the surgical approach includes video-assisted thoracoscopic surgery (VATS), medial sternotomy, or thoracotomy. Approximately 20% to 30% of emphysematous lung is removed.[73,74] The National Emphysema Treatment Trial was a randomized, controlled trial developed to evaluate medical versus medical and surgical treatment in patients with symptom limiting emphysema.[75,76] All patients were required to undergo pulmonary rehabilitation prior to randomization, followed by maintenance rehabilitation. The surgical technique was either performed through a median sternotomy or via VATS. Survival and maximum exercise capacity were the two primary outcomes. Patients with distinct upper-lobe disease and low exercise capacity benefited the most from LVRS.[73] Mortality between the two study arms was similar, but the surgical group was more likely to have an improved quality of life and exercise performance.[73] LVRS has been used independent of lung transplantation, in conjunction with lung transplantation, and following lung transplantation.

Noninvasive Positive Pressure Ventilation

Noninvasive positive pressure ventilation (NPPV) is applied to patients with acute exacerbations of COPD and respiratory failure, patients with CF, neuromuscular diseases, chest wall deformities, and OSA due to high mortality rates with intubation.[77–80] NPPV is used to assist with weaning from invasive ventilation and as bridging therapy for patients awaiting lung transplantation.[81] Increased work of breathing, inspiratory muscle weakness, and fatigue are the final common denominators for acute respiratory failure. The suggested benefits of NPPV are improvements in gas exchange (decreased PCO_2, increased PaO_2) and decreased work of breathing. Other benefits include sleep efficiency, quality of life scores, and distance walked.[78–80,82] NPPV has also been used as an adjunct during exercise and pulmonary rehabilitation.[80] Claustrophobia, recent head and neck surgeries, poor appliance fit, poor adherence to medical therapy, inability to protect the airway from aspiration, and cognitive deficits are relative contraindications to NPPV.[80]

REHABILITATION OVERVIEW

Physical Therapy for the Pulmonary Patient/ Pulmonary Rehabilitation

Pulmonary rehabilitation is defined as a multidimensional continuum of services directed to persons with pulmonary disease and their families, usually by an interdisciplinary team of specialists, with the goal of achieving and maintaining the individual's maximal level of independence and functioning in the community.[83] Therapists are important members of the interdisciplinary team. Intervention for the patient diagnosed with either primary or secondary respiratory disease covers a broad spectrum of areas. Therapeutic interventions vary from positioning recommendations for the bed bound, medically paralyzed, mechanically ventilated individual to improving exercise capacity via ambulation or even treadmill walking following an uncomplicated LVRS.

The challenges in the acute care setting are two-fold: first to prevent the complications of immobility (see Chapter 4) and second to examine and intervene in specific aspects of respiratory impairments.

Functional progression and discharge from acute care are dependent on treating respiratory impairments and dysfunction like respiratory muscle weakness or retained sections with mobility, inspiratory muscle training (IMT), and aggressive airway clearance. Physical therapy issues related to any postsurgical patient such as pain, functional mobility in relation to surgical restrictions, and problem prevention such as pressure ulcers are also considered. The examination process (Table 7–7) will guide the physical therapist in determining appropriate intervention to meet these challenges.

Therapeutic Interventions

The physical therapist must be open-minded in development of therapeutic interventions for the patient with respiratory dysfunction. The examination

Table 7-7

PULMONARY SYSTEM EXAMINATION: LOOK, LISTEN, AND FEEL

Examination Technique	Description of Technique	Examination Findings in Common Diseases/ Disorders
Posture, chest configuration, extremities	• Observe head, shoulder/scapula position (descriptors [ie, rounded, forward, protracted, winged]) • Note ratio of anterior-posterior (A-P) chest wall to lateral costal (A-P should be smaller) • Describe shape of chest wall/thorax (pectus excavatum; pectus carinatum; barrel chest; kyphoscoliosis) • Observe any muscle wasting and/or hypertrophy (accessory muscles) • Observe fingers/toes for cyanosis and clubbing	↑ **A-P diameter/barrel chest deformity:** Hyperinflation/air trapping (eg, emphysema, asthma, cystic fibrosis, chronic bronchitis) ↑ **accessory muscle hypertrophy:** Chronic respiratory disease and respiratory distress **Digital clubbing/cyanosis:** May indicate hypoxemia, poor peripheral circulation (eg, emboli, PVD, Raynaud's, vasospasm)
RR	• Measure the RR while the patient is unaware of measurement • Patients may automatically change the breathing pattern and rate with observation • Observe the rise and fall of the chest; movement of the shoulders; accessory muscle use, etc for 15, 30, or 60 seconds and multiply accordingly • Document rate, depth, accessory muscle use, rhythm, and audible sounds	↑ **RR:** Respiratory distress/failure, restrictive lung disease (eg, IPF/pneumonia), exertion/ exercise ↓ **RR:** Respiratory muscle fatigue and pending failure
Respiratory/ breathing pattern	• Observe inhalation and exhalation pattern at rest and with activity • Determine duration of **inspiration to expiration (I:E ratio)** • Note presence or absence of accessory muscle usage, nasal flaring, excessive sighing, etc	**Normal I: E Ratio: 1: 2** ↑ **I: E Ratio:** Obstructive lung disease (eg, emphysema, chronic bronchitis, asthma flare)

Note specific patterns:

- **Tachypnea:** Rapid, shallow breathing
- **Cheyne-Stokes:** Ramping depth changes in V_T with an apneic period
- **Biot's:** Slow, saw-toothed motion of V_T that has apneic periods
- **Paradoxical:** Abdomen is drawn inward during inspiration
- **Kussmaul:** Progressive increase in rate and depth of inhalation

- **Supraclavicular/intercostals/substernal retractions:** Anatomical regions are drawn inward during inspiration

	Tachypnea: ILD (eg, IPF)
	Cheyne-Stokes: Critically ill
	Biot's: Meningitis
	Paradoxical: SCI, diaphragm paralysis, respiratory muscle fatigue/pending respiratory failure
	Retractions: Respiratory muscle fatigue/pending respiratory failure

Auscultation

Breath Sounds: Use diaphragm of stethoscope; warm and clean prior to use; instruct patient to take a large inhalation and relax on exhalation; if unfamiliar with landmarks for lobes/segments–document breath sound finding with external/surface landmarks; use systematic method for comparing lung regions side to side.

Normal Breath Sounds:

- **Bronchial:** Normal breath sound heard over the midsternum and between thoracic vertebrae 4–5 cephalad; abnormal if over other areas of lung fields indicative of consolidation; harsh sounding equal quality on inhalation and exhalation
- **Normal or vesicular** (inhalation > exhalation; should be soft, low pitched); listen away from sternal areas and spinous processes

Abnormal Breath Sounds:

- **Bronchial:** Consolidation/pneumonia/above pleural effusion

(continued)

Table 7-7 (continued)
PULMONARY SYSTEM EXAMINATION:
LOOK, LISTEN, AND FEEL

Examination Technique	Description of Technique	Examination Findings in Common Diseases/Disorders
	Bronchial vesicular heard over large airways between scapula and below clavicle, medium sound, inhalation = exhalation; no break in sound between inspiration and expiration	
	Abnormal breath sounds:	
	• **Decreased/diminished:** Heard with a low inspiratory volume or minimal air movement and/or hyperinflation	**Decreased/diminished:** COPD (emphysema/chronic bronchitis), asthma flare, pleural effusion, pneumothorax, PE, muscle guarding (eg, thoracic incision pain), stroke, SCI, obesity
	• **Crackles/rales:** Popping sound heard primarily on inhalation. Often associated with fluid filled alveoli	**Crackles/rales:** Atelectasis, pulmonary edema, CF/brochiectasis, chronic bronchitis, IPF, PE
	• **Rhonchi/wheezes:** Musical sounds heard on exhalation > inspiration	**Wheezes:** Airway obstruction due to inflammation or bronchospasm (eg, COPD/asthma)
	• **Stridor:** Heard on inhalation in larger airways; related inflammatory process narrowing airway or obstruction narrowing airway (removal of endotracheal tube)	**Stridor:** Upper airway obstruction, epiglottic interference (eg, food particle in airway/inflammation postextubation)

	• **Pleural friction rub:** Rough, leathery sound heard on inhalation/exhalation • **Egophony:** "e" to "a" changes heard over a consolidation • **Whispered pectoriloquy:** Whispered words that are clearer and possibly louder heard over a consolidation • **Bronchophony:** Spoken word is clear and distinct over a consolidation	**Pleural friction rub:** Pleural inflammation
Tactile fremitus	• Place hands on each segment of the lung fields to compare right to left and have the patient inspire deeply and exhale easily • Document areas of fremitus if present/absent • **Vocal fremitus** may be felt if hands in place during patient conversation	↑ **tactile fremitus:** Retained secretions (eg, chronic bronchitis, CF/bronchiectasis, pneumonia) ↓ **tactile fremitus:** Pneumothorax, pleural effusion
Tracheal position	• Facing patient, move fingertips along clavicle from distal to proximal • At the proximal point of the clavicle, have the patient relax the neck and look down; trachea should rest midpoint between index fingers/head of clavicles	**Tracheal deviation towards** affected side: Atelectasis **Tracheal deviation away** from affected side: Large pleural effusion, tension pneumothorax
Mediate percussion	• Flatten two or three fingers against the chest wall • Tap firmly with either your knuckle or two fingers of your opposite hand between the DIP and the MIP • If consolidation or over dense area (bone, pneumonia, etc) should hear a "thud/dull" type sound • If over an area with "air" should hear a resonating type sound	**Dullness:** Lung consolidation (eg, pneumonia), pleural effusion, pulmonary fibrosis, atelectasis **Hyperresonance:** Pneumothorax, hyperinflation—COPD/asthma exacerbation

(continued)

Table 7-7 (continued)
Pulmonary System Examination: Look, Listen, and Feel

Examination Technique	Description of Technique	Examination Findings in Common Diseases/Disorders
Chest wall motion/expansion	• **Anterior/posterior:** Place hands in a "w" shape position with the thumbs at intercostal spaces 6 or 7—midaxillary line; keep the hand that borders the posterior rib cage stable and allow the hand closest to the anterior rib cage to move with inhalation; ask the patient to inspire deeply; note change in distance between the two thumbs • **Lateral/costal:** Place hands in a "w" shape position with the thumbs under breast area anteriorly and repeat posteriorly at least two intercostal spaces below the angle of the scapulae • A pliable tape measure or calipers can also be used (note surface landmarks when charting)	→ **chest wall expansion:** Consolidation/pneumonia, pleural effusion, pneumothorax
Diaphragmatic excursion	• Place slightly curled fingers with tips of fingers under each side of the rib cage • Ask the patient to "sniff" quickly and forcefully • Therapist should palpate hemidiaphragm movement equal and bilateral • To test for posterior diaphragmatic excursion: Use either mediate percussion with deep inhalation and compare side to side	→ **diaphragm excursion:** Diaphragm weakness/fatigue, ascites, pregnancy • Diaphragm may ascend into thorax with inspiration if paralyzed

| **Cough** | Have the patient attempt a cough on demand or monitor a spontaneous cough during other parts of evaluation
• Listen for quality and effectiveness of cough: should have a deep inhalation, followed by a forceful exhalation
• Describe sound: wet, dry, nonproductive, ineffective
• Describe secretions: color, quantity (1/2 teaspoon, table-spoon, cup, etc), viscosity (stickiness), and odor | **Persistent productive:** Pneumonia, CF/bron-chiectasis, bronchitis
Persistent, nonproductive: Pulmonary fibro-sis, sarcoid, pneumonitis
Hemoptysis: Pulmonary infarct, bronchiecta-sis/CF, lung cancer, tuberculosis
Purulent sputum: Bacterial infection
Frothy sputum: CHF, pulmonary edema
Blood tinged sputum: Tracheal inflammation/"suction trauma," infection |
| **Pulse oximetry (SpO$_2$)** | • Disinfect probe prior to placing on patient
• Place probe on digit (finger or toe) if clothes pin type connec-tion or use disposable probe against the bridge of the nose, ear, or forehead (precaution if allergic to adhesive)
• Validate observed pulse with palpated pulse, electrocardio-gram, or on monitor (left ventricular assist device, intra-aortic balloon pump, etc)
• Determine device limitations/measurement error: Low perfu-sion states/cold extremities, motion artifact/ambient fluores-cent lighting, excessive hand grip, finger nail polish, etc | Normal SpO$_2$: >93%
Abnormal SpO$_2$: <93%; consider supplemen-tal oxygen if SpO$_2$ <89%. |

Adapted from:

Frownfelter D, Dean E. *Principles and Practice of Cardiopulmonary Physical Therapy.* St. Louis, Mo: Mosby-Year Book, Inc; 1996.

Hillegass EA, Sadowsky HS. *Essentials of Cardiopulmonary Physical Therapy.* 2nd ed. Philadelphia, Pa: WB Saunders Co; 2001.

Irwin S, Tecklin JS. *Cardiopulmonary Physical Therapy: A Guide to Practice.* 4th ed. St. Louis, Mo: Mosby Inc; 2004.

Perloff JK. *Physical Examination of the Heart and Circulation.* 3rd ed. Philadelphia, Pa: WB Saunders Co; 2000.

Reid WD, Chung F. *Clinical Management Notes and Case Histories in Cardiopulmonary Physical Therapy.* Thorofare, NJ: SLACK Incorporated; 2004.

Seidel HM, Ball JW, et al. *Mosby's Guide to Physical Examination.* St. Louis, Mo: Mosby, Inc; 2003.

Watchie J. *Cardiopulmonary Physical Therapy: A Clinical Manual.* Philadelphia, Pa: WB Saunders Co; 1995.

findings will direct the therapist, but because of the constant changes in physiologic, motivational, and emotional conditions, flexibility is key to the plan of care. Whether the patient is being mechanically ventilated in the ICU or participating in an inpatient pulmonary rehabilitation program, goals of therapeutic exercise are directed at maximizing patient participation with the intent of improving functional ability and ultimately quality of life.

There are no established guidelines on precisely where to begin with this patient. Initial interventions are directed at functional mobilization while monitoring hemodynamic response to activity (See Chapters 3 and 4). Interventions are often focused on the activities of bed mobility, transfers, and ambulation while simultaneously monitoring BP, HR, RR, SpO_2, and rating of perceived exertion (RPE). Task-specific activities such as stair climbing or even transfers from sit to stand can be easily fatiguing. How quickly and intensely to progress a patient is dependent on several factors: individual tolerance to activity, patient's goals and motivation, anticipated short-term functional outcomes, caregiver ability, environmental obstacles in the home setting, and resource capability. If the patient is medically stable for discharge, yet hospital-based functional goals have not been achieved, the recommendation is made for some level of continued physical therapy services. The patient with respiratory failure may require some level of inpatient rehabilitation at the time of medical discharge from the hospital.[84] Continued physical therapy is clearly indicated at the time of acute care discharge because of functional limitations and decreased aerobic capacity.

The profound impact of immobility and bed rest is well documented, and confinement to bed is a common treatment for patients with chronic disease and injury. In addition, bed rest, anesthesia, and surgical invasion of the chest wall diminish pulmonary function resulting in reduced tidal volumes, decreased respiratory muscle force production, limited gas flow rates (FEV_1 and FVC), increased pulmonary shunt, and development of atelectasis. Typical body positioning alone can be an effective means of enhancing oxygen transport via improving V/Q matching in the lung.[85]

Body Positioning

As noted in Chapter 4, body positioning and mobilization are important therapeutic interventions to prevent and alleviate respiratory complications. Body positioning and mobilization are effective means to augment oxygen transport and improve arterial oxygenation.[85,86] Evidence supports sidelying with the affected lung uppermost to improve oxygenation and promote resolution of atelectasis for individuals with unilateral disease.[87,88] Prone positioning is advocated for patients who present with hypoxemia refractory to other ventilatory strategies. Prone position in the ARDS populations has been shown to lead to substantial improvements in arterial oxygenation in approximately 65% of patients.[89,90] Although the individual response is variable, improvements in PaO_2 may allow reductions in mechanical ventilator settings including the F_iO_2 to lessen the impact of oxygen toxicity and barotrauma associated with ventilator induced lung injury. Patients with early stage ARDS are more likely to respond favorably to prone positioning than patients in the later fibrotic stage.[91]

Positioning may lead to improvements in PaO_2 through improved V/Q matching via redistribution of blood flow to previous atelectatic but nondiseased regions, enhanced ventilation uniformity, and reduced pulmonary vascular resistance of previously dependent lung regions.[85,86,92,93] Upright positioning can increase PEFRs promoting a more effective cough aiding secretion clearance and may augment diaphragm excursion enabling an increased IC.

Complications associated with positioning and mobilization include inadvertent removal of endotracheal tubes, accidental removal of central venous/ arterial catheters, hemodynamic instability, abdominal wound dehiscence, and skin breakdown.[94] However, with proper planning, observation, and ongoing monitoring, positioning, and mobilization are safe and potentially advantageous maneuvers for patients with respiratory disease.[92,95]

Breathing Exercises

Breathing exercises are typically employed to alter the patient's breathing pattern by modifying the rate, depth, or distribution of ventilation. Goals include increased alveolar ventilation with resultant increased oxygenation and reductions in CO_2, reduced sensation of dyspnea, and reduced work of breathing. The breathing strategies commonly administered include diaphragmatic breathing (breathing control), pursed-lip breathing, segmental breathing, and sustained maximal inspiration breathing exercises (incentive spirometry/thoracic expansion exercises).

Diaphragm Breathing

Diaphragmatic breathing, or **breathing control**, exercises attempt to enhance diaphragmatic motion throughout the respiratory cycle resulting in reduced accessory muscle usage and a more normalized breathing pattern. Few studies have examined the impact of breathing control in the acute care setting. However, a lack of evidence does not necessarily translate to a lack of effectiveness. For example, patients with advanced COPD recovering from respiratory failure who were instructed in diaphragmatic breathing demonstrated significant increases in oxygenation along with a decrease in carbon dioxide during the breathing exercise. However, they also showed reduced chest wall coordination, increased dyspnea, and were mechanically less efficient in their breathing.[96,97] These effects were demonstrated during the diaphragm breathing trial, and there was no carry-over effect. These studies demonstrate a transient physiologic benefit with diaphragm breathing at a substantial cost. Therefore, the physical therapist needs to determine the principle goal to be achieved via the application of the breathing exercise and to determine the effectiveness of their therapeutic intervention.

Pursed Lip Breathing

PLB is believed to increase positive pressure generated within the airways and buttress the small bronchioles preventing premature airway collapse. This stenting of the airways should promote effective expiration and potentially result in a reduced functional residual capacity. This breathing pattern significantly decreases the RR and increases the V_T improving alveolar ventilation and enhances the ventilation of previously underventilated area.[98] Although these results may not be universal, PLB appears to reduce RR and increase V_T thereby

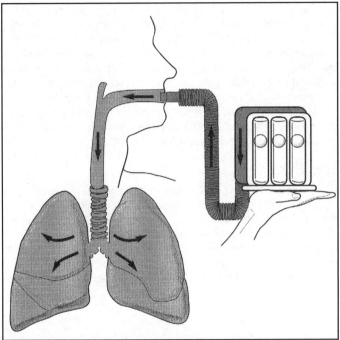

Figure 7–18. How to use an IS. (Reprinted with permission from Sheldon LK. *Oxygenation.* Sudbury, Mass: Jones and Bartlett Publishers; 2001. Available at: www.jbpub.com.)

not compromising MV. This breathing pattern is more cost effective from an energy standpoint and may reduce the work of breathing for select patients.

Segmental Breathing Exercises

Segmental breathing, also referred to as **localized expansion breathing**, assumes that inspired air can be directed to a specific area of lung by enhancing movement of the thorax overlying that lung region. Although limited research demonstrates the efficacy of these techniques, a recent study demonstrated that relative regional ventilation to the ipsilateral lung can be increased during a unilateral thoracic expansion exercise in trained individuals.[99] Various techniques have been promoted to augment regional ventilation including the use of proprioceptive neuromuscular facilitation, joint mobilization, and thoracic flexibility exercises. Anecdotally, enhanced chest wall motion, improved ventilation, increased aeration via auscultation, and more effective airway clearance have been noted as a result of these mobilization procedures.

Deep Breathing and Incentive Spirometry

An incentive spirometer (IS) is a device that encourages, through visual and/or audio feedback, the performance of reproducible, sustained maximal inspiration as noted in Figure 7–18. IS use is widely employed in the prophylaxis and treatment of respiratory complications in postsurgical patients.[100] IS and deep breathing are effective in the prevention of postoperative pulmonary complications after surgery in comparison to no physical therapy.[101] However, the current evidence does not support the routine use of IS following cardiac and abdominal surgery if these patient are engaged in physical therapy.[102–104] Physical therapy including PLB, huffing, coughing, and early mobilization has been demonstrated to improve oxygen saturation and reduce the incidence of postoperative pulmonary complication after major abdominal surgery.[105] Therefore, it is prudent all patients who are at risk for pulmonary complications should engage in an airway clearance and mobility regimen.

Inspiratory Muscle Training

Respiratory muscle dysfunction often a contributes to weaning failure and the need for prolonged mechanical ventilation. When the load placed on the musculoskeletal pump exceeds its capacity, ventilatory failure ensues.[106] Conditions that contribute to respiratory muscle dysfunction include metabolic abnormalities, sepsis, malnutrition, infection, electrolyte abnormalities (hypokalemia/hypomagnesemia), acid-base disturbances, phrenic nerve dysfunction, steroid administration, acquired neuromuscular dysfunction (steroid myopathy/critical illness myopathy and polyneuropathy), and disuse atrophy/deconditioning. Additionally, the patient in respiratory failure may present with an increased demand placed on the respiratory system due to airway obstruction (retained secretions, bronchospasm, inflammation), mechanical disadvantage (hyperinflation), reduced lung compliance (pulmonary edema/fibrosis), and decreased chest wall compliance (kyphoscoliosis/ankylosing spondylitis).[106–108]

Although IMT has been shown to increase the inspiratory muscle strength (maximal inspiratory pressure), reduce dyspnea, alter the breathing pattern, and increase exercise capacity and walking distance in patients with chronic lung disease, the implementation of this modality has not been widely used in the hospitalized or ventilator-dependent population.[109–111] Two recent studies have provided evidence that the inclusion of IMT for select patients with respiratory failure may promote successful liberation from mechanical ventilation after failed attempts at standard weaning procedures.[107,112] These studies utilized a threshold training device and emphasized a low repetition, high resistance exercise prescription.[112,113]

Range of Motion, Resistance Exercise, and Aerobic Exercises

Joint ROM for the prevention of contractures is important for any patient, particularly one whose mobility is limited and is receiving mechanical ventilation. Joint contractures and muscle tightness interfere with regaining functional mobility. Proper bed positioning, frequent turning and repositioning, use of splints and footboards, and encouragement of self-care activities supplement ROM exercises in preventing contractures. Physical constraints imposed by monitoring or life support equipment is one of the most difficult problems restricting the patient from carrying out ROM exercises. Restriction in specific joint movement occurs when mechanical ventilation tubing or IV/arterial lines, central venous pressure and pulmonary artery catheters, temporary cardiac pacemakers, traction devices, and renal dialysis cannulas are placed in arteries or veins close to involved joints (see Chapter 3).

Patients diagnosed with advanced lung disease and respiratory failure have often spent some time in the ICU, usually with an enforced bed rest. The sequelae on aerobic deconditioning and muscle atrophy and weakness (see Chapter 4) is well understood and must not be underestimated by the physical therapist.[114] Gravity alone may be sufficient resistance when initially prescribing an exercise program. Progression to manual resistance, isometric, and progressive resistance exercise (PRE) increases strength. Resistive exercise with rubberbands or weights can provide the patient with objective goals for strengthening as number of repetitions increases or band color changes.

Although aerobic training is an important intervention in the long-term management of individuals with chronic lung disease, classic aerobic conditioning has a limited role in the plan of care for the patient with acute respiratory insufficiency. The major aspects of conditioning for this population include activities aimed at improving mobility and ambulation in preparation for discharge to an acute rehabilitation facility, a skilled nursing facility, or home. Functional mobility training is normally paced with patient safety and destination after discharge in mind. Hospital-based goals are focused on independent mobility while improving aerobic capacity. The schedule for ambulation sessions must be coordinated with other activities such as bronchodilator medications and airway clearance that may reduce the work of breathing. Select patients, especially those who are functioning at a high level or were attending pulmonary rehabilitation prior to hospital admission, may benefit from use of exercise equipment including treadmills and bicycle ergometers.

Careful monitoring of the patient's vital signs, including oximetry, is imperative before, during, and after each therapy session. The most likely time of critical changes in respiratory and hemodynamic status occurs when the patient progresses from one stage of functional mobility to another, such as from supine to OOB sitting, then standing, then ambulating. The therapist must control the progression of ambulation to ensure the tolerance of one stage before a patient advances to the next.

Gait and transfer training can be performed with patients who require mechanical ventilation using a self-inflating anesthesia bag (AMBU bag) or portable ventilators with an attached oxygen source. This task is cumbersome, especially if the patient has difficulty ambulating because of weakness and balance dysfunction. Careful preparation and planning may include premedication for anxiety, airway clearance techniques including suctioning, a portable oxygen source, monitoring equipment such as an oxygen saturation and ECG monitor, assistive devices, a wheelchair, gait belt, extra tubing if on IV medications, portable suction unit for chest tubes, extra staff for guarding and transporting equipment, etc. The assistance of nursing, respiratory therapist, or an additional therapist will allow task completion. Few therapeutic interventions provide more positive feedback to the patient and medical team as walking the mechanically ventilated patient.

If ambulation, for whatever reason, is not a safe or effective means of mobility, then wheelchair propulsion should be considered because this can allow independence. When prescribing wheelchair activities, the therapist should

---

Table 7–8

CONCEPTS TO CONSIDER FOR CHOOSING
AN AIRWAY CLEARANCE TECHNIQUE

- Ongoing evaluation of initial treatment choice for effectiveness, efficiency, and adherence.
- Can the technique meet the goals of treatment without complication?
- Treatment can be done in any setting or disease state (mild to end-stage)?
- Technique can be performed with little to no assistance.
- Techniques should not fatigue the patient.
- Age and cognitive level of the individual must be considered.
- Comfort and time efficiency.
- Cost effective.
- Patient motivation.

Adapted from:
Hardy KA. A review of airway clearance: new techniques, indications, and recommendations. *Respiratory Care.* 1994;39(5):440–452.
Hardy KA, Anderson BD. Noninvasive clearance of airway secretions. *Respir Care Clin N Am.* 1996;2(2):323–345.

---

consider that UE activity imparts greater ventilatory and cardiovascular demand. This increased demand may warrant consideration of a power chair. Finally, the prescription, instruction, and performance of a home-based exercise program is an important goal for the acute care patient who will be directly discharged to home.

AIRWAY CLEARANCE IN THE ACUTE CARE SETTING

Airway clearance has been a mainstay in respiratory care for nearly 50 years.[14] Airway clearance can be as simple as assisting with a cough by splinting an incision to instruction in huffing maneuvers to performance of manual techniques such as percussion, vibration, shaking, or abdominal thrusts for spinal cord injured patients. Pulmonary complications associated with hospitalization are anticipated due to incisions, pain, chest tubes, fractures, effects of anesthesia or other medications, artificial airways, and/or muscular weakness and immobility. The primary purpose of airway clearance in the acute care setting is to mobilizing secretions improving ventilation and oxygenation. Mobilizing secretions and improving ventilation helps to prevent complications such as atelectasis and pneumonia that may prolong hospitalization. Additional benefits may include reduced work of breathing, improvements in ventilation/perfusion matching, and decreased dyspnea.[14]

The chest physical therapy or airway clearance technique administered will depend on the patient presentation and physical therapy examination findings as noted in Tables 7–7 and 7–8. Obviously, if the patient has an unstable fracture, coagulopathy, osteopenia/osteoporosis, or is hemodynamically compromised, the aggressiveness of the treatment will be tempered. Determining the degree and presumed anatomic locations of pulmonary abnormalities are keys to focusing treatment. Proper set up, timing, and administration of airway clearance techniques and medications and assistance with coughing or suctioning should be individualized.

Mobilizing secretions can be accomplished through deep breathing exercises, bronchial drainage positions, frequent repositioning, manual techniques, and early mobilization OOB including ambulation as noted in Table 7–9. Airway clearance techniques, especially manual techniques, have noted precautions, but airway clearance should not be contraindicated for the individual with retained secretions. The therapist will need to determine the most advantageous technique within the confines of the patient's presentation and comorbidities.

Bronchial or **postural** drainage refers to positioning the segment of the lung for gravity to assist secretion drainage. There is a specific position for each segment but precautions should be considered and modifications implemented as necessary. Trendelenberg, or head down positioning, should be avoided in patients with reflux disease or elevated intracranial pressures. Enteral feeding (tube feeds, gastrostomy [G] or jejunostomy [J] tubes; see Chapter 11) should be discontinued for at least an hour prior to positioning in bronchial drainage positions or vigorous manual and coughing maneuvers.

Percussion is a manual technique where the hand is "cupped" or small suction cup devices are used to transmit pressure waves through the chest wall to loosen airway secretions. A rhythmic pattern and a hollow type sound should be generated if the technique is performed correctly. A barrier should be placed between the patient's skin and the therapist's hand (eg, towel, gown). Precautions include osteopenia, osteoporosis, pain, coagulapathies, bronchospasm, and hemoptysis. Additionally, therapists should avoid percussing over bony prominences and the floating ribs.

Vibration and **shaking** are performed during the expiratory phase of respiration. These maneuvers aid the forward movement of secretions loosened by percussion and drainage positions. Vibration is a "fine" type movement whereas shaking is more vigorous. Precautions are similar to percussion.

Rib springing is an effective method to enhance ventilation, specifically inspiration. Using the respiratory sequence, a controlled thrust at the end of expiration enhances the volume of the next breath. This technique utilizes the muscle spindles of the intercostals to enhance muscular contraction. This technique is beneficial when the patient is unable to follow cues for taking a deep breath and enhances secretion clearance following percussion or vibration. Enhanced inspiratory efforts followed by expiratory maneuvers (eg, vibration, shaking, coughing/huffing/suctioning) will augment secretion movement based on the principles of collateral ventilation.

The therapist and patient are at risk for injury from repetitive movement, poor posture, and overzealous pressure during the maneuvers.

ISs are devices to practice deep breathing exercises. Visual cues provide feedback regarding inspiratory volumes. Typically, the patient is encouraged to use the IS devices hourly followed by coughing or huffing. Following inspiration, the breath is held, an inspiratory hold, which provides collateral ventilation via the pores of Kohn, Lamberts canals, etc. This technique is useful with alternative airway clearance techniques such as ACB and AD (see Table 7–9). IS can be combined with percussion, vibration, and drainage positions.

Table 7–9
Airway Clearance Techniques

Technique	Precautions
Percussion, vibration, shaking	Osteopenia/osteoporosis/bleeding disorders/ elevated intracranial pressure/spinal instability or hemodynamic instability; mechanical devices available; will need assistance to perform
Bronchial drainage (sometimes called postural drainage)	Gastric reflux/intracranial pressure/uncontrolled bleeding/spinal or hemodynamic instability
Forced expiratory technique	Easy to learn; precautions include control flow on exhalation to prevent bronchospasm/airway collapse
Autogenic drainage (AD)	Challenging to learn; patients may feel like they need to take deeper breaths
Active cycle of breathing (ACB)	Gastric reflux/intracranial pressure/uncontrolled bleeding/spinal or hemodynamic instability; if quite ill may need assistance to perform
Assistive/splinted coughing	Pain, osteopenia/osteoporosis/increased intracranial pressure/bleeding disorders/chest tubes/incisions/pain (see Table 7–10)
Suctioning	Dysrhythmias, hypoxia, vaso-vagal response, and bleeding (see Table 7–11)
Aerobic exercise	Modifications to exercise prescription must consider hemodynamics, respiratory status, psychologic factors, and clinical laboratory data
Positive expiratory pressure (PEP) devices (PEP Flutter[a], TheraPEP[b], Acapella[b], Quake[c], ThresholdPEP[d])	Positioning may alter efficacy of device (eg, flutter must be held upright)/patient's inability to generate correct expiratory pressure may impact efficacy of device (eg, TheraPEP requires 10 to 20 cm H_2O), cognitive impairments, avoid high pressure PEP due to risk of pneumothorax; claustrophobia with facemasks
High Frequency Chest Wall Oscillation (The Vest[e]; MedPulse System[f])	Must ensure proper fit—over lung not stomach/ bladder area, claustrophobia, bruising, and c/o discomfort or shortness of breath, dry mouth, hydration
Intrapulmonary Percussive Ventilator (Percussionaire[g])	Patient comfort, proper settings for delivery of medications

(continued)

Table 7–9   (continued)

AIRWAY CLEARANCE TECHNIQUES

Technique	Precautions
Cough assist[h]	Patient comfort, proper fit if artificial airway, may need assistance to set up, pneumothorax risk
PercussiveNeb[i]	Patient comfort, proper fit if artificial airway, may need assistance to set up, pneumothorax risk

[a] AxcanScandipharm Pharmaceutical Co
[b] DHD Health Care
[c] Thayer Medical
[d] HealthScan Products Inc
[e] Hill-ROM
[f] Electromed, Inc
[g] Percussionaire Corp
[h] JH Emerson Co
[i] Vortran Medical Technology 1, Inc

Adapted from:
Hardy KA. A review of airway clearance: new techniques, indications, and recommendations. *Respiratory Care.* 1994;39(5):440–452.
Hardy KA, Anderson BD. Noninvasive clearance of airway secretions. *Respir Care Clin N Am.* 1996;2(2):323–345.
Pruitt B, Jacobs M. Clearing away pulmonary secretions. *Nursing.* 2005;July:37–41.

Alternative airway clearance techniques are valuable in the acute care setting. These techniques include high frequency chest wall compression or oscillation (HFCWO), PEP devices, AD, and ACB (see Table 7–9). HFCWO has been administered in the ICU and hospital ward as an alternative to standard CPT. This device utilizes airway vibration to break up mucus and alters airflow to create "mini-coughs" that move the secretions toward the trachea. Vests should be individually sized, checked for proper fit, and the skin should be inspected for redness after treatment. Frequency is set to mobilize mucus peripherally to the more central airways. In theory, lower frequency settings (5 to 10 Hz) loosen secretions in the periphery with higher frequency ranges mobilizing secretions cephalad (10 to 15 Hz and 15 to 20 Hz). Pressure in the vest should be set by type of vest used (chest versus full vest) and patient comfort. Less than 5 is recommended for the chest vest and greater than 4 is recommended for the full size vest. Patients may complain of chest wall soreness, claustrophobia, dry mouth, and fatigue. A cotton blend shirt or other barrier should be placed between the patient's skin and the vest.

Use of PEP devices depends on the patient's ability to control the breathing pattern, maintain a good seal with the mouthpiece or face mask, and generate sufficient positive pressure for benefit of the device. There are several devices available in the United States including Therapep, Threshold Pep, Acapella,

Flutter, and Quake. The patient typically generates 10 to 15 mmHg of pressure for 5 to 10 seconds to recruit collateral ventilation and mobilize secretions. Some of the devices require the patient to generate a set flow rate, volume, pressure, and are dependent on position to be beneficial. Advantages of the PEP devices are that they are simple to learn, portable, give feedback, and in some cases are even fun. If the patient is obtunded, unable to follow directions, or requires physical assistance, PEP devices are not as beneficial as the more traditional forms of chest physical therapy or HFCWO.

AD and ACB may be difficult to initiate during an acute exacerbation because they require high levels of concentration and control of the breathing pattern. These techniques may be modified to complement segmental breathing exercises and manual techniques and improve breathing control. However, if the patient is highly anxious or unable to master the proper sequence of the breathing pattern, if the breathing pattern is too shallow or if the patients expirations are too short or obstructed, positioning and adherence to the traditional, more passive techniques (eg, percussion, vibration, high frequency chest wall oscillations) are usually recommended.

Secretion Removal

Once the secretions are mobilized they must be removed by coughing or by suctioning if the cough is ineffective. The cough sequence is logical: the patient must inhale a large volume of air, the glottis must close, a pressure gradient is created between the abdominal and thoracic cavities, and then the glottis must open with sequential contraction of the abdominal muscles causing the forceful expulsion of air.[14] The phases and effectiveness of the cough can be impacted by pain, muscle weakness, poor coordination of the sequence, incisions, chest tubes, positioning, patient cognition or alertness, artificial airways, etc. Therapists must determine which phase of the cough is impairing effective secretion removal and direct interventions to elicit a favorable outcome (eg, incision pain will limit deep inspiration; therefore, proper pain medication and pillow splinting will improve cough). A tracheal tickle is a noninvasive tool to stimulate a stronger cough. Brief pressure is applied inward and upward with the therapist's thumb just above the sternal notch and a neurogenic cough is stimulated. A tracheal tickle should be applied cautiously or avoided in children, patients with bleeding disorders, or in the presence of tracheal stenosis or malacia. This procedure should only be performed following proper demonstration and mentoring. Common assisted cough techniques are described in Table 7–10.

Suctioning is an excellent way to stimulate a cough or directly remove retained secretions. However, suctioning is an invasive procedure and may cause airway trauma, hypoxia, dysrhythmias, or a vasovagal responses (eg, bradycardia, hypotension). Suctioning should be the last intervention chosen instead of the first to assist with mucus clearance unless the airway and oxygenation are severely compromised (Table 7–11). Preoxygenation, sterile technique, proper negative pressure, duration of suctioning, catheter size, length of catheter, and catheter placement should be considered whether the patient is intubated (orally, nasally, or via a tracheostomy) or if the technique is performed blindly. Mentoring of new staff is important for proper technique.

Table 7–10
ASSISTED COUGH TECHNIQUES

Splinted cough	Used to support incision area. Patient or therapist braces the incision using a pillow, blanket, or extended hand while the patient attempts a cough. Gentle pressure is applied for bracing only.
"Quad cough" (abdominal thrust)*	Similar to Heimlich maneuver used in cardiopulmonary resuscitation (CPR). As the patient attempts a cough, the heel of the therapist's hand is thrust inward and upward above the umbilicus but below the xiphoid process. The upward thrust must be coordinated with the patient's expiration/cough. If the patient is intubated, suctioning should occur with the abdominal thrust. If the patient has a recent incision, a blanket or a towel can be used to apply pressure instead of a "heel thrust." The blanket or towel is held taunt across the abdominal area on the "cough" acting as a "brace" for the abdominal cavity during the cough cycle.
Combined "quad cough" and thoracic bracing	Use the hand/heel thrust as described in "quad" cough combined with a downward pressure across the upper anterior rib cage with the other forearm (mid to upper sternal area). There is a downward motion toward the upward thrusting hand/heel on exhalation. This should be done only when timed with an attempted cough by the patient. Precautions include fractured ribs, central lines (eg, pulmonary artery catheter [PAC], central venous pressure [CVP], dialysis ports), osteopenia/osteoporosis, innervated abdominals, and bleeding disorders.
Thoracic splinting combined with cough	Used with patients with intact spinal cord. As the patient coughs, the therapist applies firm pressure to the chest wall and can even vibrate during the cough. Thoracic splinting is coordinated with the patient's exhalation/cough.
Bilateral rib compression	Can be used with intact spinal cord. The therapist places hands on each side of the thoracic rib cage but avoids floating ribs. As the patient inspires/expires and out, the therapist gets in sequence with the patient's rib cage movements. Ask the patient to cough, and on exhalation, the therapist brings his or her hands downward and inward augmenting the movement of the rib cage. Timing is key and the therapist should practice having the patient inhale and exhale.

(continued)

Table 7–10 (continued)

ASSISTED COUGH TECHNIQUES

Cough combined with airway clearance techniques	An assistive cough can be facilitated using any of the following airway clearance techniques: vibration, shaking, PEP devices (PEP, Flutter[a], TheraPEP[b] Acapella[b] Quake[c] ThresholdPEP[d], high frequency chest wall oscillation (The Vest[e]; the therapist can either apply the "pressure" (vibration/shaking) on exhalation/cough or the patient can be instructed to "forcefully huff or cough" into the device (PEP, Flutter[a], TheraPEP[b], Acapella[b], Quake[c], ThresholdPEP[d]). HFCWO is also beneficial to perform an "assistive" cough maneuver to help brace the rib cage.
Positioning	Optimize the patient's position to enhance the cough phases: inspiration-extension of the trunk and neck, rib springing/PNF techniques; expiration–trunk and neck flexion; expiratory flow rates are increased with upright positioning.
Precautions	All assisted coughs require caution. The physical therapy examination should identify comorbidities that would modify patient positioning and the technique chosen (eg, osteopenia/osteoporosis, recent thoracic and/or abdominal surgeries, agitation, thoracic and abdominal innervation, feeding tubes/timing of supplemental feeds, corticosteroids, bleeding disorders, pain, intercranial pressure [ICP]).

[a] AxcanScandipharm Pharmaceutical Co
[b] DHD Health Care
[c] Thayer Medical
[d] HealthScan Products Inc
[e] Hill-ROM

*Pruitt B, Jacobs M. Clearing away pulmonary secretions. *Nursing.* 2005;July:37–41.

Adapted from:
Frownfelter D, Dean E. *Principles and Practice of Cardiopulmonary Physical Therapy.* St. Louis, Mo: Mosby-Year Book, Inc; 1996.
Hillegass EA, Sadowsky HS. *Essentials of Cardiopulmonary Physical Therapy.* 2nd ed. Philadelphia, Pa: WB Saunders Co; 2001.

CASE STUDY

Mrs. Andrews is a 75-year-old (y/o), right-handed woman admitted with complaints of (c/o) SOB and pain in her right hip and arm following a fall earlier today at her home. She was evaluated in the emergency department and admitted to the orthopedic service with a right hip fracture (fx) requiring open

Table 7–11

ENDOTRACHEAL SUCTIONING (VIA ARTIFICIAL AIRWAY)

Evaluate patient for ineffective cough/inability to clear secretions (auscultate lung fields):

1. Explain rationale and procedure to patient.
2. Prepare sterile work area for suctioning. Gloves, catheter, and saline (if used). Size of catheter, length of catheter should be determined by the size of endotracheal tube, size of patient, and amount/thickness of secretions.
3. Preoxygenate using 100% F_iO_2 prior to, during, and following airway suctioning.
4. Visually measure length of catheter for depth of insertion not to exceed carina (use Angle of Louis as visual landmark or second rib).
5. Insert sterile catheter until resistance is felt; withdraw 1 cm, and apply suction no longer then 8 to 10 seconds at a pressure of 80 to 100 mmHg as catheter is withdrawn from airway. (Recommend therapist hold breath to simulate patient's breath hold during suctioning.)
6. Repeat cycle depending on volume of secretions and patient's hemodynamic and respiratory responses, and note time to recovery to baseline status.
7. Document procedure, secretion color/viscosity/amount, patient hemodynamic response, any adverse reactions, and recommendations for follow-up sessions.

Considerations and precautions:

- Sterile instilled (2 to 3 cc's) saline may be beneficial for cough stimulation. Some evidence relates that instilled saline may lead to increased pulmonary infections. Use instilled saline cautiously.
- Universal precautions (goggles/ gloves/gown if indicated).

Observe for:

- Frank, red blood (hemoptysis)
- Prolonged bronchospasm or wheeze
- Dysrhythmias associated with decreased oxygen
- Vasovagal response with insertion of catheter (bradycardia, hypotension)
- Elevated blood pressure
- Transient or prolonged decline in oxygenation
- Recovery/return to baseline of VS

reduction internal fixation(ORIF), right upper extremity (RUE) radius fx that was treated by casting. Physical therapy was consulted for evaluation and treatment postoperative day 1.

Patient/Client History

General Demographics/Social History/Living Environment

Mrs. Andrews is a retired paralegal and has been married for 51 years. She lives in a two-story home with five steps to enter and a handrail. The bedroom and full bathroom are on the second floor and a half bath is on the first floor. She does not drive, but her husband is 79 and continues to drive.

General Health Status/Family History

Mrs. Andrews is overweight with a body mass index (BMI) of 38. She quit smoking 3 years ago when she was diagnosed with COPD but admits to smoking two packs per day for more than 35 years. She states she enjoys two cocktails with dinner each night, and she does not participate in any type of exercise routine. Her hobbies include playing bridge on Thursday and canasta on Saturday. She and her husband have two grown children that live locally and five grandchildren. Her family history is unremarkable.

Medical/Surgical History

Mrs. Andrews is diagnosed with oxygen dependent (2 L/minute via nasal cannula) COPD, HTN, osteoporosis, and is moderately obese. She takes Metoproplol (a beta blocker) for HTN, 7.5 mg of prednisone every other day, and uses an Albuterol inhaler 2 puffs twice a day.

Current Conditions/Chief Complaints

Mrs. Andrews c/o SOB and pain on any movement in bed. Her chest roentgenogram is suspicious for RML pneumonia. Mrs. Andrews has a Foley catheter in place for urination and to monitor output volume. She is receiving 2 liters of oxygen (O_2) via nasal cannula and has received some pain medication for 7 out of 10 pain with any movement. Her activity status is OOB as tolerated, nonweightbearing (NWB) on her right lower extremity (RLE) and partial weightbearing on RUE.

Functional Status and Activity Level

Prior to admission, Mrs. Andrews was independent with ambulation with a cane on all surfaces and ADLs. She reports she can walk around the house, but more than one block is "pushing it." She reports needing minimal assistance with IADLs such as housecleaning and food shopping. Her husband also assists with some household tasks, and they both are retired.

Systems Review

Cardiovascular/Pulmonary

Resting vital signs in supine (head of bed raised >30 degrees) are oxygen saturation (SpO_2) 93% on 2 liters via nasal cannula, RR 22, HR 110, BP 108/60, rating of perceived exertion (RPE) 2 (modified Borg Scale), and obvious accessory muscle use. In sitting Mrs. Andrews's vital signs were SpO_2 89% on 2 liters, RR 24, HR 120, BP 156/88, RPE 5, and continued accessory muscle use. Mrs. Andrews was allowed to rest and provided emotional support. Her vital signs (VS) returned to baseline after 10 minutes. While sitting IS was practiced with Mrs. Andrews only achieving 400 mL with three trials. A transfer was attempted from bed to an elevated chair. Maximal (max) assistance was required of two. Her vital signs following the transfer were SpO_2 86% on 3 liters, RR 30, HR 132, RPE 7, BP 186/92, and continued accessory muscle use. Again, her VS returned to baseline after 10 minutes. Her breath sounds were distant bilaterally and absent in the area under her right axilla. Mrs. Andrews practiced the IS and performed ankle pumps and ADLs (ie, washed her face and hands) in the elevated chair prior to transfer back to bed. She was able to sit out in the chair for 35 minutes total. ABGs on 3 liters were pH $7.34/PCO_2$ $52/PO_2$ $62/HCO_3$-32 the morning of her evaluation.

Integumentary

Mrs. Andrews was placed on a pressure-relieving, low air-loss mattress. She has been wearing pneumatic compression stockings on BLE (bilateral lower extremities) since her surgery. Her surgical wound site is not visualized secondary to the dressing. Her right forearm has some bruising areas and her skin appears quite dry.

Musculoskeletal

Gross myotome assessment of left upper extremity (LUE) and left lower extremity (LLE) reveals strength of 4/5 in all major muscle groups. Mrs. Andrews is unable to lift her RUE cast without assistance and unable to flex or abduct her RLE without assistance. AROM appears grossly within normal limits (WNL) for LUE and LLE. Her RLE was not formally assessed secondary to pain with motion and RUE limited to angle of cast and length of cast.

Neuromuscular

Sensation to light touch and gross proprioception were intact LUE/LLE and RLE.

Communication, Affect, Cognition, Language, and Learning Style

Mrs. Andrews is awake, alert, and oriented to person, place, and time. She reports feeling anxious about moving because of the fear of pain. Her primary language is English.

Tests and Measures

Aerobic Capacity and Endurance

As noted above, the patient demonstrated HTN and tachycardia with moderate drop in oxygen saturation and increase in accessory muscle use and RR. Her ABGs suggest respiratory acidosis.

Assistive and Adaptive Devices

Patient performed a stand-pivot with maximal assistance of two therapists. A bedside commode has been ordered with an elevated seat as well as a long-handled reacher.

Gait, Locomotion, and Balance

Mrs. Andrews required max assistance of two for transfer sitting on the edge of the bed and stand-pivot to chair. Gait assessment was held due to HTN, tachycardia, and oxygen desaturtion accompanied by c/o pain and SOB.

Pain

The patient reports 8 out of 10 on a 0–10 visual analog scale for pain with any movement of RLE. Rest and elevation relieve pain.

Evaluation

The patient is an older, frail female currently hospitalized secondary to a fall resulting in a femoral neck fracture, ORIF, a humeral fracture s/p cast, and a possible RML pneumonia. PMHx is remarkable for HTN, COPD, osteoporosis, and obesity.

Diagnosis

The patient presents with mobility impairments related primarily to pain with movement secondary to her fx's, impaired pulmonary function, impaired gas exchange, and increased work of breathing related to her airflow obstruction (ie, COPD) and possible RML pneumonia. Recommended treatment pattern: 6F, impaired ventilation and respiration/gas exchange associated with respiratory failure.[115]

Prognosis

Complete healing of femoral fracture (s/p ORIF) and radius fracture should allow return to previous functional mobility but most likely with the need of a different assistive device from admission. The patient will require acute inpatient rehabilitation (or a lower intensity program) upon discharge from the hospital based on current mobility deficits, pain, her challenging home environment, and the limited assistance her husband can provide. Her SOB, pain, tachycardia, anxiety, risks for falls, and possible pneumonia will slow her functional progression.

Intervention

Daily physical therapy intervention with short-term goals of increasing OOB tolerance and decreasing level of assistance required for bedside mobilization are appropriate for this patient. In addition to these functional goals, optimizing cough effectiveness and mobilizing secretions are fundamental for progressing with function. Improving her breathing pattern related to COPD and early mobilization to decrease effects of bed rest will also enhance airway clearance. Manual techniques should be utilized with caution due to the risk for rib fractures from potential steroid-induced osteopenia. Airway clearance will focus on deep breathing exercises, effective coughing, and mobilization. Her rapid shallow breathing pattern is expected and instruction in PLB and pacing during bed mobility, transfers, and gait training will decrease work of breathing as well as normalize the breathing pattern. Pain control and position changes may increase her inspiratory abilities to augment effective coughing. Interventions included ADL and functional training, assistive and adaptive device training, and therapeutic exercise. Additionally, patient education will continue including the use of pain medication prior to therapy sessions, skin integrity, IS, weightbearing restriction, bedside ROM exercise program, and the importance of airway clearance.

Reexamination

Reexamination after three treatment sessions revealed the same level of assistance for transfers OOB and continued tachycardia and HTN, but she maintained her SpO$_2$ >91% on 2 l pm. Complaints of SOB decreased (Borg scale = 4 with activity) and pain was reported to be 5 to 6 on the scale after receiving pain medication 45 minutes prior to the therapy session. The physical therapist recommended two "short" therapy sessions with getting OOB with the nurses at least one other time during the day with progressing OOB time to >2 hours.

Outcomes

Mrs. Andrews was seen by the acute physical therapy service for 7 days after the initial physical therapy exam at which point she was transferred to a skilled nursing facility. She continued using her oxygen, but the Foley catheter was discontinued, and she was transferring onto the elevated bedside commode with moderate assistance of 2. Pain and anti-anxiety medication continued to be required prior to OOB activities. The patient required moderate assistance of two for all transfers due to her difficulty with using the RUE. Once standing and her RUE was placed in the "cuff" of the rolling platform walker, she could ambulate 10 feet x 2 with moderate assistance of one. SOB, anxiety, and pain continued to limit her functional progression but was improving as noted by rating pain and SOB 1 at rest and 3 with mobility. Her RML pneumonia responded to antibiotics and airway clearance.

CHAPTER REVIEW QUESTIONS

1. Name two types of pulmonary complications following surgery.
2. What is the difference between pleural effusion and pulmonary edema?
3. Name two types of assisted cough techniques and potential patient populations that these techniques would be applied.
4. What is MV, and how does the MV change with exercise performance?
5. What is the difference between a restrictive and an obstructive pulmonary pattern as measured by pulmonary function testing?

PHARMACOLOGICAL INFORMATION: PULMONARY DISEASES AND DISORDERS PHARMACOLOGY

Medications that Promote Bronchodilation

Adrenergic Agents/Beta Agonists/Sympathomimetics/ Combination[15,16,116–120]

Action

Adrenergic agents stimulate the beta adrenergic receptors in the bronchial smooth muscle (beta$_2$ receptors) resulting in increased levels of cyclic adenosine monophosphate (cAMP). CAMP causes smooth muscle relaxation as well as inhibition of inflammatory mediator release (eg, mast cells); steroid combination incorporates alternate anti-inflammatory mechanisms; beta agonists are used chiefly as aerosol inhalants with oral and IV applications available; first line bronchodilator for acute events.

Side Effects

CNS: Muscle tremor; headaches; anxiety, dizziness, hyperactivity
CV: Tachycardia, HTN, dysrhythmias, palpitations;
GI: Nausea, heartburn, bad taste
Misc: Muscle cramps, increased mortality related to overuse of short-acting beta agonists in asthma, spacers, and reservoir devices helpful
Pulm: Increased bronchial hyperresponsive on methacholine challenge with regular use of beta 2 agonists

Common Medications

Metaproterenal sulfate (Alupent), Albuterol (Proventil, Ventolin), Salmeterol (Serevent), Pirbuterol (Maxair), Terbutaline (Brethaire), Bitolterol (Tornalate), Ephedrine, Epinephrine (Adrenalin), Racemic Epinephrine (MicroNefrin), Isoproterenol (Isuprel), Isotharine (Brokosol)
Combination: Advair Diskus (fluticasone propionate and salmeterol)
Anticholinergic Agents/Combination[15,54,117,118,120,121]

Action

Anticholinergic agents facilitate bronchodilation by decreasing acetylcholine activity. Normally, parasympathetic activation and acetylcholine release promote bronchial smooth muscle contraction. Additionally these agents may reduce bronchial secretions. Anticholinergic agents reduces intracellular concentration of cyclic guanosine monophosphate (cyclic GMP) leading to decreased calcium release from the sarcoplasmic reticulum and smooth muscle relaxation.

Side Effects

CNS: Blurred vision, confusion, dizziness, nervousness, headache
CV: Tachycardia, palpitations, cough, HTN, chest pain
GI: Dry mouth, constipation, GI upset

Misc: Reduce sputum volume without changing viscosity
Common Medications
Ipratropium bromide (Atrovent); glycopyrrolate (Robinul)

Methylxanthines[15,16,54,117–119,121–123]

Action
Xanthine derivatives (similar to caffeine) promote bronchodilation through smooth muscle relaxation. Proposed mechanisms include elevations of cAMP by inhibition of phosphodiesterase (an enzyme that breaks down cAMP), antagonisms of adenosine, enhanced release of catecholamines, and inhibition of prostaglandins. Methylxanthines also may have anti-inflammatory effects in airways and may augment respiratory muscle function and respiratory drive.

Side Effects
CNS: Tremors, headaches, insomnia, neuromuscular irritability, seizures, nervousness, fever
CV: Tachycardia, dysrhythmias, hypotension, palpitations
GI: Vomiting, nausea, hyperglycemia, hypokalemia
Misc: Narrow therapeutic range (5 to 15 µg/mL) leading to risk of toxicity

Common Medications
Theophylline (Theobid, Theolair, Theo-Dur, Slo-phyllin), Aminophylline (Phyllcontin), Oxtriphylline (Coedyl)

Medications for Treatment of Airway Inflammation

Cromolyn Sodium[15,16,54,116–119,121,122,124,125]

Action
Cromolyn sodium prevent inflammation of airway by inhibiting release of inflammatory mediators in respiratory mucosa and stabilize mast cells.

Side Effects
CNS: Dizziness, headache
GI: Nausea, abdominal pain, esophagitis, bad taste
Misc: Anaphylaxis; can be used alone or in combination with bronchodilators and anti-inflammatory steroids
Pulm: Transient cough

Common Medications
Cromolyn (Intal, Nasalcrom)

Leukotriene Modifiers[15,16,54,116–119,121,122,124,125]

Action
Leukotriene modifiers have two main actions: inhibition of leukotriene formation or antagonism of leukotriene receptors. Leukotrienes are phospholipid inflammatory mediators synthesized from arachodonic acid that promote bronchoconstriction and mucus production.

Side Effects
CNS: Headaches
CV: Cough
GI: Nausea, abdominal pain
Misc: Hepatotoxicity, useful in treatment of aspirin-intolerance in asthma

Common Medications
Zileuton (Zyflo), Zafirlukast (Accolate), Montelukast (Singulair), Pranlukast (Onon)

Corticosteroids[15,16,54,116–119,121,122,124,125]

Action
Corticosteroids are medications that inhibit inflammatory and immunologic processes. These agents are postulated to decrease the synthesis and release of a variety of mediators (eg, prostaglandins, leukotrienes, histamine) within lymphocytes, eosinophils, neutrophils, and mast cells.

Side Effects
CNS: Depression, euphoria, headache, restlessness
CV: HTN
Endocrine: Hyperglycemia
GI: Peptic ulcers, nausea, vomiting
Misc: Osteoporosis, myopathy, weight gain, skin fragility/tears, immuno-suppression, fluid retention/edema, cushingoid appearance (moonface/buffalo hump)

Common Medications
Beclomethasone (Beclovent, Vanceril), Fluticasone (Flovent), Methylpred-nisolone (Medrol), Prednisone (Prednisone, Deltasone), Prednisolone (Prelone), Budesonide (Pulmicort), Triamcinolone (Azmacort), Flunisolide (AeroBid)

Smoking Cessation Drugs[54,117,121]

Action
These agents replace nicotine by providing an influx of nicotine to help diminish cravings: nicotine receptor agonists, nicotine receptor blockers, and nonnicotine receptor agents. (Bupropion may potetiate effects of dopamine and norephrine in brain). Delivered via patch, gum, lozenge, nasal spray, and inhalers.

Side Effects
CNS: Mild headache, insomnia, dream abnormalities, dizziness
CV: Angina, dysrhythmias (avoid if recent myocardial infarction or CVA)
GI: Nausea, vomiting, anorexia, excessive salivation
Misc: Recommend counseling and social support to improve success rate, skin irritation with patch, avoid if skin sensitivities to adhesive, combination therapy now available

Common Medications
Bupropion (Zyban), Nicotine Polacrilex (Nicorette), mecamylamine (Inversine), fluoxetine (Prozac)

Medications Specific for Respiratory Secretions

Mucolytics[15,16,117,119,121]

Action
Mucolytics decrease viscosity of mucus and promote expectoration by various mechanisms. For example, pulmonary infections and secretions attract leukocytes that degenerate, releasing large volumes of DNA. N-Acetylcystein (Mucomyst) lyses mucus proteins, and Pulmozyme (DNAse) assists in the clearance of airway DNA, decreasing airway obstruction.

Side Effects
CNS: Dizziness, headache
CV: Tachycardia, hypo or HTN, chest pain
GI: Irritation of mouth and throat, nausea, vomiting
Misc: rhDNAse not proven efficacious with COPD and chronic bronchitis
Pulm: Bronchospasm, mucosal irritation, cough

Common Medications
Recombinant human deoxyribonuclease I/Dornase alfa (rhDNAse/Pulmozyme), N-Acetylcysteine (Mucomyst, Mucosil)

Expectorants[16,117,119,121,123]

Action
Expectorants facilitate mucous clearance and increase secretion of airway water, thin sputum in upper respiratory tract.

Side Effects
CNS: Dizziness, headache
GI: Diarrhea, nausea, vomiting, stomach pain
Misc: Rash

Common Medications
Guaifenesin (Anti-Tuss; Humibid)

Antitussives[16,117,119,121,123]

Action
Antitussives bind at opiate receptor site in the CNS suppressing the cough reflex. Additionally, these agents may provide pain relief.

Side Effects
CNS: Suppression of cough reflex, sedation, drowsiness, lethargy, anxiety, dysphoria, mood changes, blurred vision
CV: Hypotension, bradycardia orthostatic hypotension risk with injection, chest tightness

GI: Constipation, nausea and vomiting
Pulm: Respiratory depression

Common Medications
Hydromorphone hydrochloride (Dilaudid), Hydrocodone polistirex (Tussionex)

Neuromuscular Blocking Agents[116–119,121]

Action
Neuromuscular blocking agents impede or prevent transmission at the neuromuscular junction resulting in paralysis. Two classes are depolarizing agents or nondepolarizing agents.

Depolarizing agents react with receptors at muscle end-plate and results in overstimulation, so that the end-plate is unable to respond to further excitation. Prolonged exposure reduces receptor sensitivity manifested as flaccid paralysis. Often used for intubation.

Nondepolarizing/competitive agents bind at the muscle end-plate's acetylcholine receptors resulting in a competitive, reversible blockade. These agents inhibit excitation potentials at end-plate preventing the motor unit from reaching threshold.

Side Effects
CNS: Agents do not affect sensorium (agents are not anesthetics/analgesics), individuals are conscious and can feel pain
CV: Bradycardia, hypotension
GI: Increased gastric pressure with abdominal fasciculations
Misc: Prolonged paralysis/myopathy (associated with co-administration of corticosteroids/antibiotics/sedatives), hyperkalemia with depolarizing agents, antibiotics (eg, aminoglycosides, macrolides)
Pulm: Apnea, increased airway secretions, bronchoconstriction

Common Medications
Non-depolarizing: d-Tubocurarine (Tubarine), Vecuronium (Norcuron), Pancuronium (Pavulon), Atracurium (Tacrium)
Depolarizing: Succinylcholine (Anectine, Sucostrin)

Oxygen[119]

Action
Oxygen delivered in a higher concentration elevates alveolar oxygen tension, thereby increasing arterial oxygen content and PaO_2 to improve peripheral tissue oxygenation. Corrects hypoxemia.

Side Effects
CNS: May depress respiratory drive in carbon dioxide (CO_2) retainers (eg, patients with advanced COPD)
Pulm: Oxygen toxicity/pulmonary fibrosis, atelectasis

REFERENCES

1. Kochanek KD, Smith BL. Deaths: preliminary data for 2002. *National Vital Statistics Reports.* 2004;52(13):1–48.
2. Hospital Inpatient Statistics, 1996. HCUP-3 Research Note. Agency for Health Care Policy and Research, Rockville, Md. Available at: http://www.ahrq.gov/data/his96/clinclas.htm.
3. Petty TL. Scope of the COPD problem in North America: early studies of prevalence and NHANES III data: basis for early identification and intervention. *Chest.* 2000;117:326S–331S.
4. Mannino DM, Homo DM, Akinbami LJ, Ford ES, Redd SC. Chronic obstructive pulmonary disease surveillance—United States, 1971–2000. *MMWR Surveill Summ.* 2002;51(6):1–6.
5. Garcia-Aymerich J, Farrero E, Felez MA, Izquierdo J, Marrades RM, Anto JM. Risk factors of readmission to hospital for a copd exacerbation: a prospective study. *Thorax.* 2003;58:100–105.
6. van Schayck CP, Loozen JMC, Wagena E, Akkermans RP, Wesseling GJ. Detectin patients at a high risk of developing chronic obstructive pulmonary disease in general practice: cross sectional case finding study. *BMJ.* 2002;324:1370.
7. Stang P, Lydick E, Silberman C, Kempel A, Keating ET. The prevalence of COPD: using smoking rates to estimate disease frequency in the general population. *Chest.* 2000;117:354S–359S.
8. West JB. *Respiratory Physiology—The Essentials.* 3rd ed. Baltimore, Md: Williams & Wilkins; 1985.
9. Crystal RG, West JB, Barnes PJ, et al. *The Lung: Scientific Foundations.* New York, NY: Raven Press, Ltd; 1991.
10. West JB. *Pulmonary Pathophysiology—The Essentials.* 3rd ed. Baltimore, Md: Williams & Wilkins; 1987.
11. Cohen M, Michel TH. *Cardiopulmonary Symptoms in Physical Therapy Practice.* New York, NY: Churchill Livingstone; 1988.
12. Toews GB. Host defense. In: Albert RK, Spiro SG, Jett JR, eds. *Comprehensive Respiratory Medicine.* Harcourt Brace and Co. 1999.
13. Rubin E, Farber JL. The respiratory system. In: Rubin E, Farber JL, eds. *Essential Pathology.* 2nd ed. Philadelphia, Pa: JB Lippincott Co; 1995.
14. Frownfelter D, Dean E. *Principles and Practice of Cardiopulmonary Physical Therapy.* 3rd ed. Philadelphia, Pa: Mosby; 1996.
15. Watchie J. *Cardiopulmonary Physical Therapy: A Clinical Manual.* Philadelphia, Pa: WB Saunders Co; 1995.
16. Des Jardins T. *Clinical Manifestations of Respiratory Disease.* 2nd ed. Chicago, Ill: Year Book Medical Publishers, Inc; 1990.
17. Celli BR. Standards for the optimal management of COPD: a summary. *Chest.* 1998;113:283S–287S.
18. Clini E, Costi S, Lodi S, Rossi G. Non-pharmacological treatment of chronic obstructive pulmonary disease. *Med Sci Monit.* 2003;9(12):RA300–RA305.
19. Hajiro T, Nishimura K, Tsukino M, Ikeda A, Oga T, Izumi T. A comparison of the level of dyspnea vs disease severity I indicating the health-related quality of life of patients with COPD. *Chest.* 1999;116:1632–1637.
20. Bullock BA, Henze RL. *Focus on Pathophysiology.* Philadelphia, Pa: Lippincott Williams & Wilkins; 2000.
21. Pannettieri RA. Chronic obstructive pulmonary disease. In: Grippi MA, ed. *Pulmonary Pathophysiology.* Philadelphia, Pa: JB Lippincott Co; 1995.

22. Corwin EJ. *Handbook of Pathophysiology.* 2nd ed. Philadelphia, Pa: Lippincott Williams & Wilkins; 2000.

23. Fraser KL, Tullis E, Sasson Z, Hyland RH, Thornley KS, Hanly PJ. Pulmonary hypertension and cardiac function in adult cystic fibrosis. *Chest.* 1999;115: 1321–1328.

24. Brenckmann C, Papaioannou A, Freitag A, et al. Osteoporosis in Canadian adult cystic fibrosis patients: a descriptive study. *BMC Musculoskeletal Disorders.* 2003;4:13.

25. Sood N, Paradowski LJ, Yankaskas JR. Outcomes of intensive care unit care in adults with cystic fibrosis. *Am J Respir Crit Care Med.* 2001;163:335–338.

26. Boehler A. Update on cystic fibrosis: selected aspects related to lung transplantation. *Swiss Med Wkly.* 2003;133:111–117.

27. Cordier JF. Update on cryptogenic organizing pneumonia (idiopathic bronchiolitis obliterans organizing pneumonia). *Swiss Med Wkly.* 2002; 132:588–591.

28. Husain SJ, Irfan M, Zubairi AS, Salahuddin N. Rapidly-progressive bronchiolitis obliterans organizing pneumonia. *Singapore Med J.* 2004;45(6): 283–285.

29. Nagai S, Izumi T. Bronchiolitis obliterans with organizing pneumonia. *Curr Opin Pulm Med.* 1996;2(5):419–423.

30. Chapman HA. Disorders of lung matrix remodeling. *J Clin Invest.* 2004; 113(2):148–157.

31. Keller CA, Cagle PT, Brown RW, Noon G, Frost AE. Bronchiolitis obliterans in receipients of single, double, and heart-lung transplantation. *Chest.* 1995;107:973–980.

32. Bando K, Paradis IL, Similo S, et al. Obliterative bronchiolitis after lung and heart-lung transplantation: an analysis of risk factors and management. *J Thoracic Cardiovasc Surg.* 1995;110:4–14.

33. Husain AN, Siddiqui MT, Holmes EW, et al. Analysis of risk factors for the development of bronchiolilitis obliterans syndrome. *Am J Respir Crit Care Med.* 1999;159:829–833.

34. Raghu G. Interstitial lung disease—a clinical overview and general approach. In: Fishman AP, Elias JA, Fishman JA, Grippi MA, Kaiser LR, Senior RM, eds. *Fishman's Pulmonary Diseases and Disorders.* 3rd ed. New York, NY: McGraw-Hill; 1998.

35. Lynch JP, Toews GB. Idiopathic pulmonary fibrosis. In: Fishman AP, Elias JA, Fishman JA, Grippi MA, Kaiser LR, Senior RM, eds. *Fishman's Pulmonary Diseases and Disorders.* 3rd ed. New York, NY: McGraw-Hill; 1998.

36. Britton J. Idiopathic pulmonary fibrosis. In: Albert RK, Spiro SG, Jett JR, eds. *Comprehensive Respiratory Medicine.* Harcourt Brace and Co; 1999.

37. Moller DR. Sarcoidosis. In: Albert RK, Spiro SG, Jett JR, eds. *Comprehensive Respiratory Medicine.* Harcourt Brace and Co; 1999.

38. Cagatay T, Bilir M, Gulbaran M, Papila C, Cagatay P. The immunoglobulin and complement levels in the active pulmonary sarcoidosis. *Kobe J Med Sci.* 2003;49(5):99–106.

39. Ryu JH, Doerr CH, Fisher SD, Olsen EJ, Sahn SA. Chylothorax in lymphangioleiomyomatosis. *Chest.* 2003;123:623–627.

40. King TE, Crausman RS. Pulmonary lymphangioleiomyomatosis. In: Fishman AP, Elias JA, Fishman JA, Grippi MA, Kaiser LR, Senior RM, eds. *Fishman's Pulmonary Diseases and Disorders.* 3rd ed. New York, NY: McGraw-Hill; 1998.

41. Boughton WA, Bass JB. Tuberculosis and disease caused by atypical myocbacteria. In: Albert RK, Spiro SG, Jett JR, eds. *Comprehensive Respiratory Medicine.* Harcourt Brace and Co; 1999.

42. Onorato EM, Ridzon R. The epidemiology, transmission, and prevention of tuberculosis in the United States. In: Fishman AP, Elias JA, Fishman JA, Grippi MA, Kaiser LR, Senior RM, eds. *Fishman's Pulmonary Diseases and Disorders.* 3rd ed. New York, NY: McGraw-Hill; 1998.

43. Pillaye J, Clarke A. An evaluation of completeness of tuberculosis notification in the United Kingdom. *BMC Public Health.* 2003;3(1):31.

44. Dannenberg AM, Tmashefski JF. Pathogenesis of pulmonary tuberculosis. In: Fishman AP, Elias JA, Fishman JA, Grippi MA, Kaiser LR, Senior RM, eds. *Fishman's Pulmonary Diseases and Disorders.* 3rd ed. New York, NY: McGraw-Hill; 1998.

45. Lanken PN. Pathophysiology of respiratory failure. In: Grippi MA, ed. *Pulmonary Pathophysiology.* Philadelphia, Pa: JB Lippincott Co; 1995.

46. MacIntyre NR. Respiratory mechanics in the patient who is weaning from the ventilator. *Respir Care.* 2005;50(2):275–284.

47. Hutter DA, Holland BK, Ashtyani H. The effect of body mass index on outcomes of patients receiving noninvasive positive-pressure ventilation in acute respiratory failure. *Respir Care.* 2004;49(11):1320–1325.

48. Gattinoni L, Pelosi P, Brazzi L, Valenza F. Acute Respiratory Distress Syndrome. In: Albert RK, Spiro SG, Jett JR, eds. *Comprehensive Respiratory Medicine.* Harcourt Brace and Co; 1999.

49. Bernard GR, Artigas A, Brigham KL, et al. The American-European Consensus Conference on ARDS: definitions, mechanisms, relevant outcomes, and clinical trial coordination. *Am J Resp Crit Care Med.* 1994;149:818–824.

50. Ware LB, Matthay MA. The acute respiratory distress syndrome. *N Engl J Med.* 2000;342(18):1334–1349.

51. American Lung Association. Available at: http://www.lungusa.org. Accessed on April 2, 2006.

52. Roach HD, Davies GF, Attanoos R, Crane M, Adams H, Phillips S. Asbestos: when the dust settles-an imaging review of asbestos-related disease. *RadioGraphics.* 2002;22:S167–S184.

53. Jett JR. Malignant mesothelioma. In: Albert RK, Spiro SG, Jett JR, eds. *Comprehensive Respiratory Medicine.* Harcourt Brace and Co; 1999.

54. Hodgkin JE, Celli BR, Connors GL, eds. *Pulmonary Rehabilitation: Guidelines to Success.* 3rd ed. Philadelphia, Pa: Lippincott Williams & Wilkins; 2000.

55. Bach JR. *Pulmonary Rehabilitation: The Obstructive and Paralytic Conditions.* Philadelphia, Pa: Hanley & Belfus, Inc; 1996.

56. Prakash ES, Madanmohan. When the heart is stopped for good: hypotension-bradycardia paradox revisited. *Adv Physiol Educ.* 2005;29:15–20.

57. Vanderschueren R. Pneumothorax. In: Albert RK, Spiro SG, Jett JR, eds. *Comprehensive Respiratory Medicine.* Harcourt Brace and Co; 1999.

58. Peters JI, Sako EY. Pneumothorax. In: Fishman AP, Elias JA, Fishman JA, Grippi MA, Kaiser LR, Senior RM, eds. *Fishman's Pulmonary Diseases and Disorders.* 3rd ed. New York, NY: McGraw-Hill; 1998.

59. Schuster DP. Pulmonary edema. In: Fishman AP, Elias JA, Fishman JA, Grippi MA, Kaiser LR, Senior RM, eds. *Fishman's Pulmonary Diseases and Disorders.* 3rd ed. New York, NY: McGraw-Hill; 1998.

60. Herold CJ, Bankier AA, Burghuber OC, Minar E, Watzke HH. Pulmonary embolism. In: Albert RK, Spiro SG, Jett JR, eds. *Comprehensive Respiratory Medicine.* Harcourt Brace and Co; 1999.

61. Davignon K, Kwo J, Bigatello LM. Pathophysiology and management of the flail chest. *Minerva Anestesiol.* 2004 Apr; 70(4):193–9.

62. Fishman AP. Pulmonary hypertension and cor pulmonale. In: Fishman AP, Elias JA, Fishman JA, Grippi MA, Kaiser LR, Senior RM, eds. *Fishman's Pulmonary Diseases and Disorders.* 3rd ed. New York, NY: McGraw-Hill; 1998.

63. Via G, Braschi A. Pathophysiology of severe pulmonary hypertension in the critically ill patient. *Minerva Anestesiol.* 2004;70(4):233–237.

64. Jones A, Evans T. Pulmonary hypertension. In: Albert RK, Spiro SG, Jett JR, eds. *Comprehensive Respiratory Medicine.* Harcourt Brace and Co; 1999.

65. Sulica R, Poon M. Current medical treatment of pulmonary arterial hypertension. *Mt Sinai J Med.* 2004;71(2):103–114.

66. Vizza CD, Lynch JP, Ochoa LL, Richardson G, Trulock EP. Right and left ventricular dysfunction in patients with severe pulmonary disease. *Chest.* 1998;113:576–583.

67. Lattimore JDL, Celermajer DS, Wilcox I. Obstructive sleep apnea and cardiovascular disease. *J Am Coll Cardiol.* 2003;41:1429–1437.

68. Ferguson KA, Ono R, Lowe AA, Keenan SP, Fleetham JA. A randomized crossover study of an oral appliance vs nasal-continuous positive airway pressure in the treatment of mild-moderate obstructive sleep apnea. *Chest.* 1996;109:1269–1275.

69. Mayer P, Dematteis M, Pepin JL, Wuyam B, Veale D, Vila A, Levy P. Peripheral neuropathy in sleep apnea: a tissue marker of the severity of nocturnal desaturation. *Am J Respir Crit Care Med.* 1999;159:213–219.

70. Javaheri S. Effects of continuous positive pressure on sleep apnea and ventricular irritability in patients with heart failure. *Circulation.* 2000;101:392–397.

71. Tkacova R, Rankin F, Fitzgerald FS, Floras JS, Bradely TD. Effects of continuous positive airway pressure on obstructive sleep apnea and left ventricular afterload in patients with heart failure. *Circulation.* 1998;98:2269–2275.

72. Jokic R, Limaszewski A, Crossley M, Sridhar G, Fitzpatrick MF. Positional treatment vs continuous positive pressure airway pressure in patients with positional obstructive sleep apnea syndrome. *Chest.* 1999;115:771–781.

73. Benditt JO. Surgical therapies for chronic obstructive pulmonary disease. *Respir Care.* 2004;49(1):53–61.

74. Gelb AF, McKenna RJ, Brenner M, Epstein JD, Zamel N. Lung function 5 yr after lung volume reduction surgery for emphysema. *Am J Respir Crit Care Med.* 2001;163:1562–1566.

75. The National Emphysema Treatment Trial Research Group. Rationale and design of the national emphysema treatment trial: a prospective randomized trial of lung volume reduction surgery. *Chest.* 1999;116:1750–1761.

76. Mohsenifar Z, Lee SM, Diaz P, Criner G, Sciurba F, Ginsburg M, Wise RA. Single-breath diffusing capacity of the lung for carbon monoxide. *Chest.* 2003;123:1394–1400.

77. Clark HE, Wilcox PG. Noninvasive positive pressure ventilation in acute respiratory failure of chronic obstructive pulmonary disease. *Lung.* 1997;175:143–154.

78. Plant PK, Owen JL, Elliott MW. Non-invasive ventilation in acute exacerbations of chronic obstructive pulmonary disease: long term survival and predictors of in-hospital outcome. *Thorax.* 2001;56:708–712.

79. Anton A, Guell R, Gomez J, et al. Predicting the result of noninvasive ventilation in severe acute exacerbations of patients with chronic airflow limitation. *Chest.* 2000;117:828–833.

80. Hill NS. Noninvasive ventilation for chronic obstructive pulmonary disease. *Respir Care.* 2004;49(1):72–87.

81. Hamm H, Luterbacher T, Matthys H. Noninvasive ventilation in respiratory insufficiency. Indications-methods-limits. *Fortschr Med.* 1997;115(16):52–55.

82. Wijkstra PJ, Lacasse Y, Guyatt GH, et al. A meta-analysis of nocturnal non-invasive positive pressure ventilation in patients with stable copd. *Chest.* 2003;124:337–343.

83. Fishman AP. Pulmonary rehabilitation research. *Am J Respir Crit Care Med* 1994;149(3[Pt 1]):825–833.

84. Stewart DG, Drake DF, Robertson C, Marwitz JH, Kreutzer JS, Cifu I. Benefits of an inpatient pulmonary rehabilitation program: a prospective analysis. *Arch Phys Med Rehabil.* 2001;82(3):347–352.

85. Ross J, Dean E. Integrating physiologic principles into the comprehensive management of cardiopulmonary dysfunction. *Phys Ther.* 1989;69(4):255–259.

86. Stiller K. Physiotherapy in intensive care: towards an evidence-based practice. *Chest.* 2000;118:1801–1813.

87. Ibanez J, Raurich JM, Abizanda R, et al. The effect of lateral positions on gas exchange in patients with unilateral lung disease during mechanical ventilation. *Intensive Care Med.* 1981;7:231–234.

88. Stiller K, Jenkins S, Grant R, et al. Acute lobar atelectasis: a comparison of five physiotherapy regimens. *Physiother Theory Pract.* 1996;12:197–209.

89. Stocker R, Neff T, Stein S, et al. Prone positioning and low-volume pressure-limited ventilation improve survival in patients with severe ARDS. *Chest.* 1997;111:1008–1017.

90. Pelosi P, Tubiolo D, Mascheroni D, et al. Effects of the prone position on respiratory mechanics and gas exchange during acute lung injury. *Am J Respir Crit Care Med.* 1998;157:387–393.

91. Nakos G, Tsanagaris I, Kostanti E, et al. Effect of the prone position on patients with hydrostatic pulmonary edema compared with patients with acute respiratory distress syndrome and pulmonary fibrosis. *Am J Respir Crit Care Med.* 2000;161:360–368.

92. Pappert D, Rossaint R, Slama K, et al. Influence of positioning on ventilation-perfusion relationships in severe adult respiratory distress syndrome. *Chest.* 1994;106:1511–1516.

93. Mure M, Lindhal S. Prone position improves gas exchange, but how? *Acta Anaesthesil Scand.* 2001;45:150–159.

94. Offner PJ, Haenal JB, Moore EE, et al. Complications of prone ventilation in patient with multisystem trauma with fulminant acute respiratory distress syndrome. *J Trauma.* 2000;48:224–228.

95. Beiburg A, Aitken L, Reaby L, et al. Efficacy and safety of prone positioning for patients with acute respiratory distress syndrome. *J Adv Nurs.* 2000;32:922–929.

96. Gosselink RA, Wagenaar RC, Rijswijk H, et al. Diaphragmatic breathing reduces efficiency of breathing in patients with chronic obstructive pulmonary disease. *Am J Respir Crit Care Med.* 1995;151:1136–1142.

97. Vitacca M, Clini E, Bianchi L, Ambrosino N. Acute effects of deep diaphragmatic breathing in COPD patients with chronic respiratory insufficiency. *Eur Respir J.* 1998;11:408–415.

98. Thoman RL, Stoker GL, Ross JC. The efficacy of pursed lips breathing in patients with chronic obstructive pulmonary disease. *Am Rev Respir Dis.* 1966;93:100.

99. Tucker B, Jenkins, Cheong D, et al. Effect of unilateral breathing exercises on regional lung ventilation. *Nucl Med Commun.* 1999;20:815–821.

100. O'Donohue WJ. National survey into the use of the usage of lung expansion modalities for the prevention and treatment of postoperative atelectasis following abdominal and thoracici surgery. *Chest.* 1985;87:76–80.

101. Thomas JA, McIntosh JM. Are incentive sprirometry, intermittent positive pressure breathing, and deep breathing exercises effective in the prevention of postoperative pulmonary complications after upper abdominal surgery? A systematic overview and meta-analysis. *Phys Ther.* 1994;74:3–10.

102. Gosselink R, Schrever K, et al. Incentive spirometry does not enhance recovery after thoracic surgery. *Critical Care Medicine.* 2000;28:679–683.

103. Overend TJ, Anderson CM, Lucy SD, et al. The effect of incentive spirometry on postoperative pulmonary complications: a systematic review. *Chest.* 2001;120:971–978.
104. Crowe JM, Bradley CA. The effectiveness of incentive spirometry with physical therapy for high-risk patients after coronary artery bypass surgery. *Phys Ther.* 1997;77:260–268.
105. Oslen MF, Hahn I, Nordgren S, et al. Randomized controlled trial of prophylactic chest physiotherapy in major abdominal surgery *Br J Surg.* 1997;84:1535–1538.
106. Polkey MI, Moxham J. Clinical aspects of respiratory muscles dysfunction in the critically ill. *Chest.* 2001;119:926–929.
107. Sprague SS, Hopkins PD. Use of inspiratory strength training to wean six patients who were ventilator dependent. *Physical Therapy.* 2003;83:171–181.
108. Reid WD, Dechman G. Considerations when testing and training the respiratory muscles. *Phys Ther.* 1995;75:971–982.
109. Sturdy G, Hillman D, Green D, et al. Feasibility of high-intensity, interval based respiratory muscle training in COPD. *Chest.* 2003;123:142–150.
110. Koessler W, Wanke T, Winkler G, et al. 2 years experience with inspiratory muscle training in patients with neuromuscular disorders. *Chest.* 2001;120:765–769.
111. Sanchez RH, Montemayor RT, Ortega RF, et al. Inspiratory muscle training in patients with COPD: effect on dyspnea, exercise performance, and quality of life. *Chest.* 2001;120:748–756.
112. Martin DA, Davenport PD, Franceschi AC, et al. Use of inspiratory muscle strength training to facilitate ventilatory weaning: a series of 10 consecutive patients. *Chest.* 2002;122:192–196.
113. Johnson JL, Cowley AJ, Kinnear WJ. Evaluation of the THRESHOLD trainer for inspiratory muscle endurance training: comparison with the weighted plunger method. *Eur Resp J.* 1996;9:2681–2684.
114. Convertino VA, Bloomfield SA, Greenleaf JE. An overview of the issues: physiological effects of bedrest and restricted physical activity. *Med Sci Sports Exerc.* 1997;29(2):187–190.
115. Guide to Physical Therapy Practice. 2nd ed. *Physical Therapy.* 2001;81(1).
116. Jacob LS. *Pharmacology.* 4th ed. Philadelphia, Pa: Williams & Wilkins; 1996.
117. *Nursing 2004 Drug Handbook.* 24th ed. Springhouse, Pa: Lippincott Williams & Wilkins; 2004.
118. Casaburi R, Petty TL, eds. *Principles and Practice of Pulmonary Rehabilitation.* Philadelphia, Pa: WB Saunders Co; 1993.
119. Hillegass E, Sadowsky HS. *Essentials of Cardiopulmonary Physical Therapy.* 2nd ed. Philadelphia, Pa: WB Saunders Co; 2001.
120. *Physicians' Desk Reference.* 57th ed. Montvale, NJ: Thomason PDR; 2003.
121. DeTurk WE, Cahalin LP. *Cardiovascular and Pulmonary Physical Therapy: An Evidence-Based Approach.* New York, NY: McGraw-Hill; 2004.
122. Kallsrom TJ. Evidence-based asthma management. *Respir Care.* 2004;49(7):783–792.
123. Hodgson BB, Kizior RJ, eds. *Saunders Nursing Drug Handbook 2005.* St. Louis, Mo: Elsevier Saunders; 2005.
124. Dahlen B. Treatment of aspirin-intolerant asthma with antileukotrienes. *Am J Respir Crit Care Med.* 2000;161:S137–S141.
125. Claesson HE, Dahlen SE. Asthma and leukotrienes: antileukotrienes as novel anti-asthmatic drugs. *J Intern Med.* 1999;245(3):205–227.

Musculoskeletal/ Orthopedic Diseases and Disorders

Joseph Adler, MS, PT

The hospital-based, or acute care, physical therapist who treats orthopedic patients will work, primarily, with these main conditions: degenerative joint disease, spine pathology, and acute fracture related to trauma and its sequelae. The physical therapist responsible for the examination, intervention, and physical therapy plan of care of the patient with orthopedic pathology must be familiar with several important and common issues such as weightbearing and range of motion (ROM) restrictions, surgeon-specific activity protocols, and how to gait-train a patient with multiple fractures, as well as appropriate indications for orthotic devices. Because the acute care orthopedic patient frequently requires assistive and adaptive equipment as well as specialized education in mobility and ambulation, the physical therapist plays a vital role in the multidisciplinary team management of the patient with acute musculoskeletal dysfunction.

Elective Surgery

Protocols for postoperative orthopedic management often vary with different surgeons. When to initiate ROM activities, how much weightbearing is allowed and when, or if braces may be removed are all examples of surgeon-specific protocols encountered by the acute care therapist. Prior to mobilizing the post-operative patient, the physical therapist should be confident that activity status and restrictions are documented and orders clarified.

Primary, or first time, total joint replacements are often progressed along institutional guidelines or clinical pathways.[1-3] Guideline or pathway outcomes center on decreasing length of stay, decreasing cost, and improving function while mandating clinical activity such as number of times per day physical therapy intervention should occur and what milestones are expected on a given postoperative day. Although the average length of stay has decreased over the past decade for elective joint replacements,[4] the evidenced-based literature provides inconsistent data on the impact of these guidelines on total cost and

Table 8–1

LOWER EXTREMITY JOINT ARTHROPLASTY

	Knee Arthroplasty	Hip Arthroplasty
Primary diagnostic indications	• OA • RA • Post-traumatic arthritis	• OA • RA • Post-traumatic arthritis • Proximal hip fracture 　○ *Hemi*arthroplasty indicated
Surgical approach	• Anterior	• Posterolateral • Anterolateral • Two incisions 　○ "Minimally invasive"
Hardware	• Cobalt chrome femoral component • Metal-backed polyethelene tibial component	• Metallic femoral stem/head • Polyethelene acetabular liner
Acute care physical therapy	• Early mobilization • ROM • Education 　○ Weightbearing 　○ Gait • CPM 　○ Monitor 　○ Progress • Discharge planning	• Early mobilization • Gentle strengthening • Education 　○ Hip precautions 　○ Weightbearing 　○ Gait • Discharge planning

function at the time of discharge from the hospital.[5-7] The physical therapist may be required to document outcomes such as distance walked or ROM on special forms that become part of the medical record.

The most common joint replacements performed are **total knee arthroplasties (TKA)** and **total hip arthroplasties (THA)**. According to the American Academy of Orthopedic Surgeons (AAOS) over 260,000 TKAs and 168,000 THAs are performed annually in the United States.[8] Long-term increase in arthritic pain, decline in physical function, and lack of response to conservative management are the primary reasons degenerative joints are replaced.[9] The degenerative process could be inflammatory as in rheumatoid arthritis (RA), non-inflammatory as in osteoarthritis (OA), or related to post-traumatic arthritis as noted in Table 8–1.

RA is an autoimmune, polyarticular disease process of unknown etiology that targets the synovial membrane. The synovium hypertrophies, causing joint effusions, ligamentous damage, and eventual joint destruction. Episodes of relapse and remission are common. It is estimated between 1 and 3 million persons are affected with RA worldwide.[10]

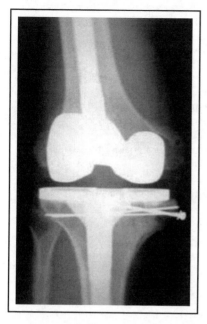

Figure 8–1. Total knee arthroplasty performed for hemophiliac arthropathy with medial tibial structural autograft and press-fit stems. (Reprinted with permission from Canale ST. *Campbell's Operative Orthopaedics.* 10th ed. St. Louis, Mo: Mosby Inc; 2003.)

OA tends to be more prevalent in individuals over 50 years of age, directly affects articular cartilage, and may be caused by either mechanical or biochemical factors. Traumatic injuries that affect joint integrity or ligamentous structures (often with accompanying vascular damage) are a cause of joint replacements. Although the predisposing conditions are different, physical therapy approach to acute TKA remains basically the same, but therapists may anticipate greater challenges in early mobilization in patients with RA if multiple joints are involved.

Total Knee Arthroplasty (Figure 8–1)

Postoperative, hospital-based physical therapy intervention focuses on early mobilization, functional training, ROM, and discharge planning. Clinically relevant issues are whether or not unilateral or bilateral replacements have been performed,[11–13] whether a clinical pathway exists and, in some institutions, management of the **continuous passive motion (CPM)** machine. Early, full weightbearing, with an assistive device, is to be expected although postoperative pain can be a limiting factor. The physical therapist can anticipate collaboration with the surgical and nursing staff whose primary acute care goals are prevention **of deep vein thromboses (DVT), pulmonary emboli (PE),** and infection, as well as reduction of swelling and pain.[4,9]

The use of a CPM machine during the immediate postoperative acute care phase is common, and the physical therapist may play an important role in the set-up, progression, and management of the device. The degrees of motion and when to increase those values are generally physician prescribed or protocol driven. CPM usage often provides early benefits of increased ROM, particularly in the absence of similar time availability of a therapist. Since greater knee ROM presumably provides greater functional ability, CPM may also impact hospital

Table 8–2

PHYSICAL THERAPY AND KNEE ARTHROPLASTY

Summary:
- Generally physical therapy begins postoperative day 1.
- Patients are usually weightbearing as tolerated with an assistive device.
- Active ROM and strengthening begins immediately and are generally accompanied by surgeon-specific protocols.
- Although not achieved by all patients, a knee ROM goal for the acute phase is 0 to 90 degrees.
- Discharge planning begins with the initial examination (see Chapter 1).
- Assist surgical and nursing team with postoperative complication prevention:
  - Breathing exercises to promote lung function (see Chapter 7)
  - Active exercise, weightbearing as indicated, and out of bed activity to prevent thromboembolic disease
- Physical therapy intervention:
  - Education
  - Mobility
  - ROM
  - Discharge recommendations

length of stay. When long-term follow-up has been performed, however, there appears to be no significant difference in ROM, pain, or function when comparing CPM as an adjunctive ROM therapy to physical therapy intervention without CPM.[14–16]

In addition to the physical therapist's focus on out of bed mobility and functional activities, therapeutic exercise and patient/family education begin immediately. Surgeon preference is often based on a combination of literature-based documented outcomes and clinical experience, which is why one surgeon may want a regimen of quad sets, active assisted ROM, and a knee immobilizer worn until the patient can perform an independent straight leg raise, while another wants no brace, no quad sets, and active motion only in sitting. Once again, the therapist should be familiar with the preferences of the patient's surgeon.

Functional goals of acute care physical therapy will diverge depending on the immediate discharge disposition of the patient.[17,18] There may be a specific institutional mechanism by which all patients status post joint replacement surgery are transferred to a skilled orthopedic rehabilitative unit. If this situation does not exist, then an early determination must be made, with the patient, whether functional goals can be achieved (eg, stair management, bathroom activities) to allow for discharge to home. In an increasingly cost-conscious health care environment, therapists are asked to make this discharge recommendation after only one or two interventions and must take into consideration factors such as safety, patient goals, insurance restrictions, and patient tolerance for ongoing therapy.

Examination of the patient after knee replacement focuses on functional mobility and knee ROM. Goniometric measurements of knee ROM are data collected throughout the hospital stay and become part of objective documented

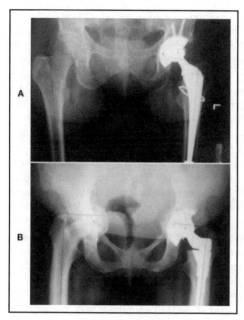

Figure 8–2. Total hip arthroplasty. Note relation of femoral neck orientation to vertical height. A. Valgus femoral neck with large vertical height. B. Varus femoral neck with large femoral offset. (Reprinted with permission from Canale ST. *Campbell's Operative Orthopaedics.* 10th ed. St. Louis, Mo: Mosby Inc; 2003.)

progress. Other baseline data to collect are skin integrity at the wound site and patient reports of pain. Ninety degrees of passive knee flexion is generally expected prior to discharge from the hospital. If, after several weeks or months, stiffness, pain, and lack of adequate ROM persist, manipulation under anesthesia may be indicated (Table 8–2).[19,20]

Total Hip Arthroplasty (Figure 8–2)

The components of total hip replacements are made from metal alloys, high-grade plastics, and polymeric materials. Implants are either cemented in place, not cemented, or a hybrid of the two. The needs and individual circumstances of each patient will determine the surgeon's choice of procedure.[8] A noncemented prosthesis has a specialized, porous surface texture that stimulates bone growth. These noncemented femoral stems have small openings allowing for bone to attach and grow through.

Because the soft-tissue capsule and musculature surrounding the hip joint must be cut and entered to replace the degenerative joint, patients are placed on what are commonly referred to as "hip precautions" postoperatively. These precautions attempt to limit excessive motion of the hip and prevent dislocation of a joint that does not have normal restraints due to the surgery. Patients are educated on these precautions,[21] which may last weeks to months depending on the surgeon, throughout their hospital stay. Specific precautions are dependent on the surgical approach. The hip is approached posterolaterally, anterolaterally, or by two smaller incisions, front and back.[9] **Posterolateral approach precautions** are no hip flexion past 90 degrees, no adduction past neutral (or midline), and no internal rotation. The **anterolateral** and **two-incision approaches** primarily restrict hip extension especially with external rotation.

Rotation at the hip joint is a relative motion created by either motion of the leg in relation to the trunk (femoral head on acetabulum) or the trunk in relation to the leg (acetabulum on the femoral head). Patients must be instructed to avoid twisting motions of the trunk such as reaching to answer the phone while lying in bed.

Some therapists may begin to encounter a two-incision, or minimally invasive, approach. Although the prosthetic components are the same as traditional approaches, two smaller incisions are made, one anterior and one posterior. The soft tissue capsule is still violated, but less muscle is incised to enter the hip joint. Proponents of this relatively newer technique report reduced hospital stays and quicker return to function.[8]

Several studies have examined the forces applied to the hip joint during functional activity, and these data often influence postoperative strengthening protocols.[22–24] Ankle pumps and quad and glut sets are usually initiated with first patient contact postoperatively as these are gentle yet active. Depending on the institution, the patient will be seen between one and three times daily according to patient tolerance. As out of bed endurance increases, supported standing exercises (in the parallel bars or at a walker) for the operated hip begin. Gentle, active, gravity-only resisted hip flexion, abduction, and extension, while maintaining specific precautions, have been an effective, hospital-based regimen at our institution. The goal of these exercises is to prevent postoperative stiffness and pain while improving functional strength for bed mobility, transfers, stair climbing, and ambulation. Unless discharged to an inpatient rehabilitation unit, the expectation is that the patient will be independent with a home exercise program, safe with all aspects of household level mobility and knowledgeable about precautions.

The weightbearing status of the patient depends on several factors: implant type, surgeon preference, and any intraoperative events or findings. Traditionally, a primary difference between cemented and noncemented prostheses was that cemented allowed for earlier, full weightbearing, whereas greater time was required for bone to attach to porous implants requiring restricted weightbearing. Long-term studies, however, have demonstrated the durability of both types of hip replacements, and therapists will treat patients who are full weightbearing, regardless of implant type. The physical therapist should expect to use a bilateral assistive device initially, regardless of implant type, to safely mobilize the patient at the bedside. Cemented implants are allowed weightbearing to tolerance yet do not generally progress to a cane until outpatient follow-up with the surgeon. Noncemented implants require more restrictive initial weightbearing, as a longer time is required for bone to attach to the implant. These patients may be partially weightbearing (approximately 50% of full), toe-touch or minimally weightbearing (approximately 10%), or nonweightbearing (NWB) depending on surgeon protocol.

In collaboration with the other health care team members (generally nurses and occupational therapists) patient education regarding the restricted motions of the hip, particularly during functional activities, are a fundamental component of postsurgical rehabilitation. Patients usually wake up in the recovery room with some type of pillow or wedge between their legs preventing adduction past mid line. Often, this is accompanied by a knee-immobilizer on the operated leg to further prevent unwanted knee and hip flexion. Use of adaptive equipment such as long-handled reachers, shoehorns, leg lifters, elevated toilet seats as well as walkers are all a part of the instruction in the acute phase. This equipment

---

Table 8–3
PHYSICAL THERAPY AND HIP ARTHROPLASTY

Summary:
- Physical therapy usually begins postoperative day 1.
- Multiple factors dictate weightbearing status; therefore, determine proper weightbearing status prior to initial examination.
- Education regarding hip precautions accompanies every session.
- Active ROM and strengthening begins immediately but may have surgeon restrictions.
- Discharge planning begins with the initial examination (see Chapter 1).
- Assist surgical and nursing team with postoperative complication prevention:
  - Breathing exercises to promote lung function (see Chapter 7)
  - Active exercise, weightbearing as indicated, and out of bed activity to prevent thromboembolic disease
- Physical therapy intervention:
  - Education
  - Mobility
  - Strengthening
  - Discharge recommendations

---

should promote successful performance while maintaining designated precautions with dressing, bathing, hygiene, and feeding.

Problems encountered with hip replacements are pain that results from loosening of the cement/prosthesis interface as well as dislocation. Remediation of these problems includes relocation under anesthesia, application of preventative dislocation braces, and surgical revision or reimplantation. Long-term follow-up, however, demonstrates excellent clinical results for most patients regardless of the type of implant used (Table 8–3).[25,26]

Total Shoulder Arthroplasty

Total shoulder arthroplasty (TSA) is the most common upper extremity (UE) arthroplasty and the third most commonly encountered joint replacement by physical therapists after TKA and THA. Surgical intervention is indicated when conservative treatments are no longer effective and pain limits functional activity to an unacceptable degree. The primary diseases affecting the glenohumeral joint are degenerative arthritis, traumatic arthritis, osteonecrosis, RA, and rotator cuff arthropathy. Shoulder replacement can include total arthroplasty or hemiarthroplasty when there is no glenoid involvement, as in proximal humeral fractures.[27]

Typical hospital length of stay after shoulder replacement is 2 to 3 days with instruction on early shoulder mobilization beginning postoperative day 1. Patients are instructed in passive forward flexion and external rotation and encouraged to perform these exercises independently several times per day. Active hand and elbow motion will maintain strength and minimize distal edema. Use of ice for pain and edema control is encouraged. Hip level activity of the involved arm is allowed but without lifting, pushing, carrying, or pulling.

Patients can expect several months of rehabilitation for TSA as they progress through several phases of strengthening and ROM exercises. Intensity of outpatient rehabilitation will, of course, be dependent on the individual goals of the patient.[27]

Spinal Surgery

The acute care therapist typically encounters three types of spinal surgery: discectomy combined with laminectomy, decompression, and fusion, all of which are encountered in both the cervical and lumbar spines (see also Tables 9–20 through 9–22). Lumbar disc disease (primarily the lower segments of L4-L5 and L5-S1) is the most prevalent cause of surgical intervention and increased morbidity in the United States, with thoracic disease accounting for <1% of herniated disc disease.[28] Annually, approximately 285,000 fusions are performed in the United States with slightly more than half in the lumbar region.[8] As with other chronic orthopedic conditions, patients seek surgical treatment when conservative measures (eg, nonsteroidal anti-inflammatory drugs, outpatient physical therapy, steroid injections) no longer are effective in controlling pain as physical function becomes impaired to an unsatisfactory degree.[29]

Sources of low back pain can be interveterbral disc herniation, stenosis of either the central vertebral canal or foramina, and degenerative disc disease with accompaning spondylolisthesis. Decompression of neural structures via excision of protruding or herniated interdiscal material (**discectomy**), removal of bone (**decompression**), and stabilization of hypermobile vertebrae (**fusion**) are primary indications for spinal surgery.[28]

Discectomy

This is the least invasive of the three types of procedures, often referred to as microdiscectomy because microscopic lenses are used to visualize the operating field. Discectomies are typically accompanied by laminectomies. In the absence of complications, patients usually require one overnight stay in the hospital. Orthotic bracing is not indicated in the acute phase.

Laminectomy

This is a more involved surgical procedure than discectomy, particularly when more than one vertebral level is involved. The term *hemi*laminectomy refers to one side of a vertebral level (left or right) that is excised. Orthotic bracing is not indicated in the acute phase.

Decompression

A procedure whereby the posterior elements of the vertebral column are removed, including lamina and spinous process, and foramen are widened to relieve pressure on neural elements.

Fusion

When vertebrae are fused, the spine can be approached either anteriorly or posteriorly. When both approaches are performed, they either occur during the same surgery or are separated by days during the same hospitalization. Fusion material is a combination of hardware (pedicle screws, cages) and bone. Bone may come from a bone bank (allograft) or from the patient (autogenous). Autogenous grafts are usually harvested from the iliac crest. This donor site is frequently painful during the postoperative hospital phase and often requires the use of either a walker or cane for several days after surgery to lessen an antalgic gait pattern.[30]

Orthotic bracing is often ordered by the surgeon after fusion to provide external support. The type of brace and wearing schedule will vary with the surgeon. When the L5-S1 junction is fused, a brace with a thigh piece extension may be prescribed and requires more intensive education and training prior to discharge. Instruction about the brace is given initially by the orthotist who fabricates the brace, but subsequent education and training during functional activities is done by the therapist. The therapist needs to have a good working knowledge of proper application and fit of the prescribed braces. The orthotist may fit the brace in supine but not sit or stand the patient. Improperly fitting braces may either be too high under the axilla/throat/neck area or too long across the hips limiting hip flexion and upright sitting. Postoperative edema may also cause a brace that was measured preoperatively to appear improperly sized. When these situations are encountered, the therapist should contact the fabricating orthotist for modifications.

Spinal Precautions

Regardless of the type of surgery, therapists will instruct patients in "spinal precautions" postoperatively. A "log rolling" technique is used to get out of bed. The hips and shoulders roll as one unit, thereby avoiding spinal rotation. Excessive trunk flexion should be avoided when sitting. Extended periods of sitting should be limited, and lifting is restricted. Clinical experience has demonstrated that spinal surgeons have different views on the necessity of some or all of these restrictions, but because they are protective and conservative in nature, surgeons are generally supportive.

Patients do not usually have weightbearing restrictions after spinal surgeries, but ambulatory assistive devices can provide stability during walking activities and give confidence to the patient. Physical therapy intervention focuses on functional mobility, patient education, pain management, and assistance with appropriate discharge planning. Therapeutic exercise that addresses strength or flexibility deficits, other than gentle active ROM of the extremities, are generally not initiated in the acute care setting and should only be applied judiciously (Table 8–4).

TRAUMA

Physical therapy intervention for the acutely injured orthopedic patient varies widely. In smaller facilities the therapist may encounter primarily isolated extremity fractures or dislocations, whereas the therapist working in a larger trauma center will encounter the patient with multiple injuries who has sustained fractures to multiple extremities, spine, and pelvis. Injuries from gun shot wounds, unfortunately, are consuming large resources of orthopedic surgery

---

Table 8–4

PHYSICAL THERAPY AND SPINAL SURGERY (SEE ALSO TABLE 9–22)

Summary:
- Therapists educate patients in:
  - Log rolling
  - Avoiding heavy lifting
  - Avoiding prolonged sitting
  - Brace application and wearing schedule (if appropriate)
- Patients are usually full weightbearing.
- Expect pain from autogenous bone graft (use assistive device as needed).
- Stair climbing is NOT contraindicated.
- Assist surgical and nursing team with postoperative complication prevention:
  - Breathing exercises to promote lung function (see Chapter 7)
  - Active exercise, weightbearing as indicated, and out of bed activity to prevent thromboembolic event
- Physical therapy intervention:
  - Education
  - Mobility
  - Discharge recommendations

---

services that work in urban trauma centers.[31,32] Often, a therapist must work under difficult circumstances related to injury and related criminal activity.

Working with orthopedic injury as a result of trauma becomes more challenging in the presence of other body–system injuries, particularly traumatic brain injury, and often necessitates recommendations for continuing levels of in-patient rehabilitation care. This section examines frequently seen orthopedic injuries associated with trauma.

Spine Trauma

When the spine is involved in acute trauma, the surgical team asked to evaluate the patient must determine whether bony and/or neurological injury has occurred, if the spine is stable, and if not, how to appropriately manage the instability. To evaluate the spine a combination of diagnostic imaging (x-ray, CAT scan, and MRI) and clinical exam is used to assess the extent of the injury. Anatomically, the spine is generally divided into three columns: anterior, middle, and posterior (Figure 8–3). When two or more columns are injured, ligamentous damage generally occurs and the spine is considered unstable. To stabilize the spine, surgical internal fixation, external rigid bracing, or both are required (Figure 8–4). The physical therapist must understand what structures are involved in the spine injury, what procedures have been performed, whether and what type of bracing is indicated, and whether the definitive plan has been clearly documented.

Transverse or Spinous Process Fractures

These are often seen in high-energy impact injuries such as motor vehicle crashes (MVC) and falls from heights. These injuries do not generally require

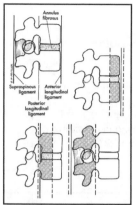

Figure 8–3. The three-column concept of spinal injury. A. Anterior column contains the anterior longitudinal ligament, the anterior half of the vertebral body, and the anterior portion of the annulus fibrosis. B. The middle column consists of the posterior long ligament, the posterior half of the vertebral body, and the posterior aspect of the annulus fibrosus. C. The posterior column includes the neural arch, the ligamentum flavum, the facet capsules, and the interspinous ligaments. (Reprinted with permission from Canale ST. *Campbell's Operative Orthopaedics.* 10th ed. St. Louis, Mo: Mosby Inc; 2003.)

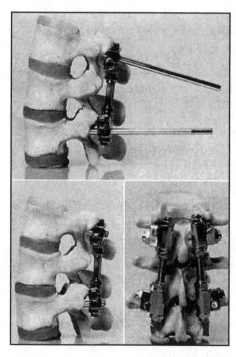

Figure 8–4. Example of Cotrel-Dubousset instrumentation for spinal fracture-dislocations and unstable burst fractures. (Reprinted with permission from Canale ST. *Campbell's Operative Orthopaedics.* 10th ed. St. Louis, Mo: Mosby Inc; 2003.)

surgical intervention or weightbearing restrictions. Pain with motion is common especially during the rotary motions associated with bed mobility. These fractures do not require bracing from a stability standpoint but may be of benefit in reducing pain and allowing greater functional mobility.

Ligamentous Injury

Ligamentous injury of the spine is more commonly seen in the cervical spine than in either the thoracic or lumbar spine. Typical orthopedic management involves rigid bracing for 6 to 12 weeks (see Table 8–10). Weightbearing

---

Table 8–5*
PHYSICAL THERAPY AND SPINAL TRAUMA

Summary:
- When the spine is injured, the therapist must be assured that the spine is "cleared" for mobility.
- When braces/orthotics are ordered, the therapist must understand the wearing schedule (ie, hours on/off, activity limitations, time in sitting).
- The therapist should be attentive to signs and symptoms of possible neurological impairment resulting from spine injury.

*See also Tables 9-21 and 9-22.

---

restrictions during ambulation are generally not required. Patient education should include proper application and wearing schedule of the brace.

Compression or Burst Vertebral Fractures

A burst fracture is a comminuted compression fracture of the vertebral body that often includes retropulsion of fragments into the spinal canal.[33] These injuries occur from pure flexion moments with little or no rotation of the spine. Compression or burst vertebral fractures are commonly seen in high-energy injuries such as falls from large heights or gunshot wounds. They often require rigid bracing and surgical intervention to maintain spinal extension and prevent further injury associated with flexion (see Figure 8–4). Weightbearing during ambulation is not restricted but can be limited by pain.

Multiple-Level Injury

When multiple levels of the spine are involved (eg, L2 to L4 or T10 to T12), clinical experience has shown pain with functional mobility usually increases. When multi-level injuries are combined with spinal instability (two-column involvement) surgical intervention is required. Depending on surgeon preference, bracing may or may not be indicated postoperatively. Pain control becomes more of a concern postoperatively, as is application of the brace over a surgical wound site (Table 8–5). Physical therapy intervention must address postoperative complication prevention (eg, infection, pneumonia, DVT, pressure ulcer).

PELVIS (FIGURE 8–5)

Injuries to the pelvis could involve several anatomical areas including the acetabulum, ilium, and pubic rami. For the sake of convenience, the sacrum will be included although, anatomically, it is not part of the pelvis proper.

Since the acetabular cup is composed of several bones fused together, fracture nomenclature often refers to either the anterior or posterior column. Small chip or non-displaced fractures often do not require surgical intervention but frequently there are weightbearing restrictions on the side of injury. Larger, displaced, or comminuted fractures (as seen in fracture/dislocations secondary to MVC where the head of the femur is posteriorly displaced) require internal

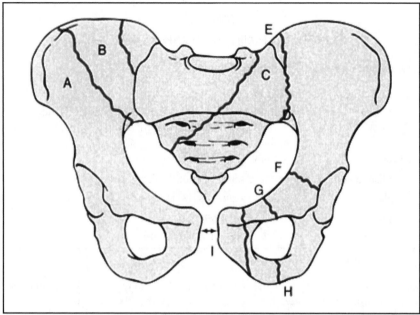

Figure 8–5. The Letournel and Judet classification of pelvic fractures. A. Iliac wing fractures. B. Ilium fractures with extension to the sacroiliac joint. C. Transsacral fractures. D. Unilateral sacral fractures. E. Sacroiliac joint fracture-dislocation. F. Acetabular fracture. G. Pubic raus fractures. H. Ischial fractures. I. Pubic symphysis separation. (Reprinted from Browner BD, Jupiter JB, Levine AM. *Skeletal Trauma: Basic Science, Management, and Reconstruction.* 3rd ed. 2003, with permission from Elsevier.)

fixation. The patients who have dislocated (whether a fracture exists) generally remain NWB acutely and are placed on the same preventative hip precautions as after hip replacement because the capsular hip ligaments have been stretched.

The superior and inferior pubic rami may be fractured individually or together. These injuries typically do not require surgical fixation or weightbearing restrictions but are very painful during functional activities. The therapist should anticipate pain with motions associated with bed mobility and standing. Cooperation with the medical and nursing team in aggressive pain management is fundamental to enable the patient maximum mobility thus preventing possible secondary bed rest-associated sequelae. Because of the anatomical position of the rami, the pain associated with movement tends not to respond to orthotic management (ie, some type of bracing that may provide compressive support).

When the sacrum is involved in bony injury, surgeons will often refer to either left- or right-sided involvement. If extension of the fracture into the sacroiliac joint exists, a weightbearing restriction usually applies. In severe injury to the sacrum, bars or a plate will be used for fracture fixation. This patient may be allowed out of bed and allowed to ambulate with an assistive device as tolerated. The immediate complication the therapist will confront is patient pain as he or she attempts to flex the trunk to attain a functional sitting

Table 8–6 FRACTURE TERMINOLOGY (SEE FIGURE 8–3)	
Open	• Violation of the skin. • Often associated with high-energy injury. • Increased risk of infection. • Stabilized with external fixation or internal fixation. • Requires immediate sterile irrigation, debridement, and antibiotics.
Closed	• No violation of the skin.
Nondisplaced	• Fracture segments not displaced relative to each other.
Displaced	• Fracture segments displaced relative to each other.
Simple	• Two fractured parts.
Comminuted	• Three or more fractured parts.

position. This inability to achieve a sitting position may necessitate dependent transfers initially and often has an impact on discharge recommendations. These types of injuries most often require two-person assist during the acute phase (for rolling, sitting, and all out of bed transfers) and usually require aggressive pain management, especially prior to therapy intervention.

When major trauma has occurred to the pelvis, disrupting the anatomical structure known as the pelvic ring, the use of external or internal fixation is generally required.[34,35] These patients are functionally limited by pain, as well as mechanically blocked by the fixation bars from achieving a functional sitting position. Dependent or assisted transfers to a reclining wheelchair that has an adjustable back angle should be employed to facilitate out of bed benefits (cardiovascular and pulmonary) and UE activity (wheelchair propulsion). When major trauma has occurred to the pelvis, the therapist should anticipate associated injuries to the perineal area that may involve painful mobility-limiting edema.

EXTREMITIES

Nearly all components of the apendicular skeleton can be fractured during trauma. This section is not meant to be an exhaustive list but rather to emphasize commonly seen fractures and how physical therapy can appropriately intervene in the acute care setting for both UE and lower extremity (LE) injuries. Common fracture terminology and hardware are provided in Tables 8–6 and 8–7 and Figure 8–6.

Upper Extremity

UE fractures include digits, carpal bones, radius, ulna, humerus, clavicle, and scapula. The physical therapist should anticipate the use of a shoulder sling, particularly with more proximal fractures, that will provide support and comfort

Table 8–7
FRACTURE HARDWARE

Dynamic hip screw	• Used commonly to stabilize intertrochanteric hip fractures. • One large screw with a side plate and several small screws.
Intermedullary rod or nail	• Generic term for a longitudinal rod placed within the medullary canal. • Stabilizes diaphyseal long bone fractures.
Intramedullary hip screw	• Combination of intramedullary rod and dynamic hip screw. • Stabilizes intertrochanteric hip fractures.
Percutaneous pin	• Pin placed through the skin. • Stabilizes bone, fracture, or joint.
Open reduction internal fixation	• Term used when skin must be opened and hardware placed to reduce and stabilize a fracture.
External fixation	• A structure of connected pins and bars inserted externally through the skin. • Generally used to stabilize high-energy, comminuted fracture with significant soft tissue damage. • Allows access for wound care.

during out of bed activities. Where indicated, the patient should be educated in removing the sling while in bed or seated and positioning the extremity to minimize the effects of gravity-induced swelling. Active or active assisted shoulder motion, when allowed, should be taught to minimize the stiffness that will accompany long-standing shoulder immobility and internal rotation. Figure-of-eight slings may be indicated for clavicle fractures or sternoclavicular dislocations. These braces are fit over both shoulders maintaining the scapulae in an adducted, retracted position.

When examining a patient with any UE fracture, there are several concerns the physical therapist must address: Is there active motion and intact sensation distal and proximal to the injured segment, and does a weightbearing restriction exist? If a restriction exists, especially in the presence of other injuries, how will this restriction impact mobility? An example to illustrate this point is presented in Table 8–8.

Humeral fractures may be splinted or casted and placed in a shoulder sling postinjury without surgical intervention. Humeral fractures are generally NWB as any axial load through the hand/wrist or forearm will be transmitted proximally. Consider this patient fully NWB through the entire UE but remember to encourage hand/wrist and elbow motion where applicable. When the dominant hand is involved, consider a consult for occupational therapy.

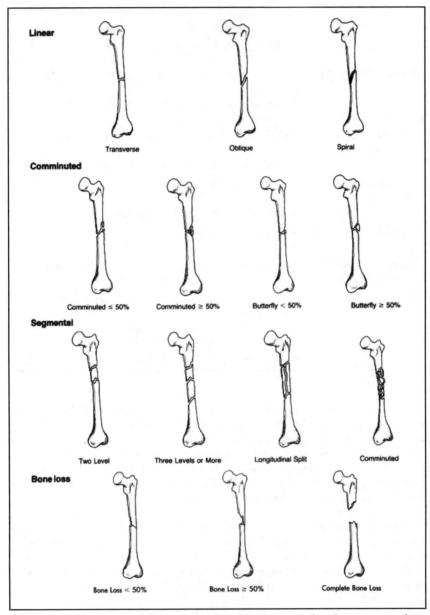

Figure 8–6. Classification of long bone fractures. (Reprinted with permission from Canale ST. *Campbell's Operative Orthopaedics*. 10th ed. St. Louis, Mo: Mosby Inc; 2003.)

<u>Table 8–8</u>

CASE EXAMPLE

A 24-year-old female is in a motor vehicle crash and sustains fractures of the left femur and the right distal radius. Both require open reduction and internal fixation (ORIF). The postoperative PT orders state NWB LLE and NWB RUE. Based on the orders as written, this patient should not be allowed to ambulate because, for most patients, it is neither safe nor feasible to maintain NWB on one LE without using both UEs. Functional goals will focus on transfers and wheelchair mobility.

Further discussion by the PT with the orthopedic surgeons, regarding weightbearing restrictions, however, changes the activity status of her RUE to include weightbearing through the proximal forearm or elbow. Now that she can use both UEs she has the opportunity to ambulate with a platform attachment on either a walker or crutch. This patient is now able to have ambulation goals. The difference between having ambulation goals and having only transfer goals often impacts discharge disposition.

Fractures of the forearm can be isolated to the radius, ulna, or both. These may be internally or externally fixated. As discussed in the case example, when the fracture is in the distal third of the forearm, regardless of type of fixation, the patient may be allowed to bear weight through the proximal third of the forearm or the elbow. This weightbearing is on a platform attachment to a crutch or walker.

Lower Extremity

The physical therapist will intervene with a wide range of LE fractures and must be scrupulous in several different areas: reliably verifying and instructing the weightbearing status, assessing wound status during functional activities, applying appropriate bracing (if indicated), and selecting the most appropriate assistive device based on weightbearing, activity restrictions, and current functional ability.

Femur

Physical therapists will treat patients who have fractured all parts of the femur: proximally at the neck or intertrochanteric line, mid-shaft, or distally with or without involvement of the knee joint.[36] Proximal fractures are most often internally fixed (ORIF) with femoral neck fractures frequently receiving hemiarthroplasty (*hemi* as opposed to *total* in the absence of degenerative joint disease and no acetabular injury). Mid-shaft and distal femoral fractures are either internally fixed, often with an intramedullary rod, or externally fixed when significant soft tissue damage is present (Figure 8–7). The femur is usually casted, whether or not surgical fixation has occurred, for distal fractures. The cast is often flexed at the knee to keep the foot off the floor and assist with NWB transfers and ambulation.

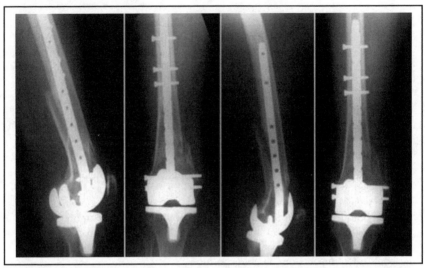

Figure 8–7. Supracondylar intramedullary nail used for fixation of femur fracture. (Reprinted with permission from Canale ST. *Campbell's Operative Orthopaedics.* 10th ed. St. Louis, Mo: Mosby Inc; 2003.)

Hip Fracture

The therapist working in acute care orthopedics should anticipate treating the elderly patient who has fallen and broken his or her hip. Much research focuses on hip fracture in the elderly, as it is a tremendous financial and societal burden.[37–40]

The common orthopedic surgical interventions for hip fractures are ORIFs and hemiarthroplasty, with determination of procedure based on several factors: prior activity level of the patient (independent community dweller versus wheelchair bound or minimally ambulatory) and quality of bone (soft osteoporotic bone does not hold screws well). When treating the elderly patient who has fractured a hip, the physical therapist encounters several challenging issues: presence of co-morbid conditions, weightbearing restrictions complicating mobility, fear and depression regarding loss of independence, and poor tolerance to narcotic pain medication, often resulting in acute delirium. Therapists working with this population, and in the sub-acute phase, are challenged to mobilize these patients quickly because much literature supports early return to ambulation as an important indicator of return to prehospital function.[41,42]

Knee

Injuries involving the knee, including patellar or quadriceps tendon ruptures or patellar fractures, are usually managed surgically and then braced, or casted, postoperatively.[43]

Postoperative immobilization includes knee immobilizers, dial lock knee braces, and cylinder-type casts made of either plaster or fiberglass with the foot and ankle left free to move. The therapist should anticipate pain if flexion occurs with weightbearing. The use of knee immobilizers and other foam and metal braces may not completely prevent unwanted knee flexion with axial loading. Clinical experience has shown that cylinder casting provides the greatest functional stabilization of full knee extension. This type of injury, once surgically fixed and externally immobilized, allows full weightbearing. The therapist should prepare for difficult sit<>stand transfers (especially in the complicated instance of bilateral involvement) because the patient is at a considerable biomechanical disadvantage while attempting to rise to a standing position. Use of hospital-bed height elevation is generally required secondary to lack of knee flexion. In fact, when considering recommendations for post-hospital discharge a hospital bed that elevates can make the difference between dependent and independent bed mobility and transfers.

Foot/Ankle

Closed fractures of the foot/ankle complex (metatarsals, malleoli, calcaneii) that require surgical fixation often have too much traumatic edema to either internally fix or cast immobilize. This patient remains splinted (posterior half cast), strictly NWB, and generally ready for discharge. If the injury is isolated and unilateral in the absence of significant co-morbidities, this patient generally has good potential for gait training. If there is bilateral involvement the patient must be instructed in NWB transfers to a wheelchair and commode. This type of transfer requires adequate UE strength to achieve independence or minimal dependence. Expect this individual to be non-ambulatory for several months and require ongoing episodes of physical therapy for ROM, strengthening, and gait training as bone healing progresses.

External Fixation

When high-energy fractures occur in combination with extensive soft tissue damage, external fixation devices are applied.[44] External fixators are made of titanium pins and rods inserted externally through the skin and connected to each other to provide fracture stabilization. External fixators of the LE can span either the length of the femur, the tibia, or cross the knee joint (Figure 8–8). Distal tibial fractures may extend from the lower third of the leg across the ankle joint.

Mobilizing patients with external fixators can be intimidating. The physical therapist should keep in mind that most individuals have never seen an external fixation device, and the sight of pins and rods protruding from the skin can be difficult. Second, the therapist is now asking that the patient, who may have difficulty even looking at this device, to become mobile. When assisting a patient out of bed, clinical experience has demonstrated that patient comfort is increased if the injured limb is moved by the rods of the external fixation device rather than by supporting the skin and soft tissue underneath.

The therapist should look for excessive or purulent drainage from the pin sites as well as pistoning (up and down motion) of the pins. Skin movement around pin sites is normal and may mimic a pistoning pin. A problem that should be attended to immediately is a loose pin that no longer provides fracture stabilization. The therapist must stop activity and contact the surgical team, as readjustment may be required.

Figure 8–8. Knee arthrodesis with biplanar external fixation secondary to persistent infection. (Reprinted with permission from Canale ST. *Campbell's Operative Orthopaedics.* 10th ed. St. Louis, Mo: Mosby Inc; 2003.)

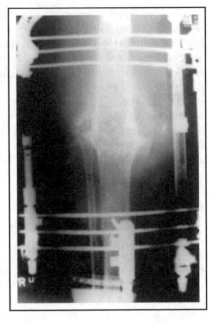

Many LE external fixators are constructed to prevent heel breakdown while in bed. Elongated pins connected to the fixators project posteriorly at the foot/ankle so the heel rests without contact when the patient is supine. Although this provides excellent prophylactic pressure relief, these pins add depth and width to the fixation device and can complicate ambulation. When lower leg external fixation devices are applied around the foot and ankle, standard practice at our institution is to custom mold a foot plate (held in place by rubber exercise band attached to the pins) with the intent of maintaining neutral dorsiflexion and preventing ankle or forefoot contractures.

INFECTION/NON-HEALING FRACTURES

With any surgical procedure, and particularly in the presence of open traumatic wounds, there is a risk of infection. A worrisome complication after joint replacement or fracture repair is persistent infection, poor healing, or nonunion with bone loss or separation (see Figures 8–6 and 8–8).[45,46] It is common in large trauma centers for the orthopedic surgery service to treat patients for nonhealing, mal-aligned, or nonunion fractures. For open fractures, risk of infection increases linearly based on size of soft tissue damage and length of time from fracture to initial debridement.[47] Acute **osteomyelitis** is an infection of bone that requires hospitalization for a variety of treatments: sterile debridements, intravenous antibiotics, hyperbaric oxygen, skin grafting, and removal of infected implanted hardware or bone.

Physical therapists will treat previously injured patients who have had some training in ambulation with an assistive device and who now return to the hospital because of infection. A new episode of hospital-based gait and mobility training may be required. Physical therapy is generally indicated prior to discharge because of a NWB status, pain, and possible acute deconditioning secondary to inactivity.

Ridding the patient of infection is the primary medical goal, and several medical/surgical approaches are taken including serial sterile debridements in the operating room, the use of implanted antibiotic beads or cement,[48,49] restricted weightbearing on the affected extremity, superficial wound management, direct current electrical stimulation,[50] and intravenous antibiotics. New hardware may have to replace infected rods, nails, or prosthetic implants.

In cases of chronic infection, where long-term antibiotic use, multiple operative procedures, and even use of bone stimulators has failed, segments of bone may need to be completely removed. These osteotomies may include fusions as are often seen at the knee and ankle. The Girdlestone procedure at the hip removes a segment of infected, or nonhealed, proximal femur and purposefully allows scar tissue to form in order to stabilize the joint.[51] Despite the lack of a true hip joint, independent ambulation is often a realistic long-term goal. The patient may present, ultimately, with a limp and require heel lifts secondary to a leg-length discrepancy.

When osteotomies are performed, surgeons may apply skeletal traction to maintain alignment. A removable pin is placed either through the proximal tibia or the distal femur with weights and pulleys hung over the foot of the patient's bed. The therapist must be aware of the activity status because this patient may be allowed to come out of traction to participate in therapy (Table 8–9).

ORTHOTICS

Important components of acute fracture and orthopedic management are support, comfort, and immobilization. Therefore, the use of orthotic devices is commonplace. The physical therapist must understand indications for use in the acute care setting, application, and implications for function.[52] The tables of this section are arranged by anatomical area and, although not an exhaustive listing, give the reader an idea of commonly used devices, frequently encountered brand names, and indications.

For any orthotic device, proper fit is essential. A brace can appear well fitting in a static position but shift during functional activities. Therapists will assist patients by educating them as to the reason for the brace, how it should be applied, when it should be worn, and how to monitor the skin underneath the brace. A frustrating complication of orthotic use is the occurrence of preventable problems, such as skin breakdown under a brace secondary to lack of vigilant observation.

When outside vendors provide service to patients in the hospital (some hospitals have their own orthotics department) interaction and collaboration can be more difficult. The therapist should attempt to coordinate fittings or adjustments with the outside vendor because this facilitates more efficient patient care.

Beside the use of orthoses, the acute care physical therapist will encounter the use of cast immobilization. Gait and mobility training is impacted by the weight of the cast and the degree to which the immobilization provides comfort. The physical therapist must be alert to complaints of a tight-fitting cast such as

Table 8–9

PHYSICAL THERAPY AND JOINT INFECTIONS

Summary
- Chronic and acutely infected joints or hardware often require hospitalization.
- Patients usually have had physical therapy in the past for gait training.
- A new episode of PT intervention is frequently required prior to discharge.
- Procedures frequently encountered:
  - Hardware removal or exchange
  - Osteotomies
  - Joint fusions/arthrodesis
  - Multiple operative debridements
  - Antibiotics (may have central intravenous line placement, eg, peripherally inserted central catheter [PICC])
- Physical therapy intervention:
  - Assess mobility/gait
  - If orthotic management required, instruct patient in use
  - Bedside exercise program if a long-term hospital stay anticipated

acute pain or parasthesias within or distal to the cast. Contact the surgical team immediately because pressure relief may be indicated. This is performed by either bivalving the cast or windowing the area in question.

Spine

As a general rule, no matter what segment of the spine requires bracing, the primary question to ask is, "Does the orthosis attempt to stabilize an unstable area or is it meant for comfort?" When stabilization is required, rigid bracing is indicated. If pain is present but no underlying anatomical structures are at risk, soft material can be appropriate. The important difference is that soft braces can be removed without risk of injury, but rigid braces should have specific wearing schedules, which the patient or caregiver must understand. The important question that requires a definitive answer is whether the brace can be removed when lying in bed or must the patient have it on continuously. Common cervical and thoracolumbar orthoses are provided in Tables 8–10 and 8–11 (see also Table 9-20).

Extremities

A wide variety of extremity orthoses exist, most that immobilize, but some that allow degrees of motion. Depending on the institution, either physical therapists or occupational therapists may be responsible for custom molding certain extremity braces. The physical therapist will be challenged to assist the patient and the surgical team with recommending the most appropriate, cost-effective device. Common UE orthoses are provided in Table 8–12 and LE orthoses are provided in Table 8–13.

Table 8–10
CERVICAL ORTHOSES

Rigid

Indications:
- Unstable cervical spine at C1 to C2

Type:
Halo
- Pins inserted externally into skull
- Pins attached to plastic and padded-lined vest

Semi-Rigid

Indications:
- Stable fractures
- Nonoperative ligamentous injury
- Postoperative
- Prescribed wearing schedule

Type:
Miami-J
- Two-piece
- Hard plastic
- Gortex liner
- Velcro strap closure
- Opening for tracheostomy

Philadelphia
- Two-piece
- Hard plastic
- Foam
- Velcro strap closure

Cervical Thoracic Orthosis (CTO) or *Cervical Thoracic Lumbar Orthosis* (CTLO)
- Any brace that has both cervical and thoracic components or extensions
- Stabilize cervical and high thoracic injury

Sternal Occipito Mandibular Immobilizer (SOMI)
- Three-piece
  - Sternal pad or yoke
  - Anterior mandibular support
  - Occiptal support
- No rolling of patient required to apply brace

Soft

Indications:
- Symptom management and pain control
- Flexible wearing schedule

Type:
- Foam and fabric with Velcro strap closure
- Indicated after trauma to control pain in the absence of bony or ligamentous injury

Table 8–11
THORACOLUMBAR ORTHOSES

Rigid

Indications:
- Stable fractures
- Non-operative ligamentous injury
- Postoperative
- Prescribed wearing schedule

Type:
Thoracic LumboSacral Orthosis (TLSO)
- Indicated for mid thoracic and lumbar injuries
- Usually two-piece
- Hard plastic
- Velcro straps
- Custom molded or prefabricated

Sternal OccipitoMandibular Immobilizer (SOMI)
- Stabilize cervical and high level thoracic injury
- No rolling of patient required to apply brace
- Mandibular and occipital attachments

Jewitt Hyperextension Brace
- Maintains extension, prevents flexion
- Used frequently for compression fractures
- Sternal and pubic anterior pads
- Posterior lumbar pad
- No lateral bars allows for lateral bending

Boston Overlap
- One piece, flexible plastic
- Velcro straps
- Opens anteriorly, at midline

Semi-Rigid

Indications:
- Combination of soft fabrics and metal or plastic
- Symptom management
- Pain control in the absence of instability

Type:
Corset
- Fabric with side and posterior metal stays, lace-up sides or front
- Often tolerated better than rigid braces, particularly in the geriatric population
- More support than soft binders

Soft

Indications:
- Symptom management
- Pain control in the absence of instability
- Flexible wearing schedule

Type:
Abdominal Binder
- Fabric with Velcro closure anteriorly

Table 8–12
UPPER EXTREMITY ORTHOSES

Rigid

Indications:
- Nonoperative fractures requiring external immobilization
- Postoperative stabilization
- Prescribed wearing schedule

Type:
Sarmiento Fracture Brace
- Stabilize proximal or mid-shaft humeral fractures
- Two-piece hard plastic
- Velcro strap closure
- Prefabricated

Custom-Molded Immobilizers "Gutter Splint"
- Static splint
- Maintains functional position
- Protects postoperative procedures (eg, skin grafts)

Wrist "Cock-Up" Splint
- Static splint
- Maintains functional wrist position
- Radial nerve palsy/paresis
- Prevents wrist contracture in presence of external fixation

Semi-Rigid

Indications:
- Components allow for static (or resting) immobilization, as well as dynamic ROM

Type:
Hinged or Dial-Lock Elbow Brace
- Lock in full extension or any degree of elbow flexion
- Foam with metal stays
- Velcro strap closures

Soft

Indications:
- Most often indicated for symptom management and pain control in the absence of instability

Type:
Shoulder Slings
- For clavicle, scapular, humeral fractures
- Used to unweight heavy splints or casts of radius/ulna and wrist fractures

(continued)

Table 8–12 (continued)
UPPER EXTREMITY ORTHOSES

Soft

- Flexible or prescribed wearing schedule
- Shoulder slings may cause shoulder stiffness and decreased ROM while maintaining shoulder in adduction and internal rotation

Figure-of-Eight
- For clavicle fractures
- Attempts to align fracture segments
- Maintains scapulae retracted and adducted

Shoulder Abduction
- Large foam wedge at hip with over-the-shoulder strap
- Used often for postoperative shoulder and humeral fractures
- Maintains shoulder/extremity in abducted, "gunslinger" position

Foot/Ankle

Orthotic shoes and braces are used to support, relieve pressure, or facilitate weightbearing at the foot and ankle.[53] Custom molded orthotic shoes that accommodate deformity are not fabricated during the acute care phase of injury and require outpatient follow-up. Despite the various, and often confusing, array of brand names, the physical therapist must focus on the goal of foot/ankle bracing. Is the orthosis for short or long term? Is support or pressure relief required? How much and where is weightbearing allowed? By answering these questions the therapist should be able to recommend the appropriate orthotic device as noted in Table 8–14.

Clinical experience has found the use of ankle air splints or casts to be effective in assisting weightbearing mobility in the appropriate patient. When the foot and ankle are injured during trauma to other limbs, ankle sprains or ligamentous injury often go unnoticed until the patient first gets out of bed and attempts to bear weight. If physical examination (eg, tenderness to palpation, painful resisted movement, ecchymosis) supports the clinical diagnosis of ligamentous injury, a recommendation for an ankle splint should be made. These splints are either air or foam filled, two-piece plastic, and have Velcro straps closure. They are designed to fit into a regular shoe or sneaker but may be limited secondary to acute edema.

ASSISTIVE DEVICES

All therapists who work in the hospital setting are familiar with the prescription of assistive devices to address mobility impairment and dysfunction. With an orthopedic population, therapists are frequently asked to train patients with various types of devices as outlined in Table 8–15. Choosing which device to

Table 8–13
LOWER EXTREMITY ORTHOSES

Rigid

Indications:
- Postoperative stabilization
- Prescribed
  wearing schedule

Type:

Hip Abduction Brace
- Usually prefabricated
- Hip spica appearance
- Indicated for acute and/or multiple hip dislocations after hip replacement
- Degree of hip flexion and abduction controlled by external hip joint locking mechanism
- Hard plastic, shoulder and waist straps, thigh cuff

Fracture Brace
- Custom molded
- Usually two-piece hard plastic with Velcro strap closure
- Often seen for the nonunion, nonhealing fracture

Semi-Rigid

Indications:
- Stabilization of fractures, either nonoperative or surgically repaired
- Ligamentous injuries of the knee
- Support for weightbearing activities
- Prescribed or flexible wearing schedule

Type:

Dial-Lock; Hinged
- Bledsoe, Exo-Tec, Don Joy
- Stabilize postoperative fracture stabilization or non-operative ligamentous injury
- Foam padding, medial and lateral metal stays
- Velcro strap closure, adjustable dial locks at knee joint
- Allows for any degree of knee flexion ROM, often locked in full extension acutely
- Indicated for more long-term use than knee immobilizer

Knee Immobilizer
- Foam, posterior metal stay, adjustable medial and lateral metal stays, Velcro strap closure
- Attempts to lock knee in full extension with no motion

(continued)

Table 8-13 (continued)
LOWER EXTREMITY ORTHOSES

Semi-Rigid	• Used frequently in acute care for multiple scenarios: 　○ Stabilize distal femoral or proximal tibial fractures 　○ Protect postoperative procedures (eg, skin grafts) 　○ Provides knee stability for weightbearing in the presence of quadriceps weakness
Soft	*Used very infrequently in acute care.*
	Ace Bandages • Compressive, elastic wrap • Holds dressings in place, provides comfort but no stability

use is often determined by several factors. The therapist must know what, if any, weightbearing restriction exists as any condition requiring less than full, LE weightbearing necessitates a bilateral device such as a walker or crutches. Since many types of walkers and crutches exist, the clinical decision to use one device instead of another is influenced by the patient's demonstrated ability to safely use the device based on the demands of the discharge environment.

Coordination, fear, prior use of device, pain, ability to learn new skills, and family/caregiver assistance are all considerations in the final recommendation. The physical therapist must determine the ability of the patient to maintain a given weightbearing restriction during functional activities and to direct intervention accordingly. Practically, this often means restricting an activity until further appropriate training can take place, possibly in settings after hospital discharge. Often an activity must wait until the weightbearing restriction is lifted. Ambulation for an older individual with a long-leg cast may not be realistic, but transferring independently to a wheelchair or bedside commode might be. The reader is referred to the table on assistive ambulatory devices for types and indications.

CONCLUSION

The hospital-based therapist who works with patients who have orthopedic impairment will treat a variety of conditions and age ranges. In the examination, evaluation, and formulation of the physical therapy plan of care, the therapist will employ many skills including patient/caregiver education, mobility training, and discharge planning.[54] Attention to surgeon-specific protocols, as well as knowledge of orthotic devices, is critical for safe and effective collaborative patient care. This chapter is meant as a guide to common, hospital-based

Table 8–14
FOOT AND ANKLE ORTHOSES

Rigid

Indications:
- In the presence of ankle dorsiflexion weakness, facilitates normal swing-through during swing phase of gait

Type:
Ankle Foot Orthosis (AFO)
- Usually prefabricated in acute care setting
- Flexible plastic
- Velcro strap closure below fibular head
- Fits inside shoe

The term MAFO refers to a molded ankle foot orthosis, which is custom made. A MAFO is a definitive, long-term brace, fabricated either in the outpatient or inpatient rehabilitation setting. NOT indicted during acute care phase secondary to wound issues, edema fluctuations and, often, evolving injury status.

Semi-Rigid

Indications:
- For minimally or non-ambulatory patients while in bed:
  - Provides heel pressure relief
  - Prevents heelcord contracture
  - Maintains neutral hip rotation
- For ambulatory patients:
  - Facilitates swing-through
  - Not a long-term device

Type:
Ankle Foot Orthosis
- *PRAFO, Multipodus Splint, Oscar Boot*
- Foam/fabric lining, flexible plastic shell, thick rubber sole

Shoes

Indications:
- For weightbearing activities
- To relieve pressure either on forefoot or hind foot
- Provide comfort and/or support
- Used to protect wounds

Type:
In general, made of durable, thick fabric with Velcro strap closure and thick crepe or hard rubber sole. Soles can be full or partial length. Height layers can be added to crepe soles.

Wide Toe Box
- *DARCO*-to accommodate metatarsal fractures or edema

(continued)

Table 8-14 (continued) **FOOT AND ANKLE ORTHOSES**	
Shoes	**Type:** *Heel Weight Bearing (Forefoot Relief)* • *Barouk Shoe*—thick heel wedge • *DARCO Wedge*—thick heel with fore-foot protective plate *Postoperative Shoe* • Usually open-toed, hard-soled, fabric, and Velcro *Cast Shoe or Boot* • Open-toed or closed • Thick sole for weightbearing

orthopedic conditions and is not an exhaustive compendium. For areas not addressed, such as spinal cord injury, the reader is encouraged to review Chapter 9 and other texts detailing acute orthopedic and traumatic conditions.

CASE EXAMPLE

Mrs. Jackson, a 58-year-old female, restrained driver sustains a head-on car collision against a pole after skidding on ice during a winter storm. This patient was transported from the scene via helicopter to a Level I Trauma center. After evaluation in the trauma bay/emergency department, she is admitted to the hospital for surgical/medical management. Three days after admission, a physical therapy consult is ordered.

Patient/Client History

General Demographics/Social History/Living Environment

Mrs. Jackson was working full time as an accountant, is married, and lives in a split-level two-story home with three steps to enter and a handrail. The bedroom and bathroom are six steps up with a family room, and the powder room is six steps down. One grown daughter lives out of state. Her husband was a passenger in the car. He was treated for multiple facial lacerations and a fractured left wrist and required a one-night hospital stay. He was discharged to home.

General Health Status/Family History

Mrs. Jackson is overweight with a body mass index (BMI) of 30. She admits to smoking a half to one pack per day and "social" drinking. She denies drug use. She does not consider herself active and has no regular exercise routine. Hobbies include movies, knitting, and travel. Her family history is unremarkable and unrelated to the current condition.

Table 8–15
COMMON ASSISTIVE DEVICES

Bilateral

Indications:
- For use with restricted LE weightbearing
- Provide stability during ambulation
- MUST be used in conditions of:
  - Non weightbearing (0%)
  - Minimal or toe-touch weightbearing (≈10%)
  - Partial weightbearing (≈50%)

Percentages (10%, 50%, etc) refer to percent of total body weight. Sometimes restrictions are given in absolute pounds, regardless of body weight.

Type:
Crutches
- Axillary
  - Most commonly issued
  - Wooden or aluminium
- Forearm or Canadian
- Lofstrand is a brand name of forearm crutches

Walkers
- Standard, no wheels
- Wheeled or rollator
- Usually front wheeled, no brakes

Forearm platforms can attach to either crutches or walkers to allow proximal weightbearing in the presence of a distal UE fracture.

Unilateral

Indications:
- Increase stability during ambulation
- Relieve pressure on contralateral side

Type:
Straight Point Cane
Wide or Large Base Quad Cane
Narrow or Small base Quad Cane

Wheelchairs

Indications:
- When ambulation is not safe or functional

When wheelchair propulsion is performed with one leg, or both, consider a shorter ground-to-seat height, referred to as "hemi-height" to get the foot closer to floor.

Type:
Standard
- 16 inch seat depth, 18 inch width
- Removable or swing-away arm rests
- Leg rests, with calf pads, usually elevating
- Rear anti-tippers
- Consider wheel-lock (brake) extensions, when one extremity has activity restrictions

Custom
- Generally not indicated during acute phase of injury or rehabilitation

Medical/Surgical History

Mrs. Jackson has hypertension (HTN), hypercholesterolemia, and is obese. She takes Metoproplol (a beta blocker) for HTN, Lipitor for high cholesterol, and a nonsteroidal anti-inflammatory for "aches and pains" as needed. Surgical history includes caesarean section, gall bladder removal (cholecystectomy), and left arthroscopic knee surgery 3 years ago.

Current Conditions/Chief Complaints

Mrs. Jackson is status post (s/p) MVC. There was loss of consciousness (LOC) requiring intubation for airway protection by the emergency medical technician (EMT) at the scene. Injuries diagnosed upon arrival to the hospital include a left-side hemopneumothorax (Hptx), a distal right lower extremity (RLE) tibial fracture, and several (L1 to L3) lumbar spinous process fractures.

A chest tube was place in the trauma bay to evacuate blood and air from the left pleural space. Orthopedic surgery performed an ORIF to stabilize the tibia fracture. The patient spent 1 day in the intensive care unit (ICU) after surgery where she was extubated without complication and received a blood transfusion for a hemoglobin (Hgb) level of 7.3 g/dL. She was transferred to the general care ward on 2 liters of oxygen via nasal cannula, with a Foley catheter, a morphine (MS0$_4$) patient controlled analgesia (PCA) pump for pain control, and a posterior, ace wrapped splint immobilizing her distal RLE. She has a chest tube in her left flank draining to a Pleurovac collection system connected to 15 cm H$_2$O suction. Her activity status is out of bed (OOB) as tolerated, NWB on her RLE.

Functional Status and Activity Level

Prior to admission, the patient was independent with all aspects of mobility and ADLs/IADLs without the use of an assistive device. Currently, the patient is NWB on the RLE, allowed out of bed ad lib, and is dependent for all mobility secondary to pain.

Systems Review

Cardiovascular/Pulmonary

Resting blood pressure (BP) is 150/78, heart rate (HR) 90, SpO$_2$ 97% on 2 lpm. Incentive spirometry (IS) averages 500 mL. Chest tubes on left draining serosanguinous fluid. Decreased breath sounds bilateral bases with no adventitious sounds. After sitting at the edge of the bed and standing to a walker, her vital signs are: BP 116/68, HR 126, SpO$_2$ 94%. Patient reports feeling lightheaded after standing and is returned to bed. Vital signs return to baseline.

Integumentary

Based on body habitus and lack of mobility, the patient has been placed on a pressure relieving, low air-loss mattress. She has been wearing a pneumatic compression stocking on her left calf. Her surgical wound site is not visualized secondary to the dressing; the chest tube site is sutured and appears clean, dry, and intact (C/D/I). Her right toes are visible, mildly edematous, and show brisk capillary refill.

Musculoskeletal

Gross myotome assessment of bilateral UEs and left lower extremity (LLE) reveals strength within functional limits (WFL) (5/5) against gravity in all major muscle groups with left UE shoulder strength limited by pain at chest tube site. Active ROM appears grossly within normal limits (WNL). RLE not formally assessed secondary to pain with motion.

Neuromuscular

Sensation to light touch and gross proprioception are intact throughout. Patient reports "tingling" sensation at the right foot/ankle, which has been elevated since surgery.

Communication, Affect, Cognition, Language, and Learning Style

Mrs. Jackson is awake, alert, and oriented to person, place, and time. She reports feeling anxious about moving because of the fear of pain. The primary language is English. She reports that she likes to be told what is going to happen prior to moving.

Tests and Measures

Aerobic Capacity and Endurance

As noted above, the patient demonstrated orthostatic hypotension (drop in BP of 20 mmHg with symptoms) with standing at the bedside. Compensatory tachycardia was noted, with mild drop in oxygen saturation.

Assistive and Adaptive Devices

Mrs. Jackson was assisted into a standing position with use of a standard walker. The patient was able to assist with bed mobility by grabbing an overhead trapeze bar. A bedside commode has been ordered as well as a long-handled reacher.

Gait, Locomotion, and Balance

Mrs. Jackson required moderate assistance to transition from supine<>sitting at the edge of the bed and maximal assistance to complete the sit<>stand transfer and maintain abbreviated standing with a standard walker. A gait assessment was not performed at this time due to symptomatic orthostatic hypotension.

Pain

Using a visual analogue scale patient reports 5/10 pain at rest (aching) and 8/10 (sharp) with moving. Rest and elevation relieve pain.

Evaluation

Mrs. Jackson is a middle-aged female currently hospitalized secondary to a MVC sustaining orthopedic and chest wall trauma. PMH is remarkable for HTN and obesity.

Diagnosis

Mrs. Jackson presents with mobility impairments related primarily to pain with movement. Orthostatic hypotension is potentially associated with opiod analgesics and blood loss secondary to Hptx and traumatic fractures. Pulmonary function is impaired by pneumothorax and subsequent chest tube insertion leading to chest wall pain and limited ventilation. Recommended treatment pattern 6A: primary prevention/risk reduction for cardiovascular/pulmonary disorders.[1]

Prognosis

Complete tibia fracture healing should allow return to independent mobility and full-time employment without the need of an assistive device. However, it is anticipated that the patient will require acute inpatient rehabilitation upon discharge from the hospital based on current mobility deficits, pain, and her challenging home environment. Additionally, the patient may require ongoing episodes of physical therapy including outpatient services once allowed to bear weight on her RLE.

Intervention

Daily physical therapy intervention with short-term goals of increasing out of bed tolerance and decreasing level of assistance required for bedside mobilization. Interventions include ADL training (eg, bed mobility, transfers, toilet and gait training, wheelchair management), assistive and adaptive device training (eg, walker, reacher), orthotic device training (eg, posterior splint), therapeutic exercise (eg, UE/LE AROM and resistive exercises), and continuing education on use of PCA, skin integrity, incentive spirometry, weightbearing restriction, bedside ROM exercise program, and smoking cessation.

Reexamination

Patient received a fluid bolus after the first physical therapy session secondary to orthostasis. Reexamination the following day revealed the same level of assistance required but an adaptive vital sign response including an elevation in HR, BP, and stable SpO$_2$ without complaint of cardiopulmonary symptoms.

Outcomes

The patient was treated for 3 days after the initial physical therapy exam, at which point she was transferred to inpatient rehabilitation. Her chest tube, Foley catheter, and oxygen were all discontinued, and she has been converted from the PCA to oral analgesics. The patient required minimal assistance to transfers from supine to sitting, moderate assistance for sit<>stand, and was ambulating 10 feet x 2 with a rolling walker and moderate assistance. Pain continued to limit her function, particularly at her lumbar spine and tibia but was successfully managed with a pain scale rating of 1 at rest and 4 with mobility.

CHAPTER REVIEW QUESTIONS

1. What are two indications for total knee and/or hip arthoplasties?
2. Compare and contrast the pathophysiology of RA versus OA.
3. Describe at least three benefits of a CPM.
4. What is the benefit of a "log rolling" technique following spinal surgery?
5. Provide physical therapy examination findings that would lead to the prescription of a walker as compared to a large-based quad cane.

PHARMACOLOGICAL INFORMATION: MUSCULOSKELETAL/ORTHOPEDIC DISEASES AND DISORDERS PHARMACOLOGY

Biphosphonates

Action
Biphosphonates are indicated for the treatment and prevention of osteoporosis, reduce bone pain and risk of fracture in patients with bone metastases and Paget's disease. These medications reduce the resorption of bone by inhibiting the activity and recruitment of osteoclasts. Additionally, biphosphonates stimulate the production of osteoblasts.

Side Effects
CNS: Headache
CV: Dysrhythmias/tachycardia, HTN
GI: Abdominal discomfort, dyspepsia, acid reflux, nausea, vomiting
Misc: Hypokalemia, muscle weakness, musculoskeletal pain

Common Medications
Alendronate (Fosamax), Etidronate (Didronel), Pamidronate (Aredia)

Corticosteroids

Action
Systemic corticosteroids are prescribed in the management of adrenocortical insufficiency and inflammatory, allergic, hematologic, neoplastic, and autoimmune diseases. These medications inhibit inflammatory and immunologic processes through a variety of mechanisms including the reduced synthesis and release of a variety of mediators (eg, prostaglandins, leukotrienes, histamine) from lymphocytes, eosinophils, neutrophils, and mast cells.

Side Effects
CNS: Depression, euphoria, headache, restlessness
CV: HTN
Endocrine: Hyperglycemia
GI: Peptic ulcers
Mis: Osteoporosis, myopathy, weight gain, skin fragility/tears, immunocompromise

Common Medications
Betamethasone, Cortisone, Dexamethasone, Hydrocortisone, Methylprenisolone, Prednisone

Disease Modifying Antirheumatic Drugs

Action

DMARDs are a varied group of medications that alter arthritic conditions by influencing mediators, metabolites, and immune responses involved in inflammation and autoimmune reactions.

Side Effects

CNS: Fatigue, headache, dizziness
CV: Chest pain, hypotension, HTN, tachycardia
GI: Abdominal pain, nausea, vomiting, constipation, diarrhea, dyspepsia
Misc: Arthralgia, myalgias, alopecia, rash
Pulm: Upper respiratory tract infections, cough

Common Medications

Anti-tumor necrosis factor (TNF): Etanercept (Enbrel), Infliximab (Remicade)
Immune modulation: Leflunomide (Arava)
Cytostatic-cytotoxic drugs: Azathioprine (Imuran), cyclophosphamide (Cytoxan), Methotrexate (Rheumatrex)
Misc: Gold preparations

Gout Agents

Action

Gout agents attempt to decrease the hyperuricemia (elevated blood uric acid concentration), local inflammation, and pain associated with the acute bouts of arthritis that typify gout. Medications may inhibit uric acid synthesis (eg, allopurinol), alter immune responses (eg, Cholcicine), and inflammation reactions (eg, NSAIDs, corticosteroids).

Side Effects

CNS: Drowsiness
GI: Diarrhea, nausea, vomiting
GU: Renal insufficiency, hematuria
Misc: Allergic reactions, bone marrow depression (leukopenia, thrombocytopenia), aplastic anemia

Common Medications

Allopurinol, Colchicine, corticosteroids (see above)

Non-Steroidal Antiinflammatory Agents

Action

NSAIDs primarily inhibit the synthesis of prostaglandins leading to their anti-inflammatory function and to a lesser extent the thrombaxanes leading to inhibition of platelets. These medications inhibit the enzyme cyclooxygenases (COX-1, COX-2) that are required for the formation of the prostaglandins and thrombaxanes from arachidonic acid. These medications are prescribed as analgesics (mild to moderate pain), antipyretics (fever reduction), anti-platelets (eg, MI), in addition to their antiinflammatory functions (eg, OA/RA).

Side Effects
CNS: Headache, dizziness, drowsiness
CV: Prolonged bleeding times, edema
GI: Erosive gastritis, peptic ulcer disease, bleeding, dyspepsia/heart burn, nausea, vomiting
GU: Diminished sodium excretion and fluid retention, renal insufficiency (azotemia, oliguria)
Misc: Allergic reactions (bronchospasm), hyperkalemia, tinnitus

Common Medications
Salicylates (Aspirin—Ecotrin, Zorprin, Bufferin), Ibuprofen (Advil, Motrin, Nuprin), Indomethacin (Indocin), Naproxen (Aleve, Anaprox, Naprosyn)
COX-2 inhibitors: Celecoxib (Celebrex), Rofecoxib (Vioxx)

Opioids

Action
Opioids are a class of medications that bind to specific receptors within the CNS leading to alterations in the perception and responses to painful stimuli. Opioids potentiate the activitiy of endogenous opiod peptides (eg, eukephalins, endorphins) by binding to receptors resulting in the efflux of potassium, hyperpolarization, and limiting calcium influx and production of cyclic AMP. The sum of these effects reduces the release of the neurotransmitters dopamine and serotonin and inhibits nociceptive peptides such as substance P, resulting in blockage of pain transmission.

Side Effects
CNS: CNS depression/sedation, confusion, dizziness, hallucinations, seizures
CV: Hypotension, bradycardia
GI: Constipation, nausea, vomiting
Misc: Flushing, sweating, physical dependence, tolerance
Pulm: Respiratory depression/apnea, bronchospasm

Common Medications
Butorphanol (Stadol), Codeine, Fentanyl, Hydrocodone, Meperidine (Demerol), Methadone, Morphine, Oxycodone (Oxycontin, Percocet (oxycodone + acetaminophen), Percodan (oxycodone + aspirin)

Skeletal Muscle Relaxants and Antispasticity Agents

Action
Skeletal muscle relaxants and antispasticity agents are a diverse group of medications that impact neuromuscular activity. Agents may act within the CNS by inhibiting release of excitatory neurotransmitters (eg, Baclofen) or presynaptic inhibition (eg, benzodiazepines). Agents may also act peripherally

by inhibiting neuromuscular transmission through inhibition of acetylcholine release by nerve terminals (eg, Botulinum toxin) or by blocking calcium release from the sarcoplasmic reticulum thereby uncoupling muscle excitation-contraction coupling (eg, Dantrolen sodium).

Side Effects
CNS: Dizziness, drowsiness, fatigue, headache
CV: Hypotension, edema, dysrhythmias
GI: Constipation, dyspepsia, nausea
Misc: Dry mouth

Common Medications
Centrally acting: Baclofen (Lioresal), Diazepam (Valium), Cyclobenzaprine (Flexeril)
Direct acting: Dantrolene sodium (Dantrium), neuromuscular blocking agents (see Chapter 9, Pharmacological Information)

REFERENCES

1. Fisher DA, Trimble S, Clapp B, Dorsett K. Effect of a patient management system on outcomes of total hip and knee arthroplasty. *Clin Orthop.* 1997;345:155–160.
2. Mabrey JD, Toohey JS, Armstrong DA, Lavery L, Wammack LA. Clinical pathway management of total knee arthroplasty. *Clin Orthop.* 1997;345:125–133.
3. Weingarten S, Riedinger MS, Sandhu M, et al. Can practice guidelines safely reduce hospital length of stay? Results from a multicenter interventional study. *Am J Med.* 1998;105:33–39.
4. Hip and knee reconstruction 2. In: Pellici PM, Tria AJ, Garvin KL eds. *Orthopaedic Knowledge Update.* Rosemont, Ill: American Academy of Orthopaedic Surgeons; 2000.
5. Pearson SD, Kleerfield SF, Soukp JR, Cook EF, Lee TH. Critical pathways intervention to reduce length of hospital stay. *Am J Med.* 2001;110:175–180.
6. Pennington JM, Jones DPG, McIntyre S. Clininical pathways in total knee arthroplasty: a New Zealand experience. *J Orthop Surg.* 2003;11(2):166–173.
7. Orest MR. Total joint replacement literature review. *Acute Care Perspectives* (American Physical Therapy Association). 2004;13(1):10–12.
8. AAOS Department of Research and Scientific Affairs. Summary and Resources for Osteoarthritis of the Hip & Knee. Available at: http://www.aaos.org/wordhtml/research/oainfo/oainfo.htm. Accessed on April 2, 2006.
9. Vaupel G, Cacanindin N, Wong J. Total knee replacement. In: Maxey L, Magnusson J, eds. *Rehabilitation for the Post Surgical Orthopedic Patient.* St. Louis, Mo: Mosby; 2001:268–287.
10. Gartland JJ. Disorders of joints. In: Brinker MR, Miller MD, eds. *Fundamentals of Orthopaedics.* Philadelphia, Pa: WB Saunders Co; 1987:122–148.
11. Lane GJ, Hozack WJ, Shah S, et al. Simultaneous bilateral versus unilateral total knee arthroplasty. Outcomes analysis. *Clin Orthop.* 1997;345:106–112.
12. Ritter MA, Meding JB. Bilateral simultaneous total knee arthroplasty. *J Arthroplasty.* 1987;2(3):185–189.
13. Bullock DP, Sporer SM, Shirreffs TG. Comparison of simultaneous bilateral with unilateral total knee arthroplasty in terms of perioperative complications. *J Bone Joint Surg.* 2003;85(10):1981–1986.
14. Lau SKK, Chiu KY. Use of continuous passive motion after total knee arthroplasty. *J Arthroplasty.* 2001;16(3):336–339.
15. Milne S, Brosseau L, Robinson V, et al. Continuous passive motion following total knee arthroplasty. *The Cochrane Database of Systematic Reviews.* 2003;2. Art No: CD004260. DOI: 10.1002/14651858.CD004260.
16. Beaupre LA, Davies DM, Jones CA, Cinats JG. Exercise combined with continuous passive motion or slider board therapy compared with exercise only: a randomized controlled trial of patients following total knee arthroplasty. *Phys Ther.* 2001;81(4):1029–1037.
17. Munin MC, Rudy TE, Glynn NW, Crossett LS, Rubash HE. Early inpatient rehabilitation after elective hip and knee arthroplasty. *J Am Med Assoc.* 1998;279(11):847–852.
18. Forrest GP, Roque JM, Dawodu ST. Decreasing length of stay after total joint arthroplasty: effect on referrals to rehabilitation units. *Arch Phys Med Rehabil.* 1999;80(2):192–194.
19. Maloney WJ. The stiff total knee arthroplasty: evaluation and management. *J Arthroplasty.* 2002;17(4):71–73.
20. Chiu KY, Ng TP, Tang WM, Tau WP. Review article: knee flexion after total knee arthroplasty. *J Orthop Surg (Hong Kong).* 2002;10(2):194–202.

21. Santavirta N, Lillqvist G, Sarvimaki A, et al. Teaching of patients undergoing total hip replacement surgery. *Intern J Nurs Stud.* 1994;1(2):135.

22. Enloe LJ, Shields RK, Smith K, Loe K, Miller B. Total hip and knee replacement treatment programs: a report using concesus. *J Orthop Sports Phys Ther.* 1996;23(1):3–11.

23. Given-Heiss DL, Krebs DE, Riley PO, et al. In vivo acetabular contact pressures during rehabilitation. Part II post acute phase. *Phys Ther.* 1992;72(10):700–705.

24. Stricland EM, Fares M, Krebs DE, et al. In vivo acetabular contact pressures during rehabilitation. Part I acute phase. *Physical Therapy.* 1992;72(10):691–699.

25. Berger RA, Kull LR, Rosenberg AG, Galante JO. Hybrid total hip arthroplasty: 7-10-year results. *Clin Orthop.* 1996;Dec(333):134–146.

26. Kavanagh BF, Wallrichs S, Dewitz M, et al. Charnley low-friction arthroplasty of the hip. Twenty-year results with cement. *J Arthroplasty.* 1994;9(3): 229–234.

27. Kelly MJ, Leggin BG. Shoulder rehabilitation. In: Iannotti JP, Williams GR, eds. *Disorders of the Shoulder: Diagnosis and Management.* Philadelphia, Pa: Lippincott Williams & Wilkins; 1999:1012–1014.

28. Lauremann WC, Goldsmith ME. Spine. In: Miller MD, Brinker MR, eds. *Review of Orthopaedics.* 3rd ed. Philadelphia, Pa: WB Saunders Co; 2000:353–378.

29. Nygaard OP, Kloster R, Solberg T. Duration of leg pain as a predictor of outcome after surgery forlumbar disc herniation: a prospective cohort stud with 1-year follow up. *J Neurosurg.* 2001;95(2 Suppl):281–282.

30. Canale ST. *Campbell's Operative Orthopaedics: Part XII Spine.* 10th ed. St. Louis, Mo: Mosby Inc; 2003.

31. Brown TD, Michas P, Williams RE, et al. The impact of gunshot wounds on an orthopedic surgical service in an urban trauma center. *J Orthop Trauma.* 1997;11(3):149–153.

32. Wright DG, Levin JS, Esterhai JL, Heppenstall RB. Immediate internal fixation of low-velocity gunshot-related femoral fractures. *J Trauma.* 1993;35(5):678–681.

33. Patel AI, Lonner BS, Hoppenfield S. Cervical spine compression and burst fractures. In: Hoppenfield S, Vasantha LM, eds. *Treatment & Rehabilitation of Fractures.* Philadelphia, Pa: Lippincott Williams & Wilkins; 2000:535–544.

34. DiGiacomo JC, Bondies JA, Cole FJ, et al. *Practice Management Guidelines for Hemorrhage in Pelvic Fractures.* Winston-Salem, NC: Eastern Association for the Surgery of Trauma; 2001. Available at: http://www.east.org/TPG/Pelvis.pdf.

35. Frakes MA, Evans T. Major pelvic fractures. *Crit Care Nurs.* 2004;24:18-31.

36. Canale ST. *Campell's Operative Orthopaedics: Part XV Fractures and Dislocations.* 10th ed. St. Louis, Mo: Mosby, Inc; 2003.

37. Craik RL. Disability following hip fracture. *Phys Ther.* 1994;74(5): 387–398.

38. Khasragi FA, Lee EJ, Christmas C, Wenz JF. The economic impact of medial complications in geriatric patients with hip fracture. *Orthopedics.* 2003;26(1):49–53.

39. Melton LJ III. Adverse outcomes of osteoporotic fractures in the general population. *J Bone Mineral Res.* 2003;18(16):1139–1141.

40. Nurmi I, Narinen A, Luthje P, Tanninen S. Cost analysis of hip fracture treatment among the elderly for the public health services: a 1-year prospective study in 106 consecutive patients. *Arch Orthop Trauma Surg.* 2003;123(10):551–554.

41. Mossey JM, Mutran E, Knott K, Craik R. Determinants of recovery 12 months after hip fracture: the importance of psychosocial factors. *Am J Public Health.* 1989;79(3):279–286.

42. Magaziner J, Fredman L, Hawkes W, et al. Changes in functional status attributable to hip fracture: a comparison study of hip fracture patients to community-dwelling aged. *Am J Epidemiol.* 2003;157(11):1023–1031.
43. Browner. *Skeletal Trauma: Basic Science, Management, and Reconstruction.* 3rd ed. Philadelphia, Pa: WB Saunders; 2003.
44. Freudigman PT, Ziran BH. Orthopedic injuries. In: Peitzman AB, Rhodes M, Schwab CW, Yealy DM, eds. *The Trauma Manual.* Philadelphia, Pa: Lippincott-Raven; 1998.
45. Levine SE, Esterhai JL Jr, Heppenstall RB, Calhoun J, Mader JT. Diagnosis and staging. Osteomyelitis and prosthetic joint infections. *Clin Orthop.* 1993;295:77–86.
46. Hayda RA, Brighton CT, Esterhai JL Jr. Pathophysiology of delayed healing. *Clin Orthop.* 1998;355(Suppl):S31–S40.
47. Esterhai JL Jr, Queenan J. Management of soft tissue wounds associated with type III open fractures. *Orthop Clin North Am.* 1991;22(3): 427–432.
48. Blaha JD, Calhoun JH, Nelson CL, et al. Comparison of the clinical efficacy and toerance of gentamicin PMMA beads on surgical wire versus combined and systemic therapy for osteomyelitis. *Clin Orthop.* 1993;295:8–12.
49. Evans RP, Nelson CL. Gentamicin-impregnated polymethylmethacrylate beads compared with systemic antibiotic therapy in the treatment of chronic osteomyelitis. *Clin Orthop.* 1993;295:37–42.
50. Brighton CT, Shaman P, Heppenstall RB, et al. Tibial nonunion treated with direct current, capacitive coupling and bone graft. *Clin Orthop.* 1995;321:223–234.
51. Lane JM, Glasser DB, Cammisa FP. Tumors. In: Steinberg, M, ed. *The Hip and Its Disorders.* Philadelphia, Pa: WB Saunders & Co; 1991:493.
52. Shurr DG, Cook TM. *Prosthetics and Orthotics.* E. Norwalk, Conn: Appleton & Lange; 1990.
53. Buonomo LJ, Klein JS, Keiper TL. Orthotic devices. Custom-made, prefabricated, and material selection. *Foot Ankle Clin.* 2001;6(2):249–252.
54. American Physical Therapy Association. Guide to physical therapy practice. *Phys Ther.* 2001;8(1).

BIBLIOGRAPHY

Craig CR, Stitzel RE. *Modern Pharmacology with Clinical Applications.* New York, NY: Little, Brown, and Co; 1997.
Deglin JH, Vallerand AH. *Davis's Drug Guide for Nurses.* 8th ed. Philadelphia, Pa: FA Davis Co; 2003.
Karch AM. *Lippincott's Nursing Drug Guide.* Springhouse, Pa: Lippincott Williams & Wilkins; 2004.
Ritter JM, Lewis LD, Mant TG. *Textbook of Clinical Pharmacology.* London, England: Edward Arnold Co; 1995

NEUROLOGIC AND NEUROSURGICAL DISEASES AND DISORDERS

Colleen Chancler, PT, MHS
Heather Dillon, MSPT, NCS

PART I: NEUROLOGY

Neurologic dysfunction encompasses many different disorders, including diagnoses based on a cluster of symptoms. The physical therapist and physical therapist assistant are commonly involved in the care of the patient from the intensive care unit (ICU) to the time of discharge to the next level of care. Fortunately, some of the interventions that are performed by physical therapy have evidence to support the use and the outcome of the patient. While examination and treatment strategies are numerous, the physiological response of the patient needs to be considered in each interaction because many neurological conditions and comorbidities arise in patient care. Progress can often be seen with direct therapy intervention and is an exciting part of the overall care of the patient.

ANATOMY AND PHYSIOLOGY

Anatomically, the **cerebral cortex** is described by dividing the surface area into the following lobes: frontal, parietal, temporal, occipital, limbic, and insular. The frontal lobe is generally described as the executor of human function. It is responsible for organizing behavior, shaping self-awareness, and controlling the actions of our bodies.[1] The parietal lobe serves as the sensory integrator for pain, temperature, detection of taste, and touch; it also coordinates the process of reading.[1] The temporal lobe contains the primary auditory center along with regions that are responsible for emotion, memory, and speech.[2,3] The occipital lobe contains the primary visual cortex and the visual association area (Figure 9–1).

Figure 9–1. Cerebral lobes. (Reprinted with permission from Gutman SA. *Quick Reference Neuroscience.* Thorofare, NJ: SLACK Incorporated; 2001:7.)

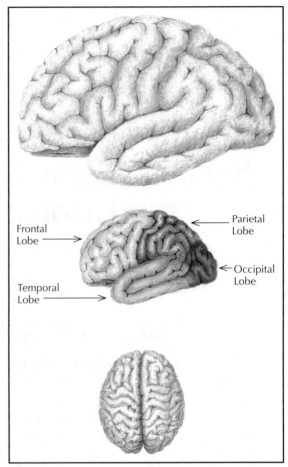

Frontal Lobe →

Temporal Lobe →

← Parietal Lobe

← Occipital Lobe

The **brainstem** is a stalk-like structure, located in the posterior cranial fossa, that forms the rostral continuation of the spinal cord; this junction is marked by the foramen magnum.[4,5] The brainstem is covered posteriorly by the cerebellum and houses the fourth ventricle.[6] It consists of the medulla oblongata, pons, and midbrain. Each region has specialized responsibilities while sharing common fiber tracts.[2,7] These tracts carry somatosensory impulses as well as voluntary motor signals.[8] In addition, all but one of the 12 cranial nerves are located within the brainstem.[3] The brainstem connects to the cerebellum by three pairs of cerebellar peduncles that enable the transmission of information.[6]

The **cerebellum** lies anterior to the medulla and pons and is separated from them by the fourth ventricle. It connects to the brainstem via the paired inferior, middle, and superior cerebellar peduncles.[3,5] The cerebellum also contains four pairs of cerebellar nuclei deep to its surface.[2] The cerebellum is responsible for coordinating movements and balance by influencing the timing and force of voluntary muscular contractions (Figure 9–2).[2,4]

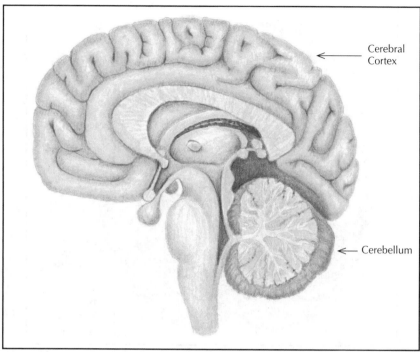

Cerebral
Cortex

Cerebellum

Figure 9–2. Midsagittal cross section of the brain. (Reprinted with permission from Gutman SA. *Quick Reference Neuroscience.* Thorofare, NJ: SLACK Incorporated; 2001:13.)

Four main arteries furnish the blood supply to the brain (Figure 9–3). They include the paired vertebral arteries, which supply the brainstem, cerebellum, and posteroinferior cerebrum, and the paired ICA, which supply the anterior, superior, and lateral cerebral hemispheres.[2,8,9]

The paired **vertebral arteries**, the first branches of the subclavian arteries, carry approximately one-third of the blood supply to the brain. Each vertebral artery has three main branches: the anterior and posterior spinal arteries and the posterior inferior cerebellar artery (PICA). All three branches supply blood to the medulla. In addition, the PICA also supplies the inferior cerebellum.[2,10] A stroke within the distribution of the vertebral artery may cause the following signs and symptoms[2,9–11]:

- **Wallenberg's syndrome**, also known as **lateral meduallary syndrome**, which involves pain, numbness, impaired sensation over half of the face, ataxia, vertigo, nystagmus, diplopia, dysphagia, muscular weakness or paralysis, numbness on the lateral side, and impaired pain and temperature on the contralateral side. This syndrome may also include ipsilateral **Horner's syndrome** (miosis, ptosis of the upper lid, elevation of the lower lid and anhidrosis on the affected side of face).[11]

- **Medial medullary syndrome** which involves ipsilateral paralysis of the tongue, contralateral paralysis of the upper extremity (UE) and lower

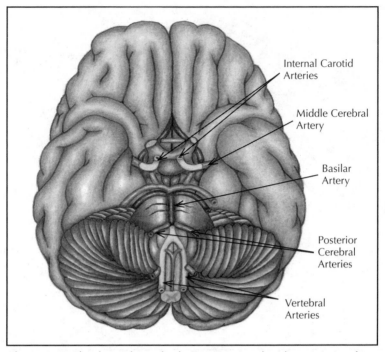

Figure 9–3. Blood supply to the brain. (Reprinted with permission from Gutman SA. *Quick Reference Neuroscience.* Thorofare, NJ: SLACK Incorporated; 2001:197.)

extremity (LE) (facial muscles typically spared) and contralateral impairment of touch and position sense.

- Pain in the face, nose or eye; ipsilateral numbness and weakness of the face, nystagmus.
- Decreased coordination, dizziness, staggering gait.
- Dysphagia and/or dysarthria.

The **basilar artery** and its branches, which include the anterior inferior cerebellar artery (AICA) and superior cerebellar artery, supply the pons and the cerebellum.[6] At the junction of the midbrain and pons, the basilar artery divides into the posterior cerebral arteries, which serve as the primary blood supply to the midbrain.[2,11] Complete occlusion of this artery may be fatal. In general, basilar artery strokes may cause the following signs and symptoms[2,9]:

- Disturbances of consciousness (often coma).
- Bilateral cerebellar ataxia.
- Decreased strength in facial, tongue, and pharyngeal muscles.
- **Locked-in syndrome,** which is characterized by the patient being alert and awake but completely paralyzed. The only functions spared are the ability to move eyes vertically and blink.

- Paralysis.
- Diplopia, paralysis of conjugate lateral and/or vertical gaze, ophthalmoplegia (paralysis of ocular musculature), and/or nystagmus.

AICA stroke, also known as **lateral inferior pontine syndrome**, may cause the following signs and symptoms[2,9–11]:

- Ipsilateral paresis of lateral conjugate gaze and or nystagmus.
- Ipsilateral **Horner's syndrome** (see description on p 319).
- Ipsilateral limb ataxia.
- Vertigo, nausea, and/or **oscillopsia** (illusory sensation of the oscillation or swinging of the visual field).
- Impaired hearing and/or tinnitus.
- Contralateral impaired pain and temperature sensation in the trunk, limbs, and face.

The **internal carotid arteries** (ICA) originate from the common carotid artery, and bifurcate into the external and ICA. The external carotid arteries divide into extracranial branches, while the ICA enter the skull through the temporal bones.[3,6] Branches of the internal carotid artery become the **posterior communicating arteries** (PCA), which join the ICA to the posterior cerebral artery.[6] Near the optic chiasm, the ICA divides into anterior and middle cerebral arteries. Internal carotid artery stroke may cause the following signs and symptoms[2,9,10]:

- Paralysis of the contralateral face, UEs and LEs.
- Sensory impairments of the contralateral face, UEs and LEs.
- Aphasia if the dominant hemisphere is affected.
- Apraxia, agnosia, and unilateral neglect if the nondominant hemisphere is affected.
- **Homonymous hemianopsia,** which involves similar visual loss in both eyes involving half of each visual field.

The **circle of Willis** (Figure 9–4) is an anastomotic ring of nine arteries: the anterior communicating, the left anterior cerebral, left internal carotid, left posterior cerebral, basilar, right posterior cerebral, right posterior communicating, right internal carotid, and right anterior cerebral artery (ACA).[6,12] Because of its communicative design, the circle of Willis serves as a potential vascular shunt. This mechanism may assist in the development of collateral circulation to the brain should one of the proximal vessels, such as the carotid or basilar, become occluded.

The three major **cerebral arteries** (anterior, middle, and posterior) have cortical branches that supply the cortex and outer white matter and deep branches that supply the central gray matter and adjacent white matter.[6,8] The **ACA** supplies the medial surfaces of the frontal and parietal lobes as well as the anterior head of the caudate nucleus, which is part of the basal ganglia.[3,6] The ACA is the least likely vessel to become occluded. The **middle cerebral artery (MCA)** divides into branches that ultimately supply the lateral surface of the frontal, parietal, temporal, and occipital lobes.[6] The branches that supply these regions,

Figure 9–4. Circle of Willis. (Reprinted with permission from Gutman SA. *Quick Reference Neuroscience*. Thorofare, NJ: SLACK Incorporated; 2001:199.)

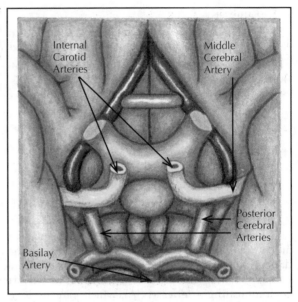

Internal Carotid Arteries

Middle Cerebral Artery

Posterior Cerebral Arteries

Basilay Artery

also known as lateral striate arteries, are frequently the site of rupture or occlusion.[6] The **posterior cerebral artery (PCA)** supplies the midbrain, thalamus, occipital lobe and sections of the medial and inferior temporal lobe.[3]

The **watershed** area represents an area of marginal blood flow on the surface of the lateral hemispheres, where small anastomoses link the distal ends of the cerebral arteries.[13] Hypotension, or hypoperfusion, may cause decreased blood flow to this area and may cause upper limb paresis and paresthesia.[8] The most common watershed cerebral infarct is between the ACAs and MCAs.[13]

PATHOLOGY

Stroke

A **stroke** or brain attack (cerebrovascular accident [CVA]) is currently the third leading cause of mortality and the leading cause of disability in the United States.[14–16] This disease process manifests as a sudden neurologic deficit, with a duration greater than 24 hours, due to a disruption of blood supply to the brain.[17] A **transient ischemic attack (TIA)** is described as a temporary focal brain or brainstem ischemia with symptoms lasting less than 24 hours. TIAs often preclude stroke.[15] There are approximately 700,000 strokes per year in which more than 300,000 individuals sustain significant disability. Stroke can be linked to the following risk factors: atherosclerosis, hypertension (HTN), vascular insufficiency, diabetes, cardiac disease, and advanced age.[16–19]

Table 9–1 provides general descriptions of the impairments that may result from damage to regions of the brain.

The pathological processes causing strokes are classified as ischemia or hemorrhage. Cerebral damage occurs secondary to reduced oxygenation of brain

Table 9–1
CEREBROVASCULAR ACCIDENT IMPAIRMENTS BASED ON CENTRAL NERVOUS SYSTEM REGION[15]

Region	Impairment
Right cerebral hemisphere	Left-sided paresis, decreased attention span, decreased awareness and judgment, memory deficits, left hemianopsia, left inattention, decreased abstract reasoning, emotional lability, impulsivity and/or decreased spatial orientation
Left cerebral hemisphere	Right-sided paresis, right hemianopsia aphasia, apraxia, decreased right and left discrimination, dysphagia, decreased initiation of tasks, increased frustration, and/or compulsive behavior
Brainstem	Bilateral paresis, unstable vital signs, decreased consciousness, and/or dysphagia
Cerebellum	Bilateral decreased coordination, ataxia, nystagmus, nausea, and/or decreased postural control

tissue, which leads to cell damage and/or death.[14,16] The location and severity of the lesion coupled with the quality of collateral blood flow influence the severity of neurologic deficits that evolve following a stroke.[14,15]

Ischemic strokes are more common than hemorrhagic strokes and account for approximately 80% of the strokes in the United States.[17] Ischemic strokes are characterized by cerebral hypoperfusion which causes tissue injury secondary to a reduced oxygen and glucose supply.[14,17] The most common cause of ischemic stroke is thromboembolic atherosclerotic disease with emboli traveling from the cervical vessels (carotid arteries or vertebrobasilar system) and/or the heart.[19] Additional causes include thrombosis, hemodynamic compromise, and vessel stenosis.[16,18]

Symptoms of ischemic stroke develop and worsen over time. Ischemic strokes occur most often in the early morning or the evening. Warning symptoms such as visual changes, cognitive impairment, slurred speech, motor dysfunction, and impaired ambulation usually precede an ischemic stroke.

Hemorrhagic strokes are characterized by abnormal bleeding of cerebral vessels. This type of stroke may occur within the brain parenchyma (intracerebral hemorrhage [ICH]) or within the meninges (subdural hemorrhage [SDH] or subarachnoid hemorrhage [SAH]).[15] Cellular destruction is caused by ischemia secondary to reduced blood flow beyond the damaged portion of the vessel and mechanical injury caused by edema and the pressure of blood collection.[17] Causes of hemorrhagic strokes include advanced age, HTN, arteriovenous malformation (AVM), closed head injury, coagulopathy, ruptured aneurysms, and drug abuse.[14,19,20]

Unlike ischemic strokes, the area of infarction association with hemorrhagic strokes does not follow vascular territories but instead may travel deep into brain structures and extend into several vascular territories causing unique clinical symptoms.[20] Vomiting, a severe headache, and/or impaired consciousness are symptoms that typically occur with hemorrhagic strokes. The sudden onset of these symptoms may help differentiate hemorrhagic strokes from ischemic strokes.[18,19]

Acute diagnosis for a stroke typically involves a thorough systems review, past medical history, physical examination, and diagnostic testing to determine the origin and the extent of the stroke.[21] Lab values, electrocardiogram (ECG), and scanning images are performed prior to the initiation of a treatment plan. Computed tomography (CT) scan, magnetic resonance imaging (MRI), and magnetic resonance angiography (MRA) to examine blood flow and vascular integrity in the neck, brain, and intracranial arteries are also typically performed. Transcranial doppler (TCD) is the use of ultrasound waves to measure blood velocity through the major intracranial arteries as well as the collateral circulation.[18] Increased TCDs may signify ischemic stroke. Acute ischemic strokes may be treated with intravenous tissue plasminogen activator (tPA) if the onset of symptoms is known to be less than 3 hours and specific criteria, including brain imaging, confirms a nonhemorrhagic event.[17] tPA is a thrombolytic agent known to be effective in reducing impairments and/or disability caused by ischemic strokes by reducing or eliminating the presence of a blood clot within the brain.[17] Functional abilities should be documented at the time of admission and monitored throughout the length of stay. The modified NIH stroke scale (mNIHSS) is an excellent tool for measuring stroke severity in the acute care setting.[22] The mNIHSS is a quantiative scale that includes motor, sensory, cognitive, speech, and visual domains (Table 9–2). This scale has established reliability and validity in clinical research.[23–25]

Neuromuscular Diseases

Parkinsonism syndrome (PS) is characterized by clinical features of tremor, rigidity, bradykinesia, changes in handwriting (micrographia), reduction in speech volume, and gait disorders.[14] Medical conditions that cause PS include toxic exposures, hypothyroidism, hypoparathyroidism, and other neurologic conditions. One of the main causes of Parkinsonism is **Parkinson's disease (PD)**.[15] PD is an idiopathic neurogenerative disorder that affects approximately 1 out of 100 people over the age of 75 years old, and 1 out of every 1,000 people over the age of 65.[9,26,27] The etiology is unknown; slightly more males than females are affected by the disease. Management of PD typically involves pharmacologic therapy with antidyskinetic agents.[13]

Clinical features include tremor at rest, rigidity, bradykinesia, and gait impairments. Tremor is characterized by "pill rolling" of the fingertips and hands. Tremor is exacerbated by conditions of stress, fatigue, or by the beginning or end of movement. **Dykinesia**, overactivity of muscles, can cause rigidity of movement patterns. Rigidity in the extremities is a "cogwheel" phenomenon, which is resistance to passive movement in a jerking fashion throughout the range of motion (ROM) or "lead pipe" phenomenon, which is resistance to passive movement throughout the entire motion. Facial rigidity, fixed trunk flexion, and loss of trunk rotation may occur as the syndrome/disease progresses. **Bradykinesia** is slowness in initiating movement or completion of tasks. Persons with PS/PD

Table 9–2
MODIFIED NATIONAL INSTITUTES OF HEALTH STROKE SCALE

	Item Name	Response
1A	Level of consciousness	0 = Alert 2 = Not alert, obtunded 3 = Unresponsive
1B	Questions	0 = Answers both correctly 1 = Answers neither correctly 2 = Answers neither correctly
1C	Commands	0 = Performs both tasks correctly 1 = Performs one task correctly 2 = Performs neither task correctly
2	Gaze	0 = Normal 1 = Partial gaze palsy 2 = Total gaze palsy
3	Visual fields	0 = No visual field loss 1 = Partial hemianopsia 2 = Complete hemianopsia 3 = Bilateral hemianopsia
4	Facial palsy	0 = Normal 1 = Minor paralysis 2 = Partial paralysis 3 = Complete paralysis
5	Motor arm	0 = No drift 1 = Drift before 5 seconds 2 = Falls before 10 seconds 3 = No effort against gravity 4 = No movement
6	Motor leg	0 = No drift 1 = Drift before 5 seconds 2 = Falls before 5 seconds 3 = No effort against gravity 4 = No movement
7	Ataxia	0 = Absent 1 = One limb 2 = Two limbs
8	Sensory	0 = Normal 1 = Mild loss 2 = Severe loss

(continued)

Table 9–2 (continued)
MODIFIED NATIONAL INSTITUTES OF HEALTH STROKE SCALE

	Item Name	*Response*
9	Language	0 = Normal 1 = Mild aphasia 2 = Severe aphasia 3 = Mute or global aphasia
10	Dysarthria	0 = Normal 1 = Mild 2 = Severe
11	Extinction and inattention	0 = Normal 1 = Mild 2 = Severe

Adapted from Kasner SE, Cucchiara BL, McGarvey ML, et al. Modified National Institutes of Health Stroke Scale can be estimated from medical records. *Stroke.* 2003;34:568–570.

demonstrate decreased ability to initiate movement and change directions (mild hypokinesia). Associated gait disorders can vary in presentation and severity. **Festinating gait** (small shuffling gait pattern), **akinesia** (decreased initiation of motion), and severe **hypokinesia** (reduction in movement) can result in instability and falls.[27] Recent studies have shown that patients with PS/PD have difficulty when trying to self-initiate a task. In gait for instance, the patient would have a more difficult time when walking across a floor because he or she has to choose the path and the sequence of the task. If presented the same task with external cueing by music or verbal commands, then the patient would be motivated by external stimulus and have less difficulty in initiation and completion of the motor task.[28]

The pathophysiology of PD is related to decreased amounts of the neurotransmitter dopamine. **Dopamine** is produced by nerve cells in the substania nigra and is responsible for smooth and balanced movement. PD causes nerve cell death that impacts the production of dopamine. Changes of dopamine receptors result in decreased binding of dopamine within the basal ganglia.[14,15] Diagnosis is often delayed because symptoms can initially mirror other neurologic conditions. There is no specific diagnostic test for PD. Rather, diagnosis of the disease is made by the physician examination, comprehensive history, activity level, and elimination of other neurologic causes for the symptom manifestation. Use of the Hoehn and Yahr classification allows for a clinical representation and staging progression of the disease process (Table 9–3).

Multiple sclerosis (MS) is an upper motor neuron disease characterized by an inflammatory process that results in the destruction of the myelin sheath within the white matter of the central nervous system (CNS).[9,29] This process disrupts neurotransmission and leaves patches of sclerotic tissue or scarring

Table 9–3	
HOEHN AND YAHR CLASSIFICATION	
Stage I	Unilateral involvement only with minimal or no functional impairment
Stage II	Bilateral or axial involvement without balance impairment
Stage III	Impaired righting reflexes; functional impairments exist, but patient remains independent
Stage IV	Able to walk but severe disability
Stage V	Confined to bed or chair and requires assistance for all tasks

Adapted from Morris ME. Movement disorders in people with Parkinson's disease: a model for physical therapy. *Physical Therapy.* 2000;80:578–596.

that contributes to the destruction of axons.[14] With prolonged scarring produced by damaged glial cells, called gliosis, the nerve fibers in that region degenerate and cause permanent disability.[5,15] Initially, neurologic symptoms typically correspond to the affected region of the CNS and disappear completely during remission.[15]

The signs and symptoms of MS are widely varied because the disease affects multiple regions within the CNS. Typical impairments include: fatigue, sensory dysfunction, motor symptoms, spasticity, ataxia, visual disturbances, and/or decreased coordination.[30] When the brainstem is involved, **Charcot triad** may emerge which includes nystagmus, intentional tremors, and staccato speech scanning.[30]

MS is the most common cause of severe physical disability in young adults; the highest rate of incidence is between 20 and 40 years of age.[2,31] The majority of persons with MS report the onset of symptoms to occur in their 30s, with women being slightly more affected than men, and whites being more affected than blacks.[15] The etiology of MS is unknown. There is no specific diagnostic test for MS. Diagnosis is primarily clinical diagnosis and supportive evidence from MRI, spinal tap, EMG, and laboratory studies.[30]

The clinical description of MS can be roughly divided into four patterns as described in Table 9–4. MS is often managed pharmacologically with the use of interferons, immunosuppressive agents, and hormones; steroids are commonly administered during exacerbations (see Pharmacological Information in Chapters 7, 10, and 14).[30]

The most common cause of acute neuromuscular paralysis is **Guillain-Barre syndrome** (GBS), also called **acute idiopathic polyneuritis**.[15] GBS strikes approximately 1 in 100,000 people annually with a 10% mortality rate.[32]

GBS is a lower motor neuron disease that involves rapid demyelination causing motor weakness, areflexia, and sensory abnormalities.[33] Symptoms typically begin distally with fine paresthesias in toes and/or hands and develop into acute motor weaknesses and sensory disturbances that ascend symmetrically to the upper body. Weakness may also involve respiratory, bulbar, and/or autonomic failure.[9,15]

Table 9–4

CLINICAL COURSE OF MULTIPLE SCLEROSIS

Type	Incidence	Description
Benign	20%	Abrupt onset with mild symptoms and few exacerbations. Remissions are near complete with minimal or no disability.
Exacerbating/remitting	20% to 30%	Increased frequency of attacks with sudden onset of symptoms; partial or complete remission of symptoms after exacerbations. Patients often go for long periods between attacks, but may be left with permanent disabilities.
Remitting-progressive	40%	Similar to exacerbating—remitting except the remissions are fewer with decreased resolution of symptoms. The disease becomes cumulative and disability increases.
Progressive	10% to 20%	Insidious onset without remission, leads to progressive loss of function and severe disability.

Adapted from:
Hickey JV. *Clinical Practice of Neurological and Neurosurgical Nursing*. Philadelphia, Pa: JB Lippincott Co; 1992.
O'Sullivan, Schmitz TJ. *Physical Rehabilitation, Assessment and Treatment*. 3rd ed. Philadelphia, Pa: FA Davis Co; 1994.
Umphred DA. *Neurological Rehabilitation*. 3rd ed. St. Louis, Mo: Mosby-Year Book, Inc; 1995.

The etiology of GBS is unknown. Approximately 40% to 60% of patients with GBS report a preceding bacterial or viral infection.[33] The predominant pathological finding is an immune-mediated inflammation of the cranial and spinal nerve roots with lymphocytic and macrophage infiltration and demyelination.[32,33] Damage to the myelin sheath reduces and/or blocks saltatory nerve conduction, causing paresis.[6] In addition, axonal degeneration has been noted in many cases, in which conduction velocity is within normal limits, but the number of motor units is decreased.[34]

At the peak of its course, which is typically 7 to 14 days, 20% to 30% of persons with GBS will require mechanical ventilation.[34] The recovery phase typically begins 2 weeks to 1 month following onset and involves remyelination that usually begins proximally and spreads distally.[33,34] Weakness that progresses chronically (longer than 4 weeks) or relapses may be considered **chronic idiopathic demyelinating polyradiculoneuropathy (CIDP)**.[33] The recovery phase for GBS may continue for many months. Approximately 80% of patients become ambulatory within 6 months following onset, with 70% to 80% of patients making a full recovery.[15] Treatment of GBS typically includes plasmapherisis and high dose immunoglobulin therapy.[9]

The most common primary disorder of neuromuscular transmission is **myasthenia gravis (MG)** with an incidence of 14 out of every 100,000 people in the United States.[35,36] MG is a chronic, progressive autoimmune disease that is characterized by weakness of the voluntary muscles, particularly those of chewing, swallowing, speaking, as well as the facial and extraocular muscles.[37] The onset of symptoms is typically gradual, with symptoms progressing over a period of 5 to 7 years.[35] The ocular, facial, and oropharyngeal muscles are often affected first, with weakness eventually extending to the extremities and diaphragm.[35] A sudden exacerbation of symptoms that involves respiratory failure is known as a myasthenic crises and often requires mechanical ventilation.[36,37]

The pathophysiology of MG is related to antibodies that bind and degrade acetylcholine (Ach) receptors located within the neuromuscular junction.[36] This process reduces the number of receptor sites interfering with the transmission of nerve impulses to the muscle and inhibiting muscle contraction.[35,36] There is currently no cure for MG. Treatment options for symptom management include cholinesterase inhibitors, immunosuppressive medications, plasmapheresis, thymectomy, and intravenous immunoglobulin.[35-37]

Amyotrophic lateral sclerosis (ALS), also known as Lou Gehrig's disease, is a rapidly progressive, fatal, degenerative disease that affects both upper and lower motor neurons.[15] In the United States, the incidence of ALS is 1.4 per 100,000 people with a ratio of three men to every woman.[2] It is characterized by an insidious onset of asymmetrical weakness. Additional symptoms include muscle cramping and fasciculations, hyperreflexia, and cranial nerve dysfunction with intact sensation and cognition.[2,35]

The etiology of ALS is unknown; however, numerous theories, including viral, toxic, defective DNA, and/or hormonal malfunction have been proposed.[2,15] ALS is characterized by massive destruction of anterior horn cells and motor cranial nerve nuclei, along with demyelination and gliosis of the pyramidal tracts.[15] ALS progresses rapidly; researchers estimate that by the time patient identifies his or her first symptom, 80% of the motor neurons in the affected region have already been destroyed.[15] Patients with an initial onset of bulbar and respiratory weakness tend to have a more rapid progression than patients who report their initial symptoms in the distal extremities.[9] The median survival time is approximately 4 years after onset of symptoms.[15] Currently, there is no cure for ALS.

Traumatic Brain Injury

According to Davies, 1.5 to 2 million traumatic brain injuries (TBIs) occur annually in the United States and up to 90,000 of these persons will experience long-term functional impairments, cognitive impairments, and emotional changes.[38] TBI is currently the number one killer and disabler of children and young adults, with child abuse accounting for 64% of infant brain injuries.[15] The most common age group for TBI is 15 to 24 years old, with the incidence in males two to three times greater than females.[2,15,38]

Motor vehicles accidents are the most common cause of TBI, accounting for 50%, falls account for 20%, violence accounts for 12%, and sports-related injuries account for 12%.[38] According to Yanko and Mitcho, there has been gradual decline of TBIs in the past 20 years, which is attributed to improvements in automobile safety standards.[39]

The pathophysiology of TBI involves primary and secondary injuries. The **primary** mechanism of injury occurs at the moment of impact and involves extracranial injury (open head injury), including skull fracture(s) and/or intracranial injury (closed head injury).[39] **Secondary** brain injuries are related to the pathophysiologic changes that occur after the primary insult to the brain. These changes include systemic hypotension, edema, respiratory complications, hypoxia, autodestructive cellular phenomena, which involves neurochemical changes that ultimately cause the destruction of neurons, and increased **intracranial pressure (ICP),** which may result in **herniation** of brain tissue.[15,39,40]

Intracranial injury often includes local brain damage caused by contusions and/or lacerations along the surface of the brain. These may occur at the location of impact (coup), directly opposite the site of impact (contrecoup), or in both regions (coup-contrecoup).[13] **Diffuse axonal injury (DAI)** is characterized by diffuse white matter degeneration, global neurologic dysfunction, and diffuse cerebral edema.[39] DAI occurs secondary to a widely scattered shearing of subcortical axons within their myelin sheaths in the presence of impact forces.[40,41] DAI remains a diagnosis of exclusion because imaging technology often fails to detect changes in the brain tissue despite clinical presentation of cognitive impairment or conscious changes.[40,42] If damage is widespread and extends into the midbrain and brainstem, it may cause cumulative effects such as coma and/or autonomic dysfunction.[40,41]

Late-occurring intracranial hematomas and/or ICHs are additional sources of secondary brain injury. Hematomas are named for the location in which they occur (epidural, subdural, or intracerebral) and by the time in which they develop (acute, subacute, or chronic).[41]

TBIs can be classified based on the location, extent, severity, and/or the mechanism of injury.[13] In addition, several clinical rating scales have been developed to standardize the descriptions of patients who have sustained brain injury. The **Glasgow Coma Scale (GCS),** as described in Table 9–5, rates the level of consciousness from 3 to 15 using the following three parameters: eye opening, motor response, and verbal response.[14] According to Jennett and Teasdale, the researchers who developed the GSC, patients who score 8 or less are classified as having severe head injuries. Scores between 9 and 12 are indicative of moderate head injuries, and those classified as mild head injuries score 13 and above. The minimum GCS score is 3, and the maximum is 15.[5,15]

The **Rancho Los Amigos Level of Cognitive Functioning (LOCF),** as featured in Table 9–6, was also designed to assess arousal by describing a predictable sequence of cognitive and behavioral recovery seen in patients with TBI.[14] A patient may plateau at any level but will typically progress through the described stages. By referring to the appropriate stage, therapists are able to complete a uniform assessment, documentation, and prediction of behavior.[14,15]

REHABILITATION INTERVENTIONS

Neurologic Evaluation

One of the most important aspects of completing a thorough neurologic examination (Table 9–7) is to first complete a comprehensive chart review. After

Table 9–5
GLASGOW COMA SCALE

Activity	Score
Eye opening (E):	
Spontaneously	4
To verbal command	3
To pain	2
No response	1
Best motor response (M):	
To verbal command:	
Obeys	6
To painful stimulus:	
Localizes pain	5
Flexion-withdrawl	4
Flexion-abnormal	3
Extension	2
No response	1
Verbal response (V):	
Oriented and converses	5
Disoriented and converses	4
Inappropriate words	3
Incomprehensible sounds	2
No response	1
Coma score (E + M + V) = 3 to 15	

Adapted from O'Sullivan, Schmitz TJ. *Physical Rehabilitation, Assessment and Treatment.* 3rd ed. Philadelphia, Pa: FA Davis Co; 1994.

the chart review, approach the patient with an observant eye. Many functional and cognitive behaviors are apparent with a brief period of observation prior to the actual examination and intervention.[43]

To assess **tone**, ask the patient to relax and allow the examiner to do the work of moving the patient's muscles. The examiner begins by passively moving each limb through all available planes of motion at a constant speed while providing support to the joints in motion.[14,44,45] Next, the examiner completes the same movements with an increased and then decreased speed to assess the effects of velocity. The characteristics of movement should be described according the muscle group(s) tested and include a bilateral comparison along with a description of how velocity affected the movement(s).[44,45]

Flaccidity refers to hypotonia or decreased/absent muscular tone. Resistance to passive range of motion (PROM) is decreased, causing the limbs to feel heavy and/or floppy to the examiner. This state can be caused by upper motor neuron lesions affecting the cerebellum or pyramidal tracts, as a temporary state following injury to the CNS, or secondary to a lower motor neuron lesion affecting the peripheral nervous system (PNS).[45]

Table 9–6
RANCHO LOS AMIGOS LEVELS OF COGNITIVE FUNCTIONING[14,15]

#	Level	Description
I	No response	The patient does not demonstrate any response to stimuli.
II	Generalized response	The patient reacts in a nonspecific and nonpurposeful way to stimuli. Responses are inconsistent and may be physiologic changes, gross movements, and/or vocalization.
III	Localized response	The patient reacts specifically but inconsistently to stimuli. Simple commands such as closing eyes or squeezing hand may be followed in a delayed inconsistent manner.
IV	Confused agitated	The patient demonstrates increased activity with bizarre nonpurposeful behavior in relation to his or her surroundings. Decreased attention, short- and long-term recall, and often with incoherent and/or inappropriate verbalization. Not able to directly cooperate with treatment efforts.
V	Confused inappropriate	The patient can follow simple commands but demonstrates nonpurposeful, random, or fragmented responses to complex commands. Highly distractible with an inability to focus on a specific task. May perform previously learned tasks with structure, but does not demonstrate ability to learn new information. Verbalization is often inappropriate and/or confabulatory.
VI	Confused appropriate	The patient is able to demonstrate goal-directed behavior but is dependent on external input or direction. Demonstrates carryover for relearned tasks such as self-care. Past memories more intact than recent. Responses may by incorrect secondary to memory problems, but they are appropriate to the situation.
VII	Automatic appropriate	Patient demonstrates appropriate behavior within the hospital and home settings, is oriented, and with structure, is able to initiate social or recreational activities. There is carryover for new learning but at a decreased rate; affect is robot-like and automatic. Judgment remains impaired.
VIII	Purposeful appropriate	The patient is aware of and response to his or her surroundings, demonstrates carryover, and is able to demonstrate new learning as well as recall and integrate past and recent events. The patient may still have difficulty when faced with stress, abstract reasoning, emergencies, and/or unusual circumstances.

Table 9–7
ACUTE NEUROLOGIC PHYSICAL THERAPY EXAMINATION

Examination Feature	Documentation	Clinical Tips
History	Prior neurological events, smoking, other stroke risk factors Social history Employment history Medical and/or surgical history	This may guide your education strategy for the patient Include set-up at discharge if known.
Chief complaint	A subjective statement from the patient	Often taken as the first statement made by the patient.
Prior level of function		Include use of assistive devices and the need for orthotics/prosthetics; any adaptive equipment at home.
Medications	All medications including over-the-counter	Include adherence to medications in the past.
Observation of the patient	Notice the self-selected positioning of the patient prior to mobilization	Neglect/inattention to hemiparetic side is often apparent.
Arousal, attention, and cognition	Use Rancho Los Amigos Cognitive Scale, GCS, Mini-Mental Status Examination (MMSE), motivation, memory, ability to follow commands	Sitting upright may stimulate the reticular activating system (RAS) and increase patient arousal.[37]
ROM and tone assessment		Consider grading a muscle with neurologic impairment means isolation movement. If increased tone is present, alternate methods of grading need to be considered. See text for full description.
Integumentary system	Inspect the skin for edema, discoloration, and breakdown	

(continued)

	Table 9–7 (continued)	
Examination Feature	Documentation	Clinical Tips
Gait and balance	Describe characteristics of gait and use of assistive devices and/or orthotics	Consider the FIM, Barthel Index, Berg Balance Test, Timed-Up-N-Go Test, Functional Reach Test, and Dymanic Gait Index.
Pain	Use 0 to 10 pain scale	
Sensation	Deep touch, light touch, vibration, proprioception	Deficits can also cause impaired motor response[11]
Medical interventions in patient care	Peripheral or central lines, catheter, drains, supplemental oxygen, mechanical ventilation	Origin and implication for treatment of lines should be known prior to movement of the patient
Physiologic readings	BP, HR, ECG, RR	May need to use mean arterial pressure (MAP).[44] Record with each session and more than one time in session. See text for full details.

Rigidity refers to nonvelocity dependent resistance that is felt in both the agonist and antagonist muscles with PROM. Two types of rigidity are typically described: **leadpipe**, which refers to constant hypertonia (increased tone), and **cogwheel,** which describes a rachetlike response to passive movement in which the tone increases and then decreases.[15] Rigidity is a characteristic of disorders within the extrapyramidal system such as PD.[14]

Dystonia refers to a condition in which tone fluctuates unpredictably from low to high with sustained and twisting involuntary movements. Dystonia results from a central deficit and may be inherited (primary idiopathic dystonia), related to neurodegenerative disorders such as PD or Wilson's disease, or secondary to metabolic disorders.[2,15]

Spasticity refers to a velocity dependent (the quicker the stretch, the stronger the resistance of the spastic muscle) increase in tonic stretch reflexes. Spasticity is felt within the muscles on one side of the joint that is being stretched and is indicative of upper motor neuron damage.[14,45] The **Modified Ashworth Scale for Grading Spasticity**, as described in Table 9–8, may be used to objectively describe the muscles demonstrating increased spasticity.[14,22]

Clinical Tips

- Position patients with low tone in positions that will preserve the correct anatomical position of their joints.[44]

Table 9–8

MODIFIED ASHWORTH SCALE FOR GRADING SPASTICITY

Grade	Description
0	No increase in muscle tone
1	Slight increase in muscle tone, detectable by a catch and release or by minimal resistance at the end range of flexion or extension.
2	Slight increase in muscle tone, detected by a catch, followed by minimal resistance throughout the remainder (less than half) of the ROM. The affected part(s) is(are) easily moved.
3	More marked increase in muscle tone through most of the ROM, but affected musculature easily moved.
4	Considerable increase in muscle tone; PROM difficult.
5	Affected musculature rigid in flexion or extension.

Adapted from Howe T. Measuring muscle tone and movement. *Nursing Standard.* 1995;9:25–29.

- To facilitate a muscular contraction, attempt a quick stretch or light strokes in the desired motion, tapping the muscle belly, high intensity vibration, and/or functional electrical stimulation.
- To reduce spasticity, complete active assistive ROM (AAROM), PROM, and stretching with slow gradual motions; avoid sudden quick movements.
- Deep pressure applied to the muscle belly and/or tendons, prolonged ice, low intensity vibration, heat, and maintained touch may inhibit muscle tone.
- Gentle rocking and rhythmic stabilization and the addition of a rotational component to the desired motion may help reduce rigidity.
- Positioning the patient in sidelying helps to reduce rigidity; complete ROM from this position when possible.[44]
- MAP may serve as a parameter for blood pressure (BP) limits as indicated by the medical team.

Normal MAP values range between 70 and 110 mmHg (see Table 3-1).[46] The parameters for patients with decreased perfusion, such as following an ischemic stroke, may involve MAPS of up to 130 mmHg. Be sure to note BP parameters in the patient's chart and confer with the patient's nurse and/or doctor if BP recordings are outside of the specified parameters.

Treatment Strategies

Focusing the activity of the patient to functional tasks that have meaning is important in any setting. Task specificity, quantity of practice, and environmental set-up enable success in the presence of neurologic injury. Common treatment strategies for the neurologic patient are provided in Tables 9–9 through 9–11.

Table 9–9

ACUTE CARE PHYSICAL THERAPY AND STROKE

Impairments	Interventions	Clinical Tips	Goals
Shoulder subluxation	• Positioning • Functional electrical stimulation (FES)[50,51]; taping techniques • Strength training • Preserve ROM especially for external rotation[51]	• Facilitate anatomic positioning to avoid stretch of the brachial plexus[48,49] • FES protocol for shoulder subluxation can be initiated in acute care[50,51] • ROM preservation is preventative for painful shoulder syndrome[51]	• Promote stability in affected musculature to prevent pain • Maintain ROM • Facilitate motor return to involved area
Sensory changes	• Tactile input to stimulate affected region • PT and family education to draw visual attention to affected region(s) and forced use of extremity[52]	• Sling may be indicated for hemiparetic arm if there is decreased awareness and potential for injury[49] • Protect affected side from injury while moving	• Improve motor control of affected region • Prevent injury to affected area
Altered communication	• Determine which method of communication works best for your patient[48] • Use short, simple commands	• Coordinate therapy with speech therapy • Use the same commands with a consistent voice tone	• Participate in therapy session • Decrease frustration

Problem	Interventions	Considerations	Goals/Rationale
Decreased endurance	• Cardiovascular exercise such as a restorator, kinetron, UBE, or treadmill[16,53,54] • Monitor physiologic response to all exercise[16,56]	• Use of the BORG scale • Consider strengthening of the "uninvolved" side as weakness is present[55] • Consider pre-existing cardiac deconditioning of the patient[16]	• Improve patient's cardiovascular condition • Initiate a lifestyle change for personal fitness program
Gait deficits	• Body weight support[57,58] • Early mobilization is beneficial[59] • Repetition of practice[60]	• Consider using the Up and Go or Lite Gait • Mass practice is more beneficial for learning of the motor task	• Early mobilization • Gait will be crucial to assist with discharge to another level of care • Upright position stimulates RAS and ensures successful intervention
Cognitive changes	• Use MMSE • Ensure arousal level is optimized	• Consider subtle cognitive deficits and referral to neuropsych for future interventions	
Neglect and/or inattention	• Draw attention to hemiparetic side[55,59]	• Position patient to attend to affected side in room and when talking with visitors	• Prevent learned disuse
Lack of knowledge related to healthy lifestyle	• Patient and family education[16,56]	• Consider use of the AHA guidelines for stroke[16,56]	• Facilitate lifestyle change for daily exercise

Table 9-10

ACUTE CARE PHYSICAL THERAPY AND PARKINSONISM

Impairments	Interventions	Clinical Tips	Goals
Postural instability	• Transfer training • Bed mobility training, turning and reaching activities	• Emphasize whole body movements and speed of action; increase the height of the chair and use of armrests[27] • Mental rehearsal and a night light[27]	• Facilitate functional mobility which requires spinal ROM[61]; prevent falls
Bradykinesia	• External cueing,[27,62,63] energy conservation compensation, muscle strengthening	• Focusing attention to task to avoid degradation	• Refocus attention of the task to decrease the slowed movement pattern[62]
ROM deficits	• Flexibility and ROM exercises, yoga, Tai Chi techniques	• Axial rotation loss is present especially as trunk flexion progresses[61]	• Preserve biomechanical alignment, preserve motion for functional tasks
Muscle strength	• Therapeutic exercise[64]	• Loss may be from insufficient neural activation and/or disuse[27]	• Prevent deconditioning and focus strengthening for targeted muscle groups
Cardiopulmonary deconditioning	• Bicycle (recumbant vs upright), kinetron, treadmill	• Encouragement of conditioning should occur with the first and every subsequent session[27,64,65]	• Prevent further decline of cardiovascular status

Gait dysfunction	• Use of treadmill training, enhanced gait training with external cueing,[27,62,63] timed walks over ground	• Consider the 6 minute walk time (MWT), Timed Up and Go,[65] bimanual tasks	• Encourage mobility for aerobic conditioning • Maintain ambulation for functional tasks
Depression	• Use Beck depression inventory[66,67]	• More prevalent in patients with akinetic rigidity than tremor dominance	• Monitor affective mood on ability to perform tasks and participate in therapy
Quality of life issues	• Use of PD quality of life (QOL) questionnaire (PDQOL 39) • Unified PD rating scale (UPDRS) motor part/part III	• UPDRS scale correlates to QOL,[66,67] depression important predictor of QOL[66,67]	• Enables therapist to ensure patient-centered goals
Cueing	• External cueing assists with improved motor performance (verbal, visual, proprioceptive)[27,62,63]	• Cues of "take longer steps" will assist to correct gait deficits[62] • Use of auditory cues successful for akinesia • Use of visual cues for hypokinesia	• Enables enhanced performance of tasks and process of the motor program
Cognitive impairment	• Use MMSE	• Score below 24 of 30[27]	• Monitor to maintain safe functional ability
Balance deficits	• Structure activity for avoidance of dual tasks, environmental set-up, balance exercises for single limb stance, rotation of the trunk, and reaching[27,68]	• Consider using Berg Balance Test, one-leg stance, step test, and external perturbation to assist in prediction of falls and tailor program accordingly[68]	• Prevention of falls • Promote functional independence in the safest environment

Table 9–11

ACUTE CARE PHYSICAL THERAPY AND NEUROMUSCULAR DISEASE AND DISORDERS

Impairments	Interventions	Clinical Tips	Goals
Changes in muscle tone	• Medications[69] • Baclofen pump[70] • Orthotics[15] • Positioning[47,71]	• See previously described tone assessment	• Prevent tonal changes from interfering with functional ability[47,71]
Altered sensation	• Tactile input, prevent injury to affected area with positioning and possible splinting[14,72]	• Visual compensation	• Prevention of injury • Increase awareness of affected area[47]
Decreased endurance	• Short bouts of therapeutic exercise with monitoring for fatigue[37,72]	• Use of assistive device may conserve energy[2,36] • Prioritization of tasks for importance to the patient[37] • Consider use of Borg scale	• Preserve cardiovascular conditioning
Fatigue	• Strengthen large muscle groups to maximize compensation strategies	• Do not overexert—this may cause exacerbation of the medical condition[15,32,37]	• Maintain balance of strengthening and precautions to enable full benefit of exercise session
Pain management	• Limitation of sensory input • Positioning and turning schedule • Maintain ROM[33,35]	• Coordination of medications[35] • Consider use of complimentary alternative medicine (CAM) and modalities	• Recognize and remediate pain for patient comfort[33]

(continued)

Table 9–11 (continued)

ACUTE CARE PHYSICAL THERAPY AND NEUROMUSCULAR DISEASE AND DISORDERS

Impairments	Interventions	Clinical Tips	Goals
Decreased ROM	• Gentle stretching, splinting, bracing and casting[33,35,72]	• Decreased ROM can increase tonal changes or cause pain syndromes[33,35]	• Preserve biomechanical alignment for best functional outcome[35]
Visual impairments	• Patch may assist with diplopia • Teach scanning techniques[15]	• Check for vestibular component by examination of nystagmus and vestibuloocular reflex (VOR)[14,15]	• Decrease symptoms that can cause nausea or impair safety[15]
Decreased balance	• Clinical test of sensory interaction and balance (CTSIB) to identify specific area of deficit[15]	• Consider affect of proprioception as deficit may cause further balance impairment[15]	• Prevention of falls • Promote functional independence in safest environment
Gait deficits	• Gradual increase of gait distance • Consider use or change of assistive device[2,36] • Consider use or change of orthotic device[14,15]	• When fatigue occurs at the end distance of gait, patients have little reserve and require immediate rest. Planning should include wheelchair follow, immediate stand-by assistance, or chairs for rests along the path	• Encourage mobility for aerobic conditioning • Maintain ambulation for functional tasks

Secondary medical conditions must be considered; coordinating interventions with medication dosing is helpful. However, the physical therapist/physical therapist assistant should not neglect teaching the patient and family strategies during periods when medication is not at peak levels.[47] Due to the chronic and progressive nature of many neurologic conditions, durable medical equipment will likely be needed to maximize the patient's functional level. Consideration should be given to rental equipment if change in the neuromuscular condition may warrant different equipment within a year.

From the acute care environment, most patients will require another level of care post-discharge. This may include inpatient rehabilitation, outpatient, home, or long-term care services. Continuation of the rehabilitation process should be considered in the plan of care for the patient.

Neurology Summary

The clinical signs and symptoms resulting from neurologic dysfunction vary greatly depending on the region of the nervous system affected. By first gaining an understanding of the anatomy and physiology of an intact system, a clinician may better understand the mechanisms underlying pathology and, thereby, provide appropriate interventions for the resulting impairments.

The two general categories of stroke are ischemia and hemorrhage; ischemic strokes are more common than hemorrhagic strokes. In both instances, cerebral damage is caused by reduced oxygenation of brain tissue, which leads to cell damage and/or death. The location and severity of the lesion coupled with the quality of collateral blood flow influence the severity of neurologic deficits that evolve following a stroke.

Similar to strokes, TBIs also involve cerebral damage; however, the pathophysiology of head injury involves primary and secondary injuries. TBI may also involve local brain damage caused by contusions and/or lacerations along the surface of the brain and/or DAI. If cellular damage is widespread and extends into the midbrain and brainstem, it may cause a dramatic cumulative effect such as coma and/or autonomic dysfunction. TBIs can be classified based on the location, extent, severity, and/or the mechanism of injury.

Neuromuscular diseases such as PD, MS, GBS, and ALS involve both upper and lower motor neuron dysfunction, which results in various impairments such as muscle weakness, fluctuations in muscle tone, impaired balance, decreased coordination, and impaired functional mobility.

In the acute care setting, a thorough chart review and understanding of the source of physiologic pathology are essential prior to mobilization of the patient. In addition, a description of the patient's prior level of function should be ascertained prior to the functional examination in order to best understand the acuity of impairment.

When examining patients with neurologic impairment, assess level of arousal, cognition, and ability to communicate first to determine the most appropriate techniques for conducting the functional assessment. When establishing the patient's plan of care, the therapist shoulder consider the estimated length of stay in acute care, the social support available for the patient, and the recommendation for the next level of care.

In treating patients with neurologic impairment, it is important to focus treatment activities to functional context. The task specification in the acute care setting is typically transfers, bed mobility, and gait training. These activities provide the patients with practice as well as the justification for continued therapy services.

Many patients and families need to cope with significant change in function and role within the family unit after neurologic impairment. Some acute care institutions offer specific support groups for patients and family members, while additional support groups and disease/disorder information can be found on the internet.

CASE STUDY

Mr. Bryant is a 68-year-old male with a past medical history including HTN, coronary artery disease (CAD), atrial fibrillation (AF), and increased cholesterol. After dinner one evening, he was having difficulty moving his left arm and leg. He thought after a good night sleep, his symptoms would resolve. His wife noticed a left-sided facial droop and garbled speech. She could not convince her husband that he required medical attention. After several hours passed, Mrs. Bryant called 911. Mr. Bryant was transported to the local hospital where he was evaluated for stroke. His MRI revealed an infarct in the distribution of the right MCA. The attending neurologist ordered that Mr. Bryant be positioned with his bed flat, intravenous fluids be administered, and that "neurological checks" be completed every 2 hours along with a recording of the patient's vital signs. Mr. Bryant was declared NPO (nothing per os, nothing by mouth) until the speech therapist assessed his ability to swallow. After spending 48 hours flat in bed, Mr. Bryant's doctor consulted physical therapy to complete an examination.

Patient/Client History

General Demographics/Social History/Living Environment

Mr. Bryant lives with his wife in a two-story home with the bathroom on the second floor. There are six steps to enter.

General Health Status/Family History

Mr. and Mrs. Bryant are both retired. They walk a mile every other day during nice weather.

Medical/Surgical History

Mr. Bryant has HTN, CAD, AF, and increased cholesterol. He had been diagnosed with HTN and AF 5 years ago and has been taking medication prescribed by his family physician. His cholesterol was being managed through diet only. His surgical history is not significant.

Current Conditions/Chief Complaints

Mr. Bryant presented with a right-sided ischemic stroke of duration >12 hours. He has no active movement in the left upper extremity (LUE) or left lower extremity (LLE) except for trace left hip flexion and extension. He has left-sided neglect as well as dysarthria. There is increased extensor tone in the LLE and flaccidity in the LUE.

Functional Status and Activity Level

Mr. Bryant's chart was reviewed, and he was found supine in bed with his head turned toward the right. Mrs. Bryant was present and provided the therapist with a description of the patient's functional level before admission and the home setting. Prior to this event, Mr. Bryant was independent with all of his activities of daily living (ADLs) and instrumental ADLs (IADLs).

Systems Review
Cardiovascular/Pulmonary

Resting vital signs supine in bed are oxygen saturation (SpO_2) 94% on 3 liters nasal cannula, HR 96, pulse irregularly, irregular, RR 18 and shallow, BP 160/86, pain was unable to be measured due to communication challenges, and breath sounds were diminished throughout lung fields. Following ROM, manual muscle test (MMT), bed mobility, transfers, and neurologic examination, his vital signs were 96% SpO_2, HR 104, RR 22, and BP 154/84. Arterial blood gases pH 7.32/PCO_2 50/PO_2 90/HCO_3- 24%.

Integumentary

Skin intact with IV line in RUE.

Musculoskeletal

MMT results for LUE and LLE revealed no active movement except trace left hip flexion and extension. ROM was within normal limits (WNL) bilateral upper extremity (BUE)/bilateral lower extremity (BLE). Maximal assistance is required for bed mobility, transfers, and static/dynamic sitting. Maximal assistance of two was required to attempt standing for <20 seconds. For all standing positions Mr. Bryant's LUE was placed in a sling to prevent injury.

Neuromuscular

There is increased extensor tone in the LLE and flaccidity in the LUE. Sensation not evaluated.

Communication, Affect, Cognition, Language, and Learning Style

Mr. Bryant's speech is dysarthric. His wife explains that Spanish is his primary language, but he is fluent in English.

Tests and Measures
Aerobic Capacity and Endurance

Mr. Bryant demonstrated blunted hemodynamic responses with bed mobility, transfers, and standing. He is at risk for aspiration pneumonia due to potential swallowing dysfunction and limited mobility. He is NPO. AF continues and may limit BP responses with functional activities. Mr. Bryant's presents with a respiratory acidosis most likely related to an altered breathing pattern and diaphragm weakness.

Assistive and Adaptive Devices

Left knee immobilizer is recommended for gait training. His left ankle should be ace wrapped to provide passive dorsiflexion, and a sling should be used for his LUE for standing activities. A hemiwalker is recommended for gait training with progression to a smaller based support device when improved functional level is obtained.

Gait, Locomotion, and Balance

Mr. Bryant's balance is poor in static sitting requiring moderate assistance. He required maximal assistance to stand and transfer onto the commode. Maximal assistance of one and moderate assistance of one was required to ambulate four steps with a left knee immobilizer donned and a supportive ace wrap on the left ankle. Moderate assistance was required to advance the LLE.

Pain

Pain is difficult to measure due to language impairment. Observe grimaces/facial expressions during treatment to qualify pain.

Diagnosis

In Mr. Bryant's examination, the therapist described his diagnosis as a right ischemic stroke resulting in left-sided hemiplegia. Recommend treatment pattern 5D: impaired motor function and sensory integrity associated with nonprogressive disorders of the CNS-acquired in adolescence or adulthood.[48]

Prognosis

The physical therapist estimated that Mr. Bryant would require daily physical therapy services until his predicted discharge in 5 days. The recommended goals were that the patient be able to roll onto his involved side and transfer from supine to a sitting position with moderate assistance. The patient will maintain static sitting balance on the edge of bed for 10 minutes with minimal assistance and BUEs support on the bed. The patient will transfer onto a commode toward his strong side with moderate assistance. The patient will stand and ambulate 25 to 50 feet with moderate assistance, a left knee immobilizer, left ankle dorsiflexion wrap, a single point cane. In the acute setting, trial bracing provides stability; however, definitive bracing orders typically occur in rehab. With supervision from the therapist, the patient's family will demonstrate proper positioning and ROM for the patient's LUE and LLE as well as the proper techniques for assisting the patient with his bedside therapeutic exercise routine.

Intervention

In order to accomplish these goals and, thereby, decrease Mr. Bryant's functional limitations, the physical therapist incorporated the following interventions into Mr. Bryant's plan of care: strength, coordination, balance, gait and perceptual training, and neuromuscular education including FES to the supraspinatus and deltoid muscles to stabilize the humeral head in the glenoid fossa. Patient/family education regarding the intervention techniques as well as long term health and social concerns for a stroke survivor were incorporated into each treatment session. The communication and documentation of Mr. Bryant's plan of care to the interdisciplinary team members was completed following evaluation.

Reexamination

Mr. Bryant is ambulating with left knee immobilizer 20 feet times two with moderate assistance of two. He still requires a sling for protection of his LUE. He is able to transfer with moderate assistance of one from a chair with arms and a mat table with maximal assistance of one. His speech is still dysarthric, and he is progressing with swallowing exercises with speech therapy. Mr. Bryant continues to be unaware of his left side and must receive continued cues for safety.

Outcomes

Mr. Bryant has been accepted to transfer to the inpatient rehabilitation hospital.

PART II: NEUROSURGERY

Intervention by the physical therapist in cases involving neurosurgery has not been well documented in acute care literature. While patients often demonstrate functional deficits that are similar in nature to the patient with neurologic deficit, there are certain unique characteristics to this patient population. As hospital length of stay decreases, intervention is often requested for discharge planning purposes, initial functional retraining, and patient/family education. Therapists need to consider the medical stability of the patient as well as the consequence of intervention in lieu of the surgical procedures performed.

ANATOMY AND PHYSIOLOGY

Spinal Region

The spinal region is responsible for carrying impulses for sensations such as pain and temperature and for the signals that command voluntary movements in the limbs, trunk, and neck.[2,8] This region includes the spinal cord, dorsal and ventral roots, spinal nerves, and the meninges.[8] Damage to the spinal region may cause paralysis and/or the loss of general sensations.

The **spinal cord** forms a cylindrical column approximately 0.5 m long (in an adult) with an estimated diameter between 1 and 1.5 cm that is located within the vertebral canal.[49] It begins as the inferior continuation of the medulla and extends from the foramen magnum to the intervertebral disc between the first and second lumbar vertebrae (Figure 9–5).[4,8] The internal structure of the spinal cord consists of white matter that surrounds a distinctive H-shaped pattern of gray matter located centrally. The **white matter** contains a large number of myelinated fibers (accounting for its white appearance) that transmit impulses superiorly or inferiorly.[3,6] The **gray matter** within the spinal cord consists

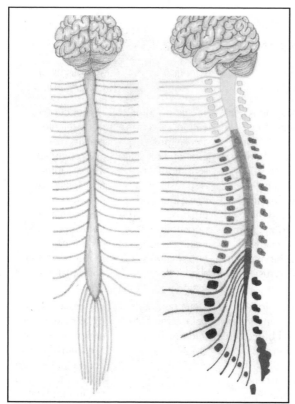

Figure 9–5. Spinal cord. (Reprinted with permission from Gutman SA. *Quick Reference Neuroscience.* Thorofare, NJ: SLACK Incorporated; 2001:35.)

largely of nerve cell bodies and interneurons; its lateral sections are divided into the dorsal, lateral, and ventral horns.[8,49] The **dorsal horns** contain groups of neurons that are largely responsible for carrying sensory information.[8] Many neurons within this region communicate with axons that enter the white matter and contribute to the **ascending tracts.**[4,8] The nuclei within the **anterior horns**, which are located between the anterior and lateral funiculi, are related to voluntary movement and are hence referred to as the "motor" part within the spinal gray matter.[4] The **lateral horns** contains cell bodies of preganglionic neurons of the sympathetic nervous system and are largely responsible for processing autonomic information.[4,8] The **ascending tracts** carry sensory information from nerve endings, and joint receptors to the cerebrum or cerebellum.[4,6] Table 9–12 provides descriptions of the ascending spinal tracts commonly assessed in clinical care.

The **descending pathways** originate in the cerebrum, cerebellum, midbrain, and brainstem and carry information responsible for voluntary motor activity, posture, tone, and coordination.[6,8] Table 9–13 provides descriptions of the descending spinal tracts commonly assessed in clinical care.

Axons relaying afferent information to the to periphery exit the anterolateral cord in small groups are **rootlets**. Ventral rootlets from a single spinal cord

Table 9–12
ASCENDING SPINAL TRACTS

Spinal Tract	Pathway	Function	Symptoms of Dysfunction
Dorsal columns (fasciculus gracilis and fasciculus cuneatus) Also called medial lemniscus or the Posterior Columns	Originates in receptors located in skin, muscle and joints. Cell bodies are located in dorsal root ganglion. **Crosses in the lower medulla**, and travels to the primary somatosensory area within the post central gyrus.	Tactile discrimination, vibration, **stereognosis**, joint and muscle sensation. Also responsible for conscious and unconscious proprioception, integrating sensory information and spatial discrimination.	Dysfunction of the fasciculus gracilis may cause **astereognosis**, loss of vibration sense, loss of two-point discrimination and/or impaired proprioception in the LE on the contra lateral side.
Lateral spinothalamic	Originates in free nerve ending receptors. Cell bodies are located in dorsal root ganglion. The impulse ascends 1 to 2 segments, **crosses**, and travels to the thalamus and somatosensory area.	Detection of pain, temperature and touch.	Decreased ability to detect pain and temperature sensations on the contra lateral side below the level of the lesion; bilateral sensory loss at the level of the lesion.
Anterior spinothalamic	Originates in light touch receptors such as Merkel's discs. Cell bodies located in dorsal root ganglion. **Crosses at level of entry** and travels to the thalamus and somatosensory area.	Detection of light touch. Also responsible for detecting pressure and crude touch from the extremities and trunk.	Bilateral destruction of this tract may result in general tactile impairment as well as reduced tickling and sexual sensations.

(continued)

Table 9–12 (continued)

ASCENDING SPINAL TRACTS

Spinal Tract	Pathway	Function	Symptoms of Dysfunction
Posterior Spinocerebellar	Originates in muscle spindles and golgi tendon organs, travels to the posterior horn and then to the cerebellum **without crossing.**	Enables the precision and smoothness of movement; provides the coordination of muscle movement and position sense, subconscious proprioception, and kinesthetic sense.	Damage to this tract causes uncoordinated postural movements on the ipsilateral side of the lesion.

Adapted from:

Parent A. *Carpenter's Human Neuroanatomy.* 9th ed. Media, Pa: Williams and Wilkins; 1996.

Hickey JV. *Clinical Practice of Neurological and Neurosurgical Nursing.* Philadelphia, Pa: JB Lippincott Co; 1992.

Adams RD, Victor M, Ropper AH. *Principles of Neurology.* 6th ed. New York, NY: McGraw-Hill Co; 1998.

Gutman SA. *Quick Reference Neuroscience for Rehabilitation Professionals. The Essential Neurologic Principles Underlying Rehabilitation Practice.* Thorofare, NJ: SLACK Incorporated; 2001.

segment coalesce to form a single ventral root.[6,8] The **dorsal root** is composed of sensory axons carrying efferent information. Each dorsal root corresponds to a dorsal root ganglion located outside the spinal cord that contains the cell bodies of sensory neurons. The dorsal and ventral roots from each segment merge to form a **spinal nerve,** which contains all of the sensory and motor axons that correspond to a single segment of the spinal cord.[3,6,8] There are 31 pairs of spinal nerves with the following distribution: cervical, 8; thoracic, 12; lumbar, 5; sacral, 5; coccygeal, 1 (Figure 9–6).[8,52]

The peripheral distribution of each spinal nerve represents an original segmental organization that relates to a specific region of skin, muscle(s), and connective tissue.[8] The region of skin supplied by the sensory fibers from an individual spinal nerve is referred to as a **dermatome.**[14] Clinical diagnosis may be aided by tracing regions with impaired sensory signals to its respective spinal cord segment (Figure 9–7).

Reflex contraction of muscles may also be used in clinical diagnosis of specific spinal segments. Hyperactivity or hypoactivity at a specific segment is often useful in forming a clinical picture of a disease process. Segmental organization

Table 9–13
DESCENDING SPINAL TRACTS

Spinal Tract	Pathway	Function	Symptoms of Dysfunction
Lateral corticospinal (Pyramidal)	Originates in the precentral gyrus, premotor cortex and/or the post-central gyrus. **Crosses in the lower medulla;** travels to the anterior horn and/or the posterior horn.	Controls voluntary skilled motor activity with a influence predominantly over the limbs.	Voluntary muscle paresis/paralysis on the contra lateral side, hyperactive reflexes and spasticity of muscles distal to the lesion.
Anterior (ventral) corticospinal (Pyramidal)	Originates in the precentral gyrus, premotor cortex and/or the post-central gyrus; travels to the anterior horn and/or the posterior horn. **Does not cross until level of termination.**	Controls voluntary skilled motor activity with a influence predominantly over the trunk and axial muscles.	Voluntary muscle paresis/paralysis on the contra lateral side, hyperactive reflexes and spasticity of muscles distal to the lesion.
Vestibulo-spinal (Extra-pyramidal)	Originates in the brainstem and travels to the anterior horn; interneurons play a role in this pathway. **This tract does not cross.**	Controls the antigravity muscles, by facilitating extensor alpha motor neurons and inhibiting the flexors. Responsible for involuntary movements of balance and coordination. Also influences sweating, pupillary dilation, and circulation.	**Decerebrate posture** (continuous extensor rigidity) which results secondary to a lack of inhibition of vestibulospinal impulses and is indicative of a poor prognosis.

Tract	Origin and Pathway	Function	Clinical Effect
Rubrospinal (Extra-pyramidal)	Originates in the red nucleus within the midbrain. **Crosses in the midbrain** and travels to anterior horn cells ending in the thoracic region. Interneurons play a role in this pathway.	Facilitates flexor alpha and gamma motor neurons and inhibits the extensors. Also influences muscle tone and posture, especially in the UEs	Altered muscle tone and posture, with increased extensor tone; may result in decerebrate posture (described previously).
Tectospinal (Extra-pyramidal)	Originates in the superior colliculus of the midbrain. **Crosses in the midbrain** and travels to anterior horn cells located with in the cervical region. Interneurons play a role in this pathway.	Integrates visual and auditory reflexes with postural reflexes (ie, causes you to turn your head toward a visual and/or auditory stimulus).	Impaired integration of visual, auditory and/or postural reflexes.
Reticulo-spinal (Extra-pyramidal)	Two divisions, the pons and medulla, that originate in the brainstem; both divisions synapse on the same interneurons with antagonistic effects and project to alpha and gamma motor neurons. **This tract does not cross.**	Facilitates or inhibits voluntary movement, muscle tone and reflex activity. Also influences respiratory and circulatory systems. Pons division increases BP and HR and facilitates tone. Medulla division decreases BP and HR and inhibits tone.	Altered muscle tone and posture, with increased extensor tone; may result in decerebrate posture. May also result in an altered cardiovascular response.

Adapted from:
Parent A. *Carpenter's Human Neuroanatomy.* 9th ed. Media, Pa: Williams and Wilkins; 1996.
Hickey JV. *Clinical Practice of Neurological and Neurosurgical Nursing.* Philadelphia, Pa: JB Lippincott Co; 1992.
Adams RD, Victor M, Ropper AH. *Principles of Neurology.* 6th ed. New York, NY: McGraw-Hill Co; 1998.
Gutman SA. *Quick Reference Neuroscience for Rehabilitation Professionals. The Essential Neurologic Principles Underlying Rehabilitation Practice.* Thorofare, NJ: SLACK Incorporated; 2001.

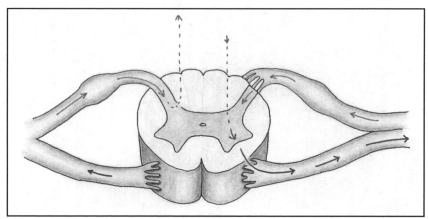

Figure 9–6. Ventral horn of spinal cord, rootlets and root. (Reprinted with permission from Gutman SA. *Quick Reference Neuroscience.* Thorofare, NJ: SLACK Incorporated; 2001:35.)

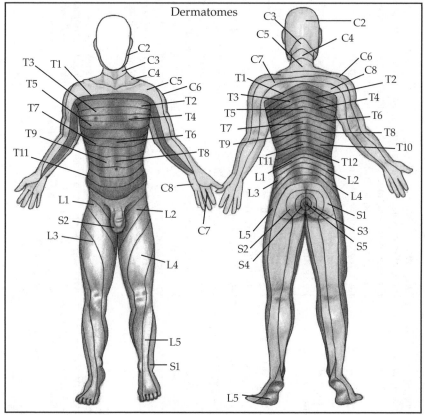

Figure 9–7. Dermatomes. (Reprinted with permission from Gutman SA. *Quick Reference Neuroscience.* Thorofare, NJ: SLACK Incorporated; 2001:37.)

for motor innervation is represented by **myotomes**. The term **myotome** refers to a group of muscles innervated by the same segmental spinal nerve.[14] Refer to Tables 9–14 and 9–15 for descriptions of spinal nerves, corresponding dermatome distribution, and the muscles that correspond to each motion. **Bolded** muscle(s) and or sensory levels within the table indicate key muscles and/or sensory levels used to identify the neurologic level of injury as defined by the American Spinal Cord Injury Association (ASIA) (Table 9–16).[50]

Meninges

Three layers of meninges cover and protect the CNS. They include the external **dura mater**, the delicate **arachnoid membrane** that lines the dura, and the innermost **pia mater** which adheres to the brain and spinal cord.[3,6] The space between the arachnoid and the pia mater, the **subarachnoid space,** is filled with **cerebrospinal fluid (CSF)**. The CSF coupled with the dura mater serve as a protective cushion between the brain and the skull as noted in Figure 9–8.[49] The **dura mater** is a dense, firm layer of connective tissue that surrounds the spinal column and the brain. The innermost layer of the dura lies superior to the arachnoid membrane and is in close contact with this region.[49]

A **subdural hematoma (SDH)** refers to bleeding within the subdural space and may be caused by the rupture of small vessels, bleeding from damaged areas of the brain, and/or a contusion of brain tissue.[2] The hemorrhage caused by a SDH is often venous blood which does not flow as rapidly as arterial blood. Therefore, the signs and symptoms may worsen over a prolonged period as the hematoma causes compression of the underlying brain tissue.[51] The manifestation of a SDH is classified as either acute (within 48 hours), subacute (from 2 days to 2 weeks), or chronic (from 2 weeks to several months) depending on the interval between injury and the appearance of symptoms.[2]

SDHs may be treated without surgical intervention if small in size because the blood may be reabsorbed. If the SDH is large, surgical evacuation is often necessary to prevent secondary damage from brain herniation and/or increased ICP.[2,13,8] Burr holes and a gentle irrigation technique can be used to drain the SDH if the hemorrhage does not coagulate. Once the SDH has solidified, a craniotomy with evacuation may be indicated.[51-53]

Skull fractures that lacerate the meningeal arteries supplying the dura may result in an **epidural hematoma (EDH),** also called an **extradural hematoma**.[2] EDH typically occurs in a younger population because the dura is more likely to rip from underlying skull in this population.[51] Symptoms develop rapidly and include a worsening headache, vomiting, altered consciousness, and/or hemiparesis.[13] Lateralizing of cranial nerve III (dilation of pupil), progressive hemiparesis, a change in mental status, and/or and decreased consciousness indicate emergent surgical evacuation.[8,13,51]

The **arachnoid mater** is a nonvascular membrane located between the dura and pia mater, with loose attachments to the dura.[6] It serves as the principal physiologic barrier that separates the CNS from the surrounding connective tissue.[49] Projections of arachnoid from the arachnoid villi allow CSF to flow into the sinuses, enabling CSF to flow into the venous system.[8]

The **subarachnoid space** surrounds the brain and conforms to its shape by forming a narrow passage in convex regions and deeper areas within the sulci.[49]

<u>Table 9–14</u>

UPPER EXTREMITY SPINAL NERVE ROOT DISTRIBUTION

Nerves	Dermatome Distribution	Motions	Muscles
C1	Vertex of the skull (top of head).	None	None
C2	Superior region of neck, posterior cheek, superior temporal region and posterior skull.	Weak cervical flexion, lateral flexion, rotation and extension.	Longus colli, partial sternocleidomastoid, and rectus capitis.
C3	Anterior and posterior neck region, and inferior temporal region.	Weak shoulder elevation and extension of head. Accessory muscles of respiration.	Partial trapezius, sternocleidomastoid and splenius capitis.
C4	Upper clavicular region and superior region of shoulders.	Respiration and full shoulder elevation.	**Diaphragm** and **trapezius**.
C5	Delton region of shoulder extending inferiorly down the arm to the base of the thumb.	Partial elbow flexion and supination. Scapular elevation and external rotation. Partial shoulder abduction, internal and external rotation.	Partial innervation of **biceps, brachialis,** and **brachioradialis**. Supraspinatus, infraspinatus, rhomboid, and deltoid.
C6	Anterior region of arm extending to and including the thumb.	Adduction, protraction and full rotation of shoulder. Strong elbow flexion and supination. Wrist extension.	Clavicular portion of pectoralis major, serratus anterior and full rotator cuff musculature. Full biceps, brachialis, supinator and brachioradialis. **Extensor carpi radialis and brevis**.

(continued)

<u>Table 9–14</u> (continued)

UPPER EXTREMITY SPINAL NERVE ROOT DISTRIBUTION

Nerves	Dermatome Distribution	Motions	Muscles
C7	Posterior lateral region of arm extending to and including the second and third digit.	Shoulder depression, adduction, internal rotation, and horizontal adduction. Elbow extension, pronation of forearm, wrist flexion, thumb extension and finger extension.	Latissimus dorsi, sternal portion pectoralis major, **triceps**, pronator teres, flexor carpi radialis, extensor pollicus longus and brevis; finger extensors.
C8 to T1	Medial region of arm and forearm extending to and including the fourth and fifth digit.	Finger flexion, full movement of thumb. Normal grasp and finger dexterity.	**Flexor digitorum profundus** (C8), finger flexors, flexor carpi ulnaris, flexor pollicus longus and brevis; **Interossei** (T1); intrinsic finger flexors.
T1 to T6	Anterior and posterior upper thorax region. (T4 corresponds to the level of the chest.)	Extension of thoracic spine. Control of inspiration and forced expiration.	Sacrospinalis and semispinalis; partial intercostal musculature.
T1 to T12	Inferior thorax region extending inferiorly to superior pelvic region. (T10 corresponds to the level of the umbilicus.) **T2-L1 sensory level** for AISA	Trunk flexion and rotation; partial pelvic elevation.	Full innervation of abdominal musculature; partial quadratus lumborum.

Adapted from:
Rohan JW, Yokichi C, Lutjen-Drecoll. *Color Atlas of Anatomy*. 4th ed. Media, Pa: Williams and Wilkins; 1998.
Lundy-Ekman L. *Neuroscience Fundamentals for Rehabilitation*. Philadelphia, Pa: WB Saunders Co; 1998.
Netter; Hislop & Montgomery; Giles.

Table 9–15
LOWER EXTREMITY SPINAL NERVE ROOT DISTRIBUTION

Nerves	Dermatome Distribution	Motions	Muscles
L1 to L2	Groin region extending anteriorly and inferiorly to the mid-thigh region.	Hip flexion and full pelvic elevation.	**Iliopsoas** and full innervation of quadratus lumborum.
L3 to L4	Anterior and posterior region of thigh extending medially to include medial ankle and dorsum of great toe.	Lumbar extension, hip adduction, knee extension and partial knee flexion.	Lower erector spinae, **quadriceps** (L3), adductor longus, brevis and longus. Partial hamstrings (semi-tendinosus, semi-membranosus, biceps femoris), and **anterior tibialis** (L4).
L5	Posterior and lateral region of thigh extending down lateral leg to the dorsum and plantar regions of the foot, including the first three digits.	Partial hip extension and abduction, ankle dorsiflexion and extension of great toe.	Partial gluteus medius and maximus. Anterior tibialis and **extensor hallicus longus.**
S1	Buttock region extending down posterior region of thigh to the lateral region of the ankle and fifth digit.	Hip internal rotation, partial plantarflexion, flexion; extension of great toe, ankle inversion and eversion.	Gluteus minimus and tensor fasciae latae; partial **gastrocnemius**, and soleus. Flexor hallucis longus; flexor digitorum, and tibialis posterior.
S2 to S4	S2 extends down the medial region of the posterior thigh terminating within the plantar aspect of the foot. S3 and S4 correspond to the perineal area. (**S2 to S5 sensory levels** for ASIA)	Full hip extension, abduction, and external rotation. Full plantarflexion and knee flexion, extension, internal and external rotation.	Full innervation of hamstrings and plantarflexors, gluteus maximus, obturator internus, piriformis, and gracilis. (**Sphincter tone** for ASIA)

Adapted from:
Rohan JW, Yokichi C, Lutjen-Drecoll. *Color Atlas of Anatomy.* 4th ed. Media, Pa: Williams and Wilkins; 1998.
Lundy-Ekman L. *Neuroscience Fundamentals for Rehabilitation.* Philadelphia, Pa: WB Saunders Co; 1998.
Netter; Hislop & Montgomery; Giles

Table 9–16

AMERICAN SPINAL CORD ASSOCIATION IMPAIRMENT SCALE[16]

Letter	Classification	Description
A	Complete	No sensory or motor function is preserved in the sacral segments S4 to S5.
B	Incomplete	Sensory but not motor function is preserved below the neurological level and includes the sacral segments S4 to S5.
C	Incomplete	Motor function is preserved below the neurological level, and more than half of key muscles below the neurological level have a muscle grade less than 3.
D	Incomplete	Motor function is preserved below the neurological level, and at least half of key muscles below the neurological level have a muscle grade greater than or equal to 3.
E	Normal	Sensory and motor function are normal.

At the base of the brain, the space between the pia and arachnoid layer enlarges, creating a subarachnoid cisternae.[6] The **lumbar cistern** extends from the conus medullaris to S2. It contains the **filum terminale** and nerve roots of the **cauda equine** and is the site most often used for a spinal tap.[2]

The **pia mater** is a highly vascular, loose connective tissue that is tightly apposed to the surfaces of the brain and spinal cord.[1,3] It is also located within the roof of the third ventricle and contributes to the formation of the **choroid plexuses** of the lateral, third, and fourth ventricles. The **denticulate ligaments**, which are extensions of the pia mater, anchor the spinal cord to the dura mater.[6]

Ventricular System

CSF, a watery, clear, and colorless substance, fills the ventricular system and the subarachnoid space (Figure 9–9). It protects the brain by serving as a cushion and provides a suitable environment for nervous tissue. It is produced by the **choroid plexuses,** which are located primarily within the lateral ventricles.[3]

CSF flows from the lateral ventricles, into the third ventricle through the interventricular foramina. Next, it passes through the cerebral aqueduct into the fourth ventricle.[3] CSF exits the ventricular system through the median and the two lateral apertures of the fourth ventricle.[3] CSF then travels within the subarachnoid space superiorly over the medial and lateral surfaces of the cerebral hemispheres and inferiorly around the spinal cord.[3] Finally, CSF is absorbed through the arachnoid villi, which project into the dural venous sinuses and direct the flow into venous blood.[3,6,8]

Figure 9–8. Meninges. (Reprinted with permission from Gutman SA. *Quick Reference Neuroscience.* Thorofare, NJ: SLACK Incorporated; 2001:33.)

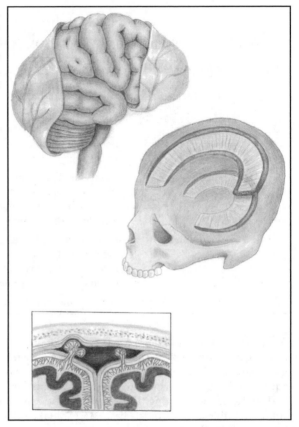

Damage or dysfunction within the ventricular system may cause a CSF leak and/or hydrocephalous. **Hydrocephalous** is related to the blockage of CSF circulation or secondary to excessive production of the fluid.[13] Hydrocephalous often causes the following symptoms: increased ICP, gait and balance impairments, frontal lobe dysfunction, and headaches.[13]

A CSF leak occurs when CSF is discharged from a body orifice and/or wound secondary to a meningeal tear. A CSF leak may occur following a lumbar puncture, neurosurgical procedure, or skull fracture. Symptoms of a CSF leak include the presence of a clear fluid leaking from a wound site or body orifice, severe headache posturally related, and/or a salty taste in the patient's mouth.[13] Medical management of a CSF leak may involve use of an epidural blood patch, repairing the dura, inserting a shunt, and/or prophylactic antibiotics.[10,39,54] Until the leak is repaired, mobility should be limited.

Venous System

The capillary bed of the brain stem and the cerebellum drain into the dural venous sinuses adjacent to the posterior cranial fossa. The cerebral veins are divided into external and internal veins, which both drain into dural venous

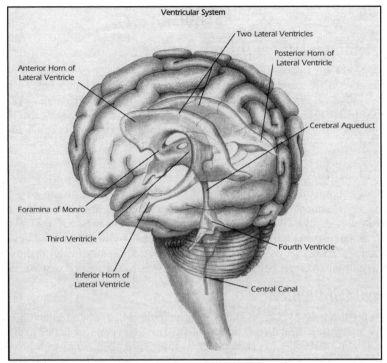

Ventricular System

Two Lateral Ventricles

Posterior Horn of
Lateral Ventricle

Anterior Horn of
Lateral Ventricle

Cerebral Aqueduct

Foramina of Monro

Third Ventricle

Fourth Ventricle

Inferior Horn of
Lateral Ventricle

Central Canal

Figure 9–9. CSF within ventricular system. (Reprinted with permission from Gutman SA. *Quick Reference Neuroscience.* Thorofare, NJ: SLACK Incorporated; 2001:27.)

sinuses.[3] The internal veins drain the cortex and the adjacent white matter and empty mostly into the superior sagittal sinus. The internal cerebral veins drain the basal ganglia, diencephalon, and nearby white matter and drain into the straight sinus. (The superior sagittal sinus and the straight sinus merge at the confluence, which forms the transverse sinus.[6]) The transverse sinus then travels anterior to become the sigmoid sinus, which ultimately drains into the internal jugular vein.[3]

Damage or dysfunction within the venous system may be secondary to an **AVM,** which is a disorganized collection of abnormally thin and dilated blood vessels that directly shunt arterial blood into the venous system.[2,13] As a result, blood flow is accelerated and the pressure is elevated within the malformed vessels of the AVM. These impairments predispose the lesion to hemorrhage in the surrounding area if the AVM leaks or ruptures.[2]

The signs and symptoms of AVMs include seizures, severe headaches, dizziness, syncope, aphasia, motor and/or sensory deficits; subjective complaints of hearing a "swishing noise in the head" may also occur.[2] Treatment options for managing AVMs include surgery to embolize the vessels, irradiation to thicken the vessel walls, and/or radiation therapy for nonsurgical candidates.[2]

PATHOLOGY

Upper Motor Neuron Disease

Upper motor neuron diseases involve lesions within the descending motor tracts, within the cerebral motor cortex, internal capsule, brainstem, or spinal cord.[10,50] Typical symptoms of upper motor neuron dysfunction include weakness of the involved muscles, hypertonicity, hyperreflexia, disuse atrophy and abnormal reflexes.[10,49] Strokes, birth injuries, MS, brain tumors, hydrocephalous, and cerebral palsy are examples of upper motor neuron disease.[10,49]

Lower Motor Neuron Disease

Lower motor neuron diseases involve lesions, which affect nerves or their axons at or below the level of the brainstem.[10,49] Typical symptoms of lower motor neuron dysfunction include flaccidity or weakness of the involved muscles, decreased tone, fasciculations, muscle atrophy, and decreased or absent reflexes.[10,49] Muscular dystrophy, poliomyelitis, ALS, tumors involving the spinal cord, trauma, and infection are examples of lower motor neuron disease.[10,49]

Spinal Cord Injury

Approximately 250,000 to 400,000 individuals in the United Stated are currently affected by spinal cord injury (SCI); with an average of 10,000 new cases annually.[56,57] According to statistics from the National Spinal Cord Injury Data Research Center, 50% of SCIs occur between the ages of 16 and 30 years; 82% of this population is male.[14,57] SCIs can be divided into two broad categories: traumatic and non-traumatic; traumatic SCIs account for roughly 80% of all cases.[14,57]

The most common cause of traumatic SCI is motor vehicle accidents. Acts of violence rank second and falls third.[14,55,56] Nontraumatic injuries are typically the result of a disease or pathologic process that compromises the integrity of the spinal cord. Some examples include transverse myelitis, syringomyelia, aterial venous malformation, spinal tumors, thrombosis, embolus, and vertebral subluxations secondary to arthritis.[14,58]

The mechanism of SCI is often acceleration—deceleration events such as hyperflexion, hyperextension, deformation, axial loading, compression, and/or rotation that produce excessive forces within the spinal column.[50,55] While the spinal cord is usually not severed at the time of injury, the damage typically occurs secondary to the inflammatory process that follows the injury.[13,50]

An overview of the sequence of physiologic events that precede SCI include hyperemia, edema, decreased BP, ischemia, hemorrhagic areas within the center of the cord, increased norepinephrine, serotonin and histamine levels, and decreased dopamine within the injured tissue.[2,11] This response causes the formation of glial and fibrotic scar tissue that may result in permanent neurologic damage.[2]

The two broad classifications of SCI include tetraplegia (quadriplegia) and paraplegia. **Tetraplegia** results from injury to the cervical spinal cord region and involves partial or complete paralysis of all four extremities and the trunk.[14,35,50] Paraplegia results from lesions of the thoracic, lumbar spinal cord, or sacral roots

Table 9–17

INCOMPLETE SPINAL CORD SYNDROMES[7,10,22]

Syndrome	Mechanisms of Injury	Clinical Description
Anterior cord	Flexion injury; damage to the anterior third of spinal cord.	Motor function, pain, temperature, and sensation are lost bilaterally below the injured segment. Poor prognosis for return of bowel and bladder function, hand function, and ambulation.
Central cord	Hyperextension injury; damage to the central gray matter. (Most common syndrome.)	More neurologic involvement of UEs than LEs; sensory deficits less than motor. Ambulation, bowel, and bladder functions typically preserved with distal UE weakness.
Posterior cord	Compression or infarction of the posterior spinal artery. (Very rare.)	Proprioception, stereognosis, two-point discrimination and vibration sense are lost below the lesion; with preservation of motor function, pain, and light touch. A wide based steppage gait pattern is common.
Brown-Sequard	Penetrating injuries (gunshot, stab wound); damage to half of the spinal cord.	Ipsilateral loss of motor function and position sense; contralateral loss of light touch pain and temperature sensation several levels below the lesion. Good prognosis for ambulation, bowel and bladder function, and hand function.
Cauda equina/ conus medullaris	Damage at L1 vertebral level and below; **lower motor neuron** lesion.	Flaccid paralysis below level of lesion without the presence of reflex activity. Loss of bowel, bladder, and sexual function.

and involves partial or complete paralysis of all or part of the trunk and both LEs.[14,35,50] Paraplegia does not apply to lumbosacral plexus lesions.[14,50]

The severity of SCI is classified based on motor function according to spinal level. The examiner indicates the most distal uninvolved segment with motor function (3/5 strength) at the intact skeletal level.[55] The ASIA Impairment Scale is used to classify the extent of the damage (see Table 9–16).

In addition to classifying SCIs by the level and degree of impairment, some incomplete lesions have distinct clinical signs and symptoms that enable further classification. Refer to Table 9–17 for a description of incomplete spinal cord syndromes.

Brain Tumors

Brain tumors account for approximately 2% of all cancer-related deaths in the United States. They are the leading cause of solid tumor deaths in children under the age of 20, the leading cause of cancer-related deaths in males from 20 to 39 years old, and the fifth leading cause of cancer-related deaths in women ages 20 to 39 years.[60] The general incidence in the United States is 14 to 15 per 100,000 persons.[59]

Classification of tumors is difficult because there are at least 100 different types of brain tumors. The current system of classification, developed by The World Health Organization (WHO), describes tumors according to the origin of the cell type.[51,60]

Clinical presentation of a person with a brain tumor varies greatly depending on the type, size, and duration of tumor. Elevated ICP symptoms such as headache, drowsiness, nausea and vomiting, seizure activity, personality change, eye weakness, speech disturbance, memory loss, and/or focal neurologic deficits may occur in the presence of a brain mass.[60] Medical work-up includes imaging scans such as a CT, MRI with or without contrast, and cerebral angiography.

Surgery is considered when a definitive diagnosis, alleviation of symptoms, and/or reduction/elimination of the tumor is possible. Nonsurgical interventions include radiation therapy, chemotherapy, and steroid medications (see Chapter 13).[60]

Intracranial Surgery

Intracranial surgery may be necessary to decrease ICP, obtain a brain biopsy, evacuate a hemorrhage, embolize an aneurysm, excise a brain tumor, repair an AVM, and/or to repair damage to the cerebrum.[13,61] Table 9–18 provides descriptions of the most common intracranial neurosurgical procedures.

Spinal Surgery

Spinal surgery is indicated to provide stability to a fractured region, correct a disc abnormality, correct a dislocation, correct spondylolisthesis or scoliosis, correct neural compression, remove osteophytes, repair a dural tear, remove a tumor, for emergent treatment of acute cauda equine syndrome, and/or to correct spinal stenosis.[50,62–65]

Table 9–19 provides descriptions of the various spinal neurosurgical procedures.

REHABILITATION INTERVENTIONS

Neurosurgical Examination and Treatment

Prior to the initiation of intervention strategies, a thorough chart review is essential. The chart review should include the following factors: the patient's symptoms prior to surgery, the nature of the surgical procedure, any complications related to the surgery, and the postoperative instructions and/or precautions. In addition, it is important to gain an understanding of the patient's social history and functional abilities prior to admission.

Table 9–18

INTRACRANIAL NEUROSURGICAL PROCEDURES[1,10,26]

Burr hole	A small hole is made in the cranium with a specialized drill. This procedure may be used to evacuate an extracerebral clot such as a subdural or epidural hematoma, access brain tissue for a brain biopsy, access the brain for placement of ICP monitoring systems, or to place stereotactic devices. A series of burr holes may be used to perform a craniectomy.
Craniotomy	Involves surgically opening the skull to provide access to the brain. This procedure may be used to remove a tumor, clip an aneurysm, and/or to repair damage to the cerebrum. A craniotomy is named according to the area of bone that is affected (ie, frontal, occipital or tempoparietal craniotomy).
Craniectomy	This surgical procedure is similar to a craniotomy except that a bone flap is removed. This procedure is often done to decompress brain tissue and/or to fight infection. The excised bone may be stored in a bone bank, or placed within the subcutaneous tissue of the abdomen in order to maintain blood supply. *Note: Patients without a bone flap should wear a helmet whenever OOB to protect the exposed area after a craniectomy.*
Cranioplasty	Involves replacing the bone flap excised during a craniectomy. The replacement flap may be the original bone removed, a graft, or acrylic material. This procedure typically takes place three to six months after a craniectomy and is indicated in order to restore the protective properties of the skull and for cosmesis.

Care of the patient with neurosurgical involvement should begin in the ICU. Knowledge of the medical management and equipment is vital to successful interventions. Often, patients will have numerous lines and monitors, but this should not deter the interventions (see Chapter 3).[65] Safety and efficacy of interventions for physical therapy have been studied.[65,66] Careful progression of the patient from supine to out of bed (OOB) can occur with coordination from the medical team. Family education and teaching regarding the patient's plan of care should begin from the onset of therapy and include discharge planning discussions, therapeutic exercise, and cognitive considerations.

Clinical Tips

- Elevating the head of the bed to 30 degrees will reduce ICP by promoting venous return from the head; this position is often required for postoperative intracranial surgery.[65–67]
- Cognitive arousal is typically best in upright positions.[5]

Table 9–19
SPINAL NEUROSURGICAL PROCEDURES

Discectomy	Refers to the decompression of nerve root material accomplished by removing intervertebral nuclear disk material, which is often indicated to treat chronic disc herniation and/or nerve root impingement. This procedure may be accomplished via a microdiscectomy or laminectomy.
Laminectomy	Involves the excision of the laminae, or posterior vertebral arch, via an anterior or posterior approach (posterior most common). May be performed independently to excise disk material or as part of a spinal fusion procedure.
Microdiscectomy	Less invasive than a laminectomy, this procedure involves the decompression of nerve root(s) and excision of extruded disk material through an incision made in the inferior aspect of the lamina.
Foraminotomy	This procedure involves the surgical enlargement of the intervertebral foramen to increase the exit space surrounding a spinal nerve in order to decompress spinal nerve root impingement. This procedure is most commonly preformed in the cervical region secondary to reduced anatomical size of the foramina in this region.
Spinal fusion	Refers to the union, or arthrodesis, of two or more vertebrae in order to immobilize specific vertebrae and strengthen the integrity of a compromised vertebral column. This procedure involves the insertion of bone graft segments between the involved vertebrae. It may or may not include instrumentation, also referred to as fixation, which may include pedicle screws, rods, and/or plates. Graft material may by autologous bone from the anterior or posterior iliac spine, nonautolgous bone, typically from a cadaver, or manufactured substitutes such as hydroxylapatite.
Posterolateral lumbar fusion (PLF)	This procedure typically involves a midline posterior incision with the potential decortication (excision) of the laminae as well as additional structures in order to reach the desired region and accomplish the objective(s) of surgery. A bone graft is implanted over the decorticated surfaces, forming a contiguous region that includes all surfaces to be fused. Instrumentation may or may not be included.

(continued)

Table 9–19 (continued)

SPINAL NEUROSURGICAL PROCEDURES

Posterior lumbar inter-body fusion (PLIF)	This procedure is similar to the procedures described for PLF, except it also involves the excision of the disc in between the involved vertebrae with subsequent placement of instrumentation (inter-body cage device) within the evacuated disc space. The available area for bone union is increased with the creation of the inter-body space.
Anterior lumbar inter-body fusion (ALIF)	This procedure involves an anterior retroperitoneal approach with disc excision and inter-body bone grafting. Because ALIFs are typically not as secure as PLIFs, many surgeons protect this type of graft by adding posterior instrumentation as well. The anterior approach is also used for cervical levels C3 to C7; called anterior cervical discectomy with fusion (ACDF).
Vertebroplasty	This procedure involves injection of cement to repair a compression fracture. Complications can include cement extravasation and rarely, complications related to anesthesia. This is a relatively new procedure started in the United States in 1993. The primary purpose of the procedure is to relieve back pain, which is reported in 84% of cases, and to decrease the duration of the immobility associated with compression fracture of the spine.

Adapted from:
Parent A. *Carpenter's Human Neuroanatomy.* 9th ed. Media, Pa: Williams and Wilkins; 1996.
Broderick JP, Adams HP Jr, Barsan W, et al. Guidelines for management of spontaneous intracerebral hemorrhage: A statement for healthcare professionals from a special writing group of the Stroke Council, American Heart Association. *Stroke.* 1999;30:905–915.
Schmidt RA, Lee TD. *Motor Control and Learning, A Behavior Emphasis.* Champaign, Ill: Human Kinetics; 1999.
Mangum; Maxey & Magnusson; Lim et al; Diamond, Champion, & Clark

- Families are often seeking ways to assist with care. Consider teaching PROM, therapeutic exercise, and positioning techniques.

Comprehensive therapy should begin. This often involves coordination with respiratory and speech therapists, nursing, orthotists/prothetists, and occupational therapists.

If the patient's activity is restricted following surgery and/or if the patient requires assistance for a certain postoperative brace, this information must be gathered at the onset of physical therapy in order to incorporate these factors into the patient's plan of care. Based on the type of brace, the interventions must

Table 9–20
COMMON ORTHOTICS FOLLOWING SPINAL SURGERY

Name of Brace	Precautions	Indication
Soft cervical collar	No sudden movement of the cervical spine; driving may be difficult.	Pain relief, reduce muscular demand to hold head upright.
Hard cervical collar (Philadelphia collar, Miami J collar)	No sudden rotation of the cervical spine is possible; no driving; heat builds up under the collar.	Pain relief, reduce muscular demand to hold head upright, restrict cervical flexion and extension.[15]
Halo	Pin care; maintain ROM of the shoulders especially for end range; monitor for swallowing dysfunction.	Maximum stability to prevent flexion, extension or rotation of the cervical spine.[15]
Thoracic lumar sacral orthosis (TLSO)	No trunk flexion beyond 90 degrees to avoid compression of the femoral nerve.	Limits trunk flexion and rotation; positions in neutral or extension for postural control or spinal stabilization.
Lumbar sacral orthosis (LSO) or corset	No trunk flexion beyond 90 degrees to avoid compression of the femoral nerve.	Pain relief, proprioceptive retraining, positions in neutral or slight extension for postural control or spinal stabilization.

All orthotics mentioned generally require the patient to limit lifting and to wear the brace at a minimum while OOB.

incorporate the precautions for movement and donning and doffing the brace. Consultation with the physician and the orthotist for mobility concerns is essential. Table 9–20 provides descriptions of common orthotics used for stabilization following spinal surgery.

The therapist should assess the patient's strength, muscular tone, coordination, and overall quality of movement. To the extent that the patient is able, examine the patient's ability to complete functional tasks such as rolling side to side, transferring from supine to sit, sit to stand, and wheelchair to mat. Document the patient's balance, postural stability, quality of movement, the impairments limiting mobility, and the types of compensatory strategies used when the patient attempts to complete the aforementioned tasks. Finally, assess and describe the patient's standing balance and gait, when applicable.

- If the patient has specific postoperative lifting and activity precautions the therapist should not break test the patient to determine his or her strength.

- If the patient demonstrates unusually decreased arousal, check with the patient's nurse to determine whether it is related to a pharmacologic response; if so, coordinate activity with medication schedules.
- Pain management is essential following surgery in order to promote early mobilization of the patient. Coordination with nursing to ensure proper management of pain often results in more efficient therapy sessions.

An orthopedic surgeon and/or a neurosurgeon can perform spinal surgery. Regardless of the attending physician, pain management should be a consideration regardless of the surgical procedure. Good outcome measures for adequate pain control include the ability to participate in the therapy session, to deep breath, and to cough. Use of the Oswestry Pain Questionnaire can provide evidence-based data related to patients' subjective pain complaints.[68]

Patient education should include postoperative precautions, procedure to don/doff brace (if applicable), and lifestyle changes such as quitting smoking.[69] Table 9-21 describes general information regarding the typical clinical presentation of a patient following spinal surgery along with a general plan of care.

SCI therapy starts with the first interaction with the patient and the family. Often, this is in the ICU but may be delayed until medical stability is certain. Much of the rehabilitation for the SCI patient will occur at another level of care; however, early intervention can enhance functional outcomes. Patients should be encouraged to continue to attempt movement of muscle groups that have been reported nonfunctional. The plan of care will need to include extensive education for the long-term deficits that may have occurred with the SCI. Skin integrity is a major concern for all patients with SCI and a goal of intact skin should be the gold standard throughout the course of the care.[70] Table 9–22 provides general descriptions of the physical therapy plan of care following SCI based on the level of injury.

When evaluating and treating a patient following neurosurgery, it is essential to first gain an understanding of the operative technique, the location and indications for surgery, as well as any intraoperative tissue injury that may have occurred.

In addition to careful monitoring of the patient for complications following surgery, such as increased ICP, mental status changes, and seizure activity, early mobilization of the patient is essential.[71] Patients and family members should be informed of the postoperative precautions following surgery and instructed on positions to avoid during the initial mobilization process. Individual treatment plans should also address impairments specific to the location of surgery, cognitive involvement, and consider the prognosis and expected course of the disease process.

For patients with a poor prognosis, careful consideration must be given to psychosocial care. Goals for this patient population may include family training for positioning and comfort as well education to understand the support resources available, such as hospice care.[15]

For patients who have intracranial surgery to remove a malignant brain tumor, it is essential to consider the additional treatment techniques that may accompany intracranial surgery and their effects on rehabilitation. Gliomas are typically located in the cerebral hemispheres and are the most common type of cancerous brain tumors in adults.[15,71] The standard treatment for this type

Table 9–21

ACUTE CARE PHYSICAL THERAPY AND SPINAL SURGERY

Type of Surgery	Impairments	Interventions	Goals
Spinal fusion, decompression, and spinal stenosis surgeries	Muscle weakness, decreased functional mobility, dependence to don/doff brace; maintenance of precautions in functional tasks and IADLs.	Limited strength training in functional tasks, abdominal strengthening and stabilization. Neural mobilization is controversial. Patient education for brace care and maintenance.	Independent transfers and gait for household distances, independent bed mobility, able to instruct or apply the orthotic device. Independence in application of precautions in functional mobility.
Discectomy and laminectomy	Muscle weakness, decreased functional mobility, maintenance of precautions in functional tasks and IADLs, sitting tolerance may be limited to 30 to 60 minutes.	Early mobilization and gentle therapeutic exercise. A soft corset may be indicated for comfort. Functional retraining which may include initiation of "back school."	Independence in all functional tasks, independent with home exercise program. Referral to outpatient therapy after follow up with MD.

Adapted from:
Danielsen JM, Johnson R, Kibsgaard SK, et al. Early aggressive exercise for postoperative rehabilitation following discectomy. *Spine.* 2000;25(8):1015–1020.
Fritz JM, Delitto A, Welch WC, Erhard RE. Lumbar spinal stenosis: a review of current concepts in evaluation, management, and outcome measures. *Archives Physical Medicine and Rehabilitation.* 1998;79;700–707.
Kjellby-Wendt G, Styf J. Early active training after lumbar discectomy. A prospective, randomized and controlled study. *Spine.* 1998;23(21):2345–2352.
Phillleps FM, Cunningham B. Managing chronic pain of spinal origin after lumbar surgery: the role of decompressive surgery. *Spine.* 2001;27(22):2547–2553.
Scrimshaw SV, Maher CG. Randomized controlled trial of neural mobilization after spinal surgery. *Spine.* 2001;26(24):2647–2652.
Wilner S. Effects of a rigid brace on back pain. *Acta Orthop Scand.* 1985;56:40–42.

of tumor consists of surgery, chemotherapy, including a localized form called Gliadel wafers, which is implanted into the surgical site, radiation therapy, and/or biologic therapy.[72] The side effects of radiation therapy and/or chemotherapy, which include fatigue, anemia, nausea, difficulty eating, skin irritation, edema, and neuropathy, must be considered during the rehabilitation process (refer to Chapter 13).[73]

Acoustic neuromas, also called vestibular schwannomas, account for approximately 8% to 10% of all intracranial tumors and usually occur in the third or fourth decade of life.[71,74] This nerve sheath tumor is typically benign, slow growing, and is often located on the vestibular portion of the eighth cranial nerve (vestibulocochlear nerve).[71] The most common intervention for this type of tumor is surgical removal.[71,74]

Because of the vestibular involvement, patients' with this form of tumor often have balance and visual impairments both pre- and postoperatively.[74] Additionally, the vestibulocochlear nerve is located within close proximity to the facial and auditory nerves; patients often have permanent or transient postoperative facial paralysis and/or hearing impairment. The most favorable outcomes for patients with this type of tumor are associated with participation in vestibular rehabilitation.[75]

The goals for vestibular rehabilitation following surgical excision of an acoustic neuroma include improve functional balance, especially during ambulation, improve visual acuity during head movements, and to decrease the sense of disequilibrium.[74] Specific treatment strategies include standing balance exercises with the eyes open and closed with changes in the base of support and support surface, vestibular reflex (VOR) x1 and VOR x2 viewing paradigms, and gait training with progression to the incorporation of head turns and changes in direction.[74,75]

- Instruct the patient to avoid any activities that may involve the valsalva maneuver, this tends to increase ICP, which is contraindicated following intracranial surgery.

- A CSF leak may present as clear fluid draining from the patient incision and/or body orifice. If detected, halt any physical activity and report findings to the MD for evaluation.[13]

- If the intracranial surgery involved removal of a portion of the patient's skull, also called a bone flap removal or craniectomy, use of a helmet or other protective measures is indicated.

- Following intracranial surgery, patients are at risk for developing deep vein thrombosis and/or a pulmonary embolism because of immobility and the contraindication of anticoagulation following surgery. Patients must be monitored carefully for any signs or symptoms of these complications.[15]

- Patients who undergo intracranial surgery may develop agitation following surgery due to head injury; this patient population must be carefully monitored for cognitive involvement.

Table 9–22

ACUTE CARE PHYSICAL THERAPY AND SPINAL CORD INJURY

Level of Injury	Impairments	Interventions	Goals
High cervical injury (C2–C3)	Ventilator dependent for respiration; dependent mobility; dependence in weight shifts; no AROM; potential for contractures, skin breakdown, spasticity and automonic dysreflexia.[15]	Breathing exercises, inspiratory muscle training and pulmonary toilet.[15] PROM and positioning; Monitor for autonomic dysreflexia. Patient/family education and strengthening exercises.	Sitting tolerance for 1 to 2 hours per day at 30 to 60 degree angle, suctioning less than every 4 hours; assistance with pulmonary techniques. Initiate education for weight shifts, pulmonary hygiene, ROM and positioning.
High cervical injury (C4)	Pulmonary compromise, may have resulted in ventilator use and/or tracheostomy. Dependent mobility, dependent for weight shifts. Potential for contractures, skin breakdown, spasticity and automonic dysreflexia	Breathing exercises, inspiratory muscle training and pulmonary toilet. PROM and positioning; Monitor for autonomic dysreflexia. Patient and family education and strengthening exercises.	Sitting for 1 to 2 hours at 60 to 90 degrees, independent with respiratory exercises, independent in requesting weight shift in all positions. Able to identify symptoms associated with need for airway/secretion clearance.
C5–T1	Dependent mobility, dependent weight shift, respiratory compromise, potential for contracture, spasticity, and autonomic dysreflexia.	Functional mobility training, positioning, weight shift training, patient and family education, and strengthening exercises, including respiratory muscles. Monitor for autonomic dysreflexia.	Strength training, including respiratory musculature (may be independent with secretion clearance). ROM but avoid stretch of finger flexors if tenodysis grip will be required. Full day sitting tolerance at 60 to 90 degree angle, assists in pushing wheelchair. Independent in requests for weight shifts in all positions.

High thoracic injury (T2–T6)	Dependent mobility, decreased sitting tolerance and angle. Respiratory compromise. Potential for contracture and autonomic dysreflexia.	Functional mobility training may include standing program. Respiratory exercise and pulmonary toilet, positioning, weight shift training, patient and family education. Monitor for autonomic dysreflexia.	Assist with functional mobility, full day sitting at a 60 to 90 degree angle, independently able to clear secretions, assist with weight shifts in all positions, improve strength and PROM with avoidance of overstretch of the back extensors. Able to identify symptoms associated with autonomic dysreflexia.
Low thoracic injury (T7–T12)	Decreased mobility, decreased sitting tolerance and angle. Respiratory compromise.	Functional mobility training including standing program. Respiratory exercise and pulmonary toilet. Weight shift training. Patient and family education.	Assist with all functional mobility, full day sitting at 90 degree angle; Independent clearance of secretions and deep breathing.
Lumber injury (L1–5)	Decreased mobility, decreased sitting tolerance, dependent for weight shifts, and decreased aerobic conditioning.	Functional mobility training including gait training, weight shift training. Patient and family education.	Assist with some functional mobility, gait for short distances with assistive devices and bracing for LEs. Full day sitting at 90 degree angle. Aerobic training on UBE, and/or kinetron.
Lumbar and sacral plexus	Decreased mobility, decreased sitting tolerance, decreased aerobic conditioning.	Functional mobility training including gait training, weight shift training. Patient and family education.	Assist with all functional mobility, gait for short distances with assistive devices and bracing for L's. Full day sitting at 90 degree angle. Aerobic training on UBE, kinetron and/or bicycle.

Adapted from:
Consortium for Spinal Cord Medicine. Autonomic dysreflexia: what you should know. *Paralyzed Veterans of America.* Washington, DC: 1997.
Fujiwara T, Hara Y, Chino N. Expiratory function in complete tetraplegics. Study of spirometry, maximal expiratory pressure, and muscle activity of pectoralis major and latissimus dorsi muscles. *American Journal of Physical Medicine and Rehabilitation.* 1999;78(5):464–469.
Massery M. What's positioning got to do with it? *Neurology Report.* 1994;18(3):11–14.

Neurosurgery Summary

When treating a patient who has recently undergone neurosurgery, the therapist should first understand the pathology of the underlying impairment that required surgery. Next, it is important to understand the nature of the surgery, any postoperative complications, and the precautions associated with activity following surgery. Prior to mobilizing the patient, it is also essential to have a clear understanding of the wearing schedule and donning/doffing technique for any braces and/or orthotics required.

The clinical presentation of a person with a brain tumor varies greatly depending on the type, size, and amount of tumor, excised and/or the residual growth that could not be surgically removed. When treating a patient with a brain tumor it is important to understand the clinical effects with respect to the specific area of the brain that is affected. This may enable a therapist to identify subtle changes in a patient that may have otherwise gone unnoticed.

Spinal surgery may be indicated to provide stability, correct a disc abnormality, correct a spinal stenosis, spondylolisthesis or scoliosis, relieve neural compression, remove osteophytes, correct a dural tear, remove a tumor, or for emergent treatment of acute cauda equine syndrome.

Spinal surgery may also be indicated to stabilize a patient's spine following a SCI. When evaluating a patient with SCI it is important to understand the ASIA impairment scale in order to correctly classify and, thereby, describe the amount of motor and sensory impairment.

When evaluating and treating a neurosurgical patient in the acute care setting, the therapist must understand the postoperative surgical protocol in order to educate the patient and family. During the first interaction with the patient postoperatively, all of the precautions and activity guidelines must be incorporated into patient care. Family education is essential for this patient population to ensure the patient consistently follows the postoperative instructions and is provided with the assistance required to continue implementing the required protocol within the home setting.

When establishing the patient's plan of care, the therapist should consider what restrictions and precautions the patient must follow after surgery, the estimated length of stay in acute care, the social support available for the patient following discharge and any activity restrictions that may affect the recommendation for the next level of care.

Case Study

Ms. Cook, a 76-year-old female, presents to her primary physician (PMD) with progressive weakness in the UEs and difficulty walking over the past 4 months. She had one fall, which did not result in injury, within the last month. Her PMD refers her to a neurosurgeon for further work-up. MRI reveals degenerative disc disease throughout the spine with a herniation at C6–C7. Following multiple consultations, Ms. Cook elects to have surgery. The neurosurgeon performs an anterior cervical discectomy and fusion (ACDF) of levels C6–C7. A physical therapy evaluation was ordered the day after the surgery.

Patient/Client History
General Demographics/Social History/Living Environment

Ms. Cook's social history reveals she was living with her daughter who works during the day. They live in a two-story house with the bedroom and bathroom on the second floor. There are six steps to enter. Both sets of stairs have a railing on the right side.

General Health Status/Family History

Ms. Cook has survived her husband by 8 years. She states her mother had some heart problems but cannot remember what they were. Other then the recent fall and weakness she reports feeling fine.

Medical/Surgical History

The chart review reveals a previous medical history of HTN, diabetes, laminectomy 10 years PTA, and a history of chest pain. Her medical conditions are managed with medications. The surgeon has ordered a Philadelphia collar to be worn at all times for 6 weeks following surgery.

Current Conditions/Chief Complaints

Ms. Cook is complaining of some neck soreness and difficulty swallowing. She is also complaining of a sore throat. She is seen bedside in her room for examination.

Functional Status and Activity Level

Ms. Cook has been limited to household ambulation recently due to a fall last month. She states that she walks to the mailbox only when her daughter is home from work. Otherwise, she stays in the house most of the day. She reports using a straight cane when needed. Prior to the onset of weakness, she was a community ambulator.

Systems Review
Cardiovascular/Pulmonary

Resting vital signs in bed (head of bed >30 degrees) HR 96, RR 18, BP 136/84, pulse regular, oxygen saturation on room air 95% (SpO_2), and pain 6/10. Her breath sounds are diminished but clear. Her cough is weak and nonproductive. Following ROM, MMT, bed mobility, and transfers her vital signs were HR 114 and a regular pulse, RR 24, BP 96/84, SpO_2 96%, and pain 8/10. She complained of lightheadedness with sitting. Laboratory findings reveal troponin 0.9 ng/mL, glucose 240 mg/dL, hemoglobin A_1c 8.9%, lactate dehydrogenase (LDH) 240 U/L, aspartate aminotrasnferase (AST)/serum glutamic-oxaloacetic transaminase (SGOT) 38 U/L, and white blood cells (WBCs) slightly elevated at 11,500.

Integumentary

Ms. Cook is wearing a Philadelphia collar. She has an anterior surgical bandage on her neck. There is no drainage noted. She does have moderate edema (2+) distal UEs and LEs.

Musculoskeletal

Ms. Cook had decreased active ROM BUEs at the end range. IADLs were assessed and she was unable to reach above her head. Her trunk strength was limited as demonstrated by decreased sitting and standing tolerance. She is dependent for bed mobility and transfers. Gait was not assessed due to her drop in BP with supine to sit transfer.

Neuromuscular

Ms. Cook had impaired proprioception distal BUEs and BLEs. She had an inability to maintain balance without visual cues. Ms. Cook also has mild dysphagia.

Communication, Affect, Cognition, Language, and Learning Style

Ms. Cook was able to speak slowly but complained of the collar bothering her chin. Her speech was hypophonic, and she was unable to complete a sentence without taking a rest.

Tests and Measures
Aerobic Capacity and Endurance

Ms. Cook had orthostatic hypotension when transferring from supine to sitting. She is deconditioned as demonstrated by her HR and RR response to activity. Some of the increase in HR may be to compensate for hypotension. Ms. Cook may have had an infarction perioperatively due to the elevation in troponin and slightly elevated WBC and AST/SGOT. The poor diabetes control, age, and sedentary lifestyle are independent risk factors for cardiovascular disease.

Assistive and Adaptive Devices

A Philadelphia collar must be worn at all times for 6 weeks. Difficulty swallowing and decreased neck ROM for functional mobility may impact wearing the color.

Gait, Locomotion, and Balance

Ms. Cook is dependent for functional activities including bed mobility, transfers, and gait. Postoperative cervical precautions include no lifting >5 pounds with the UEs and no twisting of the cervical spine. Increased time was required to complete functional tasks and ADLs. Her balance was poor in sitting.

Pain

Ms. Cook's pain increases when sitting upright.

Diagnosis

Ms. Cook has functional, cardiovascular/pulmonary, and neurological limitations related to her degenerative disc disease, subsequent surgical repair, and myocardial infarction complicated by poorly controlled diabetes. Recommend treatment pattern 5H: impaired motor function, peripheral nerve integrity, and sensory integrity associated with nonprogressive disorders of the spinal cord.[48]

Prognosis

Based on the assessment of the patient's impairments and functional limitations, the physical therapist estimated that Ms. Cook would require another level of care post discharge from the hospital. Her plan of care included daily physical therapy services until she was medically ready to be transferred to the next level of care. The following are short-term goals to be achieved by discharge from the acute setting: to demonstrate maintenance of a neutral spine via the log roll technique for bed mobility and transfer from supine to sitting with minimal assistance, will maintain static sitting balance on the edge of bed for 10 minutes with supervision and BUEs supported on the bed, will verbalize understanding of postoperative cervical precautions, and instruct others for the procedure to don/doff her Philadelphia collar. Ms. Cook will stand and ambulate 25 to 50 feet with minimal assistance and a rolling walker. With supervision from the therapist, the patient's family will demonstrate the proper technique to don/doff the patient's Philadelphia collar. Recommend vital sign monitoring with progression of exercise program.

Intervention

Strength training for the LEs and compensatory techniques for proprioception deficits, such as visual cues, balance, gait and endurance training made up the care plan. In addition, patient and family education regarding the importance of maintaining postoperative surgical precautions, the wearing schedule for the brace, and lifestyle changes that incorporate a neutral spine and proper body mechanics into daily living. Vital signs and subjective complaints are closely monitored due to the possible perioperative MI. The communication and documentation of Ms. Cook's plan of care to the interdisciplinary team members was completed. Speech therapy was consulted and the physician was informed that she was having difficulty swallowing. Social work and/or a discharge planner were consulted to arrange for the next level of care.

Reexamination

On postoperative day 4, Ms. Cook is standing with moderate assistance of one for 3 minutes. Her balance with visual cues is fair and a mirror is being used during therapy. She is using a "huff technique" instead of a cough and has no pulmonary complications. She is using a rolling walker with moderate assistance of one for 25 feet x 2. Her pain is now rated a 3/10 with activity.

Outcomes

Ms. Cook was transferred to an inpatient rehabilitation unit. Recommend outpatient rehabilitation or cardiac rehabilitation following inpatient stay on rehabilitation unit depending on functional recovery.

CHAPTER REVIEW QUESTIONS

Part I

1. Name the two types of strokes and mechanism of pathology for each. How do the clinical manifestation of each vary? Which type is more common?

2. Describe the typical impairments associated with PD. Name two treatment interventions to address these impairments.

3. Describe the difference between primary and secondary injury in TBI. Name two scales used to describe patients with TBI.

4. Which components of an acute care neurologic examination should be completed prior to mobilization of the patient? Why?

5. Name two reasons why a thorough assessment of cognition and communication are essential in an acute neurologic evaluation.

Part II

6. Which spinal tract carries pain, temperature, and touch? What are the clinical implications when this spinal tract is damaged?

7. Which spinal tract influences postural control, coordination, and smoothness of movement? What clinical manifestations may be present when this tract is damaged?

8. Explain the difference between myotome and dermatome. Describe the process for evaluating the integrity of each.

9. What factors must be considered when developing a plan of care for a patient who received intracranial surgery for excision of a brain tumor? What precautions must be considered during the acute phase of treatment?

10. Describe the impairments that typically accompany an acoustic neuroma and the treatment techniques that have been associated with optimal recovery.

PHARMACOLOGICAL INFORMATION: NEUROLOGIC AND NEUROSURGICAL DISEASES AND DISORDERS PHARMACOLOGY

Antialzheimers

Action
Antialzheimer medications inhibit cholinesterase, an enzyme, which metabolizes Ach, thereby increasing the amount of Ach within the CNS to temporarily lessen dementia.

Side Effects
CNS: Headache, depression, drowsiness, fatigue, insomnia
CV: HTN, hypotension, syncope, AF
GI: Diarrhea, nausea, vomiting, anorexia/weight loss, flatulence
Misc: Muscle cramps, arthritis, hot flashes

Common Medications
Donepezil (Aricept), galantamine (Reminyl), rivastigmine (Exelon), tacrine (Cognex)

Anxiolytics/Sedatives/Benzodiazepines

Action
Benzodiazepines are the most common group of anxiolytics and sedative hypnotics. Benzodiazepines potentiate the effect of GABA, an inhibitory neurotransmitter, within the CNS. These agents lead to hyperpolarization of cells resulting in reduced synaptic transmission.

Side Effects
CNS: Dizziness, drowsiness, lethargy, depression
CV: Hypotension, bradycardia
GI: Constipation, diarrhea, nausea, vomiting
Misc: Dependence, drug tolerance, blurred vision
Pulm: Respiratory depression, apnea, bronchospasm

Common Medications
Alprazolam (Xanax), Chlordiazepoxide (Librium), Diazepam (Valium), Lorazepam (Ativan), Midazolam (Versed), Oxazepam (Serax)

Anticonvulsants

Action
Anticonvulsants inhibit sodium channels of neurons decreasing excitability and action potential propagation; enhance the effects of GABA, a CNS inhibitory neurotransmitter, or block calcium channels. These agents attempt to raise the seizure threshold, decrease the spread of seizure activity, or depress the motor cortex.

Side Effects
CNS: Drowsiness, lethargy, delirium, incoordination
CV: Hypotension
GI: Constipation, nausea, vomiting, GI discomfort
Misc: Arthralgias, myalgias, neuralgias, allergic reactions
Pulm: Bronchospasm, respiratory depression

Common Medications
Sodium channel blocking agents: Phenytoin (Dilantin), Carbamazepine (Tegretol), Oxcaraepine, Lamotrigine (Lamictal)
GABA agonists: Gabapentin (Neurotonin)
Calcium channel blockade: Ethosuximide (Zarontin), Trimethadione
Combined effects: Benzodiazepines (eg, Clonazepam (Klonopin), Phenobarbital (Luminal), Primdone (Myosoline)

Antidepressants

Action
Antidepressants potentiate the effect of serotonin and norepinephrine in the CNS. Depression is characterized by diminished interest in normal activities, anorexia and weight loss, fatigue, insomnia, and an inability to concentrate. Mania is characterized by inflated self-esteem, poverty of sleep, and expansive mood.

Side Effects
CNS: Lethargy, sedation, reduced seizure threshold
CV: Dysrhythmias, orthostatic hypotension
GI: Constipation, diarrhea, nausea
Misc: Blurred vision, weight gain, increased appetite, tremor

Common Medications
Tricyclic antidepressants: Amitriptyline (Elavil), Nortriptyline (Pamelor), Imipramine (Imprin/ Tofranil)
Selective seotonin reuptake inhibitors (SSRI): Fluozetine HCl (Prozac), Sertaline HCl (Zoloft)
Monoamine oxidase (MAO) inhibitors (block metabolism of norepinephrine and serotonin): Phenelzine (Nardil), Tranylcypromine (Parnate), Isocarboxazid (Marplan)
Miscellaneous: Buprion (Wellbutrin), Trazadone (Desyrel), Venlafaxine (Effexor)

Antiparkinson (Antidyskinetic) Agents

Action
Antiparkinson agents attempt to either increase CNS concentrations of dopamine (eg, Levodopa), potentiate dopamines actions (eg, Amantadine, Bromocriptine), or limit its breakdown (COMT inhibitors, monoamine oxidase

inhibitors Selegiline), reduce cholinergic activity (eg, benztropine, beperiden), or diminish neuronal outlflow from the basal ganglia.

Side Effects
CNS: Involuntary movements, ataxia, anxiety, dizziness, hallucinations
CV: Orthostatic hypotension, tachycardia, palpitations
GI: Anorexia, nausea, vomiting
Misc: Dry mouth, blurred vision, leukopenia, anemia

Common Medications
Dopaminergic: Amantadine (Symmetrel), Bromocriptine (Parlodel), Levodopa (L-Dopa/Larodopa)
Catechol-O-methyl-transferase (COMT) inhibitors: Entacapone (Comtan),
MAO inhibitors (monoamine oxidase inhibitors): Selegiline (Eldepryl)
Anticholinergics: Benztropine (Cogentin), Biperiden (Akineton)

Antipsychotics

Action
Antipsychotics are used in the treatment of psychosis and schizophrenia. Psychosis refers to mental disorders characterized by diminished capacity to process information, hallucinations, delusions, incoherence, aggression, or violence. Schizophrenia is a mental disorder associated with disturbances of thinking and affect. Antipsychotic drugs primarily block dopamine receptors but may additionally impact histamine, serotonin, and alpha adrenergic receptors.

Side Effects
CNS: Tardive dyskinesia, Parkinsonism, dystonia, drowsiness, lethargy, neuroleptic syndrome
CV: Orthostatic hypotension, tachycardia
GI: Dry mouth, constipation
Misc: Impotence, infertility, blurred vision

Common Medications
Clozapine (Clozaril), Chlorpromazine, Haloperidol (Haldol), Thioridazine (Mellaril), Lithium

REFERENCES

1. Parent A. *Carpenter's Human Neuroanatomy.* 9th ed. Media, Pa: Williams and Wilkins; 1996.
2. Hickey JV. *Clinical Practice of Neurological and Neurosurgical Nursing.* Philadelphia, Pa: JB Lippincott Co; 1992.
3. Barr ML, Kiernan. *The Human Nervous System.* 6th ed. Philadelphia, Pa: JB Lippincott Co; 1993.
4. Young PA, Young PH. *Basic Clinical Neuroanatomy.* Media, Pa: Williams and Wilkins; 1997.
5. Clark DL, Boutros NN. *The Brain and Behavior: An Introduction to Behavioral Neuroanatomy.* Malden, Mass: Blackwell Science Inc; 1999.
6. Diamond MC, Scheibel AB, Elson LM. *The Human Brain Coloring Book.* New York, NY: Harper Collins Publishers Inc; 1985.
7. Rohan JW, Yokichi C, Lutjen-Drecoll. *Color Atlas of Anatomy.* 4th ed. Media, Pa: Williams and Wilkins; 1998.
8. Lundy-Ekman L. *Neuroscience Fundamentals for Rehabilitation.* Philadelphia, Pa: WB Saunders Co; 1998.
9. Greenwood R, Barnes MB, McMillan TM, Ward CD. *Neurological Rehabilitation.* New York, NY: Churchill Livingstone; 1993.
10. Adams RD, Victor M, Ropper AH. *Principles of Neurology.* 6th ed. New York, NY: McGraw-Hill Co; 1998.
11. Thomas CL. *Taber's Cyclopedic Medical Dictionary.* 17th ed. Philadelphia, Pa: FA Davis Co; 1993.
12. Netter FH. *Atlas of Human Anatomy.* 2nd ed. East Hanover, NJ: Novartis; 1997.
13. Paz JC, Panik M. *Acute Care Handbook for Physical Therapists.* Newton, Mass: Butterworth-Heinemann; 1997.
14. O'Sullivan, Schmitz TJ. *Physical Rehabilitation, Assessment and Treatment.* 3rd ed. Philadelphia, Pa: FA Davis Co; 1994.
15. Umphred DA. *Neurological Rehabilitation.* 3rd ed. St. Louis, Mo: Mosby-Year Book, Inc; 1995.
16. Gordon NF, Gulanick M, Costa F, et al. Physical activity and exercise recommendations for stroke survivors: an American Heart Association scientific statement from the Council on Clinical Cardiology, Subcommittee on Exercise, Cardiac Rehabilitation, and Prevention; the Council on Cardiovascular Nursing; the Council on Nutrition, Physical Activity, and Metabolism; and the Stroke Council. *Stroke.* 2004;35(5):1230–1240.
17. Lewandowski C, Barsan B. Treatment of acute ischemic Stroke. *Ann Emerg Med.* 2001;37:202–216.
18. Gillen G, Burkhardt A. *Stroke Rehabilitation A Function Based Approach.* St. Louis, Mo: Mosby-Year Book, Inc; 1995.
19. Jamieson DG. Acute management of the stroke patient. *Phys Med Rehabil Clin North Am.* 1991;2:437–454.
20. Broderick JP, Adams HP Jr, Barsan W, et al. Guidelines for management of spontaneous intracerebral hemorrhage: A statement for healthcare professionals from a special writing group of the Stroke Council, American Heart Association. *Stroke.* 1999;30:905–915.
21. Gilroy J, Holliday PL. *Basic Neurology.* New York, NY: Macmillan Publishing Co; 1982.
22. Williams LE, Yilmaz EY, Lopez-Yunez AM. Retrospective assessment of initial stroke severity with the NIH Stroke Scale. *Stroke.* 2000;31(4):858–862.

23. Kasner SE, Cucchiara BL, McGarvey ML, et al. Modified National Institutes of Health stroke scale can be estimated from medical records. *Stroke.* 2003;34(2):568–570.
24. Appelros P, Terent A. Characteristics of the National Institutes of Health Stroke Scale: results from a population-based stroke cohort at baseline and after one year. *Cerebrovascu Dis.* 2004;17:(1):21–27.
25. Goldstein LB, Samsa GP. Reliability of the National Institutes of Health Stroke Scale. *Stroke.* 1997;28:307–310.
26. Scandalis TO, Bosak A, Berliner JC, Helman LL, Wells MR. Resistance training and gait function in patients with Parkinson's disease. *Am J Med Rehabil.* 2001;80:38–61.
27. Morris ME. Movement disorders in people with Parkinson's disease: a model for physical therapy. *Phys Ther.* 2000;80:578–596.
28. Schmidt RA, Lee TD. *Motor Control and Learning, A Behavior Emphasis.* Champaign, Ill: Human Kinetics; 1999.
29. Chiara T, Carlos J, Martin D, Miller R, Nadeau S. Cold effect on oxygen uptake, perceived exertion, and spasticity in patients with multiple sclerosis. *Arch Phys Med Rehabil.* 1998;79:523–527.
30. Confavreux C, Vukusic S, Moreau AP. Relapses and progression of disability in multiple sclerosis. *N Engl J Med.* 2000;343(20):1430–1438.
31. LaBan MM, Martin T, Pechur J, Sarnacki S. Physical and occupational therapy in treatment of patients with multiple sclerosis. *Phys Med Rehabil Clin North Am.* 1998;3:603–614.
32. Meythaler JM. Rehabilitation of Guillain-Barre syndrome. *Arch Phys Med Rehabil.* 1997;78:872–879.
33. Ensrud ERT, Krivickas LS. Acquired inflammatory demyelinating neuropathies. *Phys Med Rehabil Clin North Am.* 2001;12(2): 321–334.
34. Worsham TL. Easing the course of Guillain Barre syndrome. *RN.* 2000;63(3): 46–50.
35. Mills VM, Cassidy JW, Katz DI. *Neurologic Rehabilitation: A Guide to Diagnosis, Prognosis, and Treatment Blanning.* Malden, Mass: Blackwell Science; 1997.
36. Cunning S. When the DX is myasthenia gravis. *RN.* 2000;63(4):26–30.
37. Lee CA. Gettting a grip on myasthenia gravis. *Nursing.* 2002;32:32–34.
38. Davies AE. Cognitive impairments following traumatic brain injury. *Crit Care Nurs Clin North Am.* 2000;12:447–455.
39. Yanko JR, Mitcho K. Acute care management of severe traumatic brain injuries. *Crit Care Nurs Q.* 2001;23:1–23.
40. Smith DH, Meaney DF, Shull WH. Diffuse axonal injury in head trauma. *J Head Trauma Rehabil.* 2003;18(4):307–316.
41. Roth P, Farls K. Pathophysiology of traumatic brain injury. *Crit Care Nurs Q.* 2001;23:14–25.
42. Andrews BT. Initial management of head injury. *Phys Med Rehabil Clin North Am.* 1992;3:249–258.
43. Maher L. A quick neurologic examination. *Patient Care.* 1999;1:19–33.
44. Davies PM. *Steps to Follow.* 2nd ed. New York, NY: Springer; 2000.
45. Howe T. Measuring muscle tone and movement. *Nurs Standard.* 1995;9: 25–29.
46. Hillegass EA, Sadowsky HS. *Essentials of Cardiopulmonary Physical Therapy.* Philadelphia, Pa: WB Saunders Co; 1994.
47. Block G, Liss C, Reines S, et al. Comparison of immediate release and controlled release carbidopa/levodopa in Parkinson's disease. A multicenter 5-year study. *Eur Neurol.* 1997;37(1):23–27.

48. Guide to Physical Therapist Practice. 2nd ed. *Physical Therapy.* 2001;81(1).
49. Greenberg MS. *Handbook of Neurosurgery.* 5th ed. New York, NY: Thieme Medical Publishers; 2001.
50. Somers MF. *Spinal Cord Injury Functional Rehabilitation.* East Norwalk, Conn: Appleton & Lange; 1992.
51. Kaye A. *Essential Neurosurgery.* New York, NY: Churchill Livingstone; 1991.
52. Sawauchi S, Marmarou A, Beaumont A, Signoretti S, Fukui S. Acute subdural hematoma associated with diffuse brain injury and hypoxemia in the rat: effect of surgical evacuation of the hematoma. *J Neurotrauma.* 2004;21(5):563–573.
53. Weigel R, Krauss JK, Schmiedek P. Concepts of neurosurgical management of chronic subdural hematoma: historical perspectives. *Brit J Neurosurg.* 2004;18(1):8–18.
54. Cousins MJ, Brazier D, Cook R. Intracranial hypotension caused by cervical cerebrospinal fluid leak: treatment with epidural blood patch. *Anesthia Analog.* 2004;98(6):1794–1797.
55. Behrman AL, Harkema SJ. Locomotor training after human spinal cord injury. *Phys Ther.* 2000;80(7):688–700.
56. DeVivo MJ. Causes and costs of spinal cord injury in the United States. *Spinal Cord.* 1997;35(12):809–813.
57. McCutcheon EP, Selassie AW, Gu JK, Pickelsimer EE. Acute traumatic spinal cord injury, 1993–2000. A population based assessment of methylprednisolone administration and hospitalization. *J Trauma.* 2004;56(5):1076–1083.
58. DeVivo MJ. Causes and costs of spinal cord injury in the United States. *J Spinal Cord Med.* 2002;25(4):335–338.
59. American Brain Tumor Association. Available at: http://www.abta.org/. Accessed on April 2, 2006.
60. Reis LG, Eisner MP, Kosary CL, et al, eds. *SEER Cancer Statistics Review, 1973– 1996.* Bethesda, Md: National Cancer Institute; 1999.
61. Wick R, Wade J, Rohrer D, O'Neil O. Use of decompressive craniectomy after severe head trauma. *AORN Journal.* 1999;69(3):517–529.
62. Wang JC, McDonough PW, Kanim LE, Endow KK, Delamarter RB. Increased fusion rates with cervical plating for three-level anterior cervical discectomy and fusion. *Spine.* 2001;26:643–646.
63. Beattie P. The relationship between symptoms and abnormal magnetic resonance images of lumbar intervertebral disks. *Phys Ther.* 1996;76:601–608.
64. Fritz JM, Delitto A, Welch WC, Erhard RE. Lumbar spinal stenosis: a review of current concepts in evaluation, management, and outcome measures. *Arch Phys Med Rehabil.* 1998;79:700–707.
65. Murdocke KR. Physical therapy in the neurologic intensive care unit. *Neurology Report.* 1994;16(3):17–24.
66. Brimioulle S, Moraine JJ, Norrenberg D, Kalin RJ. Effects of positioning and exercise on intracranial pressure in a neurosurgical intensive care unit. *Phys Ther.* 1997;77(12):1682–1689.
67. Cold GE, Holdgaard HO. Treatment of intracranial hypertension in acute injury with social reference to the role of hyperventiliation and sedation with barbiturates; a review. *Intensive Care World.* 1992;9:172–178.
68. Niskanen RO. The Oswestry Low Back Pain Disability Questionnaire. A two-year follow-up of spine surgery patients. *Scand J Surg.* 2002;91(2):208–211.
69. Anderson T, Christensen FB, Laursen M, et al. Smoking as a predictor of negative outcome in lumbar spinal fusion. *Spine.* 2001;26(23):2623–2628.
70. Goldstein B, Sanders JE, Benson E. Pressure ulcers in SCI: does tension stimulate wound healing? *Am J Phys Med Rehabil.* 1996;75:130–133.
71. Hill CI, Nixon CS, Ruemeier JL. Brain tumors. *Phys Ther.* 2002;82(5): 496–502.

72. Cancerconsultants.com oncology resource center. Available at: http://www. cancerconsultants.com. Accessed on April 2, 2006.
73. RadiologyInfo - the radiology information resource for patients. Available at: http://www.radiologyinfo.org. Accessed on April 2, 2006.
74. Herdman S. *Vestibular Rehabilitation*. Philadelphia, Pa: FA Davis Co; 1994.
75. El-Kashlan HK, Shepard NT, Arts HA, Telian SA. Disability from vestibular symptoms after acoustic neuroma resection. *American Journal of Otology*. 1998;19(1):104–111.

BIBLIOGRAPHY

Barbeau H, Visintin M. Optimal outcomes obtained with body weight support combined with treadmill training in stroke subjects. *Arch Phys Med Rehabil*. 2003;84(10):1458–1465.
Bergen JL, Toole T, Elliott RG III, et al. Aerobic exercise intervention improves aerobic capacity and movement initiation in Parkinson's disease patients. *Neuro Rehabil*. 2002;17(2): 161–168.
Broderick JP, Adams HP Jr, Barsan W, et al. Guidelines for the management of spontaneous intracerebral hemorrhage. *Stroke*. 1999;30:905–915.
Brown DA, Kautz SA. Increased workload enhances force output during pedaling exercise in persons with poststroke hemiplegia. *Stroke*. 1998;29(3):598–606.
Brown D, Kautz SA. Speed dependent reductions of force output in people with poststroke hemiparesis. *Phys Ther*. 1999;79(10):919–930.
Canning CG, Alison JA, Alllen NE, Groeller H. Parkinsons's disease: an investigation of exercise capapcity, respiratory function, and gait. *Arch Phys Med Rehabil*. 1997;78(2):199–207.
Charo J, Wolf E. Subluxation of the glenohumeral joint in hemiplegia. *Am J Phys Med*. 1971;50:139–143.
Craig CR, Stitzel RE. *Modern Pharmacology with Clinical Applications*. New York, NY: Little, Brown, and Co; 1997.
Deglin JH, Vallerand AH. *Davis's Drug Guide for Nurses*. 8th ed. Philadelphia, Pa: FA Davis Co; 2003.
Dombovy ML. Understanding stroke recovery and rehabilitation: current and emerging approaches. *Curr Neurol Neurosci Rep*. 2004;4(1):31–35.
Dromerick AW, Edwards DF, Hahn M. Does the application of constraint-induced movement therapy during acute rehabilitation reduce arm impairment after ischemic stroke? *Stroke*. 2000;31:2984–2988.
Ensrud ER, Krivickas LS. Acquired inflammatory demyelinating neuropathies. *Phys Med Rehabil Clin North Am*. 2001;12(2):321–334.
Goodman C, Boiussonnault W, Fuller KS. *Pathology: Implications for the Physical Therapist*. 2nd ed. Philadelphia, Pa: WB Saunders Co; 2003.
Hesse S, Bertelt C, Jahnke MT. et al. Treadmill training with partial body weight support compared with physiotherapy in nonambulatory hemiparetic patients. *Stroke*. 1995;26(6): 976–981.
Karch AM. *Lippincott's Nursing Drug Guide*. Springhouse, Pa: Lippincott Williams & Wilkins; 2004.
Maeshima S, Ueyoshi A, Osawa A, et al. Mobility and muscle strength contralateral to hemiplegia from stroke: benefit from self training with family support. *Am J Phys Med Rehabil*. 2003;82(6):456–462.
Marchese R, Diverio M, Zucchi F, Lettino C, Abbruzzese G. The role of sensory cues in the rehabilitation of parkinsonian patients: a comparison of two physical therapy protocols. *Movement Disorder*. 2000;15(5):879–883.

McLellan DL. Co-contraction and stretch reflexes in spasticity during treatment with baclofen. *Journal of Neurology, Neurosurgery, and Psychiatry.* 1977;40:30–38.

Moodie NB, Brisbin J, Morgan GAM. Subluxation of the glenohumeral joint in hemiplegia:evalution of supportive devices. *Physiotherapy Canada.* 1986;38(3):151–157.

Paollucci S, Antonucci G, Grasso MG. et al. Early versus delayed inpatient stroke rehabilitation: a matched comparison conducted in Italy. *Arch Phys Med and Rehabil.* 2000;81(6):695–700.

Ritter JM, Lewis LD, Mant TG. *Textbook of Clinical Pharmacology.* London, England: Edward Arnold Co; 1995

Rothstein JM, Roy SH, Wolf SL. *The Rehabilitation Specialist's Handbook.* Philadelphia, Pa: FA Davis Co; 1991.

Rowat AM. What do nurses and therapists think about the positioning of stroke patients? *Journal of Advanced Nursing.* 2001;34:795–803.

Rubinstein TC, Giladi N, Hausdorff JM. The power of cueing to circumvent dopamine deficits: a review of physical therapy treatment of gait disturbances in Parkinson's disease. *Movement Disorders.* 2002;17(6):1148–1160.

Schenkman ML, Clark K, Xie T, et al. Spinal movement and performance of a standing reach task in participants with and without Parkinson disease. *Phys Ther.* 2001;81(8):1400–1411.

Schrag A, Jahanshahi M, Quinn N. What contribuites to quality of life in patients with Aprkinsons's disease? *J Neuro, Neurosurg and Psych.* 2000;69(3):308–312.

Smithson F, Morris ME, Iansek R. Performance on clinical tests of balance in Parkinson's disease. *Phys Ther.* 1998;78(6):577–592.

Soeken KL. Selected CAM therapies for arthritis-related pain: the evidence from systematic reviews. *Clin J Pain.* 2004;20(1):13–18.

Tandberg E, Larsen JP, Aarsland D, Laake K, Cummings JL. Risk factors for depression in Parkinsons disease. *Arch Neuro* 1997;54(5):625–630.

Vuagnat H, Chantraine A. Shoulder pain in hemiplegia revisitied: contribution of functional electrical stimulation and other therapies. *J Rehabil Med.* 2003;35(2):49–54.

10

ENDOCRINE DISEASES AND DISORDERS

Christy F. Ehlers, PT, CWS
Daniel J. Malone, MPT, CCS

The endocrine system is a complex arrangement of glands that impact and regulate multiple body systems through the synthesis and secretion of hormones. Hormones can elicit local responses (paracrine or autocrine activity) or effect distal processes. The endocrine glands secrete their products directly into the circulatory system to communicate with their effector tissues and utilize the neurological and immune systems to further expand their capacity. The major glands include the hypothalamus, pituitary, thyroid, parathyroid, adrenals, islets of the pancreas, ovaries, and testes (Figure 10–1). This chapter will briefly review each gland, looking at the action(s) of its hormones, and discuss the impact of common diseases. Particular attention will be directed at diabetes mellitus (DM), the most common endocrine disease. Tables describing the general features of the gland and outlining major hormones are provided for quick reference. In addition, common signs and symptoms of endocrine disorders are provided. These tables can be used during patient/client management to determine a comprehensive examination and treatment plan for the patient/client.

HORMONES

Hormones are specialized blood-borne chemical substances that regulate and coordinate various biological functions. They are produced by the endocrine cells of various glands in response to distinct stimuli and exert their actions on specific target tissues. Initially, it was believed that hormones were only secreted by the endocrine glands. However, research has shown that many hormones are also secreted by other tissues (normal or abnormal) with resultant physiologic responses. Hormone cell structure can be an amine, peptide (protein), or steroid. This permits the hormones to bind to different cell receptors with high affinity and specificity. Peptides and amines, including the catecholamines and dopamine, bind to cell membrane receptors and initiate signaling cascades

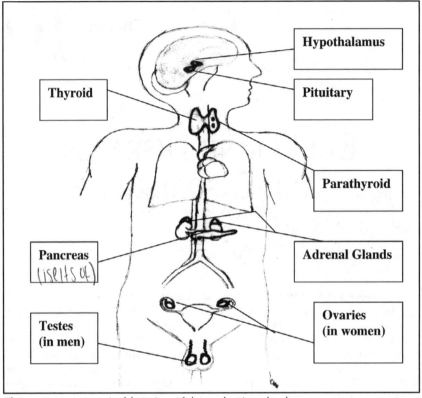

Figure 10–1. Anatomical location of the endocrine glands.

within the cell to initiate the desired responses. Steroids, which are synthesized from cholesterol, are able to penetrate the cell wall and bind to specific receptors in the cell nucleus influencing gene transcription to direct the physiologic responses.

Hormone secretion is regulated by the following:

- **Feedback mechanisms:** Chemical signals or other hormones are released into the blood resulting in hormone release or suppression. Responses can be positive (ie, high levels of a specific substance stimulate secretions and low levels suppress), negative (ie, high levels of substance suppress secretions and low levels stimulate), or complex when multiple structures and substances can stimulate or suppress the same hormone. An example of negative feedback is insulin and glucagon regulation. Insulin release is stimulated by high levels of circulating glucose, amino acids, and fats, and glucagon is depressed. As nutrients are taken up by cells, insulin secretion declines and glucagon release is enhanced.

- **Direct signaling** implies that endocrine glands are directly stimulated by other structures to secrete or suppress hormone secretion. An example is dehydration. Osmotic and pressure receptors in the heart, lung, brain, and

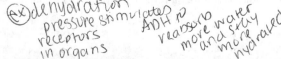

aorta signal the pituitary and hypothalamus to produce more antidiuretic hormone (ADH). ADH promotes enhanced renal reabsorption of water, maintaining fluid balance of the body.

- **Circadian rhythm:** Levels rise and fall predictably during a 24-hour period. Examples include cortisol and thyroid hormones. Cortisol levels rise early in the day, decline as the day progresses, and begin rising during sleep to peak levels upon awakening. Thyroid-stimulating hormone releases periodically throughout the day and, therefore, experiences little fluctuation.

- **Cycling:** Hormones are released at periodic times at greater than 24 hours, but it is unsure how this is controlled. Examples include luteinizing (LH) and follicle stimulating (FSH) hormones that control reproductive functions and vary to bring about the menstrual cycle.

The nervous and endocrine systems are mutually dependent on each other. Autonomic nerves control endocrine gland blood flow and hormone secretion, and hormones have a regulatory effect on nervous tissue.[1] Hormones can influence behavior and stress, and emotional states (eg, anxiety and fear) can influence hormone production. Dependent on the origin of secretion, substances can be hormones or neurotransmitters. For example, catecholamines are hormones secreted by the adrenal medulla and neurotransmitters when they are secreted by the post-synaptic cells of the sympathetic nervous system.

The immune and endocrine systems are also interrelated. Both systems use hormones and the nervous system as a means of communication allowing reciprocal regulation. Adversely, many endocrine disorders are caused by immune system dysfunction.

HYPOTHALAMUS

The **hypothalamus** is part of the diencephalon, surrounded by the cerebrum of the brain, and functions as a regulator of the autonomic nervous system and the majority of endocrine glands. The hypothalamus is described in Table 10–1. Neurotransmitters and hormones are used to carry out hypothalamic regulatory functions on body temperature, sexual behavior, appetite control, fluid balance, levels of arousal or wakefulness, and emotional expression. The hypothalamus primarily impacts the pituitary gland. Hypothalamic hormones may be stored in the pituitary (ADH/oxytocin) or act as stimulators or inhibitors of pituitary hormones. Table 10–2 lists the major hypothalamic secretions and how each functions.

PITUITARY GLAND

The **pituitary gland**, also termed the **hypophysis**, is surrounded by a bony structure, the sella turcica, and is divided into two parts. The anterior lobe, which is approximately 80% of the structure's weight, connects to the hypothalamus by the infundibular or pituitary stalk. Through this stalk runs a vein called the hypophyseal portal vascular system. The hypothalamus secretes its

---

Table 10–1
HYPOTHALAMUS AT A GLANCE

Location	• Below the thalamus and cerebral hemisphere • Anterior and superior to the pituitary gland • Behind the optic chiasm and between the optic tracts
Special features	• Connects to the pituitary gland by the infundibular or pituitary stalk • Communication with the anterior lobe is by hormone and chemical release • Communication with the posterior lobe is via neurotransmission • Utilizes the posterior lobe for storage of oxytocin and ADH also termed vasopressin • Regulates body temperature, sweating, appetite, thirst, gastrointestional secretion and motility, BP, sleep, sexual behavior, defensive reactions (eg, rage and fear), and body rhythms
Produces / secretes	• Oxytocin and ADH (also termed vasopressin) (stored in posterior pituitary) Releasing Hormones: • Corticotropin releasing hormone (CRH) • Thyrotropin releasing hormone (TRH) • Growth hormone (GH) releasing factor or somatotropin releasing hormone • Gonadotropin releasing hormone • Prolactin releasing factor Inhibiting Hormone: • Prolactin release inhibiting factor (PIF) • Somatostatin or GH inhibiting hormone
Functions	• Integrates communication between the endocrine and nervous system in conjunction with the pituitary gland • Mediates central nervous system (CNS) control input with hypothalamic hormones and neurotransmitters • Influences fluid and electrolyte balance and cell metabolism by hormone production and hormone releasing hormones
Major target	Pituitary gland

---

substances and hormones into the hypophyseal portal system for direct delivery to the pituitary. The posterior lobe, which is approximately 20% of the gland's total weight, is considered an extension of the hypothalamus. The posterior lobe consists of unmyelinated nerve fibers and terminals of axons that provide transport and storage for ADH, also termed vasopressin, and oxytocin, produced by the hypothalamus. It is called the master gland because it produces six hormones and stores two additional ones, although pituitary hormone secretion is regulated by hypothalamic function. The pituitary controls most of the endocrine

Table 10–2

HYPOTHALAMIC HORMONES AND CHEMICAL SUBSTANCES

Hormone/ Chemical Substance	Cell Structure	Target Area	Function/Action
CRH	Peptide	Anterior pituitary	• Stimulates release of adrenocorticotropin hormone (ATCH)
TRH	Peptide	Anterior pituitary	• Stimulates the release of thyrotropin (TSH) and prolactin • Can stimulate the release of GH
GH releasing factor or somatotropin releasing hormone	Peptide	Anterior pituitary	• Stimulates the release of GH
Gonadotropin releasing hormone	Peptide	Anterior pituitary	• Stimulate the release of LH and FSH
Prolactin releasing factor	Peptide	Anterior pituitary	• Stimulates the release of prolactin
PIF	Peptide	Anterior pituitary	• Suppresses the release of prolactin
GH inhibiting hormone or somatostatin	Peptide	Anterior pituitary	• Suppresses the release of GH
Dopamine	Amine	Anterior pituitary	• Prolactin inhibition

system, but it targets three specific glands: the reproductive organs (ovaries and testes), adrenal cortex, and thyroid. Specific details regarding pituitary gland functions are found in Table 10–3. Table 10–4 describes the major hormones and their impact on the body.

Disease states that occur in the hypothalamus and the pituitary are difficult to discuss separately because the two glands are interrelated. Damage to the hypothalamus impairs stimulating or inhibiting factors from reaching the pituitary, altering pituitary hormonal function. Both glands will be examined together to discuss the impact of disease.

Table 10–3
PITUITARY AT A GLANCE

Location	• Base of the brain in the sella turcica ("Turkish saddle") above the sphenoid bone
Special features	• Referred to as the "master gland" • Anterior and posterior lobes
Function	• Controls the functions of most of the other endocrine glands • Anterior lobe primarily functions to control metabolism, reproductive organ growth, body growth, and secretion of steroid hormones • Posterior lobe functions for reproduction (milk secretion/uterine contraction) and fluid balance (reabsorption of Na^+ and water by kidneys)
Secretes	• GH • Thyroid stimulating hormone (TSH) • Adrenocorticotropic hormone (ACTH) • Prolactin • FSH • LH • ADH or vasopressin • Oxytocin
Major targets	• Reproductive organs (ovaries and testes), thyroid, adrenal glands and kidneys

Most common disease states involving the hypothalamus and pituitary are tumors, elevated fluid and pressure within the brain (as seen in high blood pressure (BP) and traumatic head injuries), inflammatory diseases, infections, surgical excision of either gland (complete or partial), autoimmune disease, and ischemia (from blood clots, severe bleeding, or anemia). Hypopituitarism, deficient hormone production, can be primary (due to direct damage to the pituitary) or secondary (due to damage to the hypothalamus or to the adjoining pituitary stalk). Hyperpituitarism results in multiple problems dependent on the hormone. Specific signs and symptoms related to malproduction of pituitary hormones can be found in Table 10–5. Excessive production of growth hormone (GH) in children causes gigantism and acromegaly in adults. Excessive production of prolactin occurs with damage to the hypothalamus or pituitary stalk due to loss of hypothalamic suppression. Excessive prolactin causes galactorrhea (lactation in men or women who are not breastfeeding or recent postpartum), hypogonadism, and amenorrhea (lack of menstrual cycles in females). LH or FSH are secreted in both males and females but impact different organs (ovaries in women and testes in men) producing different end products (estrogen and progesterone in women and testosterone in men). Overproduction of LH and FSH is usually benign, but underproduction can be pathologic (see Table 10–5).

Table 10–4

PITUITARY HORMONES AND THEIR FUNCTIONS

Hormone	Cell Structure	Target Areas	Function/Action
GH ↳growth hormone	Peptide	Muscles and bones	• Regulates growth • Influences intermediary metabolism
Prolactin	Peptide	Mammary glands	• Lactation
LH ↳Luteinizing hormone ↓ glycoprotein	Peptide	Gonads (ovaries and testes)	• Reproductive control • Regulates ovarian and testicular function • Controls testosterone production in males • Stimulates production of androgen, which converts to estrogen and progesterone in females
FSH ↳Follical stimulating hormone ↓ glycoprotein	Peptide	Gonads (ovaries and testes)	• Reproductive control in males and females • Helps stimulate the production of sperm in males • Stimulates maturation of the ovarian follicles in females
TSH or thyrotropin	Peptide	Thyroid	• Regulates thyroid function
ATCH	Peptide	Adrenal cortex	• Controls glucocorticoid function of the adrenal cortex
ADH or vasopressin	Peptide	Kidney	• Controls water conservation by the kidneys • Potent vasoconstrictor • Potentiates the effect of corticotropin releasing hormone • Controls BP along with aldosterone
Oxytocin	Peptide	Uterus and mammary glands	• Stimulates milk ejection or "let down" for mammary glands • Contraction of smooth uterine muscle • Possibly stimulates prolactin release • Establish maternal behavior

<u>Table 10–5</u>

SIGNS AND SYMPTOMS OF HYPOTHALAMIC AND PITUITARY DYSFUNCTION

Hormone	Overproduction	Underproduction
GH	• Gigantism (children) • Acromegaly (adults) • Bony and soft tissue overgrowth • Enlarged hands, feet, and head • Enlarged tongue • Laryngeal hypertrophy • Sinus enlargement • Muscle weakness • Amenorrhea in women • Goiter	• Few symptoms in adults • Slow growth or Dwarfism (in children)

Prolactin	• Amenorrhea in women
	• Galactorrhea
	• Hypogonadism
	  Decreased sex drive
	  Decreased sperm production (men)
	  Impotence
	• Breast enlargement in women
	• Decreased fertility in women
		• Fatigue
		• Loss of pubic and axillary hair
		• Inability to produce breast milk

LH	• Essentially no biological effect	• Hypogonadism
		  Decreased sex drive
		  Decreased sperm production (men)
		  Impotence
		• Amenorrhea in women

FSH	• Essentially no biological effect	• Hypogonadism
		  Decreased sex drive
		  Decreased sperm production (men)
		  Impotence
		• Amenorrhea in women

(continued)

Table 10–5   (continued)

SIGNS AND SYMPTOMS OF HYPOTHALAMIC AND PITUITARY DYSFUNCTION

Hormone	Overproduction	Underproduction
TSH or Thyrotropin	• See Thyroid Gland Dysfunction	• See Thyroid Gland Dysfunction
ATCH	• See Adrenal Gland Dysfunction	• See Adrenal Gland Dysfunction
ADH or Vasopressin	• Increased water retention	• Diabetes insipidus Excessive dilute urine Polydipsia (excessive thirst)
Oxytocin		• Decreased milk ejection • Decreased uterine contraction during birth

Overproduction of ADH is one cause of diabetes insipidus (DI). DI is either a lack of ADH secretion or impaired renal responsiveness to ADH. DI creates excessive thirst and dilutes urine production potentially leading to dehydration, hypotension, and shock. ADH may be released by some lung cancers allowing ADH to be used as a marker for progress or regression of the tumor.

Diagnostic testing for hypothalamus and pituitary dysfunction includes blood serum levels for the specific hormone in conjunction with stimulation or suppression tests for more accurate descriptions. Varied patterns of hormone release add complexity to diagnosis. Computerized tomography (CT) and magnetic resonance imaging (MRI) scans provide anatomic descriptions of possible gland damage or disease.

THYROID GLAND

The **thyroid gland** possesses one of the most widespread effects of all the glands as described in Table 10–6. **Thyroid hormone (TH)** strongly influences growth, development, and metabolism. Its production is dependent on the dietary intake and circulating concentrations of iodine to convert TH into a usable form by the tissues. The kidney metabolizes TH, the iodine is cleaved from the hormone and returned to the thyroid gland. TH production begins in the hypothalamus with release of **thyroid releasing hormone (TRH)**. TRH travels to the anterior pituitary activating release of thyroid stimulating hormone (TSH). TSH travels to the thyroid gland as is illustrated in Figure 10–2. This action is termed the hypothalamus-pituitary-thyroid axis. TH is regulated by negative feedback. High levels of TH decrease pituitary secretion of TSH. Low concentrations of TH increase pituitary secretion of TSH. ($\uparrow$ TH = $\downarrow$ TSH and $\downarrow$ TH = $\uparrow$ TSH). Thyroid stimulation results in secretion of both **thyroxine** (T4)

Table 10–6
THYROID AT A GLANCE

Location	The "butterfly"-shaped thyroid consists of two lateral lobes connected by a narrow section called the isthmus and is located in the neck, in close approximation to the first part of the trachea, just below the larynx
Special features	• Right lobe is larger and more vascular than the left • The thyroid gland needs iodine to produce thyroid hormones • Innervated by the adrenergic nervous system via the cervical ganglia and by the cholinergic nervous system via the vagus nerve • Blood supply is greater than the kidney • Able to store large amounts of hormone, up to 30-day supply • Stimulated by the hypothalamus-pituitary-thyroid axis
Function	• Secretes thyroid hormones that control the body's chemical functions by influencing protein production and oxygen consumption. Thyroidhormones increase the basal metabolic rate.
Secretes	Thyroxine (T4) Thriiodothyronine (T3) Thyrocalcitonin (calcitonin)
Major target	All major body systems (see Tables 10–7 and 10–8)

*negative feedback system

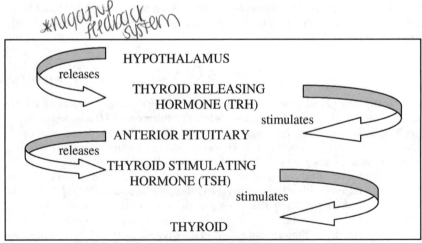

Figure 10–2. Hypothalamus-pituitary-thyroid axis.

Table 10–7

MAJOR THYROID HORMONES AND THEIR FUNCTIONS

Hormone	Cell Structure	Target Areas	Function/Action
T4	Peptide	All body tissues	• Energy metabolism • Growth and development • Metabolism speed • Control of body temperature • Maturation
T3	Peptide	All body tissues	• Energy metabolism • Growth and development • Metabolism speed • Control of body temperature • Maturation
Thyrocalcitonin (Calcitonin)	Peptide	Plasma	• Regulation of calcium and phosphate blood levels • Stimulation of bone demineralization

[handwritten annotations: "converts into" near T4; "accounts for 80%. in body hormone to extend life & metabolic state" near T3; "↓ calcium homeostasis"; "released by ↑ serum calc. levels suppressed by ↓ serum levels"]

and **triiodothyronine** (T3). Specific information on thyroid hormones can be found in Table 10–7. T4 has few effects on the body's metabolism; however, T4 can be converted to T3. T4 conversion accounts for approximately 80% of T3 in the body. T4 binding and conversion help extend the life of the hormone and maintain a metabolic steady state. T4 half-life in the bloodstream is 6.7 days; T3 half-life is about 30 hours. Only 0.04% of T4 and 0.4% of T3 are "free" in the bloodstream at any given time.[2] Adequate levels of thyroid hormone are dependent on proper functioning of the hypothalamus-pituitary-thyroid axis and proper binding and releasing of T3 and T4 to plasma proteins. **Calcitonin**, also secreted by the thyroid gland, is involved in calcium homeostasis. Calcitonin is released by increased serum calcium levels and suppressed by decreased serum calcium levels.

Thyroid function is altered by multiple factors such as gender and sex hormones, pregnancy, age, glucocorticoids, environmental temperatures, nutritional state (starvation or overeating), and nonthyroid illness (cirrhosis and chronic renal failure).[1] Signs and symptoms of hyper- and hypothyroidism can be found in Table 10–8. **Hyperthyroidism**, overproduction of thyroid hormone, is associated with Grave's disease (an immune disease), toxic nodular goiter, and secondary hyperthyroidism. Thyroid storm, an acute disproportionate production of TH, is caused by untreated or inadequately treated hyperthyroidism. The individual will develop fever, extreme weakness, restlessness, mood swings, confusion, altered mental status, and eventually coma. Thyroid storm is life threatening

Table 10–8

SIGNS AND SYMPTOMS OF THYROID DYSFUNCTION

System Affected	Hyperthyroidism (Overproduction of Thyroid Hormone)	Hypothyroidism (Underproduction of Thyroid Hormone)
Cardiovascular	• Increased heart rate (HR), palpitations • Increased cardiac output • Systolic HTN • Cardiac hypertrophy • Angina • Dyspnea on mild exercise • Increased respiratory rate (RR)	• Slowed HR • Decreased cardiac output • Varied changes in BP • Tendency to develop congestive heart failure, angina, and myocardial infarction • Dyspnea with decreased breathing capacity
Neurological	• Shakiness and tremors • Nervousness • Lability of mood • Restlessness • Personality changes of irritability and agitation • Confusion • Rapid speech	• Slowed, slurred speech • Slow movements • Decreased hearing • Carpel tunnel syndrome • Paresthesias • Confusion, forgetfulness • Depression • Lethargy • Anxiety • Dementia • Hoarse voice
Gastrointestinal	• Frequent bowel movements with diarrhea • Weight loss with increased appetite • Splenomegaly	• Constipation • Distended abdomen • Weight gain with decreased appetite
Musculoskeletal	• Weakness with proximal muscle wasting	• Muscle aches and pains
Reproductive	• Decreased libido • Impotence in men • Menstrual irregularities	• Infertility • Decreased libido • Prolonged menstrual periods
General appearance	• Swollen, reddened, bulging eyes • Hair loss • Thin, brittle nails detached from beds	• Drooping eyelids • Loss of eyebrows • Sparse, course, dry hair • Dry, scaly, thick coarse skin; raised and thickened over shins

(continued)

Table 10–8 (continued)

SIGNS AND SYMPTOMS OF THYROID DYSFUNCTION

System Affected	Hyperthyroidism (Overproduction of Thyroid Hormone)	Hypothyroidism (Underproduction of Thyroid Hormone)
General appearance	• Raised, thickened skin over shins • Premature graying • Palmar erythema • Moist warm skin • Goiter	• Decreased sweating • Puffy face
Other	• Intolerance to heat • Increased basal temperature • Increased sensitivity to stimulant drugs • Fatigue, exhaustion • Insomnia • Eyes with increased sensitivity to light	• Intolerance to cold • Increased susceptibility to infections • Anemia • Enlarged coarse tongue

and requires immediate medical attention.[3] **Hypothyroidism** (underproduction of thyroid hormone) is associated with three types of thyroiditis:

1. Hashimoto's thyroiditis (autoimmune thyroiditis)
2. Subacute granulomatous thyroiditis (usually occurs after viral illness)
3. Silent lymphocytic thyroiditis (occurs most often in women after childbirth)

and thyroid cancers including papillary, follicular, anaplastic, and medullary cancer. Hypothyroidism can also be caused from a deficiency in dietary iodine. Euthyroid sick syndrome occurs when the thyroid is functioning normally, but T4 does not convert to T3 and may result from malnutrition, illness, or surgery. Euthyroid sick syndrome typically resolves with resolution of the initiating event.

Thyroid function can be evaluated by blood tests measuring TSH (TSH is high when the thyroid is underactive and low when it is overactive) and free T4 and may be performed in conjunction with stimulation agents. Ultrasound and nuclear imaging determine the presence of anatomic anomalies. Nuclear imaging using radioactive iodine or technetium can demonstrate deficiencies in iodine uptake and hormone production.

PARATHYROID

The **parathyroid glands** are four small glands located behind the thyroid that regulate calcium and phosphate metabolism through the production and

Table 10–9
PARATHYROID AT A GLANCE

Location	Posterior surface of the thyroid gland. Sometimes it is in the mediastinum within the thyroid gland or behind the esophagus.
Special features	Usually there are two pairs of glands. There may be as few as three or as many as six.
Functions	• Calcium and phosphate homeostasis. • Production and secretion of PTH that stimulates the body to reserve its serum calcium by inhibiting formation of bone, equalizing calcium and phosphate levels and increasing calcium absorption in the intestinal mucosa.
Secretes	PTH
Major targets	Bone, kidney, and intestinal mucosa

Table 10–10
MAJOR PARATHYROID HORMONE

Hormone	Cell Structure	Target Area	Function/Action
PTH	Peptide	Bone, kidney, and intestinal mucosa	• Regulates calcium and phosphate metabolism • Regulates bone metabolism. • Maintains serum/calcium concentration • Regulates Vitamin D synthesis

secretion of **parathyroid hormone (PTH)**. The parathyroid gland is described in Tables 10–9 and 10–10. Parathyroid regulation is a negative feedback loop and responds to serum calcium levels. The parathyroid gland is free of hypothalamic and pituitary control. Increased serum calcium inhibits PTH secretion, and decreased serum calcium stimulates PTH secretion. PTH has three main targets: bone, kidney, and intestinal mucosa. PTH stimulates osteoclasts and inhibits osteoblasts in bone, resulting in enhanced serum calcium levels. PTH stimulates renal reabsorption of calcium and increases the excretion of phosphate to provide equilibration of calcium to phosphate by limiting renal losses of calcium. In the intestinal mucosa, PTH stimulates Vitamin D, which increases calcium absorption in the small intestine. PTH and calcitonin are antagonistic allowing for precise maintenance of calcium homeostasis. As noted in Chapter 2, calcium is vital for bone formation, cell division and growth, blood coagulation, muscle

Table 10–11

CLINICAL SIGNS AND SYMPTOMS OF PARATHYROID DYSFUNCTION

Hyperparathyroidism	*Hypoparathyroidism*
Gastrointestinal:	**Neurological:**
Constipation	Paresthetias seizures
Indigestion, nausea, vomiting	Organic brain syndrome
Peptic ulcers	Cataracts
Pancreatitis	Calcification of basal ganglia
Anorexia	Tetany
Kidney:	**Cardiac:**
Renal Stones	Prolonged QT interval
Nephrocalcinosis	Congestive heart failure
Polyuria (increased urine)	**Bone:**
Polydipsia (increased thirst)	Shortened digits, especially fourth and
Uremia	fifth fingers
Bones:	**Reproductive:**
Osteitis fibrosa with bone cysts, osteo-	Infertility in males
clastomas, subperiosteal resorption	Oligomenorrhea in females
Radiologic osteoporosis	**Skin:**
Osteomalacia or rickets	Dry and flaky
Arthritis	Brittle nails
Mental:	
Lethargy, fatigue	
Depression	
Memory loss	
Psychotic paranoia	
Confusion, stupor, coma	
Other:	
Proximal muscle weakness	
Itching	

contraction, and release of neurotransmitters. Profound hypoparathyroidism and resultant hypocalcemia can lead to tetany and death.

Disease states affecting the parathyroid gland are **hyperparathyroidism** (causing hypercalcemia) and **hypoparathyroidism** (causing hypocalcemia). Primary causes of hyperparathyroidism are adenomas, carcinomas, and hereditary diseases. Secondary causes are related to diseases that stimulate excessive secretion of PTH including renal disease and nutrition deficiencies of calcium or Vitamin D. Clinical signs and symptoms of parathyroid dysfunction are noted in Table 10–11.

Diagnostic testing is accomplished with PTH immunoassay blood studies. These studies may distinguish the major cause of hyper- or hypocalcemia.

Table 10–12
ADRENAL GLANDS AT A GLANCE

Location	• Superior or medial to the upper poles of the kidneys
Special features	• Composed of the adrenal cortex and adrenal medulla • Influenced by the hypothalamic-pituitary and autonomic nervous systems
Function	• Impacts multiple organ systems • Metabolic (carbohydrate, protein, fat metabolism) • Cardiovascular (HR, BP) • Renal (salt and potassium levels)
Secretes	• Aldosterone (mineralocorticoid) • Cortisol (glucocorticoid) • Catecholemones (epinephrine and norepinephrine and dopamine) • Androgens
Major targets	• Kidney, gastrointestinal, cardiovascular, and reproductive organs

---

Additionally, evaluation of nutritional history emphasizing intake of vitamin D and calcium is an important aspect of diagnosis.[4]

ADRENAL GLANDS

The matched **adrenal glands** sit atop the kidneys and are detailed in Table 10–12. Each gland is composed of an outer cortex surrounding the inner medulla. The cortex is separated into three zones producing the glucocorticoids (cortisol, corticosterone), mineralocorticoids (aldosterone), and androgens: Zona glomerulosa (produces aldosterone), Zona fasiculata (produces cortisol and androgens), and Zona reticularis (produces cortisol and androgens). Zona fasiculata and reticularis are regulated by adrenocorticotropin hormone (ACTH). Hormones excreted by the adrenal cortex respond to different stimuli. Aldosterone is regulated by serum concentrations of potassium ions (increased serum potassium elevates aldosterone) and angiotensin II. Corticotropin releasing hormone (CRH) from the hypothalamus stimulates the secretion of ACTH from the anterior pituitary gland regulating androgens and glucocorticoid production.

The adrenal medulla consists of clumps of chromaffin cells that can be considered modified sympathetic ganglia synthesizing and storing the catecholamines epinephrine, norepinephrine, and dopamine. Sympathetic nervous system stimulation releases the catecholamines into the bloodstream. Like other hormones, catecholamines exert their effects by binding to specific receptors and activating signaling pathways in their target cells.[2] The cellular responses associated with catecholamines depend upon the receptors activated (eg, the alpha [α] and beta [β] receptors). Specific hormone targets and functions are outlined in Table 10–13.

<u>Table 10–13</u>

MAJOR ADRENAL HORMONES AND THEIR FUNCTIONS

Hormone	Cell Structure	Target Area	Function/Action
Aldosterone (mineralocorticoid)	Steroid	Kidney	• Regulates sodium and potassium levels by promoting renal sodium conservation and potassium secretion • Controls BP by maintenance of extracellular volume
Cortisol (glucocorticoid)	Steroid	Gastrointestinal	• Affects excretion of digestive enzymes • Catabolic effect on cellular proteins • Regulates carbohydrate, fat, and protein metabolism • Maintenance of normal excitability of the myocardium and catecholamine action • Anti-inflammatory agent • Decreases capillary permeability • Maintenance of emotional well-being
Androgen	Steroid	Testes and ovaries	• Increase masculinization, axillary and pubic hairs in females and pubic hair in males
Catecholamines (epinephrine and norepinephrine)	Amine	Cardiovascular and metabolic system	• Stress response (ie, fight or flight) • Increase rate and force of cardiac contraction • Constricts blood vessels • Dilates airways/bronchioles • Increases metabolic rate • Blocks insulin secretion/stimulates glucagon release • Activates glycogen breakdown (glycogenolysis)

[handwritten annotation: Stimulated by potassium ions serum concentration and angiotensin II]

Disease states involve over- and underproduction of the various hormones that the adrenal glands secrete. A deficiency of corticosteroids causes **Addison's disease**, while corticosteroid overproduction or overexposure can result in **Cushing's syndrome**. Excessive amounts of androgen can cause virilization (exaggerated masculine features in men and women). Hyperaldosteronism is a condition that affects the blood levels of sodium, potassium, bicarbonate, and chloride when aldosterone is elevated above normal. Pheochromocytoma is a tumor that arises from the adrenal glands chromaffin cells and causes an overproduction of catecholamines.[3] Specific signs and symptoms for each of these conditions can be found in Table 10–14.

Diagnostic testing is done with blood and urine samples depending on the suspect hormone. CT or MRI scans can help discover any physical abnormalities or growths, but some situations may require exploratory surgery to determine the problem.

REPRODUCTIVE SYSTEM (OVARIES AND TESTES)

The endocrine glands of the reproductive system are the ovaries or testes, also termed the gonads. This system is mainly regulated by the gonadotrophins (LH and FSH), released from the anterior pituitary and the androgens (testosterone, progesterone, estrogens) from the ovaries and testes. Gonadotrophin release is regulated by the hypothalamic delivery of GnRH. LH and FSH are glycoproteins that stimulate the production of the steroid-based androgens. In men, testosterone is synthesized in the Leydig's cells of the testes. In women, LH and FSH stimulate maturation of the ovarian follicles containing the oocyte producing estradiol. The corpus luteum formed from the evacuated follicle is a transient endocrine structure. The corpus luteum primarily secretes progesterone and is essential during the first trimester of pregnancy. LH and FSH secretions follow a cycling rhythm to bring about the menstrual cycle. Specific functions of the gonadotrophic hormones are outlined in Table 10–15.

Disease states in the gonads will interfere with puberty and normal growth and development in children. In adults, problems often lead to infertility.

Much of the diagnostic testing of the gonad system can be obtained through physical examination and serum levels of the specific hormone. Reproductive hormones are typically measured repeatedly due to the cyclic rise and falls.

PANCREAS

The **pancreas** is located within the left upper abdominal quadrant, and performs both endocrine and exocrine functions. The exocrine portion secretes digestive enzymes while the endocrine portion participates in glucose, fat, and protein homeostasis. The islets of Langerhans are responsible for the endocrine functions as outlined in Table 10–16. The islets contain four cell types, and each is responsible for secreting different hormones. The alpha cells secrete glucagon, beta cells secrete insulin, delta cells secrete somatostatin, and the gamma cells are responsible for gastrin. Elevated levels of blood glucose are the primary stimulus for insulin release and result in enhanced cellular uptake of glucose. Insulin

Table 10-14

SIGNS AND SYMPTOMS IN ADRENAL HORMONAL DYSFUNCTION

Hormone	Overproduction	Underproduction
Androgen	**Eg, Adrenogenital Syndrome** • Hairiness of the face and body • Baldness • Acne • Deepening of the voice/ increased muscularity • Increased sex drive • In women, uterus shrinking, clitoris enlarges, breasts shrink, amenorrhea —irregular periods	
Aldosterone (mineralocorti-coid)	**Hyperaldosteronism** • Weakness • Tingling muscle spasms • Paralysis • Polydipsia (increased thirst) • Increased urination	**Hypoaldosteronism** • Hypotension • Cardiac failure • Low blood glucose levels • Fatigue • Decreased tolerance to stress
Cortisol (glucocorticoid)	**Eg, Cushing's Syndrome** • Altered distribution of body fat • Large round face ("moon facies") • Obesity • Increased fat of torso/ "Buffalo hump" • Muscle wasting/ weakness • Thinned skin • Increased bruising • Poor wound healing • Increased BP • Osteoporosis • Decreased resistance to infection • Diabetes • Kidney stones	**Eg, Addison's Disease** • Weak, tired, dizzy on standing • Skin darkens overall • Black freckles over face and shoulders • Lethargy • Weight loss • Dehydration • Loss of appetite • Muscle aches • Nausea, vomiting, and diarrhea • Decreased blood glucose levels • <u>Untreated</u>: Profound weakness, extremely low BP, kidney failure, shock

(continued)

Table 10–14 (continued)
SIGNS AND SYMPTOMS IN ADRENAL HORMONAL DYSFUNCTION

Hormone	Overproduction	Underproduction
Castecholamines (epinephrine and norepinephrine)	• High BP • Fast, pounding HR • Excessive sweating • Lightheaded on standing • Increased RR • Severe headaches • Nausea and vomiting • Visual disturbances • Tingling fingers • Cold and clammy skin • Chest and stomach pain	

Table 10–15
MAJOR HORMONES OF THE REPRODUCTIVE SYSTEM

Hormone	Cell Structure	Target Area	Function/Action
Testosterone	Steroid	Pituitary	• Regulation of gonadotropic secretions • Spermatogenesis • Maintains muscle mass and bone tissue in the adult male
Estrogen	Steroid	Uterus, mammary glands	• Affects uterine growth • Causes thickening of the vaginal mucosa • Thinning of cervical mucus • Develops ductile system of breasts • Alter lipid profiles and exert vascular effects to help prevent CVD
Progesterone	Steroid	Uterus, mammary glands	• Induction of secretory activity in the endometrium preparing for egg implant in the uterus • Inhibits uterine contraction • Increases viscosity of cervical mucus • Glandular development of breasts • Increases basal body temperature

Table 10–16

PANCREAS AT A GLANCE

Location	• In the abdomen, behind the stomach, and anterior to the first and second lumbar vertebrae
Special features	• Performs both endocrine (hormones) and exocrine (digestive) functions • Attached to duodenum by the pancreatic ducts • Islets of Langerhans are discrete clusters of cells scattered throughout the pancreas • Linked to autonomic nervous system
Functions	• Glucose homeostasis • Secreting its hormones into the bloodstream that diffuse to neighboring and distal cells to exert its actions
Produces/secretes	• Insulin • Glucagon • Somatostatin
Major target	• Liver, duodenum, and all major body systems

Insulin stores glycogen (from glucose) = ↑ aa transport across hepatic, muscle, and adipose tissue

stimulates the liver and skeletal muscle to store glucose in the form of glycogen and increases amino acids transport across hepatic, muscle, and adipose tissues. Additionally, insulin stimulates protein and fatty acid (lipogenesis) synthesis in the liver and adipose tissues. Blood glucose is a readily available energy source, but without insulin, a number of the body's cells are unable to absorb glucose. These cells will principally use fatty acids as an alternative energy source. The brain, however, does not require insulin for glucose uptake but solely relies upon blood glucose for metabolism. The CNS is extremely sensitive to deficient circulating blood glucose levels.

Insulin ↑ building or making of protein and fatty acid (lipogenesis) in liver & fat tissue

Glucagon is a catabolic hormone and functions in opposition to insulin to maintain a euglycemic (normal) state. Low blood glucose levels stimulate the secretion of glucagon from the pancreas. Glucagon augments the breakdown of glycogen (glycogenolysis) and amino acids resulting in glucose formation (gluconeogenesis). The major hormones secreted by the pancreas and their actions are summarized in Table 10–17. *Glucagon can form glucose w/ breakdown of glucogen & a.a.*

The most common pancreatic disease is DM. However, the acute care therapist may encounter other hormonal abnormalities of pancreatic origin. Hyperinsulinemia is regularly caused by an insulin-secreting tumor (insulinoma) or an overdose of insulin. Blood glucose levels drop precipitously leading to shock. Hypoglycemia, or low blood glucose, develops when blood glucose levels fall resulting from too much insulin secretion, too high a dose of insulin, or meals not taken in a timely manner after an insulin dose. This will be covered further in the section on diabetes. Glucagon deficiencies or excess are rare and typically develop from cancers of the alpha cells called glucagonomas.

Diagnostic testing for abnormalities of the pancreas includes blood sampling to determine specific levels of hormones or blood glucose. CT and MRI are

Table 10–17

MAJOR HORMONES OF THE PANCREAS

Hormone	Cell Structure	Target Area	Function/Action
Glucagon	Peptide	Liver	• Enhances adipose tissue lipolysis • Raises blood glucose levels • Stimulates hepatic glycogenolysis and gluconeogenesis • Raises serum glucose levels
Insulin	Peptide	All body systems	• Promotes cellular uptake and storage of ingested carbohydrates (glucose), fats, and amino acids • Reduces serum glucose levels
Somatostatin	Peptide	Pancreas	• Inhibition of insulin and glucagon

performed to identify abnormal growth or lesions. Specific testing for diabetes is discussed later in this chapter and in Chapter 2.

DIABETES MELLITUS

DM is one of the most common endocrine diseases. DM results in impaired carbohydrate metabolism because of deficient insulin secretion or increased insulin resistance. There are multiple types of DM, but all develop similar complications as a result of the disease. Classifications are type 1, type 2, and gestational DM (usually resolves after delivery of the baby). Pancreatic disease, hormonal abnormalities, drug or chemical side effects, and genetic syndromes can also precipitate DM. There are many individuals with impaired glucose metabolism, but have yet to develop the signs and symptoms of DM. Type 1 and type 2 are the more common forms of DM.

Type 1 DM, also termed insulin-dependent or juvenile diabetes, accounts for approximately 5% of the DM population. It is theorized to be an autoimmune reaction triggered by an environmental factor such as a virus or nutritional deficiency.[5] The pancreatic beta cells of the islets of Langerhans are destroyed and insulin production is substantially reduced or nonexistent. Type 1 DM onset is before the age of 30 and progresses rapidly. Clinical features of an acute diabetic exacerbation include metabolic acidosis, increased appetite (**polyphagia**) with weight loss, fatigue, frequent urination (**polyuria**), excessive thirst (**polydipsia**), dehydration, and electrolyte imbalances. Severe dehydration can lead to mental confusion, drowsiness, seizures, and eventually coma.

Missed injections or poor glucose control can lead to **diabetic ketoacidosis**. In ketoacidosis, fatty acids and proteins are the predominate fuel source resulting in enhanced ketone formation. Normally, ketones are produced in small quantities and are completely metabolized by extra-hepatic tissues so negligible amounts enter the blood or urine. However, when carbohydrate metabolism is disturbed and glucose can no longer be utilized as a fuel substrate, ketone formation increases and excess ketones enter the blood, **ketonemia**, and urine, **ketonuria**, leading to ketoacidosis.

Type 2 DM is also referred to as adult onset or non-insulin dependent DM (NIDDM), although individuals may require exogenous insulin as the disease progresses. Type 2 DM is the more common form of DM and affects 8.6% of people age 20 or older and 20.1% of people age 65 or older.[5] Type 2 DM has been found in children but usually occurs after the age of 30. Obesity is an important risk factor for type 2 DM. Race and ethnic backgrounds have also shown patterns in prevalence supporting the theory that type 2 DM is hereditary. American Indians and Alaskan Natives account for 15.1%, 10.2% of Hispanic/ Latino Americans, 13% of non-Hispanic blacks, and 7.8% of non-Hispanic whites have type 2 DM.[5] Type 2 DM is associated with failure of the beta cells to meet an increased demand for insulin due to enhanced peripheral insulin resistance. Cells are unable to respond to circulating insulin leading to elevated blood glucose levels. The signs and symptoms may take several years to be expressed. Clinical features of an acute exacerbation or poor glycemic control are similar to type I DM. NIDDM patients do not develop ketoacidosis due to their continued production of insulin. However, the type 2 DM patient can develop hyperosmolar hyperglycemic nonketotic (HHNK) coma.

Chronic Complications of Diabetes Mellitus

Prior to the development of exogenous insulin, survival was limited after the diagnosis of DM. Exogenous insulin has led to long-term survival and the development of chronic manifestations of DM including neuropathy, cardiovascular disease (CVD), nephropathy, retinopathy, impaired wound healing, and elevated infection risk. These abnormalities are generally related to the severity and chronicity of the hyperglycemia.

Diabetic neuropathy is one of the most common complications of DM and is characterized by pain and impaired sensation with eventual progression to motor dysfunction in the extremities (peripheral neuropathy) and autonomic dysfunction centrally. The etiology of neurologic derangement is poorly understood, but may be related to neural microvascular abnormalities and genetic and environmental factors. Peripheral neuropathy can increase the risk of ignoring trauma to the distal extremities leading to the development of ulcers and may play a role in the development of joint derangements. Autonomic neuropathy may cause esophageal dysfunction with difficulty swallowing, delayed gastric emptying, constipation, or diarrhea. Orthostatic hypotension, frank syncope, cardiac arrest, and sudden death have all been attributed to autonomic neuropathy.[4]

Heart disease is the leading cause of death in persons with diabetes (especially in type 2 disease). Adults with diabetes have heart disease death rates about two to four times higher than adults without diabetes.[5] Arteriosclerosis of the large and medium-sized arteries of the heart and peripheral circulation occurs earlier and more extensively and appears to be accelerated in the diabetic patient leading to coronary artery disease (CAD) and peripheral vascular disease. Autonomic neuropathy in the setting of CAD can lead to the development of silent myocardial infarctions (MI) and silent orthostatic hypotension. The person will experience little to no physical warning signs, such as chest pain, tightness, or dizziness, until cardiac failure or near loss of consciousness.

Hypertension (HTN) and stroke is also more prevalent possibly due to atherosclerotic changes in the large and small vessels. About 73% of adults with diabetes have BP greater to or equal to 130/80 mmHg or use prescription medications for HTN. Risk for stroke is two to four times higher in individuals with DM.

Diabetes is the most common cause of end-stage renal disease and is the leading reason for kidney transplantation. **Nephropathy** is associated with glomerular destruction (glomerulosclerosis) and protein in the urine (proteinuria). Progression of renal destruction leads to uremia, nausea, lethargy, acidosis, anemia, and worsening HTN.

Diabetes is a leading cause of blindness in adults aged 20 to 74 years.[5] **Retinopathy** is related to vascular abnormalities leading to neovascularization, micraneurysms, hemorrhage, and ischemia. Additional visual changes include visual blurring, glaucoma, cataracts, and macular degeneration.

Wound Healing and Infection Risk

Vascular changes include the atherosclerotic changes in the larger vessels but also includes the microcirculation. Abnormalities of the mircovascular circulation include basement membrane thickening, amyloid deposition (hyalin arteriosclerosis), increased platelet aggregation, and impaired fibrinolysis. Amyloid refers to protein deposits with common pathologic features (structural and staining characteristics). The abnormalities lead to impaired tissue perfusion and wound healing. These microvascular changes lead to the renal and visual alterations associated with DM.

Poorly controlled blood glucose levels can lead to higher risks of infection. Hyperglycemia leads to leukocyte dysfunction (impaired phagocytosis and chemotaxis) and blunted immune responses while also providing an optimum environment for proliferation of bacteria. Circulatory abnormalities limit immune responsiveness and transit to sites of infections. Sensory changes resulting from peripheral neuropathy and retinopathy increase the incidence of skin lesions.

Medical Management

Medical management of DM involves pharmacologic, dietary, and exercise therapies. Injectable insulin is indicated for type 1 diabetics and some type 2 diabetics. Insulin is prescribed in multiple forms with each type possessing varying duration and peaks of action (see Pharmacological Information). Different types can be combined to provide full-day coverage for the body's circadian changes (rises and falls over a 24-hour period) in glucose levels. Insulin pumps, an implantable delivery system, provide a continuous infusion of insulin for prolonged coverage and avoids repeated injections. Diet and exercise are the initial medical management therapies for type 2 diabetes. Diabetic diets generally consist of a balanced plan with lowered carbohydrates and meeting daily caloric needs for that individual. If blood glucose levels continue to remain high, oral medications can be prescribed. Oral medications stimulate the pancreas to release insulin or enhance insulin sensitivity and include Glipizide, Glyburide, Tolbutamide, and Chlorpropamide. Metformin helps increase the body's response to its own insulin.[3] The oral medications can be given alone or when greater glucose control is needed partnered with injectable insulin.

Physical Therapy Consideration in Diabetes Mellitus

The physical therapist/physical therapist assistant must remember that CVD is the leading cause of mortality in the diabetic population. Patients may present with atypical symptoms ("silent" ischemia) secondary to autonomic neuropathic changes and the therapist should be aware of **angina equivalents** including nausea/vomiting, dizziness, and shortness of breath. These patient symptoms may be hallmarks of ongoing ischemia. Patients with DM have an increased incidence of dysrhythmias after a MI. Therapists should monitor the hemodynamic status of the DM patient extensively and should include measures of perceived exertion as this may relate to angina equivalents (see Table 1-2). Additionally, **postural hypotension** may be encountered in DM patients. The therapist needs to assess orthostatic vital signs and to instruct the individual in adequate warm-up and cooling down exercises before and after strenuous activity to help prevent these problems.

Peripheral neuropathic pain usually comes and goes and can last for months or even years. Sensation can suddenly disappear, and loss occurs more often in the feet than hands. Individuals may not lose complete sensation, and deep pressure tends to be preserved the longest. **Protective sensation** alerts the individual to problems such as tight-fitting shoes, pebbles in shoes, shin contacting a coffee table, or water temperature too hot and is generally absent first. Protective sensation can be assessed using a 5.07 monofilament that applies 10 grams of pressure when used correctly. The fact that not all elements of sensation are lost confuses many patients/clients to believe they have no problems. Injury can be sustained with little forewarning because of a lack of protective sensation. Peripheral neuropathies in diabetics are believed to be the largest contributor to excessive callous, foot wounds, impaired wound healing, and lower extremity (LE) amputation. Assessment should include sensation testing by monofilament (specifically 5.07), followed by foot inspections for areas of callous or inflammation. Thickened callous or callous with dark red to black staining should be debrided by a trained health care professional to determine if an ulcer exists underneath and, if not, to prevent the callous from cracking and providing access to opportunistic infections. Shoes should be assessed for proper fit and the person educated in proper foot care with daily inspections, proper shoe fit, and utilization of shoes anytime the feet are on or near the ground. If the individual is wheelchair bound, shoes are imperative to provide protection to the feet while trying to maneuver in tight spaces.

Muscle **weakness** occurs in peripheral neuropathy and is usually preceded by loss of sensation. This weakness can be assessed in mobility and gait activities and may be the cause for "clumsiness" and foot drop or foot slap increasing trauma and breakdown of the forefoot.

Visual acuity needs to be closely assessed from a functional standpoint in each individual. Example: proper foot inspections can result in lower incidences of LE amputations. Will this individual be able to see small areas of trauma, like blisters, or subtle shades of erythema seen in the initial phases of wounding? If not, alternative solutions will need to be explored to provide adequate care (spouse, relative, or friend with adequate vision). Assistive devices for gait might be helpful in increasing safety with ambulation by helping identify barriers before falling over them or providing extra support for surprise changes in terrain. Patients with **retinopathy** are instructed to avoid isometric exercise, valsalva maneuvers, and head down/Trendelenburg positioning since excessive BP may lead to hemorrhage of fragile blood vessels (neovascularization). Activities that increase systolic BP >170 mmHg are typically avoided.

Peripheral vascular disease, especially small vessel diseases, is one speculative cause for peripheral nerve damage. Atherosclerotic changes in the small vessels may limit the information obtained from blood flow studies unless toe cuff pressures are also obtained to assess if adequate distal blood flow exists. **Ankle brachial index (ABI)** is often performed to assess peripheral circulation. The systolic pressure of the brachium is divided into the systolic pressure of the ankle obtained by using a Doppler and BP cuff. ABIs of 1.0 and greater are considered normal, 0.8 indicates mild disease, and 0.4 is considered severe blood flow obstruction (see Table 15–2).

Wound infections are common in patients with DM. Blood glucose levels greater than 200 mg/dL will impair and paralyze the macrophage. The macrophage is one of the key cells in wound debridement and repair (see Chapter 15). This paralysis of WBCs leads to decreased immune responses allowing infections opportunity to thrive and multiply.

Charcot foot (Figure 10–3) develops when blood glucose levels remain elevated. The blood shunts from the bone causing the bone to soften and, with repeated trauma, fracture and crumble. The only clinical signs of Charcot foot may be diffuse foot pain, mild edema, and possibly erythema. The tarsal bones of the foot and the calcaneous collapse leading to severely misshapen feet at higher risk for further skin breakdown. Poor **wound healing** has also been attributed to small vessel disease but is likely due to a combination of elevated blood glucose and peripheral neuropathies. Wound contraction is paramount to wound closure, and loss of protective sensation eliminates normal protection of the wound area. The individual will continue to fully weightbear regardless of the wound. Wound areas need to be removed from weightbearing or off loaded. Total contact casting is the optimal choice to alleviate pressure in the wound area and promote weightbearing at intact areas. Partnering total contact casting with assist devices can further encourage decreased weightbearing and increase ambulation safety and stability. Other off loading options exist in the form of total contact cast boots, modified cast walking boots, and, as a temporary option, modified postoperative shoes. Educating the individual in nonweightbearing or hopping should be closely assessed. Diabetes is a systemic disease, and problems encountered in one limb can easily occur in the other. Improper care of LE wounds can easily lead to LE amputation. Sixty percent of nontraumatic lower-limb amputations in the United States occur among people with diabetes according to the CDC National Diabetes Fact Sheet.[5]

Hypoglycemia, blood glucose levels less than 70 mg/dL, is a condition that can occur in both Types 1 and 2 DM. This can occur when a meal is late or missed, especially if timed insulin or oral medications have been taken or with

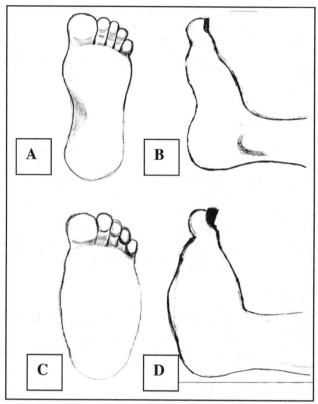

Figure 10–3. A and B are plantar and lateral views of a normal foot, respectively. C and D are plantar and lateral views of a Charcot foot.

illness impacting the gastrointestinal tract. Additionally, the therapist must consider the insulin-like effect of exercise. Hypoglycemia results in activation of the sympathetic nervous system and adrenal medulla and common symptoms include sweating, nervousness, quivering, faintness, palpitations, and sometimes hunger. Severe hypoglycemia causes dizziness, confusion, fatigue, weakness, headaches, and abnormal behavior mistaken for inebriation, inability to concentrate, vision abnormalities, seizures, and coma. Prolonged hypoglycemia can lead to permanent brain damage.[3] Persons with diabetes are recommended to keep hard candies, glucose tablets, glucagons, or high carbohydrate snacks available to counteract episodes of hypoglycemia. Fifteen grams of carbohydrate can remedy symptoms for approximately 15 minutes until an appropriate meal can be ingested.

Diagnostic testing is performed by blood tests. Two methods are recommended to make a diagnosis of DM:

1. After overnight fasting venous plasma glucose levels ≥7.8 mmol/L or 140 mg/dL on two separate occasions

2. After ingestion of 75 grams of glucose venous plasma glucose ≥11.1 mmol/L or 200 mg/dL at 2 hours and on at least one other occasion with the same test[4]

Normal blood glucose range is 70 to 110 mg/dL with an increased risk for complications at >126 mg/dL. Individuals with diabetes are also recommended to have quarterly blood testing of their $HgbA_{1c}$. This gives an average range of the individual's blood glucose over approximately a two-month period. Normal range $HgbA_{1c}$ is considered 4% to 6.7%, which corresponds to 70 to 110 mg/dL (see Table 2-17).

CASE STUDY

Mr. Close, a 56-year-old male admitted to the hospital because of a non-healing ulcer of his first metatarsal head. He has type 2 DM and uses oral medication. Blood glucose levels on admission were 240 mg/dL, and his $HgbA_1c$ was 9.6. Blood flow studies revealed decreased flow just below the popliteal fossa with an ABI of 0.6. After admission, a cardiac catheterization revealed >75% blockages of three coronary arteries. Coronary artery bypass (CABG) surgery was performed, and the patient returned to the floor after a 3-day stay in ICU. Bypass grafting of the LE is postponed until full recovery is achieved from the CABG. Physical therapy is consulted to evaluate and treat.

Patient/Client History

General Demographics/Social History/Living Environment

He lives with his wife and three children in a two-story home with 12 steps to enter from the outside and a bathroom on each level. He is employed as a manager of a grocery store.

General Health Status/Family History

Mr. Close's father and brother died at age 46 and 52, respectively, from heart attacks. He states he walks around the store all day at work, but does not participate in a formal exercise program.

Medical/Surgical History

The patient has been diagnosed with type 2 DM for 10 years. He also has a history of HTN, obesity, elevated cholesterol, and quit smoking last week prior to admission to the hospital. He has a 60-pack/year history. His tonsils and adenoids were removed as a child.

Current Conditions/Chief Complaints

Mr. Close is seen at bedside complaining of pain in his right foot and in the middle of his chest.

Functional Status and Activity Level

Prior to admission, Mr. Close was using a cane and rocker shoe to ambulate. He was staying on the first floor of his house because the climb to the second floor master bedroom made him "winded" and uncomfortable in his neck.

Other Clinical Tests

Laboratory results revealed a normal electrolyte panel and complete blood cell count. Noted abnormalities included a blood glucose 240 mg/dL, $HgbA_1c$

was 9.6, and ABI of 0.6. Arterial blood gases in the ICU prior to extubation were pH 7.34/PCO_2 38/PO_2 94/HCO_3^- 20.

Systems Review

Cardiovascular/Pulmonary

Resting vital signs sitting at the edge of the bed were oxygen saturation (SpO_2) 96% on 2 liters nasal cannula oxygen, HR 88, pulse regular, RR 18, BP 106/86, and pain 2/10. Following examination of range of motion (ROM), manual muscle test (MMT), bed mobility, transfers, and gait his vital signs were 88, RR 26, BP 88/84, and pain 4/10.

His cough was dry and nonproductive with splinting instruction. Auscultation of breath sounds revealed crackles at bilateral bases and heart sounds were normal S1, S2, and no appreciated S3.

Integumentary

Mr. Close has a surgical dressing in the middle of his thorax and a small bandage on his right forearm where he says his "IV" was. He has a dressing around his right foot and one on the inside of his left LE with some red-brownish drainage on the edges. He has mild edema in left > right LE.

Musculoskeletal

Mr. Close's ROM is within normal limite (WNL). MMT is grossly 4–/5 in the upper extremities (UEs) and 4/5 in the LEs. He needs minimal assistance of the bedrail for bed mobility, moderate assistance of one for transfer sit<>standing from an elevated surface without handrails, and gait required moderate assistance of one with rolling walker 10 feet. He was able to stand independently using a rolling walker.

Neuromuscular

Sensation testing by 5.07 monafilament demonstrated diminished findings in right > left LE. His dynamic balance was normal in sitting but decreased in standing. Proprioception was also decreased in bilateral UE (BUE)/bilateral LE (BLE).

Communication, Affect, Cognition, Language, and Learning Style

Mr. Close uses English as his primary language. Sternal precautions and functional precautions were reviewed with him due to his high risk for falling. He was able to repeat the precautions and the rationale.

Tests and Measures

Aerobic Capacity and Endurance

Mr. Close demonstrated a blunted BP/HR response to position change and ambulation. This may reflect autonomic neuropathy or medication effect. Crackles on auscultation are probably related to postoperative atelectasis.

Assistive and Adaptive Devices

Mr. Close will need to continue to use a rocker shoe to lessen weightbearing on his nonhealing ulcer. He will benefit from a rolling walker instead of a standard walker to decrease the lifting with sternal precautions.

Gait, Locomotion, and Balance

Gait and balance are both impacted by his poor endurance, possible peripheral neuropathy, pain, and limited ROM from surgery.

Pain

Mr. Close had increased pain with the examination and will benefit from pain medication prior to therapy sessions.

Diagnosis

Mr. Close presents with vascular, neurological, and autonomic complications from diabetes. His laboratory findings support poorly controlled diabetes, with large vessel involvement, and also an uncompensated metabolic acidosis possibly representing impaired renal function. Recommend treatment pattern 6D: impaired aerobic capacity/endurance associated with cardiovascular pump dysfunction or failure.[6]

Prognosis

The physical therapist estimated that Mr. Close would require daily physical therapy services until discharge at day 4 post ICU transfer. The recommended goals are to be independent with transfers, bed mobility, and gait with rolling walker 75 feet times 3. He also needs to be independent in activities of daily living (ADLs) and sternal precautions.

Intervention

Mr. Close was seen daily to progress gait, transfers, patient education, incentive spirometry hourly with splinted coughing, therapeutic exercise to enhance ROM and MMT. Wound care was also delivered to promote healing of right LE (RLE).

Reexamination

After 4 days, Mr. Close continued using a rolling walker for balance and was able to walk 35 feet times 2, required standby assistance for transfers due to continued blunted BP response, bed mobility was independent, but he required minimal assistance with ADLs, especially lower body dressing and bathing. Mr. Close was not able to climb up two steps without increasing discomfort in RLE and chest wall. Also, the vascular consultants recommend limiting stair climbing due to excessive pressure on the RLE since the longstanding DM had compromised the vascular bed resulting in a chronic wound.

Outcomes

Mr. Close was transferred to inpatient rehabilitation to alleviate his functional limitations allowing independence in his home. He will be scheduled for vascular surgery to restore adequate blood flow to his ischemic RLE.

SUMMARY

The endocrine system is a very complex network of glands that utilize hormones, the CNS, and the immune system to perform and alter its functions. These small glands can secrete hormones that can impact most every tissue in the body. Endocrine diseases and disorders are commonly caused by the immune system, and damage can be permanent. Although many of these processes are treated pharmacologically, rehabilitation may be oriented to managing the enduring functional limitations and disabilities.

CHAPTER REVIEW QUESTIONS

1. What is the main difference between type 1 and type 2 DM?
2. What is the most common endocrine disease?
3. Name two other major systems that impact the endocrine system.
4. What is the master gland and why is it called that?
5. Which of the glands are directly connected to the nervous system?

Pharmacological Information: Endocrine Diseases and Disorders Pharmacology

Antidiabetics: Oral Hypoglycemics

Sulfonylureas and Meglitinides

Action
Sulfonylureas and meglitinides are medications that stimulate release of insulin from functioning beta cells from the islets of Langerhans. These agents increase the influx of calcium leading to enhanced insulin secretion.

Side Effects
CNS: Confusion, dizziness, flushing, headache
CV: Palpitations, tachycardia
GI: Nausea, vomiting, constipation, dry mouth
Misc: Hypoglycemia, allergic reactions

Common Medications
Suflonylureas: Glymepride (Amaryl), Glipizide (Glucotrol), Glyburide
Meglitinides: Nateglinidine (Starlix), Repaglinide (Prandine)

Alpha-Glucosidase Inhibitors

Action
Alpha-glucosidase inhibitors reduce the gastrointestinal absorption of monosaccharides and glucose by inhibition of the intestinal enzyme alpha-glucosidase (alpha glucoside hydrolases).

Side Effects
GI: Abdominal pain, diarrhea, flatulence
Misc: Hypoglycemia

Common Medications
Acarbose (Precose), Miglitol (Glyset)

Biguanides

Action
Biguanides are used in noninsulin dependent diabetics to control serum glucose levels. Biguanides decrease glucose absorption from the GI tract, enhance peripheral insulin sensitivity leading to improved cellular glucose uptake and inhibits hepatic gluconeogenesis.

Side Effects
GI: Abdominal discomfort, diarrhea, nasuea, vomiting
Misc: Hypoglycemia, metallic taste, lactic acidosis

Table 10–18
INSULIN PREPARATIONS AND ACTIVITY CHARACTERISTICS

	Onset (Hr)	Peak (Hr)	Duration (Hr)
Rapid acting (regular)	• 0.5 to 1	• 2 to 4	• 6 to 8
Intermediate acting (Lente; NPH)	• 1 to 3	• 6 to 12	• 18 to 26
Long acting (Ultralente; human)	• 4 to 8	• 12 to 18	• 24 to 28

Common Medications
Metformin (Glucophage)

Thiazolidinediones

Action
Thiazolidinediones increase cellular insulin sensitivity promoting greater cellular uptake of serum glucose. These agents act as insulin receptor agonists.

Side Effects
CV: Edema
Misc: Hypoglycemia, weight gain, hypercholesterolemia, anemia

Common Medications
Pioglitazone (Actos), Rosiglitazone (Avandia)

Insulin Therapy (Table 10-18)

Insulin Preparations

Action
Insulin increases the cellular uptake of serum glucose, promotes the conversion of glucose to glycogen and amino acids to proteins while inhibiting the release of fatty acids. Formulations of insulin are available in ratios of short and longer lasting preparations (eg, Humulin 70/30). Insulin may be conjugated with protamine and zinc to prolong its duration of action. Insulin can be extracted from ox or pig or be created by recombinant technology (rDNA).

Side Effects
Misc: Hypoglycemia, rebound hyperglycemia (Somogyi Effect), allergic reactions, lipidystrophy (disappearance of subcutaneous fat at injection sites), redness/swelling at injection site

Common Medications
Insulin rDNA: Humalog, Novolog
NPH/Regular Insulin: Humulin, Novolin
Insulin zinc suspension: Lente insulin, Humulin L, Novolin L
Insulin zinc suspension, extended: Ultralente, Humulin U, Novolin U

Thyroid Hormones

Thyroid Preparations

Action
Thyroid preparations are medications that resemble the hormones T4 and T3. These medications are prescribed for patients with hypothyroidism.

Side Effects
CNS: Insomnia, irritability, headache
CV: Tachycardia, dysrhythmias, HTN
GI: Abdominal discomfort, diarrhea, vomiting
Misc: Weight loss, heat intolerance

Common Medications
Levothyroxine sodium (Levothroid, Synthroid, Levoxine)

Thyroid Hormone Inhibitors

Action
Thyroid hormone inhibitors are indicated for the treatment of hyperthyroidism/thyrotoxicosis (eg, Graves disease, toxic adenoma, thyroiditis). Medications may inhibit thyroid hormone production and secretion (eg, thiourea, iodides), reduce the amount of functional thyroid tissue by ablation (eg, radioiodine), or control symptoms of hyperthyroidism (eg, beta blockers).

Side Effects
CV: Dysrhythmias
GI: Diarrhea
Misc: Skin rash, arthralgia, myalgia, drug fever, hypothyroidism, goiter, hyperkalemia

Common Medications
Thioureas: Propylthiouracil, Methimazole (Tapazole)
Iodides (Pima, Lodopen)
Radioiodine (Iodine 131 [^{131}I])

Parathyroid

Parathyroid Hormone

Action
PTH is primarily regulated by plasma calcium concentration ($\downarrow$ Ca^{++}/$\uparrow$ PTH). PTH influences bone health through it stimulatory effect on osteoclasts and

bone resorption, renal reabsorption of Ca^{++} and enhanced intestinal Ca^{++} absorption.

Side Effects
CV: Edema
GI: Nausea
Misc: Tenderness at injection site, allergic reactions

Common Medications
Paroidin

Calcitonin

Action
Calcitonin (CT) secretion is regulated by plasma calcium concentration ($\uparrow Ca^{++}/ \uparrow CT$). These medications are primarily indicated for the treatment of hypercalcemia, osteoporosis/osteopenia and Paget's disease.

Side Effects
CNS: Headache
CV: Edema
GI: Nausea, vomiting
Misc: Tenderness at injection site, allergic reactions

Common Medications
Calcimar, Cibacalcin

Biphosphonates

Action
Biphosphonates are indicated for the treatment and prevention of osteoporosis, reduce bone pain and risk of fracture in patients with bone metastases and Paget's disease. These medications reduce the resorption of bone by inhibiting the activity and recruitment of osteoclasts. Additionally, biphosphonates stimulate the production of osteoblasts.

Side Effects
CNS: Headache
CV: Dysrhythmias/tachycardia, HTN
GI: Abdominal discomfort, dyspepsia, acid reflux, nausea, vomiting
Misc: Hypokalemia, muscle weakness, musculoskeletal pain

Common Medications
Alendronate (Fosamax), Etidronate (Didronel), Pamidronate (Aredia)

Adrenocortical Hormones

Action
The adrenal cortex is divided into three functional zones producing several hormones: zona glomerulosa (mineralcorticoid: adlosterone, fludrocortisone), zona fasciculata (corticosteroids: cortisol [hydrocortisone]), and zona reticularis (androgens). Corticosteroids are indicated in the treatment of adrenal insufficiency, inflammatory processes, leukemia, and for immunosuppression (see Pharmacological Information in Chapters 7 and 14).

Hypothalamus and Pituitary Hormones

Growth Hormone/Somatotroponin; Somatostatin

Action
GH or somatotroponin is inhibited or released from the anterior pituitary secondary to hypothalamic production of GH releasing hormone and GH release inhibiting hormone (somatostatin). GH stimulates lipolysis and release of free fatty acids, increases blood glucose levels and promotes protein synthesis. A deficiency of GH leads to dwarfism, while excessive secretion results in gigantism and acromegaly.

Common Medications
GH/Somatotroponin: Genotropin, Humatrope, Norditropin, Nutropin, Protropin

Side Effects
CV: Edema
Misc: Hyperglycemia, insulin resistance, hypothyroidism

Common Medications
Somatostatin: Octreotide (Sandostatin)

Side Effects
CNS: Dizziness, drowsiness, fatigue
CV: Edema, orthostatic hypotension, palpitations
GI: Anorexia, nausea, vomiting, abdominal pain, gallstones
Misc: Reduced insulin secretion/impaired glucose tolerance

Antidiuretic Hormone/Vasopressin

Action
ADH (also called vasopressin) is released from the posterior pituitary in response to increases in plasma osmolarity or decreases in BP. ADH acts on the kidneys and results in increased permeability of the collecting ducts leading to water retention and enhanced blood volume. Additionally, ADH promotes vasoconstriction leading to increased BP.

Side Effects
CNS: Dizziness, headache
CV: MI, angina
GI: Abdominal cramps, nausea, vomiting, heartburn
Misc: Fever, allergic reactions

Common Medications
Pitressin, Pressyn

Reproductive Hormones

Estrogens and Progestins

Action
Common estrogens and progestins include estradiol, estrone, estriol, and progesterone. These steroid hormones are produced in the ovaries of non-pregnant, premenopausal women. During pregnancy, the fetal-placental unit produces these hormones. The testes in men produce small amounts of progesterone. These hormones are under the influence of hypothalamic secretion of gonadotrophin-releasing hormone (GnRH) that stimulates the anterior pituitary to release leutinizing hormone and follicle-stimulating hormone. Estrogens and progestins are primarily prescribed for oral contraception, as replacement hormones for menopause, hypogonadal disorders, for osteoporosis and less commonly as neoplastic agents.

Side Effects
CNS: Headaches, lethargy
CV: Thromboembolic disease, CHF, edema, HTN
GI: Nausea, vomiting, increased appetite
GU: Endometrial cancer
Misc: Weight gain, gynecomastia (men)

Common Medications
Estropipate (Ogen, Estrone sulfate), ethinyl estradiol/desogestrel/ drospirenone/ethynodiol/levonorgestrel/norgestrel/norethindrone (Allesse, CyclessaDesogen, Levlen, Mircette, Nelova, Nortrel, Ovrette, Ortho-cept, Ortho Evra, Ovral, Norplant, Preven), Progesterone (Crinone, Prometrium)

Testosterone and Androgens

Action
Testosterone, produced by the testes, is the principal circulating androgen in men. Additional androgens include androstenedione, produced by the adrenal cortex and testes, and dehydroepiandrosterone (DHEA) produced by the adrenal glands. Testicular androgen synthesis is primarily influenced by hypothalamic production of GnRH and anterior pituitary release of leutinizing hormone. Testosterone and androgens are prescribed for hypogonadism, delayed puberty, and androgen-responsive breast cancer.

Side Effects
CV: Edema
GI: Nausea, vomiting
Misc: Deepening of voice, decreased breast size (women), gynecomastia (men), acne, facial hair

Common Medications
Testosterone (Andro, Andronate, Testamone, Depotest, Testex)

Antiandrogens

Action
Antiandrogens inhibits the production of testosterone (Finasteride) or the uptake of testosterone (flutamide). Antiandrogens are often prescribed for prostate cancer, benign prostatic hypertrophy, and hair loss.

Side Effects
CNS: Fatigue, lethargy, depression
GI: Nausea, vomiting, abdominal discomfort
Misc: Leukopenia, thrombocyopenia, gynecomastia, impotence, reduced libido

Common Medications
Cyproterone, Finasteride (Propecia, Proscar), Flutamide (Eulexin)

References

1. Haas LB. Endocrine system. In: Lewis SM, Collier IC, eds. *Medical-Surgical Nursing, Assessment and Management of Clinical Problems.* 3rd ed. St. Louis, Mo: Mosby Year Book; 1992.
2. Greenspan FS, Strewler GJ. *Basic & Clinical Endocrinology.* 5th ed. Stamford, Conn: Appleton & Lange; 1997.
3. Berkow R, Beers MH, eds. Hormonal disorders. In: *The Merck Manual of Medical Information, Home Edition.* New York, NY: Pocket Books; 1997.
4. Jameson JL. Endocrinology and metabolism. In: Kasper DL, Braunwald E, Fauci AS, et al, eds. *Harrison's Principles of Internal Medicine.* 13th ed. New York, NY: McGraw-Hill, Inc; 1994.
5. CDC. *National Diabetes Fact Sheet.* Atlanta, Ga: National Center for Chronic Disease Prevention and Health Promotion; 2002.
6. Guide to Physical Therapist Practice. 2nd ed. *Physical Therapy.* 2001;81(1).

Bibliography

Barrat Solomon BL, Choate Loriaux T, Drass JA. Endocrine and metabolic systems. In: McFarland GK, Hirsch JE, Tucker SM, Thompson JM, eds. *Clinical Nursing.* St. Louis, Mo: The CV Mosby Co; 1986.

Craig CR, Stitzel RE. *Modern Pharmacology with Clinical Applications.* New York, NY: Little, Brown, and Co; 1997.

Deglin JH, Vallerand AH. *Davis's Drug Guide for Nurses.* 8th ed. Philadelphia, Pa: FA Davis Co; 2003.

Greenspan FS, Gardner DG. *Basic & Clinical Endocrinology.* 6th ed. New York, NY: Lange Medical Books/McGraw-Hill; 2001.

Karch AM. *Lippincott's Nursing Drug Guide.* Springhouse, Pa: Lippincott Williams & Wilkins; 2004.

Ritter JM, Lewis LD, Mant TG. *Textbook of Clinical Pharmacology.* London, England: Edward Arnold Co; 1995

West JB. The hypothalamic-pituitary control system. In: Brobeck JR, Taylor NB, Best CH, eds. *Best and Taylor's, Physiological Basis of Medical Practice.* 12th ed. Baltimore, Md: Williams & Wilkins; 1991.

Chapter 11

GASTROINTESTINAL DISEASES AND DISORDERS

David Fichandler, MSPT
Daniel J. Malone, MPT, CCS

THE GASTROINTESTINAL SYSTEM

Physical therapy is not commonly sought for referral related to pathology in the gastrointestinal (GI) system. However, GI dysfunction is often difficult to manage medically and/or surgically leading to impairments, physical limitations, and disability. Additionally, GI issues may be a secondary diagnosis that the acute care practitioner needs to consider as the physical therapist creates the plan of care. The underlying GI process may complicate a patient's ability to perform therapeutic interventions leading to challenging rehabilitation management.

Anatomy

The GI system is a complex set of organs and glands that provide the many nutrients, electrolytes, vitamins, minerals, and fluids necessary for cellular and organ function (Figure 11–1). The normal GI tract provides the optimal environment for nutrient absorption through the coordination of motor, neural, and secretory functions.[1] For the purposes of this chapter, the GI system will be separated into the upper GI, lower GI, and glands/organs of the digestive system (Table 11–1).

Function

The primary function of the GI system is that of digestion and absorption. Digestion begins in the mouth and runs through the alimentary canal, terminating in the anus.[2]

THE UPPER GASTROINTESTINAL TRACT

The upper GI tract contains all parts of the alimentary canal from the mouth through the esophagus to the pyloric valve of the stomach. The most common set

Figure 11–1. Anatomy of the digestive system. (Reprinted from National Digestive Diseases Information Clearinghouse. Available at: www.niddk.nih.gov.)

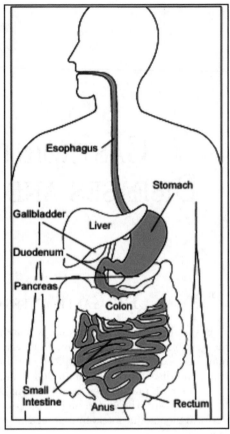

Esophagus

Stomach

Gallbladder

Liver

Duodenum

Pancreas

Colon

Small Intestine

Anus

Rectum

Table 11–1
GASTROINTESTINAL ANATOMY

Upper GI	*Lower GI*	*Glands Organs*
• Mouth	• Small intestine	• Liver
• Esophagus	• Duodenum	• Kidney
• Stomach	• Jejunum	• Gall bladder
	• Ileum	• Pancreas
	• Large intestine/colon	• Spleen
	• Ascending colon	
	• Transverse colon	
	• Descending colon	
	• Sigmoid	
	• Rectum	

of diseases effecting the upper GI tract are hyperacidity diseases. The extent and location of the disease is usually dependent upon the direction, intensity, and duration of acid flow most commonly involving the stomach and esophagus.[3]

Anatomy

The **esophagus** is a long hollow muscular tube, which originates at the distal pharynx and ends at the lower esophogeal sphincter (LES) of the stomach, about the level of T-1. It runs parallel and posterior to the trachea.[3,4] The primary functions of the esophagus include transport of materials from the oral cavity to the stomach, prevention of material from entering the trachea (upper esophageal sphincter [UES]), and limiting the reflux of gastric contents (LES).[5,6]

The **stomach** begins at the LES and terminates at the pyloric valve, which controls the entry of the food bolus into the duodenum. Major anatomical landmarks include the greater and lesser curvatures as well as the cardia, fundus, body, pylorus, and pyloric canal. The stomach stores liquids and solid foods prior to passage into the duodenum, continues the digestive process through the secretion of acids and gastric enzymes, and mixes and grinds the ingested meal (trituration). The stomach has local exocrine and endocrine functions. Exocrine function promotes digestion through the secretion of acids, pepsin, bicarbonate, and mucous as well as producing intrinsic factor that is necessary for the absorption of vitamin B_{12}.[6,7] Endocrine functions of the stomach include the release of the hormone gastrin that initiates the release of various digestive enzymes from the duodenum, pancreas, and liver.

COMMON ACID-BASED DISEASES OF THE UPPER GASTROINTESTINAL TRACT

Gastroesophageal Reflux Disease/Reflux Esophagitis

Gastroesophageal reflux disease (GERD) is the term applied to the symptoms and tissue damage associated with the reflux of gastric contents (acid/pepsin/bile from duodenum) into the esophagus and is the most common form of esophagitis.[8–10] It is estimated that 5% to 7% of the world's population is affected by GERD, and approximately 20% of Americans suffer from reflux symptoms every week.[10] GERD often goes untreated or is self-managed by over-the-counter medications. GERD is principally related to dysfunction of the LES. Weakness, inappropriate relaxation, or damage to this muscular ring allows movement of gastric contents into the esophagus. Other causes include direct irritants to the LES, disruption of the normal gastric defense mechanisms by nonsteroidal anti-inflammatory drugs (NSAIDs), alcohol, infectious agents (eg, Heliobacter Pyloris, Salmonella), smoking, decreased mucous production, as well as excessive amounts of peptic acids at the espho-gastric junction.[4,10] Common signs and symptoms of GERD are listed in Table 11–2.

The diagnosis is suggested by patient symptoms, but diagnostic testing may include endoscopy with biopsy, barium swallow, or pH monitoring.[10] Treatment is dependent on the extent of damage and dysfunction. Symptom control is often

Table 11–2
SIGNS AND SYMPTOMS OF GASTROESOPHAGEAL REFLUX DISEASE

- Heartburn
- Regurgitation
- Esophagitis
- Dysphagia
- Pain (substernal [non-cardiac], mid thoracic)
- Hoarseness or sore throat
- Occult anemia
- Hematemesis

Table 11–3
LIFESTYLE MODIFICATIONS TO REDUCE GASTROESOPHAGEAL REFLUX DISEASE

- Elevating the head of the bed
- Weight reduction for obese people
- Avoidance of fatty foods that promote reflux
- Avoidance of bedtime snacks
- Eliminate alcohol and tobacco use
- Avoidance of chocolate
- Use of thickened liquids

accomplished with lifestyle modifications as listed in Table 11–3.[4,10,11] If lifestyle modifications fail, medications prescribed include antacids and anti-ulcer agents.[9]

Barrett's Esophagus

Barrett's esophagus is the metaplastic transformation of the normal esophageal squamous epithelium to columnar epithelium in response to chronic gastroesophageal reflux.[7,10] Barrett's esophagus presents similar to GERD but carries a 30 to 125 times higher risk of developing esophageal adenocarcinoma.[4] Barrett's esophagus affects nearly 700,000 people yearly in the United States, occurs most frequently over the age of 60, and affects men and women equally. It is associated with regular alcohol consumption and smoking.[10] Diagnosis is confirmed by endoscopic evaluation with biopsy, demonstrating the pathologic changes to the lining of the esophagus.[9] Initial treatment consists of lifestyle modifications and medications similar to GERD. If the dysplasia or metaplastic changes are severe or if adenocarcinoma is present, surgical intervention becomes an option.

Esophageal Carcinoma

The majority of esophageal cancers is squamous carcinoma and is associated with alcohol consumption; smoking; diets lacking fresh fruits, vegetables, and animal protein; **achalasia** (impaired esophageal peristalsis with failure of LES to relax during swallowing); and esophageal stricture. Adenocarcinoma arises in Barrett's epithelium.[10] Further information regarding cancer can be found in Chapter 13.

SURGERY

Thoracoscopy and **mediastinoscopy**, the introduction of an endoscope into the thorax, allow visualization of the entire thoracic cavity (esophagus, trachea, azygos vein, aorta, pericardium, lungs, and diaphragm) and permits tissue sampling or excision. **Laparoscopy** is useful in evaluation and biopsy of the peritoneal cavity and abdominal organs and may be performed in conjunction with thoracoscopy. Stents may be applied to bridge esophageal obstructions allowing luminal patency to control saliva and oral nutrition. Endoscopic ablative therapy via thermal, chemical, or mechanical methods have been used for metastatic or dysplastic tissue. After tissue removal, regeneration of squamous epithelium promotes healing of the surgical site. **Esophagectomy**, either partial or complete excision, involve multiple surgical approaches depending on surgeon preference and anatomic location of the lesion. Common approaches include a left-sided thoracoabdominal incision, posterior lateral thoracotomy, and upper-midline abdominal and cervical incisions. After a portion of the esophagus is removed a conduit must be established for alimentary continuity. The stomach, colon, and jejunum have all been successfully used as esophageal substitutes and these structures are mobilized from their usual anatomic location and "pulled-through" the diaphragm into the thorax. Common complications postesophageal surgery include incisional pain, respiratory insufficiency, sepsis, and anastomotic leak.[12,13]

COMMON CLINICAL DISORDERS OF THE STOMACH

Dyspepsia

Dyspepsia is defined as imperfect or painful digestion and is usually a symptom of other GI disorders. It is characterized by vague abdominal discomfort, a sense of fullness after eating, heartburn, nausea, vomiting, flatulence, and loss of appetite.[8]

Gastritis

Gastritis is inflammation of the inner layer of the stomach, the mucosa. **Acute gastritis**, also termed **acute erosive gastritis, acute stress erosion,** or **acute gastric ulcer** occurs in the setting of severe trauma, surgery, or medical illness (Table 11–4).[10,14] While similar in presentation to GERD the symptoms of gastritis tend to be more intense and restraining.[5] Gastritis is caused by several factors including direct parasitic infection (eg, Salmonella), gastric ischemia (eg, trauma), and excessive acid production with an impaired mucosal lining of the stomach (eg, NSAIDs, aspirin, ETOH). While there is variability, the most common symptoms are listed in Table 11–5.

Clinically, the primary indicators are symptoms, medical history, and presentation. Endoscopy with biopsy can evaluate the exact status of the disease. Treatment is similar to that of GERD. Additional measures include prevention of the spread

---

Table 11–4

RISK FACTORS FOR THE DEVELOPMENT OF STRESS GASTRITIS

- Mechanical ventilation >48 hours
- Coagulopathy
- Increased intracranial pressure
- Sepsis
- Trauma
- Renal failure
- Liver failure
- Multiple organ system failure

Table 11–5

SIGNS AND SYMPTOMS OF GASTRITIS

- Epigastric pain
- Hematemesis
- Temperature
- Nausea
- Hemorrhage
- Anorexia

---

of infections, hydration, and allowing the stomach to rest. Gastric rest is accomplished by placement of a nasogastric (NG) tube to relieve pressure, maintaining the patient nothing per os (NPO or nothing by mouth) while providing parenteral nutrition and IV hydration. Medications commonly include antacids, anti-ulcer agents, anti-emetics, and antibiotics.[2,15]

Peptic Ulcer Disease

Peptic ulcers are disruptions of the gastric or duodenal mucosa. They occur in approximately 10% of the population and are responsible for more than 1 million hospitalizations and 2 billion dollars spent annually.[4,16] Peptic ulcers result from an imbalance between the protective mechanism of the stomach (the mucosal barrier, bicarbonate production, and maintenance of adequate blood flow) and the hypersecretion of stomach acids or pepsin. Mucosal breakdown is associated with the presence of *Heliobacter Pylori* (*H. Pylori*) and the use of NSAIDs. *H. Pylori* is often found with esophagitis and gastritis in addition to those with ulcers of the GI tract. Additional irritants to the peptic lining include alcohol, drugs, certain foods, and stress.[8,14,16] Common signs/symptoms are listed in Table 11–6.

Clinically, the primary indicator is symptoms and presentation. Endoscopy with biopsy can determine disease severity and rule out carcinoma. Patients may present with anemia or bloody emesis or stool warranting assessment of blood work (complete blood count [CBC]) and fecal blood content.[2,5] A breath test is used to measure the CO_2 and halitosis produced from *H. Pylori* metabolism.[11]

Table 11-6

SIGNS AND SYMPTOMS OF ULCER DISEASE

- Burning or gnawing pain
- Reduction of pain with eating (reduction lasts 2 to 3 hours)
- Burping
- Nausea and or vomiting

In severe cases:
- Bleeding
- Perforation
- Obstruction
- Malignancy

Medical treatments of peptic ulcer disease (PUD), like many other esophageal and stomach disorders, involves anti-ulcer agents to decrease acid production and antibiotics to counter infectious agents in order to promote symptom relief and allow the stomach to heal.

THE LOWER GASTROINTESTINAL TRACT

The lower GI tract consists of the entire intestinal canal from the duodenum to the anus. The intestines begin at the pyloric valve, where the stomach meets the duodenum, and terminates at the anus. The intestinal canal includes the **small intestine**, consisting of the duodenum, jejunum, and ileum, and the **large intestine,** including the cecum, ascending colon, transverse colon, descending colon, sigmoid colon, and rectum.

Motility, or movements of foods through the intestinal tract, occurs via **segmentation** and **peristalsis**. Segmentation is contraction of intestinal circular smooth muscle into parts or "segments" that provide prolonged mixing of the food bolus (chyme) with intestinal secretions to aide absorption. Peristalsis is the coordinated smooth muscular contractions creating the forward flow of materials and prevents food and toxic substances from regurgitating.[2,3,6]

Function

The intestines are the primary location for digestion and absorption of nutrients with assistance from the liver and pancreas. Additional functions include the movement of intestinal contents (motility), feedback regulation of gastric and hepatobiliary function, and immune defense. Each intestinal division plays specific roles in the absorption and excretion function of the GI tract. The small intestine is approximately 5 meters long and consists of three segments—the duodenum, the jejunum, and the ileum. The large intestine consists of the cecum and attached appendix; the ascending, transverse, descending, and sigmoid colon; the rectum; and the anus. The processes of digestion are completed in the small intestine, where the nutrients are absorbed by finger-like projections of the

Table 11-7

SIGNS AND SYMPTOMS OF IRRITABLE BOWEL SYNDROME

Signs and Symptoms

- Alternating loose stools and constipation
- Bloating
- Abdominal pain
- Cramping
- Mucous and or blood in stool

The criteria to test positive for IBS includes[26]:
- Abdominal pain for greater than 12 weeks over the past 12 months
- Pain that is relieved by bowel movement
- A change in the frequency of bowel movements
- A change in the appearance of stool

epithelial lining, the villi.[7] The large intestine produces solid wastes and mucus and is a primary site of water absorption.

COMMON DISEASES AND DISORDERS OF THE INTESTINES

For this chapter, intestinal disorders and disease will be divided into three categories: irritable bowel diseases, malabsorption diseases, and other diseases of the intestine.

Irritable Bowel Syndrome

Irritable bowel syndrome (IBS) is a disorder that interferes with the normal function of the colon. It is estimated that some 20% of Americans have IBS, women greater than men, the typical onset being in the 20s.[9,17,18] While no known cause exists for IBS, research suggests that it is due to colonic sensitivity to specific food and stresses. The disease causes a spasmodic motility pattern, decreased absorptive capacity resulting in nutritional deficiencies and loose stool. Common signs and symptoms are listed in Table 11-7.

IBS is primarily a diagnosis of exclusion from other diseases (eg, Crohn's disease, diverticulosis, and ulcerative colitis [UC]) and common testing includes bloodwork, computed tomography (CT) scan with contrast, and colonoscopy. Treatment for IBS is multifactorial. Lifestyle modification including stress reduction, increased exercise, change in diet, and adequate sleep have shown to be helpful in treatment. Medications are provided to stabilize the motility of the colon and increase absorption. Medications include: Alosetron Hydrochloride (Lotronex) and Tegaserol Maleate (Zelnorm). Additional medications include Lomotil (anti-diarrhea) and possibly steroids to decrease inflammation.[3,5] The diet change is usually called the BRAT diet. That acronym stands for banana, rice, apple, and tea or toast. These foods are nontoxic and nonirritating to the

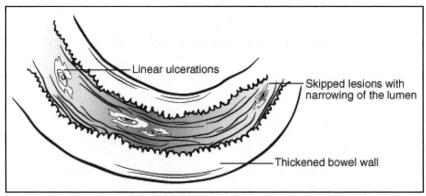

Figure 11–2. Crohn's disease of the ileum showing narrowing of the lumen, bowel wall thickening, and linear ulcerations of the mucosal surface. (Reprinted with permission from Crutchlow E, Dudac P, MacAvoy S, Madara B. *Pathophysiology.* Sudbury, Mass: Jones and Bartlett; 2002. Available at: www.jbpub.com.)

GI tract with IBS. Ancillary treatments that can promote symptom reduction include fiber supplementation, laxatives, anti-diarrhea medications, tranquilizers, and antidepressants. Patients with IBS are told to avoid:

- Large meals
- Wheat, rye, or barley
- Milk
- Alcohol
- Caffeine

Crohn's Disease (Ileitis, Enteritis)

Crohn's disease is a progressive, discontinuous inflammatory process of unknown etiology involving all layers of the intestinal wall (transmural) (Figure 11–2 and Table 11–8).[10] Crohn's disease may result from a hypersensitive immune reaction to certain viruses or bacterium resulting in extensive inflammation. Crohn's disease can occur in any location from the mouth to the anus but most commonly occurs in the terminal ileum and colon.[19] The inflammatory process results in rigidity, loss of peristalsis, and ulcerations causing right lower quadrant pain, fever, malaise, and diarrhea.[10,19] Intestinal obstruction, fistulas, and bleeding may develop.[10] It occurs equally in men and women and is not age discriminate. However, younger patients often have worse occurrences.[4,18,20]

Diagnosis is difficult because it is hard to differentiate Crohn's disease from other irritable bowel diseases such as UC and IBS. Testing includes blood work, fecal blood testing, upper GI series (x-rays with barium), and possibly colonoscopy.[4,11,15] Treatment depends on the location and severity of disease. Treatment goals include inflammation control, symptom relief, and elimination of nutritional deficiencies. Treatment may include long-term use of drugs, nutrition supplements, diet modification, and/or surgery. Medications include anti-inflammatory agents, immunosuppressives, antidiarrheal agents,

---

Table 11–8
SIGNS AND SYMPTOMS OF CROHN'S DISEASE

- Abdominal pain
- Diarrhea
- Occasional rectal bleeding
- Weight loss
- Small bowel obstruction
- Fistula formation (especially bladder, vagina, rectum, and skin)
- Nutritional deficiencies

Table 11–9
SIGNS AND SYMPTOMS OF ULCERATIVE COLITIS

- Abdominal pain
- Bloody diarrhea
- Fatigue
- Weight loss
- Rectal bleeding
- Loss of nutrients
- Electrolyte deficiencies
- Depression

---

and antibiotics. Surgery is palliative due to the progressive nature of Crohn's and includes surgical resection of diseased portions with colostomy.[12,19] Crohn's disease is variable in its presentation, intensity, and frequency of occurrence. The variable pattern of disease may result in inconsistent treatment effectiveness over time.[9]

Ulcerative Colitis (Colitis, Proctitis)

UC is a diffuse inflammatory disease of the colon and rectum. The difference between UC and Crohn's disease is that UC affects only the mucosa layer (inner region) of the intestinal lining, resulting in intestinal pain, recurrent diarrhea, rectal bleeding, and increased mucous production evident in stool.[10,19] UC generally occurs equally in men and women between the ages of 15 to 40 years old. Like many of the inflammatory bowel diseases, there is no known cause for UC, but autoimmune and hypersensitivity reactions to viral or bacterial pathogens are considered. Common signs and symptoms are listed in Table 11–9. Diagnosis is difficult secondary to the similar nature to other irritable bowel diseases. Common testing includes blood tests, colonoscopy or sigmoidoscopy, and lower GI series (barium enema with x-ray). Medications include anti-inflammatory agents, immunosuppressives, antibiotics, and antidiarrheal agents.[5,11] Medications can manage the symptoms for many patients. However, surgery can lead to a cure for UC. Twenty-five to 50% of patients require surgery

---

Table 11–10

SIGNS AND SYMPTOMS OF WHIPPLE'S DISEASE

- Abdominal pain
- Weight loss
- Incomplete breakdown of intestinal materials
- Diarrhea
- Intestinal bleeding
- Fatigue and weakness

---

and common surgical procedures include proctocolectomy with the formation of an ileal reservoir (ileum is sewn to the upper anal canal and a pouch is created), colon resection with ileostomy, and ileo-anal pull through. Surgery may be performed in stages. Complications after abdominal surgery include respiratory insufficiency, incision discomfort, stenosis or intestinal obstruction, skin irritation, odor with ostomies, and diarrhea with loss of water and electrolytes due to absence of colonic absorption.[12,19,21]

MALABSORPTION DISEASES

The major function of the GI system is digestion and absorption of nutrients. This complex process involves secretions from the salivary glands, stomach, pancreas, and liver as well as coordinated gastric motility (segmentation/ peristalsis) all which rely upon hormonal, mechanical, and neurologic inputs. Dysfunction in any component can lead to impaired GI function. Malabsorption is a general term used to describe multiple disorders where essential nutrients are inadequately absorbed. Malabsorption can be caused by many diseases of the small bowel (eg, Crohn's disease, HIV, celiac/tropical sprue, lactose intolerance), pancreas (eg, pancreatitis, cystic fibrosis), the liver (eg, liver cirrhosis) and biliary tract (eg, biliary tumors, primary sclerosing cholangitis [PSC], primary biliary cirrhosis [PBC]), and stomach (eg, gastritis, gastric resection).[22]

Whipple's Disease

Whipple's disease is a malabsorptive disease caused by the bacterium Tropheryma Whippelii. The bacterium creates lesions and scar tissue along the mucosal lining blocking the villi's ability to absorb nutrients. This disease primarily affects 30- to 40-year-old men, and common signs and symptoms are listed in Table 11–10. Diagnosis is accomplished by symptoms and endoscopy with biopsy. Treatment consists of antibiotics and nutritional supplementation including iron, folate, vitamin D, calcium and magnesium.[4]

Short Bowel Syndrome

Short bowel syndrome (SBS) is a secondary disorder that occurs in patients who have had abdominal surgery with removal of greater than 50% of their small intestines (eg, Crohn's, IBS, UC, or trauma). Normally the small intestine's

Table 11–11

SIGNS AND SYMPTOMS OF SHORT BOWEL SYNDROME

- Malnourishment and dehydration
- Weakness
- Fatigue
- Depression
- Weight loss
- Diarrhea
- Cramping
- Bloating
- Heartburn

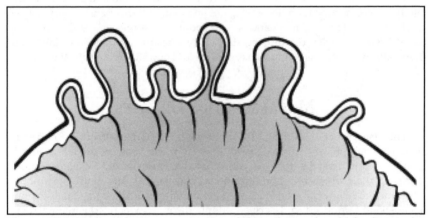

Figure 11–3. Figure shows a cross-section of the colon and multiple diverticula. (Reprinted with permission from Crutchlow E, Dudac P, MacAvoy S, Madara B, *Pathophysiology.* Sudbury, Mass: Jones and Bartlett; 2002. Available at: www.jbpub. com.)

absorptive capacity exceeds the need, but in SBS the lack of available intestinal surface area causes a malabsorption syndrome. Common signs and symptoms are listed in Table 11–11. Medical interventions include rehydration, total parenteral nutrition (TPN) or other parenteral nutrition, and small bowel transplant in select individuals.[3]

Diverticulosis and Diverticulitis

Diverticulosis is small outpouchings or herniations of the inner intestinal lining (mucosa and submucosa) through the intestinal wall (Figure 11–3).[8,14] Diverticulum are normal occurrences in 30% to 50% of people over 60 years old and nearly 100% in people over the age of 80. Infection or inflammation due to retained fecal material of diverticuli leads to **diverticulitis.** Diverticulitis can potentially cause intestinal necrosis and perforation. Diverticulitis occurs in 10%

Table 11–12

SIGNS AND SYMPTOMS OF DIVERTICULITIS

- Abdominal pain
- Fever and chills
- Nausea and vomiting
- Cramping
- Constipation
- Fistula formation

---

to 25% of people with diverticulum.[10] Common signs and symptoms of diverticulitis are listed in Table 11–12. Physical examination is suggestive and confirmed by endoscopy, blood analysis for infection, and CT with contrast.

Medical management focuses on the underlying cause. Important factors for treatment include diet modification, infection or inflammation control, intestinal rest, and minimizing further complications. Diet modification includes increasing fiber intake. Fiber keeps stool soft and lowers the internal colonic pressure. Additionally, patients are discouraged from eating nuts, popcorn, and seeds that are small enough to get lodged within the diverticulum.[18] To promote intestinal rest, patient activity is limited, a nasogastric tube is inserted, a liquid diet is initiated, and pain management medications are prescribed. Surgical intervention is necessary with severe obstruction, intestinal necrosis, and perforation (eg, laparotomy or bowel resection).[3,4,18]

COLON CANCER

Colon cancer is the second leading cause of cancer related deaths in the United States and has an annual incidence of 147,500 new cases. Colorectal polyps are masses of tissue that project into the lumen (Figure 11–4). Polyps are often an adenoma (adenomatous polyps, tubular adenoma, villous adenoma, adenomatoous polyposis coli, Gardner syndrome) and most colon cancers arise from pre-existing polyps.[10] Risk factors for colon cancer include the following:

- Age—Greater than 50
- Diet—High in fat, low in fiber
- History of polyps
- Other personal medical history
- Familial medical history
- UC (5% of people with UC develop colon cancer)

Common signs and symptoms of colon cancer are listed in Table 11–13 and staging of the disease is found in Table 11–14. Diagnosis includes a thorough history and physical examination. Diagnostic testing includes digital rectal exam and palpation of abdominal masses, fecal blood testing, radiologic studies, and proctosigmoidoscopy/colonoscopy. Treatment includes chemotherapy, radiation therapy, and immunotherapy (see Chapter 13). Surgical interventions

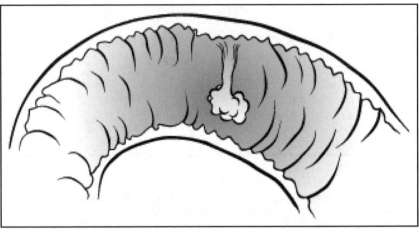

Figure 11–4. Adenomatous polyp and adenocarcinoma of the colon. (Reprinted with permission from Crutchlow E, Dudac P, MacAvoy S, Madara B. *Pathophysiology.* Sudbury, Mass: Jones and Bartlett; 2002. Available at: www.jbpub.com.)

Table 11–13
SIGNS AND SYMPTOMS OF COLON CANCER

- Changes in bowel habits
- Diarrhea
- Blood in the stool
- Narrow stools (ribbon like)
- Constant fatigue
- Weight loss

Table 11–14
STAGING OF COLON CANCER

0 = Present in the innermost lining only
1 = Present on the inner wall of the colon
2 = Present outside the colon, but not the liver
3 = Metastasis to the liver
4 = Metastasis to other parts of the body (usually liver and/or lungs)

---

vary depending on the resectability and site of lesion and distribution of lymphatic tissue. Anastomosis of remaining bowel or colostomy may be performed following resection. Surgical approaches involve abdominal or perineal incisions.[21]

INTESTINAL STOMAS/OSTOMIES

Ostomies are surgically created openings from the intestine or bowel to the outside via the abdominal wall and are common surgical interventions for intestinal disease or carcinoma. Stomas can be temporary or permanent depending on the condition, and the location may vary. Stoma placement is above the waistline and should not limit clothing or other ADLs. Common patient questions include the following: Can I exercise? Can I swim? Can I have sex? The answer to all of these is yes, but timing of these activities should be discussed with a stoma expert (enterostomal therapist).[18]

Ileostomy is common after removal of colon and rectum (proctocolectomy/ UC) and the ileum is externalized. Ileostomies drain fairly continuously and an appliance is worn at all times. **Continent ileostomy** involves the creation of a reservoir or pouch that must be evacuated periodically.

With a **colostomy**, the rectum is removed and distal colon is attached to the abdominal wall. The **Ileo-Anal Reservoir Surgery (Ileo-Anal Pull Through [IAPT])** is a two-stage process:

1. Colon and rectum are removed except for the outer muscles of the rectum. An ileostomy is placed.

2. Ileostomy closed and distal small intestine is attached to the remaining rectal muscle. This creates an internal pouch, which allows for normal elimination.

HERNIA

Hernias are an abnormal protrusion of intra-abdominal tissue through a fascial defect in the abdominal wall.[9,21] Common herniations include inguinal, femoral, umbilical, ventral, and incisional. Groin hernias account for 75% of all hernias and include an **inguinal hernia**, the bulging of intestine through a weakened area of the groin, usually in the area of the inguinal canal, and a **femoral hernia**, a protrusion into the femoral canal.[9,10,21] Risk factors for hernias include obesity, heavy lifting, straining during bowel movements, ascites, pregnancy, postoperative infection and pulmonary complications, delayed wound healing, impaired nutrition, placement of drains, and general debility.[21] Symptoms of inguinal hernias include groin pain, palpable or pulsatile lump in the groin, and bowel obstruction at the point of herniation (strangulated bowel). If the physical examination is inconclusive, additional studies may include radiology with contrast. Treatment depends on the severity of the herniation. On occasion, applying pressure to the intestinal portion can reduce the hernia. Surgery to reduce herniations include:

- **Herniorrhaphy:** After the hernia is reduced, the abdominal or inguinal wall is reinforced.

- **Hernioplasty:** A herniorrhaphy with the reinforcement of mesh or steel wire.

- Bowel resection is necessary if the loop of intestine becomes strangulated or obstructed.

Hemorrhoids

Hemorrhoids are a normal part of aging and involve the swelling and stretching of veins in and around the anal canal. Hemorrhoids normally occur in greater than 50% of people over the age of 50 and develop because of increased anal pressure (eg, straining during bowel movements, chronic constipation, or pregnancy/childbirth). Hemorrhoids cause pain, discomfort in sitting, itching, and bleeding. There are two types: internal, which are within the anal canal, and external, which are outside the rectum.[3] Diagnosis is usually confirmed by physical examination and endoscopic procedures include anoscope/sigmoidscope. Treatment goals include elimination of constipation (if present), creams (eg, Preparation H, Anusol, witch hazel pads), and a Sitz bath (which is a seated bathing tool to irrigate and cleanse the perianal region and promote muscular relaxation). Diet modification includes increasing fluid and fiber intake and stool softeners. The use of rubber, inflatable donuts used to be a common treatment. However, the donut increases the vascular pressure around external hemorrhoids by compression and promotes venous stasis.[3,4] Surgical interventions include:

- **Sclerotherapy:** Injection of inflammatory agent leading to fibrosis and scarring

- **Banding:** Placement of rubber bands leading to ischemic necrosis

- **Hemorrhoidectomy:** Surgical cauterization and removal of involved veins and tissue

The Liver and Gall Bladder

The liver is the largest organ in the body and accounts for 2% of body weight in adults (Figure 11–5).[2] It has many important metabolic and digestive functions that are essential and hepatic abnormalities impact on multiple organ systems (see Table 11–17). Interestingly, the liver possesses tremendous resilience and regenerative ability if resected or traumatized.[22] The gall bladder, on the contrary, is very susceptible to damage, injury, or dysfunction.

Anatomy

The liver is located in the right upper quadrant of the abdomen (RUQ). More specifically, it is under the diaphragm and within part of the rib cage, while protruding into the epigastrium. The liver has two lobes, right and left, which can be subdivided into lobules each of which has their own arterial, venous, and biliary supply. Hepatic blood supply arises from two sources, the hepatic artery (branches from aorta) and the hepatic portal vein (arising from mesenteric and splenic veins). On the posterior inferior surface of the liver lies the gall bladder. The gall bladder lies within a groove separating the right and left hepatic lobes and has direct connections to each of the liver lobes (biliary ducts) as well as to the duodenum and the pancreas (ampulla of Vater).[2]

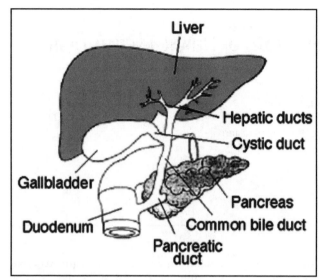

Figure 11–5. Anatomy of the liver, gall bladder, and bile duct. (Reprinted from National Digestive Diseases Information Clearinghouse. Available at: www.niddk.nih.gov.)

Function

Hepatic function can be clinically defined in four categories:

1. **Synthetic:** Production of plasma albumin, globulins, alpha-1 antitrypsin, and coagulation factors

2. **Excretory:** Production of bile (plus bilirubin, cholesterol, urobilogen, and bile salts)

3. **Metabolism: Fats** (specifically triglycerides, cholesterol, and phospholipids) are synthesized in the liver; **carbohydrates**—the primary source of blood glucose is from the liver and it is the main storage site for glycogen; **protein**—the liver is the primary organ for protein catabolism and synthesis of urea that is transported to the kidney for excretion

4. **Detoxification:** The liver detoxifies many noxious compounds found in chemicals and drugs making them less harmful[1,6]

The **gall bladder** stores and concentrates bile synthesized in the liver. Bile is delivered to the duodenum via contraction of the gall bladder passing through the common bile duct and the sphincter of Oddi. Bile is an emulsifier that facilitates the digestion of fats and stimulates intestinal peristalsis.[1,6]

COMMON SYMPTOMS OF LIVER DISEASES

Jaundice

Jaundice is due to excessive deposition of bile pigments resulting from an elevation in plasma bilirubin (>0.8 mg/dL—**hyperbilirubinemia**). The bile pigments create the yellow discoloration of the skin, eyes, and fingernails and account for dark, foul-smelling urine. Jaundice may result from obstruction of

---

Table 11–15
SIGNS AND SYMPTOMS OF HEPATIC ENCEPHALOPATHY

- Altered mood/inappropriate behavior
- Hypersomnia
- Impaired judgment/delirium
- Sluggish speech
- Flapping tremors of the hands (asterixis)
- Ataxia

Severe cases include:
- Seizures
- Coma
- Death

---

the bile passageways such as the common bile duct by a gall stone (**obstructive jaundice**), disturbances in hepatic functioning as in cirrhosis of the liver, or excessive destruction of red blood cells as seen in hemolytic anemia. Bilirubin is a by-product of hemoglobin catabolism. The liver metabolizes bilirubin allowing normal excretion and elimination from the body.[1,6]

Encephalopathy

Encephalopathy or hepatic coma is a reversible decrease in neurologic function due to shunting of blood away from the portal circulation or hepatic failure resulting in accumulation of noxious metabolic by-products.[23] Hepatic dysfunction leads to excessive amounts of ammonia and other toxic substances in the blood stream which modify cerebrovascular permeability, interfere with normal cerebral energy metabolism, disrupt cell integrity, and alter the normal balance of neurotransmitters creating the typical signs and symptoms listed in Table 11–15.[9,24] **Asterixis ("liver flap")**, a sign of hepatic encephalopathy, is the alternating flexion-extension of the hands observed when the patient is asked to dorsiflex the wrist with the arms extended.

Ascites and Peripheral Edema

Ascites, the presence of fluid in the peritoneum or swelling of the abdomen, is caused by an increase of fluid across the peritoneal membrane of the liver. The mechanisms for causing both peripheral edema and ascites are the same, an alteration in the Starling forces that regulate fluid balance. Fluid balance is generally a function of osmotic, arterial, venous, and tissue pressures. Ascites results from the synergistic relationship between an elevated portal venous pressure and low serum osmotic pressure due to hypoalbuminemia. Albumin is the most common protein of the body and is synthesized in the liver. Albumin maintains the osmotic pressure of the blood and facilitates absorption of fluid into the vasculature.[1,6] If albumin concentrations are diminished (**hypoalbuminemia**) as seen in hepatic disease, osmotic pressures are low and fluid leaks out of the blood vessels. In addition, portal hypertension creates excessive pressure in the venous system that also favors capillary leakage. The sum of these forces results in the movement of fluid across the peritoneal membrane into the abdomen.

Portal hypertension is caused by elevated venous pressure in the portal vein (>12 mmHg). The underlying cause may be multifactorial including portal vein thrombosis, neoplasm, or other form of obstruction (eg, PBC). However, the most common cause of portal hypertension is **cirrhosis**.[10,23] Cirrhosis causes fibrosis of liver tissue and restriction of portal circulation. Long-term dysfunction may lead to other disorders such as variceal bleeding, ascites, splenomegaly, right heart dysfunction, and pulmonary edema.[10,23]

Esophageal Varices

The portal veins carry blood from the upper GI tract, spleen, pancreas, and gall bladder through the liver to the heart. Portal hypertension, a sustained increase in portal venous pressures, results in elevated perfusion pressures and congestion in the spleen, stomach, and esophagus. Collateral vessels develop which become distended and varicose especially in the stomach and esophagus. In advanced liver disease, varices may burst, leading to upper GI bleeding and **hematemesis** (coffee ground vomitus).[25]

Hepatomegaly and Splenomegaly

Hepatomegaly is enlargement of the liver and is a common finding in primary and secondary hepatic disease. The usual lower border of the liver is percussed or palpated at or slightly below the right costal margin. **Splenomegaly**, enlargement of the spleen, results from passive venous congestion and is often associated with portal hypertension.[10,23]

COMMON DISEASES OF THE LIVER

Cirrhosis

Cirrhosis is the replacement of normal liver tissue with fibrotic/scar tissue and nodule formation and is the end result of hepatocellular injury.[10] This alteration in liver architecture blocks normal blood flow throughout the liver, causing many of the symptoms listed in Table 11–16. Cirrhosis is the twelfth leading cause of death in the United States, killing approximately 25,000 annually.[26] Cirrhosis is a secondary complication of multiple liver diseases including:

- Alcoholic liver disease
- Hepatitis (B, C, D)
- Autoimmune hepatitis
- Wilson's disease
- Biliary duct blockage
- Drugs and infections
- Cryptogenic liver disease

Patient presentation is variable depending upon inciting cause, but common symptoms of hepatic dysfunction are listed in Tables 11–15 and 11–16 with

---

Table 11–16
CLINICAL FEATURES OF HEPATIC DYSFUNCTION

System	Signs and Symptoms
Hematology	Anemia, coagulopathy, toxin/drug excretion
Cardiovascular	Tachycardia, hypotension/hypertension, peripheral edema, portal hypertension
Pulmonary	Hepatopulmonary syndrome, dilated pulmonary vascular bed, ventilation/perfusion mismatch, hypoxemia, ⇑ work of breathing
Neurological	Encephalopathy
GI	Varices, risk for bleeding, ascites
Musculoskeletal	General weakness/muscular atrophy, overstretched abdominal muscles (may have associated back pain), abdominal adhesions
Metabolic	Poor drug and toxin excretion, electrolyte abnormalities
Integumentary	Poor healing, brittle skin/hair
Other	Malnutrition/anorexia, hypoalbuminemia, electrolyte abnormalities

Adapted from Bishop Lindsay KL, Galantino ML, Huber F, Wells CL. Handout: Management of Medically Complex Patient. APTA Combined Sections Meeting: Pre-Conference Program. October 1997.

---

encephalopathy, ascites, and jaundice being the most frequent. Patients frequently experience exhaustion, fatigue, and weakness.

After establishing the cause of the underlying disease, the extent of scarring can be assessed through the combination of CT scan, ultrasound, and liver biopsy. Treatment is dependent on the underlying disease process, but there is no cure or reversibility of cirrhosis except liver transplantation. Many of the symptoms of cirrhosis and its counterparts can be managed with medication (eg, Lactulose) and lifestyle changes for a period of time.

Hepatitis

Hepatitis is an inflammatory process within the liver. Symptoms may vary from a minor flu-like illness to fulminant, fatal liver failure. The major causes of hepatitis are viral infections (common: HBV A/HBV B/HBV C/HBV D; rare: CMV, yellow fever) and toxic agents, specifically alcohol. Patients typically present with many of the signs and symptoms listed in Table 11–16, and diagnosis is a combination of a thorough history, physical examination, and laboratory testing (liver function tests—AST/ALT). Clinical recovery from viral hepatitis is complete in 3 to 16 weeks in most cases. However, chronic hepatitis may develop in non-HBV A infected individuals and drug side effects. The pathogenesis of chronic hepatitis is obscure, but may be related to an autoimmune mechanism.[3,4,9]

Treatment

There is a tremendous variation in presentation and progression of symptoms. Acute viral hepatitis usually is self-limiting and much of the treatment is supportive, while chronic hepatitis may progress to cirrhosis and liver failure. Ultimately, the only cure for advanced stages of the disease is liver transplantation (see Chapter 14).

Primary Sclerosing Cholangitis

PSC is a rare disease process where there is inflammation, fibrosis, and stricture of the bile ducts. Bile is prevented from passing into the gall bladder (**obstructive jaundice**) resulting in liver damage (**biliary cirrhosis**).[10] Progressive liver damage ensues leading to liver failure and death. More men than women are affected by PSC, usually between the ages of 30 to 60.[23,24] There is an increased incidence of PSC in patients with UC. The cause of PSC is unknown. However, sensitivity to bacterium or virus may account for the combined presentation of PSC and UC. The progression of PSC is gradual, and prognosis is poor. Common symptoms include jaundice, pruritus, fatigue, anorexia, and indigestion.

Common diagnostic procedures include:

- Cholangiography-x-ray with dye injection into the bile ducts
- Endoscopic retrograde cholangiopancreatography ([ERCP] an endoscopic evaluation of the bile ducts)
- MRCP (MRI retrograde cholangiopancreatography)
- Liver biopsy[4,5]

Treatment centers on symptom management. Specifically, patients are often deficient in fat-soluble vitamins (A, D, E, K) because of the bile duct obstruction and limited gut absorption. Surgical management may include balloon dilatation, stent placement, and eventual liver transplantation.

Primary Biliary Cirrhosis

PBC is an insidious chronic disease noted by progressive destruction of the biliary duct wall interfering with bile transport (**cholestasis**) and digestion. It commonly occurs in 40- to 60-year-old women (nearly 90%) and is often found as a secondary diagnosis (thyroiditis, rheumatoid arthritis, scleroderma, Sjögren syndrome, systemic lupus erythematosus).[10] The cause of PBC is unknown. However, it is believed to be an autoimmune disease with hepatic lymphocytes and plasma cells destroying the biliary ducts. Common signs and symptoms include the following:

- Jaundice
- Pruritus
- Edema
- Cholesterol deposits on the skin (xanthomas)
- Dry eyes and/or mouth
- Hepatosplenomegaly

Patients with PBC develop osteoarthritis, osteoporosis, portal hypertension, xanthomatous neuropathy, and thyroid problems. Diagnostic testing includes the following:

- Cholangiography x-ray with dye injection into the bile ducts
- ERCP
- MRCP
- Liver biopsy
- Assessment of thyroid function

Treatment

Treatments include vitamin and calcium supplementation, medications for symptom management, and hormone therapy (for hypothyroidism and for women who are menopausal). If treatment fails or the disease process continues to progress, a liver transplant is recommended.

Wilson's Disease

Wilson's disease is an autosomal recessive disorder resulting in an excess absorption of copper from the small intestine with limited hepatic excretion leading to end organ dysfunction.[4] Chronic elevations of copper in the bloodstream leads to copper deposition in the liver, brain, corneas, and kidneys. Wilson's disease usually affects children between 6 and 20 years old and if left untreated can be fatal.[5,9,22]

The hallmark sign of Wilson's disease is the **Kayser-Fleisher ring**, a brownish ring that presents around the cornea. Other signs are dependent upon which organs are involved. It is not uncommon to have hepatomegaly, splenomegaly, portal hypertension, and neurological symptoms such as dysarthria, ataxia, resting tremors, and rigidity (parkinsonian symptoms).

The pathognomonic sign, the Kayser-Fleisher ring, is unique to Wilson's disease. Other important diagnostic tools include blood and urine analysis and liver biopsy to determine the concentrations of copper.[4,5] Neurological testing is important if symptoms are present. Often, CT or MRI in conjunction with EMG is done to assess the neuromuscular component of the disease process. Treatment includes drug therapy along with diet modification. D-Penicillamine and Trientine Hydrochloride are both drugs that help remove copper from the bloodstream. Zinc acetate aids in blocking intestinal absorption of copper, thus promoting excretion. Patients take Vitamin B_6 and eat a diet low in copper. A low copper diet includes avoidance of mushrooms, nuts, chocolate, dried fruit, liver, and shellfish.[4] Treatment for Wilson's disease is life-long and prognosis is good for patients who are successfully managed before liver or brain damage has occurred. The only cure is liver transplantation. Anecdotally, if a patient with Wilson's disease is given a new liver via transplantation, his or her original liver is acceptable in another recipient.

DISEASES OF THE GALLBLADDER

Cholelithiasis (Gallstones, Biliary Calculi)

Gallstones are a common event, occurring in nearly one in 12 Americans. Most gallstones are asymptomatic; however, excruciating pain may be experienced. Risk factors for developing stones include women more than men, obesity, diabetes mellitus, and age over 40 years. Culturally, Native American, Mexican, and South American peoples are at an increased risk.[3,4,22]

Pathophysiology

Gallstones are the most prevalent cause of disorders of the gallbladder and biliary tract. There are two different types of gallstones based on their chemical composition: cholesterol and bilirubin stones. Cholesterol stones are due to an increase in cholesterol concentration, decrease in bile salts, or delayed emptying of the gallbladder. Bilirubin stones are rare. They generally occur in chronic forms of anemia such as sickle cell anemia or thalassemia. Obstruction to flow of bile into the duodenum causes distension of the bile ducts, impairs digestion, and may result in spillage of bile pigments into the circulation causing obstructive jaundice.[27]

Signs and Symptoms

- Severe pain in the epigastric region or RUQ
- Referred pain under the right scapula
- Indigestion after eating fatty foods
- Nausea and/or vomiting

Diagnosis and Testing

The gold standard for diagnosing symptomatic gallstones is an abdominal ultrasound. Other tests that can be performed include CT scan, MRCP, ERCP, and blood tests. Differential diagnosis for acute cholelithiasis includes MI, appendicitis, ulcers, IBS, hiatal hernia, and pancreatitis.

Treatment

The most common treatment for acute cholelithiasis is a cholecystectomy (excision of the gall bladder), which can often be done laproscopically. Other treatments include medications such as Chenodial, Monoctanoin, and Ursodiol.

THE PANCREAS

The pancreas is a complex organ, possessing both endocrine and exocrine functions. Endocrine function involves insulin and glucagon production, and the regulation of lipids, protein, and carbohydrates is discussed in Chapter 10. For purposes of this chapter, only the exocrine functions will be presented.[3]

Anatomy

Anatomically, the pancreas is a large, flat, finely lobulated gland associated with the duodenum. It is located posterior to the stomach along the posterior abdominal wall in the left upper quadrant. The pancreatic ducts carry the exocrine secretions and connect with the bile duct at the **ampulla of Vater**, also termed the hepatopancreatic ampulla, before entering the duodenum. Rings of smooth muscle form sphincters, the **sphincter of Oddi**, that close the ampulla until stimulated to relax by emptying of the gastric contents into the duodenum and production of hormones including cholecystokinin.[1,2,6]

Function

The **pancreas** secretes 2 to 2.5 liters per day of a bicarbonate fluid containing digestive enzymes. Regulation of pancreatic secretions involves both hormonal and neural factors and is related to the chemical composition of the meal.[6] **Secretin** and **cholecystokinin**, hormones released from the small intestine, and neural reflex arcs involving the vagus nerve regulate pancreatic secretion production. The primary stimulants of duodenal secretin production are fatty acids. Cholecystokinin is released from the duodenum in response to fatty acids and protein digestive products—peptides and amino acids.[1,6,28]

DISORDERS OF THE EXOCRINE PANCREAS

Pancreatitis

Pancreatitis is an inflammation of the pancreas. The extent of which the disease is present is variable, from mild symptoms to severe complications with risk of death. Pancreatitis can be acute or chronic. The acute form of pancreatitis is usually sudden in onset, of short duration, and self-limited. Chronic pancreatitis results in progressive destruction of pancreatic tissues.

Pancreatitis is usually caused by excessive alcohol consumption or by the presence of choleliathiasis. Gallstones block the pancreatic ducts resulting in the "escape" of activated pancreatic enzymes into surrounding tissues. Additional causes include hypercalcemia, hyperlipidemia, abdominal trauma, ESRD, bacterial and viral infections, medications (thiazides, sulfonamides) as well as structural anomalies. Common signs and symptoms are listed in Table 11–17.

Diagnosis and Testing

Acute pancreatitis can not be confirmed by a specific laboratory test. Multiple tests are used to support the diagnosis including blood testing (eg, elevations in serum amylase and lipase concentrations, white blood cells (WBCs), hematocrit (Hct), blood glucose and bilirubin; reduction in calcium). CT scans or abdominal ultrasound can be ordered to assess anatomy of the pancreas and to check for the presence of gallstones.

Treatment

Treatment is quite variable and dependent on the severity and chronicity of the symptoms. Acute pancreatitis will often resolve spontaneously in several

Table 11–17

SIGNS AND SYMPTOMS OF PANCREATITIS

- Abdominal/episgastric pain (worse with eating/walking/supine), often radiating to the back
- Abdominal swelling
- Nausea and/or vomiting
- Fever
- Dehydration
- Hypotension

days with pancreatic rest. Pancreatic rest includes withholding foods and liquids by mouth, bed rest, and possible NG suction. If symptoms are more progressive, admission to the intensive care unit (ICU), along with aggressive rehydration and electrolyte replacement, antibiotics for confirmed infections, and NG decompression are instituted. Careful observation for organ failure and other systemic complications is maintained. If the underlying cause of pancreatitis is gallstones, surgery may be warranted. Long-term treatments include a high carbohydrate and low fat diet as well as digestive enzyme supplementation.[22,28,29]

PHYSICAL THERAPY IMPLICATIONS

As stated previously, patients with GI diseases and disorders are not a common source of referral to physical therapy. However, GI complaints, especially abdominal discomfort, are common patient symptoms, and many hospitals include physical therapy in GI surgery postoperative management. Table 11–18 provides a survey of common examination procedures and findings associated with GI pathology, and Table 11–19 reviews the anatomic location of the viscera and reviews anatomic pain correlates. Therapists should recognize the potential in hospitalized patients for an **acute abdomen**, a sudden nontraumatic disorder whose chief manifestation is abdominal pain. Initial examination should determine the location, mode of onset, progression, and character of the pain.[21,30] This information is critical because an acute abdomen requires rapid recognition, diagnosis, and potential early surgery to optimize outcomes.[21,31] Examination finding may trigger consultation with the patient's nurses and physicians to initiate a more thorough examination.

Generally, there are no contraindications for patients with GI disease and disorders to participate in physical therapy. The examination process will guide therapeutic interventions (see Chapter 1 and Table 11–20). The high prevalence of PUD makes recognition important. Patients may have active bleeding or anemia making close monitoring of lab values and observation of hemodynamics necessary. Peptic ulcers are associated with chest or mid-thoracic back pain that may mimic cardiac disease (see Table 6–9). Additionally, exercise tends to increase acid secretion, which may exacerbate symptoms. Esophageal and stomach disorders in acute care can be limiting but are usually quick to resolve with proper medical and lifestyle interventions.

Table 11–18

Gastrointestinal System/Abdominal Examination

Examination Technique	Description of Technique	Examination Findings in Common Diseases/Disorders
Common questions/history	• Abdominal pain: Note onset, duration, character (eg, sharp, dull, stabbing), location/radiation to other areas • Vomiting: Color, fresh blood, "coffee grounds" • Stool characteristics (eg, color/consistency/ frequency/presence of blood–fresh blood vs black/tarry in appearance; diarrhea/constipation; incontinence • Urine characteristics (eg, color/amount/frequency/ presence of blood; incontinence–associated with activity/cough/sneeze, see Table 12–6)	**Pain characteristics:** • Burning (eg, peptic ulcer) • Cramping (eg, gastroenteritis) • Knifelike (eg, pancreatitis) • Gradual onset (eg, infection) **Anatomic Location of Pain,** see Table 11–19 **GI bleeding:** **Hematemesis:** Bloody vomitus, may be fresh, bright red blood or dark, grainy digested blood with "coffee ground" appearance **Melena:** Black, tarry, and foul-smelling stools caused by digestion of blood
Inspection of abdomen	Note general appearance and contour of the abdomen • Surface motion–pulsations/visible peristalsis • Scars/striae • Rashes/lesions • Ascites (the accumulation of fluid in the peritoneal cavity)/organomegaly/visible hernia • Presence of masses	**Abdominal distension:** Intestinal obstruction **Ascites:** Prominent abdomen or bulging flanks in supine (eg, liver disease/cirrhosis/portal hypertension) **Incisional hernia:** Protrusion of abdomen through incisional scar **Umbilical hernia:** Protrusion of navel (eg, common during pregnancy, ascites)
Palpation of abdomen	Note tenderness: Deep, superficial, guarding, rebound, or rigidity	**Local tenderness:** Intestinal obstruction/appendicitis/ cholecystitis/diverticulitis

Palpation: Always begin palpation lightly in a region where pain is NOT suspected and gradually move toward painful regions/quadrants

Rebound: Hold hand at 90-degree angle to abdomen, then press gently followed by a rapid withdrawal

Guarding: Voluntary contraction of the abdominal muscles due to tenderness, fear, or anxiety (eg, appendicitis, intestinal torsion [volvulus], fibrous adhesions)

Rebound: Abdominal tenderness that increases when the palpating fingers are quickly removed (eg, peritoneal inflammation/gastric and duodenal ulcers)

Rigidity: Involuntary contraction of the abdominal muscles due to peritoneal inflammation (eg, cholecystitis/gastric ulcer)

- Localized percussive tenderness suggests peritoneal inflammation
- Diffusely tympanic abdomen suggests intestinal obstruction
- Upward displacement of liver: liver atrophy, abdominal fluid, abdominal mass
- Downward displacement of liver: hepatomegaly, COPD/hyperinflation

↑ **Bowel sounds:** Hunger/gastroenteritis/diarrhea/diverticulitis

↓ **Bowel sounds/absent bowel sounds**

Peritoneal inflammation/paralytic obstruction or ileus

High-pitched ("tinkling") bowel sounds: Intestinal (mechanical) obstruction

Abdominal bruit: Aortic aneurysm/dissection; aneurysm or dissection of splenic, renal or iliac arteries

(continued)

Percussion of abdomen

Percussion should be performed in all four quadrants

- Note that the abdomen should have both tympanic regions (eg, stomach/gastric air bubble), gas filled bowel, and dull areas (eg, fluid filled bowel, liver)
- Percussion can be used to determine the span of the liver (~6 to 12 cm; upper border around the fifth to seventh intercostal space and lower border at or slightly below the costal margin

Auscultation

Bowel sounds ~ 5 to 34/minute; low pitch and "gurgling" in nature

Vascular sounds: Listen over aorta (midline/superior to umbilicus), renal (midclavicular line/superior to umbilicus), iliac (midclavicular line/inferior to umbilicus), and femoral arteries

Table 11–18 (continued)

GASTROINTESTINAL SYSTEM/ABDOMINAL EXAMINATION

Examination Technique	Description of Technique	Examination Findings in Common Diseases/Disorders
	Consider review of Clinical Laboratory Data (see Chapter 2, Tables 2–1, 2–13, 2–14, 2–15): • ALT/AST • Bilirubin • Amylase/Lipase • Albumin/prealbumin • Thrombin/prothrombin time • Platelet count	↑ AST/ALT: Hepatocyte inflammation/damage (eg, acute and chronic hepatitis/alcoholic cirrhosis, hepatic tumors, drug induced hepatotoxicity, MI) ↑ Bilirubin: hepatic damage, hemolytic anemia, biliary obstruction. ↓ Albumin: Advanced liver disease/cirrhosis ↑ Prothrombin time: Advanced liver disease, vitamin K deficiency, drugs (eg, warfarin) ↓ Platelets: Advanced liver disease, splemomegaly ↑ Amylase/Lipase: Pancreatitis, pancreatic and bile duct obstruction ↓ Amylase/Lipase: Chronic pancreatitis, pancreatic cancer, liver disease

Adapted from:
Fischbach FT, Dunning MB. *A Manual of Laboratory and Diagnostic Tests.* Philadelphia, Pa: Lippincott Williams & Wilkins; 2004.
Huether SE, McCance. *Understanding Pathophysiology.* St. Louis, Mo: Mosby-Year Book Inc; 1996.
Perloff JK. *Physical Examination of the Heart and Circulation.* 3rd ed. Philadelphia, Pa: WB Saunders Co; 2000.
Seidel HM, Ball JW, et al. *Mosby's Guide to Physical Examination.* St. Louis, Mo: Mosby, Inc; 2003.
Smith GC, Paterson-Brown S. The acute abdomen and intestinal obstruction. In: Garden OJ, Bradbury AW, Forsythe I, eds. *Principles and Practice of Surgery.* 4th ed. New York, NY: Churchill Livingstone; 2002.

Table 11–19

ANATOMIC REGIONS AND ABDOMINAL PAIN

Right Upper Quadrant

Anatomic structures:
- Liver and gall bladder
- Duodenum
- Head of pancreas
- Right adrenal gland
- Portion of right kidney

Causes of pain:
- Hepatitis
- Hepatomegaly
- Duodenal ulcer
- Cholecystitis
- Biliary stones
- Pneumonia

Left Upper Quadrant

Anatomic structures:
- Left lobe of liver
- Spleen
- Stomach
- Body of pancreas
- Portion of left kidney
- Portions of transverse and descending colon

Causes of pain:
- Splenic injury/ rupture
- Gastric ulcer
- Aortic aneurysm
- Perforated colon
- Pneumonia

Right Lower Quadrant

Anatomic structures:
- Lower pole, right kidney/ right ureter
- Cecum/ appendix
- Ascending colon

Causes of pain:
- Appendicitis
- Renal/ureteral stone
- Meckel diverticulum
- Regional ileitis

Left Lower Quadrant

Anatomic structures:
- Lower pole, left kidney/left ureter
- Sigmoid colon
- Portion of descending colon

Causes of pain:
- Sigmoid diverticulitis
- Renal/ureteral stone
- Perforated colon
- UC
- Regional ileitis

Umbilical and Epigastric Regions

Anatomic structures:
- Pyloric end of stomach
- Duodenum/jejunum/ileum
- Pancreas
- Portion of liver
- Omentum
- Mesentary

Causes of pain:
- Intestinal obstruction
- Acute pancreatitis
- Aortic aneurysm
- Diverticulitis
- Mesenteric thrombosis
- Hiatal hernia

Adapted from:
Huether SE, McCance. *Understanding Pathophysiology.* St. Louis, Mo: Mosby-Year Book Inc; 1996.
Seidel HM, Ball JW, et al. *Mosby's Guide to Physical Examination.* St. Louis, Mo: Mosby, Inc; 2003.

Table 11–20

EXAMPLE OF COMMON THERAPEUTIC INTERVENTIONS
FOR THE GASTROINTESTINAL PATIENT

Breathing Exercises:

- Deep breathing/inspiratory holds
- Incentive spirometry
- Huffing/directed cough
- Chest percussion/vibration

Early Mobilization:

- Log-rolling/bracing with pillow
- Transfer/gait training
- Progressive ambulation

Patient Education:

- Lifestyle modifications
- Ostomy care

Multidisciplinary Communication:

- Pain assessment and control
- Ostomy care
- Report increased pain/fever/nausea/vomiting/bloating/change stools/ diarrhea/signs of wound infection
- Discharge planning/recommendations

Patients with IBS and malabsorptive diseases can be malnourished, cachectic, and have frequent bouts of diarrhea. These side effects have the potential to leave patients dehydrated and deficient in essential nutrients, vitamins, and minerals. Nutritional deficiencies increase the risk for osteoarthritis, osteoporosis, kidney and gallstones, liver dysfunction, and muscular weakness and atrophy.

Medications must also be considered. Patients with Crohn's disease and UC are often prescribed corticosteroids for prolonged periods of time. The long-term effects of these medications include hyperglycemia and diabetes, fluid retention, muscle wasting, and peripheral neuropathies.

Abdominal surgical interventions, including esophageal procedures, require significant attentiveness by the therapist. Postoperative pulmonary complications are a major cause of morbidity and mortality after abdominal surgery resulting in prolonged hospitalization and admission into the ICU.[32] The incidence of postoperative complications ranges from 4.5% to 80% of patients after upper abdominal surgery.[33,34] Postoperative pain, drugs, CNS suppression via anesthesia, immobilization, and pre-existing lung disease all play a major role in the development of complications including atelectasis and pneumonia. It has been shown that physical therapy including deep breathing exercises, huffing, coughing, and early mobilization can improve oxygen saturation and reduce the incidence of postoperative pulmonary complication after major abdominal surgery.[35,36] In summary, patients who have undergone abdominal surgery are at risk for pulmonary complications, and all should be involved in an airway clearance and mobility regimen.

Early ambulation decreases postoperative complication rates, stimulates peristalsis, decreases the need for pain control, increases bladder pressures allowing removal of the Foley catheter and normal elimination, provides DVT prophylaxis, and may reduce overall hospital length of stay. If appropriate, allow patients to use a rolling walker. Rolling walkers may enhance dynamic standing balance but eliminate the need to lift and be unsupported while in transition. Additionally, patients frequently report reduced discomfort with a forward leaning posture.

Postoperative pain is often difficult to manage, and it is prudent for the physical therapy practitioner to coordinate pain management and the therapy session. Splinting of the incision with a pillow or the addition of an abdominal binder for transfers and gait training and instruction in "log rolling" for bed mobility tasks may lessen discomfort.

Patient education should include abdominal protection. In general, activity restrictions include no driving, swimming, or active abdominal exercise for 4 to 6 weeks postoperatively, and minimize lifting anything greater than 5 to 10 pounds. However, the therapist must collaborate with the surgeons to determine appropriateness of all activity restrictions.

Finally, the therapist must consider the psychosocial aspect of GI disease and dysfunction. Acceptance of defecating into an ostomy bag is often difficult. Always ensure that the colostomy bag is properly attached around the stoma to prevent accidental displacement and spillage. Coordination with an ostomy specialist may allow the performance of ostomy care, providing needed practice for the patient. Many GI conditions are chronic in nature, difficult to diagnose, and present with a perceived social stigma that may challenge the patient psychologically.

THE ENVIRONMENT AND PATIENT SUPPORT EQUIPMENT

Performing examinations and interventions of patients with GI disease is often a challenge to the physical therapist/physical therapist assistant. Patients may have multiple IV lines, catheters, and drains. Below is a list of common patient support equipment that may be encountered during therapeutic interactions with the postoperative GI patient.

- **IV fluids**: Clear, sterile water or saline solutions with varying degrees of dextrose and other essential electrolytes (ie, D5 ½ NS, lactated ringers). The primary function of these fluids is for rehydration, blood volume expansion, and correction of electrolyte abnormalities (see Pharmacological Information, Chapter 12).

- **TPN**: TPN is the delivery of food and nutrients intravenously. TPN bypasses the alimentary canal allowing the intestines to rest or heal, or if there are absorption deficiencies, it provides missing nutritional elements to the patient. The formula is customized for each patient and is based on basic nutritional elements as well as height, weight, and desired nutritional needs.

- **Enteral nutrition**: Unlike TPN, enteral feedings are delivered into the alimentary canal directly via the stomach or small intestine. Examples of these are percutaneous enteral gastrostomy (PEG), gastrostomy (G-tube), jejonostomy (J-tube), and on a temporary basis, nasogastric (NG) tube. Food is delivered at a specific rate and is calculated for the amount of calories a patient will require per day.

- **PRBC/FFP**: Packed red blood cells (PRBCs) or fresh frozen plasma (FFP) are two common transfusions in the postoperative patient. Often in GI or other types of surgery, there is preoperative, intraoperative, or postoperative bleeding. When this occurs (or occurs in conditions that cause bleeding [eg, ulcers, UC, esophageal varices] or anemia), PRBC is ordered to increase the oxygen carrying capacity of blood (reflected by an increase in the Hct/Hgb) or FFP is infused to expand blood volume. While these blood products are infusing, therapy is generally withheld due to close observation for deleterious transfusion reactions.

Non-Intravenous Equipment

Beyond IVs, there are several things that a therapist may encounter when examining the patient. Postoperatively, the patient may have devices that drain excess blood and/or fluids from the wound, either mechanically or manually. Examples of those include the following:

- **Jackson-Pratt drains (JP):** These small, grenade-like looking drains are surgically placed into the wound to aid in the removal of fluids. They create a small vacuum that draws fluid into the receptacle.

- **Sump drains:** These larger drains are surgically placed into the wound and are then connected to a suction device to mechanically remove the contents from the wound.

These drains are common in the management of fistulas and nonhealing open wounds.

- **Foley catheter:** The Foley catheter is placed directly into the bladder to assist or provide urine removal. When a patient undergoes general anesthesia, the entire body, including the muscles of the bladder, is medically paralyzed. The Foley catheter allows elimination of urine as well as an accurate assessment of body fluid output.

Case Study

Mr. Taylor is a 52-year-old (y/o) male with a 25+-year h/o GERD and Barrett's esophagus. The patient underwent an esophagectomy with gastric pull-up following an annual endoscopy, which revealed esophageal carcinoma. Physical therapy was consulted to initiate ambulation and assist with discharge planning on postoperative day 1.

Patient/Client History
General Demographics/Social History/Living Environment

Mr. Taylor is married and lives in a second floor apartment and has one son who is 10. He is a manager in an automotive parts store.

General Health Status/Family History

Mr. Taylor denies smoking and limited ethonal (ETOH) use.

Medical/Surgical History

Mr. Taylor is a 52 y/o male with >25 year h/o GERD and Barrett's esophagus and recent diagnosis of esophageal carcinoma. He underwent a 6.5-hour esophageal pull-up and is 1 day postsurgery.

Current Conditions/Chief Complaints

Mr. Taylor is awake and complaining of pain and soreness in his stomach area and along the incision on a scale of 6 out of 10. He has a nasal cannula running at 3 liters/minute, a nasal gastric tube, a right upper extremity (RUE) intravenous (IV) line for fluids and antibiotics, and a Foley catheter.

Functional Status and Activity Level

Mr. Taylor was independent in functional activities prior to surgery. He states that he has not participated in any type of exercise program since playing spring and summer softball 5 years ago.

Other Clinical Tests

Abnormal laboratory findings: CBC revealed hemoglobin=10.4 g/dL, WBCs >11,500/mm^3, and electrolytes were sodium <130 mEq/L and potassium of 3.3 mEq/L.

Systems Review
Cardiovascular/Pulmonary

Resting vital signs in bed (head of bed raised > 40 degrees) are oxygen saturation (SpO$_2$) 95% on 3 liters nasal cannula, heart rate (HR) 96, respiratory rate (RR) 20, blood pressure (BP) 110/85, and pain 6/10. Range of motion (ROM), manual muscle test (MMT), bed mobility, and transfers revealed a vital sign response of SpO$_2$ 96%, HR 102, RR 24, BP 100/85, and pain 8/10. Mr. Taylor is hoarse and his breath sounds are diminished at his bases with decreased chest expansion. His cough is poor and nonproductive. Gait with a rolling walker of 50 feet demonstrated a vital sign response of SpO$_2$ 96%, HR 124, RR 24, BP 146/85, and pain 8/10. The nurse was informed of his complaints of pain and coordination of pain medication was discussed prior to future therapy sessions. Mr. Taylor also complained of some nausea and "dry heaves" prior to the therapy session.

Integumentary

Mr. Taylor has a nasal gastric tube in place held by adhesive tape, RUE IV line, a Foley catheter, and a large thoracoabdominal surgical dressing with two drains. His skin appears to be dry and intact, and there is +2 edema in both ankles.

Musculoskeletal

Strength by MMT was 5/5 in all extremities, trunk not assessed due to surgical dressing/incision. ROM was within normal limits. Bed mobility supine to sit and transfers sit to stand was minimal assistance of one. He was able to ambulate with the rolling walker 50 feet with assistance of contact guard to minimal assistance of one.

Neuromuscular

Sensation was intact with point soreness over upper abdomen, scalenes/sternocleidomastoid (SCM), and upper trapezius.

Communication, Affect, Cognition, Language, and Learning Style

Mr. Taylor is awake, alert, and oriented times 4. His primary language is English, but he can understand Spanish.

Tests and Measures

Aerobic Capacity and Endurance

Mr. Taylor demonstrated appropriate vital responses for being 1 day following surgery and not being regularly active prior to surgery. His initial drop in BP with upright activities could be related to pain medications or prolonged bed rest and should improve with continued out of bed (OOB) activities. His tachycardia is expected secondary to pain. His cough, diminished breaths sounds, and poor chest expansion signify risk for pulmonary complications following GI surgery. Laboratory findings suggestive of either infection or related to cancer. Hypokalemia and low sodium and edema suggest hypervolemic hyponatremia and may be related to IV fluids, GI loss, diminished intake, or underlying disease. The therapist should monitor the ECG secondary to electrolyte abnormalities.

Assistive and Adaptive Devices

Recommend Mr. Taylor continue to progress his functional level using a rolling walker that allows him to maintain his forward leaning posture, reducing his pain.

Gait, Locomotion, and Balance

Mr. Taylor was able to ambulate with the rolling walker 50 feet with contact guard assistance to minimal assistance of one. His static and dynamic balances were diminished without the assistive device in standing and during ambulation primarily related to a forward leaning posture.

Pain

Mr. Taylor had an increase in pain level with activity that was expected. Recommend coordinating therapy with pain medication delivery.

Diagnosis

The patient presents with mild to moderate impairments related to sedentary lifestyle prior to surgery and the effects of a large thoracoabdominal surgical procedure for removal of cancer and Barrett's esophagus. Recommend treatment pattern 6B: impaired aerobic capacity/endurance associated with deconditioning.[37]

Prognosis

Mr. Taylor should progress rapidly with therapy in conjunction with pain management and airway clearance. Discharge from the hospital to home is expected.

Intervention

The plan of care included breathing exercises such as incentive spirometry and splinted coughing as well as ambulation TID (three times a day). He was instructed to sit OOB for a minimum 6 hours (including meal times) per day. Mr. Taylor was seen three times per week to advance his mobility program, determine effectiveness of airway clearance, and assess stair climbing prior to discharge home.

Reexamination

Following three physical therapy sessions the NG, Foley, and IV access have been removed. Mr. Taylor reports decreased abdominal and thoracic discomfort and rates his pain at 2–3/10. He is independent with bed mobility, transfers, and ambulates >150 feet TID with supervision and no assistive device. He ascends/descends 12 steps with one rail with supervision.

Outcomes

The plan is to discharge him from the hospital to his home with no additional therapy services.

CHAPTER REVIEW QUESTIONS

1. What are the primary functions of the GI system?
2. Describe the pathophysiology of GERD, and provide risk factors for the development of this GI disorder.
3. Why do gastric acids not erode the stomach and lead to the development of ulcers?
4. What are at least two precipitating factors for development of acute gastritis?
5. What are some implications pertaining to physical therapy when treating a patient with Crohn's disease?

Surgical Information: Obesity and Gastric Bypass Surgeries

Esther H. Bae, MPT
Robin Stott-McNulty, MPT

Prevalence

The prevalence of obesity is increasing every year in the United States. According to the Centers for Disease Control and Prevention, obesity has increased by more than 60% in the past 10 years, and approximately 59 million adults are obese.[38] According to National Health and Nutrition Examination Survey (NHANES), the prevalence of obesity among the adult United States (US) population was 65.7% between 2001 and 2002. The prevalence of obesity was estimated to be 30.6%, and extreme obesity was estimated at 5.1%.[39] In the United States, about 300,000 deaths a year are attributed to obesity, making it second only to smoking as the most common preventable cause of death.[40] Obesity affects society in many different aspects such as the cost and quality of health care and risk factors for other diseases.

The World Health Organization (WHO) uses the body mass index (BMI) to classify body overweight and levels of obesity as noted in Table 11–21. BMI is defined as weight in kilograms divided by height in meters squared (kg/m^2).

Causes of Obesity/Risk Factors

Obesity is caused by many factors such as genetics, physiology, behavior, environment, culture, and socioeconomic status. Studies have shown that the severely obese population has a significantly higher intake of total fat and report lower activity levels than the normal weight population.[41] In 2000, 27.0% of US adults did not engage in any leisure-time physical activity and another 28.2% were not regularly active.[42] Inadequate amounts of physical activity and exercise are associated with requiring more medications, visiting physicians more often, and being hospitalized more frequently. Research has shown that obesity increases the risk of developing various health conditions including Type 2 diabetes mellitus, hypertension, coronary heart disease, stroke, colon cancer, postmenopausal breast cancer, endometrial cancer, gall bladder disease, osteoarthritis, asthma, and obstructive sleep apnea.[43,44] As weight increases, so does the prevalence of health risks (Table 11–22). In addition, higher BMIs are associated with reduced life expectancies.[45]

Obesity is not only a risk factor for developing devastating illnesses, it also impacts the individual's health-related quality of life (HRQL). Overweightness is associated with poorer functional status such as walking, climbing stairs, and working, as well as pain, a negative health perception, and restricted activity.[40] Studies demonstrate that obesity is associated with a significant likelihood of disability, pain-associated activity restrictions, and depressive symptoms.[46,47]

Table 11–21

CLASSIFICATION OF WEIGHT USING BODY MASS INDEX

BMI (kg/m²)

	BMI (kg/m²)
Underweight	<18.5
Normal range	18.5 to 24.9
Overweight	25.0 to 29.9
Obese Class I	30.0 to 34.9
Obese Class II	35.0 to 39.9
Obese Class III	>40.0

Adapted from Must A, Spadano J, Coakley EH, et al. The disease burden associated with overweight and obesity. *JAMA*. 1999;282:1523–1529.

Impact on Health Care System

Obesity affects the cost of health care not only in direct medical cost but also in indirect costs. In 2000, the total cost of obesity in the United States was estimated to be $117 billion. Included in the $117 billion were $61 billion for direct medical costs and $56 billion for indirect costs.[38] Direct medical costs include preventive, diagnostic, and treatment services. Indirect costs include value of income lost from decreased productivity, restricted activity, absenteeism, and value of future income lost by premature death. In 2003, obesity-attributable medical expenditures were estimated at $75 billion in the United States with $17 million financed by Medicare and $21 million financed by Medicaid.[48]

Weight Reduction

Weight reduction is associated with an improved HRQL. Weight loss induced by surgical intervention improves HRQL as measured by the SF-36. Studies have demonstrated that severely obese people who lose weight from surgical interventions tend to begin or return to work. Additionally, modest weight reduction using lifestyle modification of moderately obese people can enhance HRQL.[40]

The goals for treatment are to achieve and then to maintain clinically significant weight loss. Weight loss reduces the risk of obesity-related diseases, impairments, and functional limitations, and weight losses of 5% to 10% of initial body weight produce health benefits.[49] There are many different weight management techniques in treating obesity including proper nutrition, regular physical activity and exercise, behavior modification, pharmacological agents, and surgery. The method for losing weight depends on the individual's needs.

Prescribing exercise for the obese individual will be different than for a normal weight individual. The goal for the obese individual is to increase caloric expenditure at the low end of the target HR range for a longer duration. The adult should aim to expend 300 to 500 kcal per session and 1000 to

Table 11–22

CLASSIFICATION OF RISK FOR METABOLIC COMPLICATIONS OF OBESITY*

BMI CATEGORY* (kg/m²)

Waist Circumference	18.5 to 24.9	25.0 to 29.9	30.0 to 34.9	35.0 to 39.9	≥40
<40" for men <35" for women	—	Increased	High	Very high	Extremely high
>40" for men >35" for women	Increased	High	Very high	Very high	Extremely high

*Waist circumference is measured midway between the lowest rib and the iliac crest; acceptable waist circumference is less than 40" (102 cm) in a man and less than 35" (88 cm) in a woman.

From World Health Organization: Measuring obesity: classification and description of anthropometric data. Copenhagen: WHO; 1989. From Sleisenger & Fordtran's *Gastrointestinal and Liver Disease*. 7th ed. 2002. With permission from Elsevier.

2000 kcal per week. The exercise program should progress to increasing the intensity to bring the target HR to the higher range. Different modes of exercise can include walking, cycling, and water exercise. Exercise precautions include activities that exacerbate pain, avoiding excess stress on joints and any restrictions prescribed by the individual's physician.[50]

Bariatrics (Medical Treatment of Obesity)

Clinically severe obesity is defined as an individual with a BMI of 40 kg/m² (Obese Class III), which is estimated as 100 pounds overweight (see Table 11–21). An increasing number of people in the United States are falling into this category. Between 2001 and 2002 the prevalence of obesity with BMI greater than 40 kg/m² was estimated at 5.1%, which is a significant increase from 2.9% from 1988 to 1994.[40,51] More people are turning to surgical intervention for long-term weight control. The age of gastric bypass patients range from mid 20s to mid 60s with about 70% being female.[52]

The NIH has established criteria for bariatric surgery patients in 1998. The criteria states that patients must be selected carefully and must have clinically severe obesity. Clinically severe obesity is defined as a patient with a BMI of 40 or greater (approximately 100 pounds overweight) or 35 or greater with obesity related co-morbidities (such as diabetes, high BP, sleep apnea). The patient must have failed less invasive weight loss measures and be at risk for obesity-associated illness.

Comprehensive preoperative screening and patient education ensure that appropriate candidates are considered for surgery. The initial consultation with the surgeon includes a complete history and physical examination,

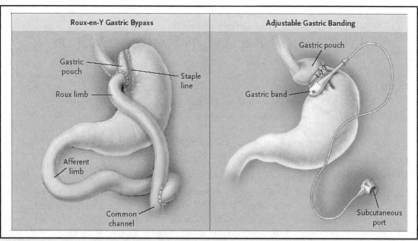

Figure 11–6. Commonly used bariatric surgical procedures. (Adapted from Steinbrook R. Surgery for severe obesity. *N Engl J Med*. 2004;350:1078.)

nutrition screening, and education regarding the surgical procedure. Other consultants may include a psychologist and nutritionist. In addition, patients must be cleared medically by a combination of internal medicine, cardiology, endocrinology, and pulmonary medicine. Periodically, patients must undergo a physical therapy evaluation prior to surgery. Some patients are also seen by vascular surgery to have an inferior vena cava (IVC) filter placed at the time of surgery to prevent blood clots from traveling to the lungs. The time frame from initial visit until surgery can take up to 2 months.

Surgical Procedures

Common surgical procedures include vertical banded gastroplasty and open gastric bypass with roux en Y anastamosis as noted in Figure 11–6. Both procedures can be performed laparoscopically, hand-assisted, or using an open technique.

The gastric bypass with roux en Y anastamosis has become the gold standard for bariatric surgery in the United States. This surgery includes the creation of a small gastric pouch attached to a limb of small intestine. This creates a restrictive component (patients can only consume a small amount of food) and a malabsorbtive component (the duodenum is bypassed). This combination results in excellent weight loss and resolution of co-morbidities.

The vertical banded gastroplasty is a version of bariatric surgery that is an option for some patients who are not candidates for gastric bypass surgery (due to technical complexity or existing medical conditions). This procedure consists of the creation of a small stomach pouch with a band placed at the distal aspect. This results in restriction of the amount of food one can consume and, thus, subsequent weight loss.

Table 11–23
COMORBIDITY IMPROVEMENTS FOLLOWING SURGERY

Diabetes	95%
Hypertension	92%
Cardiac function	95%
Osteoarthritis	82%
Sleep apnea	75%
Elevated cholesterol	97%
Gastroesophageal reflux	98%
Stress incontinence	87%

The table lists the percentage of patients whose health problems related to obesity resolve or improve within 5 years of surgery.
Adapted from Wittgrove AC, Clark GW. Laparoscopic gastric bypass Roux-en-Y—500 patients: technique and results with 3–60 month follow-up. *Obesity Surgery.* 2000;10:233–239.

Postoperative Process

After the procedure, patients remain in the hospital for approximately 4 days. This population has unique issues with cardiovascular, pulmonary, and thromboembolic complications postoperatively. Postlewait and Johnson found that the mortality rate in obese patients was 6.6% compared with 2.6% in nonobese patients undergoing GI surgery. Patients with clinically severe obesity have a higher incidence of comorbidities, including diabetes mellitus, hypertension, left ventricular hypertrophy, and gastroesophageal reflux. They experience an increase in cardiopulmonary complications such as obesity-hypoventilation syndrome, obstructive sleep apnea syndrome, pulmonary hypertension, and right ventricular failure. All of these factors make this patient population high risk.[53]

Bariatric patients can experience postoperative complications such as pain, hypoxemia, and atelectasis. In these patients, postoperative pain limits mobility and the ability to breathe deeply. As a result of atelectasis, 75% of patients will exhibit arterial oxygen pressure <60 mmHg after open gastric bypass surgery.[54] For these patients, early mobilization and encouraging deep breathing or the use of the incentive spirometer is vital.

Follow-up visits are scheduled for 1 week, 2 months, 6 months, and annually following surgery. These visits are a combined meeting with the nurse practitioner, surgeon, and nutritionist. Patients are also encouraged to continue attending support groups postoperatively because both they and patients new to the group benefit from this social interaction.

Surgical interventions are effective and safe for weight loss. Not only do patients, on average, lose 70% of their excess body weight 12 to 18 months following surgery, but patients' obesity-related health problems (such as

type 2 diabetes, obstructive sleep apnea, asthma, hypertension, elevated cholesterol, and degenerative joint disease)[55] are significantly improved or resolved
within 1 to 5 years from surgery (Table 11–23). A significant proportion of
gastric bypass patients are able to discontinue or decrease medications to treat
obesity-related co-morbidities.[51] Long-term survival rates are favorable. One
study documented a 91% 10-year survival rate after a bariatric procedure.[56]

Patients also experience a significant improvement in their quality of life.
Between 3 and 6 months following surgery, patients often describe a sudden
increase in energy. With this newfound energy, they are able to participate in
family activities and enjoy more productive careers.

Prejudice and Attitude

Clinically obese people often experience discrimination and abuse in society. However, most obese patients do not expect mistreatment by health care
professionals.[57] Obese people might believe that health care professionals better understand the factors contributing to obesity and would be more sensitive
to their condition. A study by Harvey and Hill noted that attitudes toward the
obese by physicians were neutral to negative.[58] Physicians have noted that they
spend less time with obese patients and are more likely to attribute medical
problems to the patient's obesity as a "catch-all" etiology.[59] Past studies have
also shown that health care professionals associated obese patients with poor
hygiene, hostility, and laziness.[60]

Hebl and Xu found that physicians discussed weight loss and nutrition
issues with less than 45% of obese and overweight patients, believing that
many could not lose weight.[60] One study showed that while many health care
professionals are supportive of the conditions of obese patients, the majority
do not have appropriately sized gowns, sphygmomanometers, examination
tables, or chairs for their obese patients. Despite the fact that the patients in
this study were not blatantly discriminated against, the lack of easily attainable equipment for obese patients shows a lack of consideration and may be
considered prejudicial.[58] Making simple accommodations may make obese
patients feel more comfortable and more likely to seek health care.[61]

The negative attitudes of health care professionals may initiate a vicious
cycle for obese patients. Health care professionals treat obese patients less
favorably causing obese patients to treat themselves poorly. Obese patients
may respond negatively toward this unfavorable treatment, in turn reinforcing
the negative attitudes of health care professionals. Obese patients may avoid
seeking any health care based on their negative experiences contributing to the
elevated mortality rate of this population.[62]

If physical therapists realize that they have biases and that they are affecting the quality of care delivered, then they may be able to change the way they
act toward obese patients. A method that physical therapist can use to evaluate
whether his or her biases are affecting treatments is the use of patient satisfac-
tion surveys.

The Role of Physical Therapist

Managing and supporting patients who undergo gastric bypass surgery takes a collaborative multidisciplinary team approach starting at the initial examination, continuing throughout the hospital stay and recovery. It is important that a physical therapist is involved in each phase of bariatric care. The evaluation of preoperative functional status is critical for identifying those patients who may require more intensive physical therapy. Patients who are wheelchair dependent, already using assistive devices, limited to household mobility, or have joint problems inhibiting mobility have preoperative safety risks, experience a longer recovery phase, have more postoperative pulmonary complications, less postoperative mobility, and could require further rehabilitation after acute care. A physical therapist who examines and evaluates these patients preoperatively can make immediate recommendations for appropriate assistive devices to improve safety and teach therapeutic exercises to strengthen muscles and improve mobilization in preparation for surgery.

Postoperative examinations by a physical therapist are suggested on all gastric bypass patients. The goal of the physical therapist is to assess patient needs, develop a plan of care, facilitate safe mobilization, and identify discharge recommendations.

The physical therapist collects the following information on the initial evaluation:

Social History

- **Support systems:** Identify who are the patient's significant others and what role they will play in his or her recovery.
- **Living environment:** House or apartment, location of stairs inside and outside the home, and other factors such as presence of stair railings, spiral, width and height, and covering of stairs.
- **Personal hygiene:** Location of and ability to use bathrooms or availability of commode. Identify patient's bathing habits at home and ability to use shower or tubs or sponge bathing.
- **Functional status:** Identify assistive devices used preoperatively and performance of ADLs preoperatively. Ability to manage outside the home and normal means of transportation.
- **Sleep habits:** Identify where patient slept preoperatively (eg, bed, couch, recliner chair), use of Bipap machine, hours he or she slept, and use of medications for sleep.

Past Medical History

The physical therapist performs a thorough chart review identifying health history, medication history, and psychosocial factors. This information is used to direct the physical assessment performed, planning and monitoring of interventions, and development of plan for patient education.

Systems Review

- **Cardiovascular/pulmonary assessment:** Measure the resting HR, BP, and RR to obtain a baseline status prior to mobilization. Oscillometric BP cuffs that encircle at least 75% of the arm should be used.[63] Reliable BP readings can also be obtained from the wrist or ankle.[64] This is important because most standardized BP cuffs will not fit properly around the bicep of bariatric patients. Auscultate heart and lung sounds and compare to previously documented assessments. Document and report any changes or concerns.

- **Musculoskeletal:** Assess gross ROM and range of strength. Identify bony or soft tissue restrictions and any abnormal movement patterns.

- **Neuromuscular:** Assess and identify any abnormalities with sensation. Static and dynamic balance should also be assessed in sitting and standing positions. Mobility is assessed as well including transfers and ambulation. This assessment will be performed over multiple treatment sessions based on patient's ability to mobilize.

- **Integumentary:** The excessive body weight puts this patient population at risk for increased injury to the skin over pressure areas and nerve injuries during the operative and postoperative time periods. Brachial plexus and sciatic nerve palsies have been reported. Stretch injuries may be caused by either extreme abduction of the arms or the excessive upright positioning of the patient's outstretched arms, both of which can put stress on the brachial plexus. The sciatic nerve, the lateral femoral cutaneous nerve, and the ulnar nerve are also susceptible to traction injuries. Ulnar neuropathy has been associated with increased BMI. In a retrospective analysis from Mayo clinic, 29% of patients with ulnar neuropathy in their series had a BMI >38 kg/m^2.[64] A neurology consultation should be obtained when a nerve injury is suspected. Most postoperative nerve injuries will resolve spontaneously. Perform careful inspection of the skin to identify ulcers, tears, and pressure areas. Skin folds need to be inspected for break down and infections. Assess drains sites, wounds, and areas of edema. Edema is often mistaken for adipose tissue.

Tests and Measures

Important tests and measures for this population include aerobic capacity and endurance such as pre- and postactivity vital signs since the patient will not be able to tolerate a standardized exercise test protocol. The therapist should also observe the patient for cardiovascular and pulmonary signs and symptoms of increased oxygen demand such as dyspnea, increased respiratory rate, patient's perception on exertion scales (eg, Borg scale), and patient reports of lightheadedness, angina, excessive perspiration, or sudden pallor.

Anthropometric characteristics may be helpful in evaluating the patient to compose a plan of care. There measurements include weight and height to obtain a BMI and objective assessments of edema.

Table 11–24

THINGS TO CONSIDER BEFORE GETTING THE PATIENT OUT OF BED

- When was the last time the patient was medicated for pain?
- Would an overhead trapeze help the patient to maneuver in bed?
- Is there an air mattress on the bed?
- Do you have the appropriate chair to place the patient into, and will he or she fit?
- Is the chair too low to the ground, making it difficult for the patient to get out of it?
- What if the patient has to go to the bathroom? Could you get the patient to the bathroom or is there a commode in the room?
- How long should the patient be OOB?
- What is the plan for getting the patient back to bed? Who will be available to assist?

Pain should always be assessed at rest and with activity. The pain analog scale (rating pain from 0 to 10) is useful to objectify the patient's pain. Location of the pain should be documented as well to differentiate between incisional pain, referred pain, or any new complaints of pain.

Mobilization

Early mobilization is critical in this patient population, but it can be very challenging and time consuming, requiring a team approach, including involvement of the patient. Based on the examination and evaluation, the therapist identifies a plan for mobilization and secures the proper resources. The therapist must discuss the treatment plan with the patient, listen to suggestions or concerns of the patient, and modify the plan as appropriate. The key to early mobilization is to develop a trusting relationship with the patient, minimize patient anxiety, and to experience a successful treatment session for both the patient and the care team.

Safety for the staff and the patient is a primary concern. Securing the proper number of professional staff and having appropriate equipment is very important. The number of staff and type of equipment needed should be based on the patient's preoperative functional status, weight, BMI, and current clinical condition. The physical therapist acts as the team leader directing the other staff and must be trained in the use of the equipment.

Mobilization and ambulation should begin as early postoperatively as possible with the goal of having the patient at baseline functional status at time of discharge. Common considerations and suggestions to aide in the mobilization of the obese patient are provided in Tables 11–24 through 11–27.

Table 11–25

ASSISTING THE PATIENT FROM SUPINE TO SITTING POSITION

Always utilize available equipment. If the patient is in a bed that converts into a chair, place bed in sitting position. Have the patient come forward and make sure the feet can touch the ground.

Minimal assistance: If the patient is able to get to the edge of bed with minimal assistance, then the air mattress should be deflated prior to mobilization to allow the patient to move more easily. Use of cloth under pads or draw sheets is often necessary to assist the patient to get in a sitting position.

Moderate to maximum assistance: When the patient requires this level of assistance, the therapist must utilize good body mechanics to reduce the chance of injury. Encourage the patient to assist with mobility. The therapist must make sure the patient does not attempt to pull on any of the care providers. Place bed in semi-fowlers position, one person assists in moving legs to side of bed while another person uses a gait belt to bring the patient to a sitting position. Weight of fat and skin around midsection may alter the center of gravity with a forward motion, so the therapist must be positioned in front to support the patient. Caution: If the patient is brought to a sitting position too far near the foot of the bed, some beds may tip.

Table 11–26

ASSISTING THE PATIENT FROM SITTING TO STANDING

Before getting the patient to a standing position, the therapist must assess the height of the patient and the lowest height of the bed. The patient's feet have to completely touch the floor so the patient can successfully return his or her buttocks back on the bed surface. If the patient is too short, the therapist will need to have the patient stand on a stool that can support the body weight.

Place gait belt around the lower back or mid buttocks, take up the slack, and secure a tight grip.

Follow the 90/90 rule. You must maintain hip, knee, trunk ratio to prevent a potentially dangerous situation. Always have the patient scoot forward at the hip—avoid having the patient slide his or her hips forward.

Minimal assist: Place walker in front of patient, therapist and another staff on either side of patient, each gripping an end of the gait belt. Assist patient to standing position.

Moderate to maximum assistance: Same as above except an additional therapist is needed to block the knees to prevent buckling.

Perform sit to stand transfer three times before proceeding to ambulation.

If the patient is a total dependent transfer, use a total lift machine designed to support the weight of the patient.

Table 11–27

Assist the Patient With Transfer/Ambulation

- Have the patient march in place several times using the walker.
- Have the patient take two or three steps with the walker while the therapist assesses the gait. Progress to stand pivot transfer. Make sure the patient has a chair to transfer to and avoid chairs that are too low to the ground. Getting the patient out of the chair will often be more challenging than getting him or her OOB. Be sure to have at minimum the same team/resource available to return the patient to bed.
- While patient is up, make sure he or she is in upright position have him or her complete therapeutic ex program (eg, UE D1 and D2 PNF patterns with breathing exercises incorporated for pulmonary issues).

Monitoring the Patient During the Physical Therapy Session

Vital signs (HR, BP, RR, SpO_2, and perceived exertion) must be monitored throughout the session because it may influence the physical therapist's decision about physical therapy intervention. If the patient complains of dyspnea or presents with signs of respiratory compromise, proceed cautiously during physical activities. "Central adiposity may be responsible for mechanical restrictions of breathing particularly in sitting or supine positions, even in the absence of pulmonary disease."[29] The physical therapist should be aware of patterns of pain or postural dysfunction that are consistent with long-term stress on weightbearing joints in patients who are obese.[29]

Education

Educating the patient on pressure-relieving techniques is important in this population. Patients should be educated on the frequent performance of deep breathing or incentive spirometry and lower extremity (LE) exercises. Education should include limiting activities that cause friction and shearing of skin. Patients should be advised to begin an exercise regimen including a walking program prior to discharge.

Conclusion

Obesity is a chronic health condition that is reaching epidemic proportions especially in the United States. The impact on an individual, the health care system and society becomes more evident everyday. The number of bariatric surgical procedures is increasing and success depends on a multidisciplinary approach to the care of these patients. Physical therapists are an integral part of this team. Physical therapists must understand that they will be caring for obese patients in every health care setting and must develop multiple strategies for treating this patient population.

PHARMACOLOGICAL INFORMATION: GASTROINTESTINAL DISEASES AND DISORDERS PHARMACOLOGY

Antidiarrheals

Action
Antidiarrheals provide control and symptomatic relief from chronic and acute nonspecific diarrhea. These medications slow GI motility, enhance absorption of intestinal fluids, or provide bulk to stools.

Side Effects
CNS: Dizziness, confusion, drowsiness, headache
CV: Tachycardia
GI: Constipation, fullness, urinary retention
Misc: Allergic reactions

Common Medications
Loperamide (Kaopectate/Immodium/Maalox), diphenoxylate/atropine (Logen/Lomotil, Lonox); bismuth subsalicylate (eg, Pepto-Bismol) and colloidal bismuth subcitrate (eg, De-Nol); polycarbophil (FiberCon/Fiberall)

Antiemetics

Action
Antiemetics manage nausea and vomiting associated with motion sickness, surgery, anesthesia, chemo/radiation therapy treatment. Drugs may act by antihistamine, anticholinergic, or serotonin blockage with subsequent CNS depression.

Side Effects
CNS: Sedation, confusion, disorientation, fatigue
CV: Brady/tachycardia, hyper/hypotension, palpitations
GI: Constipation, dry mouth
Misc: Allergic reactions, rash, photosensitivity

Common Medications
Prochlorperzine (Compazine), Promethazine (Anergan, Phenazine, Phenergan), Dimenhydrinate (Dimetabs/Dramamine), Granisetron (Kytril), Ondansetron (Zofran)

Antacids

Action
Antacids promote healing of gastric ulcers by neutralizing gastric acid. Other proposed benefits include stimulation of mucus and bicarbonate secretion, binding of bile salts, enhanced gastric blood flow, and inhibition of pepsin

activity. The treatment of PUD with antacids generally is less convenient, less palatable, and less effective for the long-term control of gastric acidity.

Side Effects
GI: Belching, abdominal fullness or distension, diarrhea (magnesium salts), constipation (aluminum salts)
Misc: Alkolosis, hypermagnesemia (magnesium salts), hypophosphatemia (aluminum salts)

Common Medications
Magnesium and aluminum hydroxide (eg, Maalox, Mylanta), calcium carbonate (eg, TUMS, Rolaids)

Proton Pump Inhibitors

Action
The parietal cells of the gastric mucosa produce gastric acid through the action of the proton pumps on the cell membrane. The PPIs are a class of drugs that decrease gastric acid secretion through inhibition of the proton pump.

Side Effects
CNS: Dizziness, drowsiness, fatigue, weakness, headache
CV: Chest pain
GI: Abdominal pain, constipation, diarrhea, nausea, vomiting, flatulence
Misc: Itching/rash, dry mouth

Common Medications
Omeprazole (Prilosec), esomeprazole (Nexium), lansoprazole (Prevacid), pantoprazole (Protonix), and rabeprazole (Aciphex)

Histamine–Receptor Blockers

Action
Histamine$_2$ (H$_2$) receptors are found in the heart, blood vessels, brain, and stomach. Stimulation of stomach H$_2$ receptors leads to enhanced gastric acid secretion. H$_2$ antagonists or blockers inhibit the action of histamine at the H$_2$ receptors of the stomach, inhibiting gastric acid secretion and reducing total pepsin output.

Side Effects
CNS: Dizziness, somnolence, headache, confusion, hallucinations, peripheral neuropathy, symptoms of brain stem dysfunction (dysarthria, ataxia, diplopia)
CV: Cardiac arrhythmias, arrest, hypotension (IV use)
GI: Diarrhea
Hematologic: Increases in plasma creatinine, serum transaminase
Misc: Impotence (reversible with drug withdrawal), gynecomastia (long-term treatment), rash, vasculitis, pain at IM injection site

Common Medications
Cimetidine (tagamet), famotidine (Pepcid), nizatidine (Axid), ranitidine (Zantac)

Prostaglandin Analogs

Action
Inhibit gastric acid secretion, stimulate mucus, and bicarbonate secretion from the GI mucosa, and increase mucosal blood flow.

Side Effects
CNS: Headache
CV: Frequent diarrhea, abortifacient actions
GI: Abdominal pain, diarrhea, dyspepsia, nausea, vomiting

Common Medications
Misoprostol (Cytotec)

Laxatives

Action
Laxatives provide short-term relief of constipation and prevent straining; used to evacuate the bowel for diagnostic procedures and to remove ingested poisons from the lower GI tract. These medications increase the water content of stool and increase intestinal peristalsis.

Side Effects
CNS: Weakness
CV: Dizziness
GI: Excessive bowel activity, perianal irritation, abdominal cramps, fullness
Misc: Weakness, cathartic dependence

Common Medications
Lactulose, polycarbophil (FiberCon/Fiberall), Psyllium (Metamucil), bisacodyl (Fleet), docusaate (Colace, Correctol), magnesium chloride/citrate

REFERENCES

1. Guyton AC, Hall JE. *Textbook of Medical Physiology.* Philadelphia, Pa: WB Saunders Co; 2000.
2. Moore KL. *Clinically Oriented Anatomy.* Baltimore, Md: Williams and Wilkins; 1995.
3. American College of Gastroenterology. Available at: www.acg.gi.org. Accessed in June 2004.
4. The National Institute of Diabetes & Digestive & Kidney Diseases of the National Institutes of Health. Available at: www.niddk.nih.gov. Accessed in June 2004.
5. Chandrasoma P, Taylor C. *Concise Pathology.* Norwalk, Conn: Appleton & Lange; 1999.
6. Rhoades RA, Tanner GA. *Medical Physiology.* Baltimore, Md: Lippincott Williams & Wilkins; 1995.
7. Junqueira LC, Carneiro J. *Basic Histology Text and Atlas.* 10th ed. New York, NY: McGraw-Hill Co; 2003.
8. Tierney LM, McPhee SJ, Papadakis MA. *Current Medical Diagnosis and Treatment.* Norwalk, Conn: Appleton & Lange; 1994.
9. Friedman SL, McQuaid KR, Grendell JH. *Current Diagnosis and Treatment in Gastroenterology.* 2nd ed. New York, NY: Lange Medical Books; 2003.
10. Rubin E, Farber JL, eds. The gastrointestinal tract. In: *Essential Pathology.* 2nd ed. Philadelphia, Pa: JB Lippincott Co; 1995.
11. Merahn S. *PDxMD—Gastroenterology.* Philadelphia, Pa: Elsevier Science; 2003.
12. Zwischenberger JB, Alpard SK, Orringer MB. Esophagus. In: Townsend CW, ed. *Sabiston Textbook of Surgery. The Biological Basis of Modern Surgical Practice.* 16th ed. Philadelphia, Pa: WB Saunders; 2001.
13. Kahrilas PJ, Pandolfino JE. Gastroesophageal reflux disease and its complications, including Barrett's metaplasia. In: Feldman M, Friedman LS, Sleisenger MH, eds. *Sleisenger & Fordtran's Gastrointestinal and Liver Disease Pathophysiology/ Diagnosis/Management.* 7th ed. Philadelphia, Pa: WB Saunders Co; 2003.
14. Berkow R. *The Merck Manual of Diagnosis and Therapy.* Rahway, NJ: Merck Sharp & Dome Research Laboratories; 1987.
15. Conner CEHS. *The SAGES Manual. Fundamentals of Laparoscopy & GI Endoscopy.* New York, NY: Springer Verlag; 1999.
16. Stotland BR, Ginsber GG. Upper gastrointestinal bleeding. In: Lanken P, ed. *The Intensive Care Unit Manual.* Philadelphia, Pa: WB Saunders Co; 2001.
17. Prantera C, Korelitz BI. *Crohn's Disease.* New York, NY: Marcel Dekker Inc; 1996.
18. Becker JM. Surgical therapy for ulcerative colitis and Crohn's disease. *Gastroenterol Clin North Am.* 1999;28:2.
19. Veronesi J. Inflammatory bowel disease. *RN.* 2003;66:38–46.
20. Kornbluth A, Sachar DB. Ulcerative colitis practice guidelines in adults. *Am J Gastroenterol.* 1997;92:2.
21. Way LW. *Current Surgical Diagnosis and Treatment.* Norwalk, Conn: Appleton & Lange; 1991.
22. McNally PR. *GI/Liver Secrets.* 2nd ed. Philadelphia, Pa: Hanley and Belfus; 2001.
23. Feldman M, Friedman LS, Sleisenger MS. *Sleisenger & Fordtran's Gastrointestinal and Liver Disease.* 7th ed. St. Louis, Mo: WB Saunders Company; 2002.
24. Arias IM. *The Liver—Biology and Pathobiology.* 4th ed. Philadelphia, Pa: Lippincott Williams and Wilkins; 2001.
25. Starr S, Hand H. Nursing care of chronic and acute liver failure. *Nursing Standard.* 2002;16:47–56.

26. Gines P, Cardenas A, Arroyo V, et al. Current concepts: management of cirrhosis and ascites. *N Engl J Med.* 2004;350:1646–1654.
27. Howard DE. Non-surgical treatment if gallstone disease. *Gastroenterol Clin North Am.* 1999;28(1).
28. Glazer G, Ranson HC. *Acute Pancreatitis.* London, England: Balliere Tindall; 1998.
29. Banks PA. Practice guidelines in acute pancreatitis. *Am J Gastroenterol.* 1997;92(3):377–386.
30. Seidel HM, Ball JW, Dains JE, et al. *Mosby's Guide to Physical Examination.* 5th ed. St. Louis, Mo: Mosby, Inc; 2003.
31. Smith GC, Paterson-Brown S. The acute abdomen and intestinal obstruction. In: Garden OJ, Bradbury AW, Forsythe J, eds. *Principles and Practice of Surgery.* 4th ed. New York, NY: Churchill Livingstone; 2002.
32. Lawrence VA, Hilsenbeck SG, Mulrow DC. Incidence and hospital stay for cardiac and pulmonary complications after abdominal surgery. *J Gen Intern Med.* 1995;10:671–678.
33. Aldren CP, Barr LC, Leach RD. Hypoxaemia and posteropative pulmonary complications. *Br J Surg.* 1991;78:1307–1308.
34. Schmidt GB. Prophylaxis of pulmonary complications following abdominal surgery, including atelectasis, ARDS, and pulmonary embolism. *Surg Annu.* 1977;9:29–73.
35. Oslen MF, Hahn I, Nordgren S, et al. Randomized controlled trial of prophylactic chest physiotherapy in major abdominal surgery. *Br J Surg.* 1997;84:1535–1538.
36. Thomas JA, McIntosh JM. Are incentive sprirometry, intermittent positive pressure breathing, and deep breathing exercises effective in the prevention of postoperative pulmonary complications after upper abdominal surgery? A systematic overview and meta-analysis. *Physical Therapy.* 1994;74:3–10.
37. Guide to Physical Therapist Practice. 2nd ed. *Physical Therapy.* 2001;81(1).
38. Preventing Obesity and Chronic Diseases through Good Nutrition and Physical Activity. National Center for Chronic Disease Prevention and Health Promotion Website. 2003 Available at: http://www.cdc.gov/nccdphp/pe_factcheets/pe_pa.htm. Accessed on June 25, 2004.
39. Hedley AA, Ogden CL, Johnson CL, et al. Prevalence of overweight and obesity among US children, adolescents, and adults, 1999–2002. *JAMA.* 2004;291:2847–2850.
40. Fontaine KR, Barofsky I. Obesity and health-related quality of life. *Obesity Reviews.* 2001;2:173–182.
41. Richards MM, Adams TD, Hunt SC. Functional status and emotional well-being, dietary intake, and physical activity of severely obese subjects. *J Am Diet Assoc.* 2000;100:67–74.
42. Mokdad AH, Bowman BA, Ford ES, et al. The continuing epidemics of obesity and diabetes in the United States. *JAMA.* 2001;286:1195–1200.
43. Must A, Spadano J, Coakley EH, et al. The disease burden associated with overweight and obesity. *JAMA.* 1999;282:1523–1529.
44. Mokdad AH, Ford ES, Bowman BA, et al. Prevalence of obesity, diabetes, and obesity-related health risk factors, 2001. *JAMA.* 2003;289:76–79.
45. Thompson D, Edelsberg J, Colditz GA, et al. Lifetime health and economic consequences of obesity. *Arch Intern Med.* 1999;159:2177–2183.
46. Okoro CA, Hootman JM, Strine TW, et al. Disability, arthritis, and body weight among adults 45 years and older. *Obesity Research.* 2004;12:854–861.
47. Marcus DA. Obesity and the impact of chronic pain. *Clin J Pain.* 2004;20:186–191.

48. Finkelstein EA, Fiebelkorn IC, Wang G. State-level estimates of annual medical expenditures attributable to obesity. *Obesity Research.* 2004;12:18–24.
49. Racette SB, Deusinger SS, Deusinger RH. Obesity: overview of prevalence, etiology, and treatment. *Phys Ther.* 2003;83:276–288.
50. *ACSM's Guidelines for Exercise Testing and Prescription.* 5th ed. Baltimore, Md: Williams & Wilkins; 1995.
51. Flegal KM, Carroll MD, Ogden CL, Johnson CL. Prevalence and trends in obesity among US adults, 1999–2000. *JAMA.* 2002;288:1723–1727.
52. Papasavas PK, Hayetian FD, Caushaj PF, et al. Outcome analysis of laparoscopic Roux-en-Y gastric bypass for morbid obesity. *Surgical Endoscopy.* 2002;16: 1653–1657.
53. Postlewait RW, Johnson WD. Complications following surgery for duodenal ulcer in obese patients. *Arch Surg.* 1972;105:438–440.
54. Taylor RR, Kelly TM, Elliott CG, et al. Hypoxemia after gastric bypass surgery for morbid obesity. *Arch Surg.* 1985;120:1298–1302.
55. Livingston EH. Obesity and its surgical management. *The American Journal of Surgery.* 2002;184:103–113.
56. Flum DR, Dellinger EP. Impact of gastric bypass operation on survival: a population-based analysis. *Journal of the American College of Surgeons.* 2004;199:543–551.
57. Kaminsky J, Gadaleta D. A study of discrimination within the medical community as viewed by obese patients. *Obesity Surgery.* 2002;12:14–18.
58. Harvey E, Hill A. Health professionals views of overweight people and smokers. *International Journal of Obesity.* 2001;25:1255–1261.
59. Hebl M, Xu J, Mason MF. Weighing the care: patient perceptions of physician care as a function of gender and weight. *Intern J Obesity.* 2003;27:269–275.
60. Teachman B, Brownaell K. Implicit anti fat bias among health professionals. Is anyone immune? *Intern J Obesity.* 2001;25:1525–1531.
61. National Task Force on the Prevention and Treatment of Obesity. Medical care for obese patients: advice for health care professionals. *Am Family Physician.* 2002;65:81–88.
62. Hebl M, Xu J. Weighing the care: physicians' reactions to the size of a patient. *Intern J Obesity.* 2001;25:1246–1252.
63. Abir F, Bell R. Assessment and management of the obese patient. *Crit Care Med.* 2004;32:87–91.
64. Deusinger SS, Deusinger RH, Racette SB. The obesity epidemic: health consequences and implications for physical therapy. *PT Magazine.* 2004;12:82–98.

BIBLIOGRAPHY

Deglin JH, Vallerand AH. *Davis's Drug Guide for Nurses.* 8th ed. Philadelphia, Pa: FA Davis Co; 2003.

Karch AM. *Lippincott's Nursing Drug Guide.* Springhouse, Pa: Lippincott Williams & Wilkins; 2004.

Ritter JM, Lewis LD, Mant TG. *Textbook of Clinical Pharmacology.* London, England: Edward Arnold Co; 1995.

Spechler SJ. Peptic ulcer disease and its complications. In: Feldman M, Freidman LS, Sleisenger MH, eds. *Sleisenger & Fordtran's Gastrointestinal and Liver Disease.* 7th ed. Philadelphia, Pa: Elsevier Science; 2002.

Chapter 12

GENITOURINARY DISEASES AND DISORDERS

David Fichandler, MSPT
Daniel J. Malone, MPT, CCS

Similar to the gastrointestinal (GI) system, the genitourinary (GU) system is not a common source for acute care physical therapy referral. While many of the diseases and conditions that result from a GU disorders are curable and often transient, the aggressive nature of symptoms and acute onset may require physical therapy for assistance with basic functional activities. The goals of this chapter are to introduce the more common GU pathologies with a special emphasis on renal disease, describe the diagnostics and medical management, and illustrate the roles of physical therapy in the management of these patients/clients in the acute care setting.

OVERVIEW

Once food and nutrients are digested, waste products are left behind. While the bowel handles solid wastes, the urinary system is the primary excretion system for metabolic waste products within the bloodstream.[1] The primary components of the genitourinary system include:

- Kidneys
- Ureter
- Bladder
- Urethra

Secondary components of the genitourinary system include:

- Prostate
- Pelvic floor muscles
- Genitals

ANATOMY AND PHYSIOLOGY OF THE
GENITOURINARY SYSTEM

The urinary system functions by removing **urea** from the bloodstream. Urea is the primary waste product of protein metabolism and is toxic. Urea is delivered to the *kidneys*, which filter the urea out of the blood. Urea and other waste products form urine, which is transported out of the kidneys via the *ureter*, a long muscular, contractile tube. The ureters empty the urine into the *bladder* for storage until elimination. The bladder accumulates up to 2 cups of urine in a healthy human before it contracts and releases urine for excretion via the *urethra*. The urethra then excretes urine out of the body via the *genitalia*.[2–4]

Renal System

The kidney is a complex and multifunctional organ. The kidney is responsible for maintaining the volume and composition of the body's fluids through reabsorption of water, sodium, and other compounds; regulates electrolytes and acid-base status; produces and secretes hormones (eg, erythropoietin/activated vitamin D [calcitriol]/renin/aldosterone); regulates arterial blood pressure (BP); and allows for the excretion of metabolic products and foreign substances.[5–7] Kidney dysfunction impacts most organ systems in the body as listed in Table 12–1. Anatomically, the kidneys are paired organs that are located along the posterior wall of the abdomen along either side of the vertebral column. The kidney can be divided into an outer region, the cortex, and an inner region, the medulla as shown in Figure 12–1. The cortex and medulla contain the nephrons, the functional unit of the kidney. Each kidney contains approximately 1.2 million nephrons where the functions of filtration, absorption, secretion, and excretion occur.[7] Renal blood flow is approximately 25% of the cardiac output (CO) highlighting the important functioning of the kidneys for homeostasis. The collecting ducts of the nephrons drain into the ureters leading to the bladder.[5–7]

Common disorders of the renal system that are frequently encountered in the acute care setting are detailed below.

Glomerulonephritis

The glomerulus is a specialized tuft of capillaries that is essential for the filtration of fluid as blood passes through the arterioles of the kidney. **Glomerulonephritis** is caused by a myriad of factors including immunologic abnormalities (eg, Berger's disease, Goodpasture syndrome), infections (eg, streptococcal organisms, endocarditis), drugs and toxins (eg, cyclosporin), vascular disorders (eg, atherosclerosis, thrombus), and systemic diseases (eg, systemic lupus erhythematosus [SLE], hepatitis B).[8] Glomerulonephritis is the most common cause of chronic and end-stage renal disease (ESRD) and can be categorized in multiple ways including progression (acute, rapidly progressive, chronic, diffuse) or pathologic lesion (diffuse, focal, segmental, mesangial, membranous, sclerotic, proliferative, crescentic).[8,9] Glomerulonephritis leads to alterations in capillary permeability and renal blood flow modifying glomerular filtration and renal function. Diagnosis of glomerulonephritis is confirmed by urinalysis (UA) (proteinuria, hematuria, WBCs) and renal biopsy.

Table 12–1

CLINICAL MANIFESTATIONS OF RENAL FAILURE

- **General:** Nausea, vomiting, weakness, lethargy, hiccups
- **GI:** Anorexia, ulceration of GI tract, hemorrhage
- **Cardiovascular:** Hyperkalemic electrocardiogram (ECG) changes, HTN, pericarditis, pericardial effusion, pericardial tamponade
- **Respiratory:** Pulmonary edema, pleural effusions, pleural rub
- **Neuromuscular:** Fatigue, sleep disorders, headache, lethargy, muscular irritability, peripheral neuropathy, seizures, coma
- **Metabolic and endocrine:** Glucose intolerance, hyperlipidemia, sex hormone disturbances causing decreased libido, impotence, amenorrhea
- **Fluid, electrolyte, acid–base disturbances:** Usually salt and water retention but may be sodium loss with dehydration, metabolic acidosis, hyperkalemia, hypermagnesemia, hypocalcemia/hypercalcemia, hyperphosphatemia
- **Dermatologic:** Pallor, hyperpigmentation, pruritus, ecchymoses, uremic frost-crystallization of urea on skin
- **Skeletal abnormalities:** Renal osteodystrophy resulting in osteomalacia
- **Hematologic:** Anemia, defect in quality of platelets, increased bleeding tendencies, white blood cell (WBC) dysfunction-immunocompromise
- **Psychosocial functions:** Personality and behavior changes, alteration in cognitive processes

Urinalysis

Urine output is approximately 1200 mL and is composed primarily of water, urea from the degradation of proteins and amino acids, and small amounts of organic and inorganic chemicals. Urine is generally clear, and color may vary from pale yellow ("straw-colored") to dark amber. The color of urine is a general indication of the patient's fluid status with the darker the urine indicating a more concentrated urine. Milk or cloudy urine usually indicates abnormal constituents such as red blood cells (RBCs), WBCs, or bacteria. A UA determines the properties of urine including color, odor, turbidity, specific gravity, and concentrations of glucose, ketones, RBC, WBC, bilirubin and urobilinogen, protein, and nitrites. Collection often lasts 24 hours and therapists must remember that ascertaining the entire output volume is important for the final analysis.

Nephrotic Syndrome and Proteinuria

Proteinuria is excessive amounts of protein (3.5 g or more/day) in the urine. The normal nephron of the kidney filters the blood at the glomerulus. The filtrate is termed an ultrafiltrate and is devoid of protein. **Nephrotic syndrome** is characterized by increased permeability of the nephron capillaries resulting in increased protein movement into the urine. Trace quantities of protein are

Figure 12–1. Structure of the kidney. (Reprinted from Koeppen BM, Stanton B. *Renal Physiology*. 3rd ed. Philadelphia, Pa: Mosby Inc; 2001. With permission from Elsevier.)

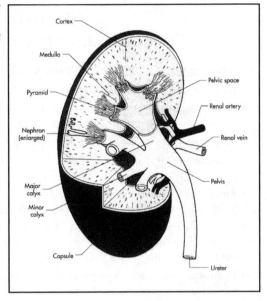

normal in the urine, but abundant concentrations are indicative of kidney dysfunction.[2,3,10] Common diseases that cause proteinuria include diabetes mellitus, hypertension (HTN), kidney failure, and cardiovascular disease. Patients with proteinuria are at increased risk of developing **nephroliathiasis**, kidney stones.

Proteinuria results in foamy urine and with continued protein excretion, peripheral edema will develop due to impaired vascular absorption of body fluids. The liver compensates for the protein loss by increasing production of albumin and other hepatic proteins, triglycerides, and cholesterol. Unfortunately this leads to hypercoagulability states and atherosclerosis. Proteinuria is diagnosed by UA, and blood testing will be performed to assess creatinine and blood urea nitrogen (BUN) levels as indicators of kidney function. Treatment for proteinuria is directed at the underlying cause and may include diuretics, steroids, and albumin replacement. Dietary modifications include fat and salt restriction.

Acute Renal Failure

Acute renal failure (ARF) is a syndrome resulting in the sudden decline in renal function and is often associated with an increase in BUN and creatinine, oliguria (less than 500 mL urine/24 hours), hyperkalemia, and sodium retention. **Azotemia** means increased serum urea levels and results from **renal insufficiency** (renal function ~25%; normal glomerular filtrate rate (GFR) = 25 to 30 mL/min) or **renal failure** (renal function <10% normal).[8] **Uremia** is a syndrome of renal failure and includes elevated blood urea and creatinine levels and is accompanied by fatigue, anorexia, nausea, vomiting, pruritis, and neurologic changes (see Table 12–1).[8,11] The pathophysiology and clinical manifestations of ARF are diverse and are determined by the inciting events. ARF can be divided into three categories:

Table 12–2
COMMON CAUSES OF CHRONIC RENAL FAILURE

- HTN, prolonged and severe
- Diabetes mellitus
- Glomerulopathies
- Interstitial nephritis
- Hereditary renal disease, polycystic disease
- Obstructive uropathy
- Developmental/congenital disorder

---

1. **Prerenal** causes result from conditions that decrease renal blood flow (hypovolemia, shock, hemorrhage, burns, impaired CO, pulmonary emboli [PE], and diuretic therapy). This condition typically presents with hypotension, oliguria/anuria, dryness of mucous membranes, and decreased tissue turgor.

2. **Postrenal** causes arise from obstruction or disruption to urine flow anywhere along the urinary tract including kidney stones, neoplasms (tumors of cervix/prostate, bladder), benign prostate hypertrophy (BPH), and blood clots.

3. **Intrarenal** causes result from injury to renal tissue and are usually associated with intrarenal ischemia, toxins, immunologic processes, and systemic and vascular disorders.[12–14]

Common diagnostic testing includes:

- UA: Reveals proteinuria, hematuria, casts
- Rising serum creatinine and BUN levels; ratio as high as 40:1
- Urine chemistry examinations to distinguish various forms of ARF
- Renal ultrasonography: For estimate of renal size and to exclude a treatable obstructive uropathy

Chronic Renal Failure

Chronic renal failure (CRF) is a progressive deterioration of renal function arising from any cause of renal dysfunction (Table 12–2). The kidneys demonstrate significant reserve capabilities, allowing maintenance of homeostasis. However, when renal function falls to approximately 80% of normal, signs and symptoms of renal insufficiency are evident. Ultimately, CRF ends fatally in uremia (an excess of urea and other nitrogenous wastes in the blood) and its complications unless dialysis or a kidney transplantation is performed.

Diagnosis

- Complete blood count (CBC)—anemia (a characteristic sign)

- Elevated serum creatinine, BUN, phosphorus
- Decreased serum calcium, bicarbonate, and proteins, especially albumin
- Arterial blood gases—metabolic acidosis, low blood pH, low CO_2, low bicarbonate (HCO_3)
- 24-hour urine for creatinine, protein, creatinine clearance

Common Management Strategies for Renal Failure

Goal: Conservation of renal function as long as possible.

1. Detection and treatment of reversible causes of renal failure (eg, diabetes control, treat HTN)

2. Dietary regulation—low-protein diet supplemented with essential amino acids or their keto analogues to minimize uremic toxicity and to prevent wasting and malnutrition

3. Treatment of associated conditions to improve renal dynamics

   a. Anemia—recombinant human erythropoietin (eg, Epogen), a synthetic hormone
   b. Acidosis—replacement of bicarbonate stores by infusion or oral administration of sodium bicarbonate
   c. Hyperkalemia—restriction of dietary potassium; administration of cation exchange resin
   d. Phosphate retention—decrease dietary phosphorus (chicken, milk, legumes, carbonated beverages); administer phosphate-binding agents that bind phosphorus in the intestinal tract

4. Maintenance dialysis or kidney transplantation (see Chapter 14) when medical/surgical management fails

Dialysis and Ultrafiltration

Renal failure results in abnormalities of the chemical and metabolic constituents of the fluids of the body. Dialysis attempts to perform the normal functions of the kidney by passing blood across a semi-permeable membrane allowing the metabolic waste products to diffuse into a correction fluid, or **dialysate**. Dialysis promotes the correction of fluid and electrolyte abnormalities, removal of toxic materials, and maintenance of acid-base balance. There are three modes of dialysis

1. Hemodialysis (HD)
2. Peritoneal dialysis (PD)
3. Continuous renal replacement therapy (CRRT)[15]

Hemodialysis

HD circulates the patient's blood in a series of semi-permeable tubes that are bathed in the diasylate in the artificial kidney or **dialyzer**.[16] Blood is accessed through an **arterial-venous (AV) fistula**, the creation of a vascular communication by suturing a vein directly to an artery; **arterio-venous graft**, an arteriovenous connection consisting of a tube graft made from autologous

---

Table 12–3
PHYSICAL THERAPY IMPLICATIONS OF DIALYSIS

- Therapeutic exercise and airway clearance may be performed as indicated, but mobilization activities are relatively contraindicated during HD and the inflow or outflow of the dialysate during PD.

- Assess fluid and electrolyte status prior to physical therapy interventions; expect fluid and electrolyte imbalances and modify the plan of care (see Chapter 2).

- Expect potential dehydration, hypovolemia, hypotension, and patient complaints of fatigue post dialysis.

- Monitor hemodynamic status and vital signs closely secondary to potential hypovolemia and electrolyte disorders.

- Avoid placement of BP cuff over arterio-venous fistula.

---

saphenous vein or from polytetrafluoroethylene (PTFE); or **central venous catheters (CVC)**, a direct cannulation of veins (subclavian, internal jugular, or femoral). AV fistulas and AV grafts allow repeated access with high flows to the dialyzer, minimize clot formation, and limit recurrent infections. CVC are usually placed in the femoral or subclavian veins and are usually temporary modes of access.[17,18]

Peritoneal Dialysis

PD uses the peritoneum as the semi-permeable membrane and the diasylate is infused into the abdomen. The peritoneum is highly vascularized allowing waste products and fluids to pass from the blood into the dialysis solution. The diasylate is infused into the abdomen and allowed to remain for several hours prior to drainage.[19]

Continuous Renal Replacement Therapy

CRRT consists of **continuous veno-venous or arterio-venous hemodialysis (CVVHD/CVAHD)**. These procedures take place in the intensive care unit (ICU) and involve the use of an extracorporeal blood circulation through a small-volume, low-resistance filter to provide continuous removal of solutes and fluid.[20,21] Patients are critically ill, often sedated, and medically paralyzed, and physical therapy is usually contraindicated except for careful application of airway clearance techniques, range of motion (ROM) exercise programs, and positioning recommendations. Patency of arterial and venous access and blood flow is critical.

Common precautions and implications associated with HD are listed in Table 12–3.

COMMON DISEASES OF THE GENITOURINARY SYSTEM

Urinary Tract Infections

Urinary tract infections (UTIs) are a common infection of adult women and the elderly and account for nearly 9 million infections annually. Moreover, one in every five women is susceptible to UTI, and the prevalence of UTI increases with age. Increased risk of UTI is associated for those with indwelling catheters in the bladder, patients with diabetes, and those with abnormalities of the urinary tract. Recurrence is the rule following UTI, and approximately 20% of women with acute UTI will experience a recurrence.[22]

Pathophysiology

UTIs are most commonly due to bacterial infections (eg, *E. coli*). The entire urinary system is at risk of invasion by bacteria following infection and the bacteria may ascend to the bladder, **cystitis,** and to the kidneys, **pyelonephritis.**[22] Other less common causes, such as sexual transmission (chlamydia and mycoplasma), may cause local infection.[19,23,24] Common signs and symptoms of UTI are listed in Table 12–4.

Standard in testing for UTI is UA. UA can detect the presence of bacteria, pus, or infection and will allow directed antibiotic treatment.[25]

UTIs are generally successfully treated and begin to resolve within 1 to 2 days, although the course of treatment is commonly 1 to 2 weeks of antibiotics (see Chapter 5, Pharmacological Information). Ancillary treatments include an increased fluid intake as well as the intake of foods that act to cleanse the bladder (eg, cranberry juice).

Hematuria

Hematuria is the presence of RBCs in the urine. Often, this is not discernible to the human eye. However, gross hematuria is visible in the urine. Hematuria is usually the symptom of an underlying disease process within the GI or GU system. Examples include liver and/or kidney disease, bladder dysfunction, kidney stone, BPH, and GU tumors. Hematuria is diagnosed via UA, **intravenous pyelogram (IVP)**, an injection of a radiopaque dye followed by x-ray of the renal pelvis and ureter, or **cystoscopy,** a direct visual of the bladder. Treatment depends on the underlying cause of hematuria.

Nephrolithiasis

Kidney stones are one of the most common GU disorders resulting in pain, obstructions, and secondary infections.[12,23] There are greater than 1 million episodes of kidney stones each year in the United States. It is estimated that 10% of Americans will have a kidney stone at some point in their lives. Kidney stones affect men more than women and usually occur between the ages of 20 and 40.[4]

Kidney stones form due to crystallization of calcium (80% to 90%), uric acid, magnesium-ammonium acetate, or cysteine in the urine. Stones may form anywhere along the urinary tract. Microscopic crystal formation is normal, and these crystals easily pass though the urinary tract. Renal and urinary

---

Table 12–4

SIGNS AND SYMPTOMS OF COMMON RENAL DISORDERS

Urinary Tract Infection:

- Frequency of urination/urinary urgency
- Painful urination
- Burning feeling in the bladder
- Milky or cloudy urine
- Reddish or bloody urine (hematuria)
- Fever
- Back pain

Renal Calculi:

- Severe back/flank pain
- Nausea and vomiting
- Hematuria
- Burning sensation with urination
- Fever or chills

---

calculi are concretions consisting of an increased mass of crystals with an organic matrix. Multiple factors may contribute to stone formation including diets high in calcium oxalate, limited fluid intake and low urine volume, genetic factors (cystinuria is an autosomal recessive disorder), hyperparathyroidism, sedentary lifestyle and bed rest, and geographic influences (high temperatures and humidity). Additional factors include chronic UTIs, kidney dysfunction, and diabetes mellitus (DM). Common signs and symptoms of urinary calculi are noted in Table 12–4. Diagnostic testing may include abdominal x-rays, renal sonogram, IVP, and blood and urine analysis.

Treatment

Acute medical management includes administration of intravenous (IV) fluids, antibiotics, and pain control. Patients may be asked to strain their urine to determine stone passage and allow determination of its chemical composition. Pharmacologic treatments include Allopurinol, diuretics (eg, Thiazides), and Thiola. Additional medical and surgical procedures include:

- **Extracorporeal shockwave lithotripsy:** Noninvasive ultrasound is used externally to disrupt stones and allow passage through the ureter.
- **Percutaneous nephrolithotomy:** A surgical technique in which a tunnel is made directly to the kidney and the stone is surgically removed or destroyed via ultrasonic wave.
- **Uteroscopic stone removal:** A uretoscope is fed into the ureter and the stone is removed manually.[4]

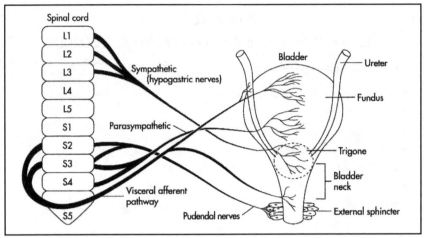

Figure 12–2. Anatomy of the lower urinary tract and its innervation. (Reprinted from Koeppen BM, Stanton B. *Renal Physiology.* 3rd ed. Philadelphia, Pa: Mosby Inc; 2001. With permission from Elsevier.)

Kidney stone recurrence is frequent and prevention may include diet modifications, increase of daily water intake, and prophylactic medications.[25]

Cystocele

Cystocele or fallen bladder occurs in women and is defined as the bladder protruding into the vagina. The common causes of cystocele include heavy lifting, straining during bowel movements, decreased estrogen concentrations, and childbirth. The severity of the dropped bladder can be graded as follows:

- Grade 1—Bladder drops into the vagina.
- Grade 2—Bladder has sunk into the opening of the vagina.
- Grade 3—Bladder protrudes from the vaginal opening.[4]

Diagnosis for grades 2 and 3 cystoceles is confirmed by physical examination. Additional testing may include a cystourethrogram, a x-ray using contrast media that shows the anatomy of the bladder and urethra during bladder contraction and voiding. Treatment for grade 1 cycstoceles includes avoidance of heavy lifting and possibly estrogen replacement therapy in post-menopausal women. Grades 2 and 3 cystoceles may require surgical repositioning and stabilization of the bladder.

Neurogenic Bladder and Urinary Incontinence

Neurogenic bladder is disruption of the complex interactions of voluntary and involuntary smooth muscle, the autonomic nervous system, and cerebral control that allow controlled micturation (Figure 12–2). Neurogenic bladder can lead to recurrent infections, urinary frequency, incontinence, or partial/complete urinary retention. **Urinary incontinence** is the involuntary loss of urine

Table 12–5
TYPES OF URINARY INCONTINENCE

Type	Description	Common Etiologies
Stress incontinence	• Intermittent leakage of urine due to increased abdominal pressure, such as coughing, sneezing, or straining.	• Indicates weakness of pelvic floor and sphincter muscles in women, and damage to the internal sphincter mechanism (usually from prostatic surgery) in men.
Urge incontinence	• Sensation of the need to urinate followed by sudden, involuntary loss of urine.	• Neurologic disease affecting the bladder, acute or chronic irritation of the bladder wall, and the effects of prolonged bladder outlet obstruction.
Overflow incontinence	• Loss of urine caused by overdistention of the bladder; associated with complete urinary retention.	• Prostate obstruction, DM, SCI, MS.
Functional incontinence	• Loss of urine due to functional impairment that causes difficulty in ambulation or dexterity in getting to the bathroom and positioned to void.	
Total incontinence	• Continuous leakage of urine from the bladder.	• Occurs with injury to the sphincteric mechanisms, bladder neck, and urethra.
Enuresis	• Involuntary voiding during sleep.	• May be physiologic during early childhood; thereafter, may be functional or symptomatic of obstructive or neurogenic disease (usually of lower urinary tract) or dysfunctional voiding.

and may be due to pathologic, anatomical, or physiologic factors affecting the urinary tract. Table 12–5 describes the types of urinary incontinence.

Pathophysiology

Neurogenic bladder is rarely caused by a hereditary malformation. It is often due to trauma (spinal cord injury [SCI], traumatic brain injury [TBI]), demyelinating diseases (MS, amyotrophic lateral sclerosis [ALS]), CVA, CNS tumors, lead poisoning, DM, and chronic UTIs.

The underlying mechanism is disordered neurologic control of the muscles of the bladder. This lack of impulse coordination often results in reflexive relaxation and discharge of urine.[3,4]

Signs of neurogenic bladder include:

- Urination on exertion
- Urination without sensation
- Chronic UTIs
- Inability to actively control bladder and urination (incontinence)

Diagnosis and Testing

Diagnosis is a two-phase process involving testing of both the muscular and neurological systems. Testing utilizes an electroencephalogram (EEG) of the brain and an electromyography (EMG) of the bladder. Additionally, a bladder ultrasound, computed tomography scan (CT scan) with bladder contrast, and a postresidual void (PRV) test (ie, a catheter is placed into the bladder after the patient has voided to assess residual urine volume) are done.[4,24]

Treatment

Treatment for a neurogenic bladder is truly dependent on the underlying cause. In cases of SCI, TBI, or other traumatic injury to the bladder or brain, a catheter is introduced to evacuate the bladder or a suprapubic indwelling catheter is inserted through the abdomen. Patients may be taught self-catheterization. If incontinence is due to muscular problems of the bladder, pharmacologic treatments include the following:

- Bladder relaxants—Propantheline, flavoxate (Urispas), dicyclomine (Bentyl), oxybutynin (Ditropan), tolterodine (Detrol)
- Antidepressants—Imipramine (Tofranil)
- Estrogen replacement therapy is another possibility

Physical therapy interventions include exercise, electrical stimulation, biofeedback, timed voiding, and instructed catheterization. Surgery is a final option.[26]

Therapuetic interventions for neurogenic bladder include the following:

- Kegel exercises strengthen and retrain pelvic floor and sphincter muscles, aiding in the prevention of urinary leakage. Examples of Kegel exercises include attempting to contract the urethra, attempting to start and stop urine in mid stream, and for women with stress incontinence, the use of weighted cones. (See Chapter 13 and Table 13–8.)
- **Electrical stimulation:** Electrodes are placed within the vagina or rectum to stimulate pelvic floor muscles. This aids in stabilizing overactive muscles while stimulating contraction of the urethral muscles.
- **Biofeedback:** Biofeedback uses electronic waves to track the contraction of the bladder and urethral muscles. Visualization of the waveforms facilitates improved coordination of contractile and relaxation activity of the involved muscles.

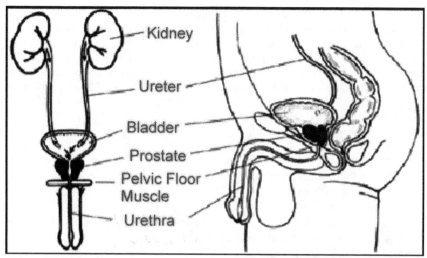

Figure 12–3. Anatomy of the male bladder, prostate, and urethra. (Reprinted from www.niddk.nih.gov.)

- **Timed voiding or bladder training:** Techniques that use a chart of voiding and leaking. As patterns are identified, scheduled voidings/emptyings are instituted. This technique works in conjunction with biofeedback and muscle conditioning to slowly increase the time scale for voiding.[4]

Benign Prostate Hypertrophy

The prostate is a small, male reproductive gland located under the bladder, anterior to the rectum, and surrounding the urethra. The prostate begins to enlarge at about 25 years of age. **BPH** can become evident after the age of 40 years and affects nearly 90% of men 70 years or older, requiring almost 400,000 hospital admissions yearly.[4,10,24]

Pathophysiology

The etiology of BPH is unclear. Theories include hormonal alterations including diminished testosterone and elevated estrogen concentrations stimulating prostatic growth.[4] Prostate enlargement exerts pressure on the urethra (Figure 12–3). Urethra compression stimulates reflexive bladder contraction regardless of urine volume and leads to bladder wall thickening and distension.

Common symptoms of BPH include:
- Hesitancy or a weak stream of urine
- Urinary urgency
- Leaking or dribbling
- Urinary frequency, especially at night

Interestingly, the amount of hypertrophy does not correlate to the severity of symptoms.

Diagnostic testing attempts to differentiate BPH from prostate cancer. Physical examinations include digital rectal exam allowing palpation of the prostate to determine size and texture. Diagnostic testing may include prostate biopsy or prostate specific antigens (PSA) testing. PSAs are present in the bloodstream, and elevated PSA concentrations are indicative of prostate cancer. Normal values are <4 ng/mL, elevated values are 4 to 10 ng/mL, and abnormal values are 10 to 20+ ng/mL.[3,10,26] Additional testing includes urine flow studies, rectal ultrasound, IVP, and cystoscopy.

Treatment

Treatment for BPH includes medications and surgical management. Medications include the following:[6]

- Finasteride (Proscar): Inhibits DHT (a hormone that promotes prostate enlargement)

- Terazosin (Hytrin); Doxazosin (Cardura); or Tamsulosin (Flomax): Relaxes smooth muscle of bladder and prostate to increase flow

Surgical treatments include:

- **Transurethral microwave thermotherapy (TUMT)** uses microwaves to heat and destroy excessive prostate tissue while protecting the rest of the urinary system by providing a coolant through the urethra.

- **Transurethral needle ablation (TUNA)** system delivers a low-level radio frequency that burns away selected prostate tissues with a shield to protect the urethra.

- **Transurethral resection of the prostate (TURP)** is performed through the urethra using a resectoscope. The resectoscope has a light and irrigator and contains an electrical loop to shave away tissue. TURP is the most common surgical intervention and accounts for 90% of all prostate surgeries.

- **Transurethral incision of the prostate (TUIP)** focuses on widening the urethra by making incisions in the bladder neck and prostate.

- **Suprapubic** and **retropubic prostatectomy** are more invasive and involve direct resection or excision of prostate tissue.

- Newer treatment options include **transurethral laser ablation** and **balloon dilatation**.

Postoperative treatment includes continuous bladder irrigation, antibiotics, and pain control with early ambulation.

GENITALIA

Male and female genitalia play important roles in both the excretion of wastes and in reproduction. However, these multiple functions leave the human genitalia susceptible to infection and disease (eg, UTI). The genitalia have an extensive vascular tree and robust arterio-venous blood flow. This leaves the external genitalia, specifically the labia and scrotum, vulnerable to edema formation. **Labial edema** is rare and often exclusively caused by liver disease and hypoproteinemia; **scrotal edema** is more common. Scrotal edema is associated with hereditary disease, liver disease and transplantation, inguinal herniation, lymphedema of the lower extremity (LE), and prostate disease. Scrotal edema secondary to liver diseases and/or transplantation is associated with portal HTN and hypoproteinemia. Inguinal herniation and lymphedema involve obstruction of arterial, venous, or lymphatic flow out of the genitalia resulting in scrotal edema.

Signs and symptoms of external genitalia edema include the following:

- Large, pitting edema

- Shiny and discolored skin

- Warm to touch

- Difficulty or inability to walk

Edema is identifiable during the physical examination. Additional testing usually consists of blood and UA, CT scan, and/or ultrasound analysis to determine the underlying cause. Interventions are determined by the underlying cause of the genital edema. Lymphedema is responsive to manual lymphatic decompression therapy and referral to a lymphedema specialist can lead to significant reductions in edema.

PHYSICAL THERAPY IMPLICATION
OF GENITOURINARY SYSTEM

While diseases and disorders of the GU system do not often present specific implications for physical therapy, there can be many challenges while treating this population. The physical therapist/physical therapist assistant may be one of the first health care practitioners who patients confide in and relate GU complaints. Although the GU physical examination is not performed by physical therapists unless they have undergone specialized training (eg, urinary incontinence, lymphedema), common questions during the history may allow a more specific description of the patient's complaints and referral to other health care professionals (Table 12–6). Additionally, the therapists need to consider that patients with advanced renal disease are typically physically inactive with reduced exercise capacity prior to hospitalization. Enforced or voluntary bed rest will exacerbate these problems, potentially challenging the acute care therapist.[28] The reason for the debility of patients with ESRD and dialysis is far from clear. The anemias of chronic renal disease, peripheral edema, and the systemic effects of uremia as well as disuse atrophy have a significant impact on the physical functioning and quality of life of these patients.[27,28] The limited exercise capacity and poor physical functioning has been linked to low quality of life and high mortality in this population. Patients with kidney disease and those receiving dialysis may often demonstrate fluid, electrolyte, and glucose abnormalities necessitating close observation of laboratory values to determine values that impact on physical therapy examination/interventions (see Chapter 2). Renal dysfunction is often associated with DM and cardiovascular disease. Patients will present with peripheral neuropathies, intrinsic weakness of the hand and feet, Charcot joint changes, coronary artery disease (CAD) and HTN necessitating close observation of hemodynamic profiles, and ECG. Patients with

Table 12-6

Genitourinary System Examination

Examination Technique	Description of Technique	Examination Findings in Common Diseases/Disorders
Common questions/history	• Abdominal pain: Note onset, duration, character (eg, sharp, dull, stabbing), location/radiation to other areas. Note anatomic location of pain (see Tables 11–18 and 11–19). • Urine characteristics (eg, color/amount/frequency/presence of blood; incontinence associated with activity/cough/sneeze (see Table 12–5). **Urgency:** Strong desire to urinate. Often related to inflammation of bladder/prostate/urethra; infection. **Frequency:** Short duration between urination. **Nocturia:** Voiding at night **Dysuria:** Burning or pain with urination, difficulty voiding (eg, pyelonephritis, cystitis, urethritis, vaginitis). **Hematuria:** Blood in urine (eg, UTI, renal disease, renal/bladder stones, GU cancer). **Frothy urine:** Proteinuria (eg, glomerulonephritis/nephrotic syndrome). • Fluid intake (eg, how many glasses of water, caffeine). • Characterization of pelvic pain (eg, onset, duration, location, character, severity, exacerbating or relieving factors). • Vaginal or penile discharge (eg, amount, color, odor).	**Pyelonephritis:** Fever, chills, increased urgency and frequency, thoracic pain, cloudy urine. **Cystitis:** Frequent urination, urinary incontinence, hypogastric/pubic pain, cloudy/foul-smelling urine. **Urethritis:** Dysuria, urethral discharge, usually no complaints of frequency or urgency. **Vaginitis (eg, candidiasis/trichomonisasis):** Pain, soreness, itching of vagina, foul-smelling vaginal discharge, pain/discomfort with sexual intercourse. **Kidney stone:** Flank tenderness, radiating pain to groin; hematuria. **Prostatitis:** Perineal pain (region between scrotum and anus), dysuria, urethral discharge. **Testicular cancer:** Testicle swelling/hard mass or lump in testicle; gradual onset of pain. **Inguinal hernia:** Groin pain, scrotal swelling—increases with standing/decreases with lying down; palpable mass in scrotum or inguinal canal.

- Premenstrual complaints (eg, headaches, weight gain, edema, breast tenderness, mood changes).
- Menopausal complaints (eg, mood changes, hot flashes, post-menopausal bleeding).

Inspection/ observation	Observation of lower abdomen and/or genitalia.

- Rashes
- Lesions
- Masses
- Hernia

Examination for edema of the extremities (see Table 1–7)

Consider review of Clinical Laboratory Data (see Chapter 2 and Tables 2–2 through 2–11, 2–15):

- Serum creatinine
- Creatinine clearance
- BUN
- Electrolytes (Na, K, Cl, Ca, Mg)
- ABG

Genital herpes: Viral infection leading to superficial, small red vesicles.

Condyloma acuminatum (genital warts): Human papillomavirus (HPV) infection; flesh/white or reddish lesions.

Epididymitis: Inflammation of the epididymis, often associated with UTI, erythema and swelling of scrotum; pain relieved with scrotal elevation.

Peripheral edema: Due to excessive loss of protein in urine (proteinuria) leading to a decrease in osmotic pressure within the vasculature (eg, nephrotic syndrome) or inability to excrete sodium and metabolic wastes (eg, renal failure) leading to excessive water retention.

Liver disease: Due to portal HTN or hypoalbuminemia (see Chapter 11).

Adapted from:
Fischbach FT, Dunning MB. *A Manual of Laboratory and Diagnostic Tests.* Philadelphia, Pa: Lippincott Williams & Wilkins; 2004.
Seidel HM, Ball JW, Dains JE, et al. *Mosby's Guide to Physical Examination.* St. Louis, Mo: Mosby, Inc; 2003.

nephroliathiasis commonly have referred low back and flank pain with difficulty in supine. Proper positioning in the bed (hooklying, propped on pillows) may assist in alleviating pain.

All patients who have undergone a surgical intervention need to be engaged in an airway clearance and mobility program due to the increased incidence of postoperative pulmonary complications (see Chapter 11). Additionally the coordination of pain management strategies will optimize physical therapy interventions.

Patients with prostate diseases are generally in the seventh decade, and it is common to encounter pre-morbid gait, balance, and postural dysfunction.

Kegel exercises can be prescribed for bladder and pelvic floor dysfunction that can alleviate pain and strengthen those muscles to prevent further dysfunction and potential embarrassment (see Table 13–8).

Initiate lymphedema management or refer patients to outpatient physical therapy with LE or genital lymphedema.

Case Study

Mrs. Noresh is a 44-year-old (y/o) female with history of (h/o) Crohn's disease x 20 years. Patient was admitted to the hospital with nausea, vomiting, abdominal pain, fever, and material draining from her vagina. Upon further examination, the material was found to be feces and the patient was diagnosed with a recto-vaginal fistula.

Patient/Client History

General Demographics/Social History/Living Environment

Mrs. Noresh lives in a first floor apartment with three steps to enter. She lives with her husband who has had four myocardial infarctions (MIs) in the past 2 years. Mrs. Noresh has been on disability secondary to the diagnosis of Crohn's disease.

General Health Status/Family History

Mrs. Noresh has complaints of chronic fatigue and lack of energy. She has difficulty sleeping more then 3 hours at a time. Her mother and father are still alive but were placed in a nursing home last year due to dementia and heart failure, respectively.

Functional Status and Activity Level

Mrs. Noresh does not use any assistive devices to ambulate but needed the handrail to enter her home. She also had a tubrail installed in the bathroom 4 months ago.

Current Conditions/Chief Complaints

Patient was admitted emergently and underwent an 8-hour exploratory laparotomy, colon resection with colostomy, and closure of the recto-vaginal fistula. Mrs. Noresh spent 5 days in the ICU for close observation and weaning from the ventilator. Her temperature is 100.1 degrees. On POD #5, she was transferred to the floor and physical therapy was consulted.

Medical/Surgical History

Mrs. Noresh required chronic Prednisone therapy use resulting in HTN, muscle weakness (myopathy), depression, and chronic UTIs.

Systems Review

Cardiovascular/Pulmonary

Resting vital signs (with head of bed raised 30 degrees) were oxygen saturation 91% (SpO_2) on 2 liters nasal cannula oxygen, heart rate (HR) 102, pulse regular, respiratory rate (RR) 24 and shallow using accessory muscles, BP 156/94, and pain was 5/10. Following manual muscle test (MMT), ROM, bed mobility, transfers, and gait her vital sign response was 94% SpO_2, HR 116, RR 32, BP 168/96, and pain 10/10. Her breath sounds were absent bilateral bases and coarse anteriorly. Her cough was weak, wet sounding, but nonproductive. Laboratory values revealed a decreased RBC, hemoglobin, and an elevated WBC. Chest x-ray shows a patchy infiltrate of the right lower lobe (RLL)/left lower lobe (LLL).

Integumentary

She had IV fluids, total parenteral nutrition (TPN), patient controlled analgesia (PCA), Foley catheter, and sump drain to abdominal wound. She appears thin and presents with +2 edema of BLE.

Musculoskeletal

Mrs. Noresh's ROM was within normal limits (WNL) except for bilateral ankles to neutral dorsiflexion (DF)/plantar flexion (PF) and minimal inversion/ eversion. Her strength was bilateral upper extremity (BUE) 3/5 and bilateral LE (BLE) 3+/5 except for tibialis anterior, posterior, and peroneal mm. at 2-/5.

Neuromuscular

Mrs. Noresh had diminished sensation in a "stocking-glove deformity" with specific hyposensitivity plantar surface of the feet.

Communication, Affect, Cognition, Language, and Learning Style

English is the primary language. She is alert, awake, and oriented x 4.

Tests and Measures

Aerobic Capacity and Endurance

Mrs. Noresh appears malnourished and is potentially deconditioned as demonstrated by the cardiovascular and pulmonary response to minimal activity. She is at risk for pulmonary complications due to the nature of the surgery and her present pulmonary findings. Her pain management must be addressed immediately because she is unable to have a productive cough and secretions are audible. Her oxygen saturation improved with mobility, and once a threshold of pain control is achieved, she should be able to progress with gait training as well as improve her airway clearance. Laboratory findings indicative of possible anemia related to her chronic disease and elevated WBC may indicate a possible infection which is supported by her low grade temperature.

Assistive and Adaptive Devices

Mrs. Noresh ambulated 15 feet with rolling walker and moderate assist x 1 on level surfaces.

Gait, Locomotion, and Balance

Mrs. Noresh's bed mobility required moderate assist x 1 to roll and transfer supine to sit at the edge of the bed. Mrs. Noresh ambulated 15 feet in a flexed posture and a steppage gait pattern. It is noted that she has limited dorsiflexion of BLE and presents with bilateral foot drop on the right > left.

Pain

Mrs. Noresh rated her pain at 10/10. She appears to understand the use of the PCA and used it prior to mobilization.

Diagnosis

Mrs. Noresh presents with limited pulmonary reserve, gross musculoskeletal weakness, altered sensation, intolerable pain, and impaired functional mobility related to her Crohn's disease, subsequent surgery, BLE "drop-foot," and perioperative bed rest. Recommend treatment pattern 4C: impaired muscle performance.[29]

Prognosis

Many patients with Crohn's disease or other inflammatory bowel disease use corticosteroids (ie, Prednisone) as a primary means of controlling inflammation and pain. Unfortunately, these drugs have many potential side effects as noted in the medical history. Her BLE "drop-foot" is a new finding and may have been caused by improper LE positioning during the 5 days in the ICU. The physical therapist recommended daily therapy to meet the goals of independence with gait using an assistive device, ascending/descending three steps, donning/doffing standard ankle foot orthosis (AFO), improve pain control, and improve airway clearance and a productive/effective cough.

Intervention

Mrs. Noresh therapy 5 times/week to progress gait, transfers, airway clearances (incentive spirometry, breathing exercises, and splinteded coughing), therapeutic exercise to enhance extremity ROM and strength, and education regarding postoperative pulmonary complications, AFO training, and ambulation safety secondary to the "drop-feet." Patient education also supported the teachings of the stoma care nurse.

The physical therapist recommended referrals to an orthotist, occupational therapy, clinical dietician, and social work for custom AFOs, ADL retraining, nutrition assessment, evaluation for depression-like symptoms, and discharge planning.

Reexamination

Two weeks after surgery Mrs. Noresh had all lines removed and her reported pain is 3/10. AROM is unchanged from initial examination, but LE passive ROM (PROM) with 3 degree increase in DF. Her strength has improved to 4/5 throughout except, tibialis anterior (TA), tibialis posterior (TP) and peroneals at 3-/5. Bed mobility-supine<> sit minimal assist x 1, transfers- sit<>stand minimal assist x 1, ambulation- 35 feet x 3 with rolling walker and 5-inch wheels. Her temperature is normal and she has an effective cough. Breath sounds are clear throughout.

Outcomes

Mrs. Noresh was recommended for acute rehabilitation.

CHAPTER REVIEW QUESTIONS

1. What are the primary components of the genitourinary system?
2. What is the primary waste product of protein metabolism?
3. What is ARF?
4. What are some common precautions when treating a patient on hemodialysis?
5. Name at least three different therapeutic interventions for a neurogenic bladder.

PHARMACOLOGICAL INFORMATION: GENITOURINARY DISEASES AND DISORDERS PHARMACOLOGY

Diuretics

Action
Diuretics increase tubular secretion or inhibit reabsorption of electrolytes (Na^+, K^+, C^-) within the loop of henle or distal tubule leading to enhanced renal excretion of electrolytes and water. Diuretics are prescribed for HTN, pulmonary edema and effusions, and hypervolemia states.

Side Effects
CNS: Dizziness, headache
CV: Hypotension (hypovolemia)
GI: Dry mouth, constipation, dyspepsia
Misc: Electrolyte abnormalities including hyper/hypokalemia, hyponatremia, hypochloremia, hypomagnesemia; metabolic alkalosis; muscle cramping

Common Medications
Loop Diuretics: Bumetanide (Bumex), Furosemide (Lasix), Toresemide (Demadex)
Osmotic Diuretics: Mannitol
Potassium-Sparing Diuretics: Amiloride (Midamor), Spironolactone (Aldactone)
Thiazide Diuretics: Hydrochlorothiazide

Electrolyte/pH/Mineral Modifiers and Replacement Solutions

Sodium Bicarbonate

Action
Alkalinizing agents are indicated to manage metabolic acidosis, neutralize gastric acid, and aid in the secretion of certain drugs (eg, phenobarbital, aspirin). These agents release bicarbonate ions, an important physiologic base, to raise serum pH by buffering excess H^+ ions.

Side Effects
CV: Edema
GI: Flatulence, gastric distension
Misc: Metabolic alkalosis, hypernatremia, hypokalemia, hypocalcemia

Common Medications
Sodium Bicarbonate (baking soda, soda mint), Sodium Citrate (Bicitra, Oracit)

Sodium Chloride

Action
Sodium chloride is primarily indicated for hydration and to supplement NaCl in deficiency states. 0.9% (normal saline) is primarily used for fluid replacement to expand extracellular fluid volume and maintenance of homeostasis. 0.45% (half normal saline) is a hypotonic solution and may be used in hyperosmolar states (eg, diabetes). Hypertonic saline (3%, 5%) is used for rapid replacement of sodium and removal of excess intravascular fluid volume.

Side Effects
CV: CHF, pulmonary edema, edema
Misc: Hypernatremia, hypervolemia, hypokalemia, irritation at IV site

Calcium Salts

Action
Calcium salts are used to treat hypocalcemia and adjunct therapy for osteoporosis and peptic ulcer disease.

Side Effects
CNS: Tingling
CV: Cardiac arrest, dysrhythmias
GI: Constipation, nausea, vomiting, calculi (stones)

Common Medications
Calcium acetate (Calphron, PhosLo), Calcium carbonate (Alka-mints, Amitone, Calcitel, Caltrate, Maalox, Tums), Calcium citrate (Citrical), Calcium gluconate (Kalcinate)

Magnesium Salts

Action
Magnesium salts are indicated for the treatment of hypomagnesemia, used as a laxative or bowel evacuant, and as antacids.

Side Effects
CV: Bradycardia, hypotension
GI: Diarrhea
Misc: Flushing

Common Medications
Magnesium chloride (Slo-Mag), magnesium citrate, magnesium gluconate, magnesium hydroxide (Phillips Milk of Magnesia), magnesium oxide, magnesium sulfate

Potassium and Sodium Phosphates and Potassium Supplements

Action
Potassium and sodium phosphates are indicated in states of phosphate depletion, to prevent urinary calculi, and as adjunctive therapy for UTIs.

Potassium supplements are indicated in hypokalemia and in the treatment of dysrhythmias due to digoxin toxicity.

Side Effects
CNS: Confusion, weakness, flaccid paralysis
CV: Dysrhythmias, cardiac arrest
GI: Diarrhea, abdominal discomfort
Misc: Hypocalcemia, hyperkalemia

Common Medications
Neutra-Phos, K-Phos, K-Lyte, Klorvess, Kaylixir, Kolyum

Ringers and Lactated Ringers

Action
These isotonic solutions closely resemble the electrolyte composition of normal blood serum and are used to replace K^+, Na^+, Cl^-, and Ca^{++}. These solutions do not provide calories or free water.

Dextrose and Saline Solutions

Action
These solutions are composed of varying tonicities (isotonic, hypotonic, and hypertonic) and contain free water (W) or saline (NS). Isotonic solutions allow for daily maintenance of body fluids as noted under sodium chloride (see above). Hypertonic solutions promote osmotic diuresis and removal of intra-vascular fluid volume, and hypotonic solutions are indicated for hydration. Dextrose solutions provide calories for nutrition, but do not correct electrolyte disturbances.

Common Medications
Hypotonic solutions: one-half NS – 0.45%NaCl
Isotonic solutions: 0.9% NS; D5W – 5% Dextrose in water; D5 one-fourth NS – 5% Dextrose and 0.2NaCl
Hypertonic solution: 3% NS; D10W – 10% Dextrose in water; D5 one-half NS – 5% Dextrose and 0.45NaCl; D5LR – 5% Dextrose in Lactated Ringers; Dextran, TPN

REFERENCES

1. Moore KL. *Clinically Oriented Anatomy.* Baltimore, Md: Williams and Wilkins; 1995.
2. Merahn S. PDxMD—*Renal and Genitourinary Disorders.* Philadelphia, Pa: Elsevier Science; 2003.
3. Weiss R, Nicholas G Jr, O'Reilly PH. *Comprehensive Urology.* London, England: Mosby; 2001.
4. The National Institute of Diabetes & Digestive & Kidney Diseases of the National Institutes of Health. Available at: www.niddk.nih.gov. Accessed in September 2004.
5. Guyton AC, Hall JE. *Textbook of Medical Physiology.* Philadelphia, Pa: WB Saunders Co; 2000.
6. Rhoades RA, Tanner GA. *Medical Physiology.* Baltimore, Md: Lippincott Williams & Wilkins; 1995.
7. Koeppen BM, Stanton BA. *Renal Physiology.* St. Louis, Mo: Mosby, Inc; 2001.
8. Huether SE, McCance. *Understanding Pathophysiology.* St. Louis, Mo: Mosby-Year Book Inc; 1996.
9. Spargo BH, Haas M. The kidney. In: Rubin E, Farber JL, eds. *Essential Pathology.* 2nd ed. Philadelphia, Pa: JB Lippincott Co; 1995.
10. Teichman JMH. *20 Common Problems in Urology.* New York, NY: McGraw Hill; 2001.
11. Jones-Kalota SM, Greene LF, Parsons SL. Evaluation of the urologic patient. In: Stein BS, Caldamone AA, Smith JA, eds. *Clinical Urologic Practice.* New York, NY: WW Norton Co; 1995.
12. Tierney LM, McPhee SJ, Papadakis MA. *Current Medical Diagnosis and Treatment.* Norwalk, Conn: Appleton & Lange; 1994.
13. Brenner BM. *Brenner & Rector's: The Kidney.* 7th ed. Philadelphia, Pa: WB Saunders Co; 2004.
14. Agrawal M, Swartz R. Acute renal failure. *Am Family Physician.* 2000;61:2077–2088.
15. The National Kidney Foundation. Available at: www.kidney.org. Accessed in September 2004.
16. Mallick NP, Gokal R. Hemodialysis. *The Lancet.* 1999;353:737–742.
17. Murphy GJ, White SA, Nicholson ML. Vascular access for hemodialysis. *Br J Surg.* 2000;87:1300–1315.
18. Work J. Hemodialysis catheters and ports. *Semin Nephrol.* 2002;22:211–220.
19. Gokal R, Mallick NP. Peritoneal dialysis. *The Lancet.* 1999;353:823–828.
20. Dirkes SM. Continuous renal replacement therapy: dialytic therapy for acute renal failure in intensive care. *Nephrol Nurs J.* 2000;27:581–590.
21. Patton ME. Continuous renal replacement therapy: slow but steady. *Nursing.* 2003;33:48–50.
22. Kreiger JN. Urinary tract infections in women: causes, consequences, and clinical management. In: Stein BS, Caldamone AA, Smith JA, eds. *Clinical Urologic Practice.* New York, NY: WW Norton Co; 1995.
23. Preminger GM. Nephrolithiasis: pathogenesis, diagnosis, and medical therapy. In: Stein BS, Caldamone AA, Smith JA, eds. *Clinical Urologic Practice.* New York, NY: WW Norton Co; 1995.
24. MD Consult: clinical information for physicians. Available at: www.mdconsult.com. Accessed on April 2, 2006.
25. Delgin JH, Vallerand AH. *Davis's Drug Guide For Nurses.* Philadelphia, Pa: FA Davis Co; 2003.

26. Physician's Desk Reference Online. Available at: www.PDR.net. Accessed in September 2004.
27. Sagiv M, Rudoy J, Rotstein A, Fisher N, Ben-Ari J. Exercise tolerance of end-stage renal disease patients. *Nephron*. 1991;57(4):424–427.
28. Painter P, Messer-Rehak D, Hanson P, et al. Exercise capacity in hemodialysis, CAPD, and renal transplant patients. *Nephron*. 1986;42(1):47–51.
29. Guide to Physical Therapist Practice. 2nd ed. *Physical Therapy*. 2001;81(1).

BIBLIOGRAPHY

Craig CR, Stitzel RE. *Modern Pharmacology with Clinical Applications*. New York, NY: Little, Brown, and Co; 1997.

Deglin JH, Vallerand AH. *Davis's Drug Guide for Nurses*. 8th ed. Philadelphia, Pa: FA Davis Co; 2003.

Karch AM. *Lippincott's Nursing Drug Guide*. Springhouse, Pa: Lippincott Williams & Wilkins; 2004.

Ritter JM, Lewis LD, Mant TG. *Textbook of Clinical Pharmacology*. London, England: Edward Arnold Co; 1995

Chapter 13

ONCOLOGICAL DISEASES AND DISORDERS

Lora Packel, MS, PT

Cancer rehabilitation is an important adjunct to cancer treatment. As the science of cancer and its treatment progresses, the focus of care is shifting to incorporate issues of survivorship. Rehabilitation specialists, notably physical therapists and physical therapist assistants, are uniquely qualified to address the musculoskeletal, neurological, and cardiopulmonary ramifications of cancer treatment and empower people to return to an active lifestyle. This chapter will focus on the acute management of the person with cancer as well as provide an overview for the role of physical therapy across the trajectory of disease.

BIOLOGY OF CANCER

Cancer cells have unique characteristics that differentiate them from healthy cells. Normal cells have a defined life span, **senescence**, with a balance between the number of new cells formed and those that die. Cancer cells, however, lack this preprogrammed life span and can continuously divide with adequate nutritional support. Cancer cells also lack **contact inhibition,** or the signal to stop dividing when there is contact with an adjacent cell. This disrupts the orderly architecture of normal tissue, resulting in a mass of unorganized cells. Finally, cancer cells can divide without being attached, or anchored, to a surface, which plays a role in metastasis.[1]

The mechanism of metastatic spread continues to evade researchers. The present theoretical framework purports that cancer cells release factors that enhance the formation of new blood vessels, **angiogenesis**, bringing needed nutrition for cell growth. These cells then break off from their original source and travel through the vascular system to a distant site, which is called **metastasis**.

Table 13–1
TNM STAGING SYSTEM

T = Tumor size
T_0 = No evidence of primary tumor
T_{1-4} = Increasing size of tumor

N = Regional lymph nodes
N_0 = No lymph node involvement
N_{1-3} = Increasing involvement of regional lymph nodes

M = Presence of distant metastasis
M_0 = No distant metastasis
M_1 = Distant metastasis

Adapted from:
Groenwald S, et al. *Cancer Nursing Principles and Practice.* 3rd ed. Jones and Bartlett Publisher; 1993:187–189.
National Cancer Institute. Available at: http://cis.nci.nih.gov/fact/5_32.htm.

STAGING SYSTEMS

Various clinical staging systems are used to denote a consistent description of a disease. The most widely used system is the TNM system—T indicates tumor size, N describes the nodal involvement, and M denotes the presence of metastases (Table 13–1).

PERFORMANCE SCALES

Oncologists utilize performance scales to describe the functional capacity of their patients. These scales are used as part of the inclusion/exclusion criteria for clinical trials to help denote which regimens may be too intensive for a debilitated patient. Two main systems are utilized: Eastern Cooperative Oncology Group Performance Scale (Table 13–2) and the Karnofsky Performance Scale (Table 13–3). These scales can be used in conjunction with a physical therapy assessment to communicate functional status to the oncologist.

CANCER TREATMENTS AND REHABILITATION IMPLICATIONS

Oncologists use a variety of clinical tests to determine a diagnosis of cancer. These tests may include biopsy, biochemical markers, genetic testing, imaging, and physical examination. Once a definitive diagnosis is determined, the oncologist and patient must consider many factors that influence the treatment plan.

- Type and stage of cancer

    What is the location?

Table 13–2
EASTERN COOPERATIVE ONCOLOGY GROUP PERFORMANCE SCALE

ECOG Scale	Details
0	Normal activity
1	Symptoms demonstrated, but the patient remains ambulatory and able to perform self-care
2	Ambulatory >50% of the time and requires occasional assistance
3	Ambulatory <50% of the time and requires nursing care
4	Bedridden
5	Death

Table 13–3
KARNOFSKY PERFORMANCE SCALE

100: Normal, no complaints, no evidence of disease
90: Able to carry on normal activity, minor symptoms of disease
80: Normal activity with effort, some symptoms of disease
70: Cares for self, unable to carry on normal activity or work
60: Requires occasional assistance but is able to care for needs
50: Requires considerable assistance and frequent medical care
40: Disabled, requires special care and assistance
30: Severely disabled, hospitalization is indicated, death not imminent
20: Very sick, hospitalization necessary, active treatment necessary
10: Moribund, fatal processes progressing rapidly

What size is the tumor?

Has it metastasized?

Is it a fast or slow growing tumor?

- What is the general health of the patient?

Can he or she tolerate intensive treatment?

What is his or her performance status?

- What is the patient's present and future quality of life?

Will the treatment significantly increase the patient's quality of life?

Will the side effects of treatment significantly decrease quality of life?

- What is the known effectiveness of each treatment?

- What financial strains will this place on the family/patient?
- Does the patient have adequate social support and psychological health to ensure follow through with the treatment plan? Can the family support the patient during and after treatment?

The goals for cancer treatment include cure, prevention of recurrence or metastasis, to control the cancer as long as possible or palliation of symptoms. These goals may be achieved through surgery, radiation, chemotherapy, or hormonal therapy (see Pharmacological Information).

Surgery

Surgery, in combination with other modalities, is the most common type of treatment for cancer. Goals of surgery include the following:

- Debulking a tumor
- Diagnosing a tumor (**biopsy**)
- Removing precancerous lesions
- Resecting a tumor
- Correction of life-threatening conditions caused by cancer
- Palliation

The rehabilitation implications after surgery depend on the particular procedure and will be discussed in the following sections. Common rehabilitation themes for the postsurgical patients include early mobilization, pulmonary hygiene, gait training, and training in activities of daily living (ADLs). Early mobilization assists in the prevention of complications such as pneumonia, ileus, deep vein thromboses, and the loss of lean body mass. Pulmonary hygiene in the form of splinted coughing, diaphragmatic and deep breathing exercises, and posture education play an important role in preventing postoperative pulmonary complications. Finally, gait training and ADL training may be appropriate if surgery included an amputation, if there is a weightbearing restriction, if pain is limiting functional mobility, or if fatigue is impeding mobility.

Radiation Therapy

A second modality used in cancer treatment is radiation. Radiation is a nonselective **localized treatment** that destroys cells by damaging DNA and impairing cell replication or by disrupting the milieu in which these cells thrive.[1] Cancer cells are often more susceptible to radiation when they are in the mitotic stage of cell division. Therefore, radiation affects tissues that normally have a high rate of division or turnover such as the gastrointestinal tract, hair follicles, and skin.

Goals for radiation include:

- Cure
- Control of cancer
- Decrease tumor size
- Palliation
- Prevention of fracture

Table 13–4

COMMON SIDE EFFECTS OF RADIATION THERAPY

1. **Immunosuppression**
   - Radiation to long bones, iliem, sternum.

2. **Skin changes**
   - Fragile skin.
   - Erythematous skin.
   - Tissue fibrosis (acute or chronic), myofascial adhesions.

3. **Gastrointestinal changes**
   - Vomiting/diarrhea which can result in impaired nutrition, protein deficiency, and muscle catabolism.

4. **Fatigue**[68]
   - Fatigue is cumulative over the course of radiation therapy.
   - Fatigue may resolve when radiation is complete or last 6 months to 1 year post-radiation.

5. **Avascular necrosis**
   - AVN is the loss of blood supply to an area resulting in necrosis of tissue. The most common area is the hip, potentially resulting in femoral head collapse and fracture.
   - Symptoms include pain with weightbearing, ache in the groin and anterior thigh, minimal relief with rest.

6. **Radiation myelitis**
   - Radiation may damage small blood vessels in the spinal column resulting in loss of blood flow, necrosis, and demyelination. Symptoms include sensory dysfunction and motor weakness. Time of onset is typically 4 to 12 months after the completion of radiation.

Radiation therapy does not discriminate between normal and abnormal tissue. The severity of side effects from radiation depends on dosing and the area being irradiated. Improved shielding techniques and conformal 3-D radiation therapy are recent advances that attempt to diminish radiation effects to surrounding tissues. The side effects that may impact rehabilitation are noted in Table 13–4.

Preventative and restorative stretching should be prescribed in anyone receiving radiation therapy. Radiation can cause acute and chronic changes in the skin and underlying tissue that can affect range of motion (ROM) and posture. The potential to develop fascial tightness after radiation needs to be considered. Exercises should continue for up to 6 months after the course of radiation is completed. One must also consider the risk for lymphedema if lymphatic beds are included in the radiation field. Patients should receive lymphedema education regarding the signs and symptoms of this condition. The issues of fatigue and the use of modalities during and after radiation will be discussed separately.

Table 13–5
COMMON SIDE EFFECTS OF CHEMOTHERAPY

1. **Immunosuppression** (Decrease in function of the components of the immune system. Patients may develop anemia or thrombocytopenia. In addition, there is a decrease in the white blood cell count [WBC] resulting in a diminished ability to resist infections.)
2. **Organ damage** (heart failure, liver toxicity, renal damage, see Table 13–6)
3. **Nausea and vomiting**
4. **Alopecia** (hair loss)
5. **Diarrhea**
6. **Mucositis or mouth sores**
7. **Sterility**
8. **Peripheral neuropathy**

Motor symptoms:
- Sense of heaviness in legs
- Tripping due to motor weakness of anterior tibialis
- Difficulty holding or manipulating objects
- Shaky handwriting

Sensory symptoms:
- Sensation of pins and needles
- Cold extremity
- Burning sensation
- Sharp "electrical" shooting pain

Autonomic symptoms:
- Orthostasis
- Feeling flush
- Tachycardia

Chemotherapy

Chemotherapy is a **systemic treatment** that does not distinguish between healthy and diseased tissue **(nonselective)**. Goals for chemotherapy include the following:

- Cure
- Slow the cancer's progression
- Shrink the tumor for palliation
- Shrink the tumor to enable surgical resection

Chemotherapy is administered using a combination of drugs. Combination therapy helps to decrease toxic side effects, lower the chances of drug resistance, and increase anti-neoplastic effectiveness. Chemotherapy has a higher kill rate for rapidly dividing cells. Thus, the side effects of chemotherapy are a result of the destruction of cells with rapid turnover such as those cells found in the bone marrow, gastrointestinal tract, and hair follicles as noted in Table 13–5.[1] Certain

Table 13–6
CHEMOTHERAPEUTIC AGENTS AND COMMON SIDE EFFECTS

Chemotherapeutic Agents	*Common Side Effects*
Cisplatin (eg, testicular, prostate, ovarian, uterine, head and neck, lung cancers)	Ototoxicity, hypokalemia, hypomagnesemia, peripheral neuropathy
Ifosfamide (eg, ovarian, breast, testicular, lymphoma, lung cancers)	Myelosuppression, lethargy, cerebellar toxicity
Cytarabine (eg, leukemia, lymphoma)	Cerebellar toxicity
Methotrexate (eg, breast, uterine, leukemia, head and neck, uterine, cervical cancers)	Myelosuppression, pulmonary fibrosis, transverse myelitis, osteoporosis, cerebellar dysfunction
Doxorubicin (eg, breast, gastric, liver, bladder, prostate, sarcoma, lymphoma, multiple myeloma, leukemia)	Myelosuppression, cardiomyopathy
Vincristine (eg, lymphoma, breast, lung, leukemia)	Paraesthesia, ataxia, foot drop, cranial nerve palsies, loss of deep tendon reflexes
Tamoxifen (breast)	Hot flashes, uterine bleeding, fluid retention
B-interferon (eg, leukemia, renal, melanoma, leukemia)	Myalgia, hypotension
Taxol	Myelosuppression, peripheral neuropathy

chemotherapy agents may also affect the musculoskeletal system and the central nervous system (CNS) as listed in Table 13–6.

The side effect profile of particular chemotherapeutic agents includes peripheral neuropathy as noted in Table 13–5. Nerves or a group of nerves can demonstrate motor, sensory, or autonomic dysfunction, resulting in a host of physically impairing symptoms. Symptoms of chemotherapy-induced peripheral neuropathy often resolve or lessen within 6 to 12 months after the completion of the chemotherapy regimen. However, some may have long-term numbness or tingling in the distal extremities.[2] Treatment interventions for peripheral neuropathy may include the use of medications such as Carbamazepine and gabapentin for pain relief.[2] In addition to medical therapy, physical and occupational therapy can be utilized for restorative and preventative therapy including fall precautions, ADL training, bracing, strengthening, and gait and balance training. There have been case reports that indicate the possible usefulness of contrast baths, massage and TENS for management of peripheral neuropathy pain.

Patients undergoing chemotherapy should be provided with education regarding the musculoskeletal side effects of their drug regimen. In addition, patients should be provided with an aerobic program to prevent loss of endurance and to mediate cancer-related fatigue. This program should be adjusted to the person's age, stage of disease, and intensity of his or her chemotherapy regimen. In addition, adjustments should be made for changes in his or her blood counts such as anemia and thrombocytopenia. Please refer to the section on Exercise for the Person with Cancer and review Chapter 2 (see Tables 2–12 and 2–13) for a more detailed discussion.

Bone Marrow Transplantation

Bone marrow transplantation (BMT) is a modality that is presently being used to treat leukemia, myelodysplastic syndrome, lymphoma, and aplastic anemia. Autologous transplants are being tested in clinical trials for ovarian, multiple myeloma, and colon cancers. BMT attempts to rid the body of diseased marrow and replace it with healthy functioning marrow from the patient themselves **(autologous or autogeneic BMT)**, or from a donor **(allogeneic BMT)**.[3] The treatment includes high dose chemotherapy and radiation **(conditioning regimen)**, followed by stem cell or bone marrow rescue. The purposes of the conditioning regimen are to eliminate the cancer cells as well as create anatomical space in the marrow for new, healthy cells to thrive. The mortality and morbidity associated with BMT is high, due to prolonged immunosuppression, side effects of high dose chemotherapy, and graft versus host disease (GVHD).

There are two main types of BMT: autogeneic and allogeneic. In autogeneic transplants, the patient's own stem cells or marrow are used as the rescue source. Stem cells are pleuripotent cells that have the ability to mature into any of the cells in the blood cell line including monocytes, neutrophils, erythrocyte, and platelets. The BMT process begins by using chemotherapy to induce clinical remission **(induction chemotherapy)**. At this time, stem cells are collected from either the patient's marrow or from his or her peripheral bloodstream through apheresis. Peripheral blood stem cell transplants are often used in those who have residual disease in their marrow or who have hypoplastic marrow from previous treatments for their cancer. Once the patient has recovered from induction chemotherapy, he or she is ready for an autologous transplant. Patients are given a second round of high dose chemotherapy to irradicate any lingering disease and then reinfused with their stem cells. These cells then migrate to the marrow and begin producing normal, healthy cell lines. While awaiting recovery of their blood counts, patients are provided with intensive medical support as they experience the side effects of chemotherapy which include neutropenia, thrombocytopenia, anemia, electrolyte abnormalities, and nausea/vomiting.

In allogeneic transplants, the patient is rescued with cells from a **human leukocyte antigen (HLA)** matched sibling or from a donor registry (**matched unrelated donor [MUD]**). The selection of the donor is one of the most critical components of the transplant. If the donor and recipient have a high degree of HLA compatibility, meaning they have a high degree of genetic similarity on the surface of their cells, there is a lower probability of developing GVHD, a condition associated with high morbidity and mortality. Similar to an autogeneic transplant, patients are given a combination of high dose chemotherapy and radiation. These doses would be lethal if the patient was not provided with the marrow rescue. The donor marrow cells are then infused and the patient is supported by blood and platelet transfusions, antibiotics, and immunosuppressants to control GVHD. While awaiting engraftment, patients are at risk for many potentially life-threatening illnesses including infection, pulmonary hemorrhage, and graft failure.

GVHD can occur either in the acute (first 100 days) or chronic phase (>100 days) of allogeneic BMT.[4] GVHD occurs when the donors cells (graft) recognize the patient's body (host) as foreign and mount an immunological attack. This process is mediated by the donor T lymphocytes and is more likely to occur when there are HLA mismatches. Controlled GVHD may be beneficial to the leukemic patient, as the immunological attack may help with a graft versus leukemia affect, essentially helping to increase the kill rate of leukemic cells.[1] However, uncontrolled GVHD is associated with high morbidity and mortality.[1] GVHD typically attacks three body systems: skin, liver, and gut. GVHD skin appears as a rash in the acute phase and soft tissue fibrosis in the chronic phase. Physical therapy can play an important role in providing a flexibility program to prevent and treat the loss of ROM with changes in the distensibility of soft tissue. In the chronic phases of GVHD of the skin, soft tissue mobilization may also help to restore ROM and flexibility. GVHD liver causes right upper quadrant pain and hepatic dysfunction with resultant elevated liver function tests, confusion/ encephalopathy, and jaundice. Finally, GVHD of the gut often results in sloughing of the intenstinal lining leading to poor absorption of nutrients, nutritional deficits, vomiting or diarrhea, and loss of lean body mass. The treatment for GVHD includes increasing immunosuppressive drugs, such as corticosteroids, to diminish the immunological attack on the host. As the doses and chronicity of these medications increase, there is a higher likelihood of steroid myopathy and osteopenia, both of which respond to physical therapy interventions. Steroid myopathy often presents with proximal hip weakness, manifesting in a difficulty with transfers and stairs. This may often go unnoticed, as walking is only impaired in later stages. A second manifestation of steroid myopathy is shoulder girdle weakness. Treatment for steroid myopathy should include weight bearing exercises and core strengthening exercises.

Therapy intervention is important during and after bone marrow, because there are many factors that can contribute to the loss of strength and endurance during hospitalization. Most BMT units place the patient in a single room for isolation during allogeneic transplants. Being confined to a room for a period of 4 to 6 weeks places the patient at risk for loss of endurance, imbalance, and postural hypotension (see Chapter 4 and Table 4–1). In addition, chemotherapy, steroid regimens, malnutrition, and limited mobility due to illness can all contribute to progressive weakness. Instruction and demonstration of a daily exercise routine that includes both aerobic and strengthening components is essential. Aerobic exercise, such as stationary biking, should be tailored to the patient's individual fitness levels and frequently modified to account for changes in his or her blood counts and overall medical condition.[5,6] Patients should also be provided with a home exercise program to restore strength and endurance.

The following sections will briefly describe a variety of cancer types with the salient implications for the acute care therapist.

BREAST CANCER

Breast cancer is the most common type of cancer in American women, with a higher incidence as one ages. The vast majority of breast cancers occurs in the ducts or lobes and is staged in the following manner:

- Stage I: Localized disease

- Stage II: Axillary node involvement

- Stage III: Advanced regional disease without metastasis

- Stage IV: Distant metastases

Staging is determined through the use of any or all of the following tests: mammogram, breast ultrasound, fine needles aspiration, skeletal survey, lymph node dissection, or sentinel lymph node biopsy.

Sentinel node biopsy: To avoid the morbidity associated with extensive axillary node dissections, sentinel lymph node biopsies are performed for those with small localized tumors to determine if cancer cells have entered the lymphatic system.[7] A radioisotope is injected around the tumor and is followed to the first node or nodes which are deemed the sentinel nodes. The sentinel node(s) is colored blue by the radioisotope for easy identification by the surgeon and removed for further evaluation. If the sentinel nodes are negative for cancer cells, no further axillary dissection is warranted. If the biopsy is positive for cancer cells, the patient must return for a full axillary dissection to help accurately stage the disease.

Treatment of breast cancer depends on the stage of disease. Most patients with Stage I or II breast cancer are treated conservatively with a lumpectomy or mastectomy followed by radiation therapy.

Lumpectomy or partial mastectomy is the removal of a suspicious breast lump and a small area of surrounding healthy tissue (clean margin). Lumpectomy is indicated for tumors <4 cm.

Mastectomy is the removal of breast tissue. Mastectomy is performed if the tumor is >4 cm, if there are multiple tumors or if the person chooses not to undergo radiation therapy. Types of mastectomy are listed below.

- **Simple mastectomy**: Removal of the entire breast, skin, and nipple.

- **Modified radical mastectomy (MRM)**: Removal of the entire breast, skin, nipple, and lining over the pectoralis muscles, with axillary node dissection.

- **Skin-sparing mastectomy**: Removal of the entire breast and nipple. The skin overlying the breast is left to allow for breast reconstruction. Axillary lymph nodes may also be removed.

- **Radical mastectomy**: Removal of the entire breast, pectoralis major and minor, fatty tissues, and axillary lymph node dissection.

Patients undergoing breast surgery should be instructed in a progressive shoulder ROM program and postural exercises and provided with lymphedema education. Practices regarding rehabilitation vary between facilities. Exercises are recommended to begin after removal of the drains, around postoperative day 7 to 10. Studies have reported fewer seroma formations when exercises are delayed without a significant impact on long-term shoulder function.[8,9]

Exercises should focus on all planes of motion including flexion, extension, ab/adduction, and rotation. In addition, postural exercises, which include pectoralis stretching and strengthening of posterior shoulder musculature, should also be emphasized. Demonstration of exercises should begin preoperatively if possible, when patients are pain free and able to focus on proper form. In addition to exercises, patients should be instructed to avoid splinting their arm, avoid repetitive motions and heavy lifting in the first few weeks after surgery to allow for wound healing. Finally, patients may experience tingling along the proximal medial aspect of the arm due to manipulation of the intercostobrachial nerve during surgery. These sensations usually resolve within 6 months; however, some patients are left with residual numbness.

Many women are now opting for immediate breast reconstruction with skin sparing mastectomies. The most common types of reconstruction are implants and **transverse rectus abdominus myocutaneous flaps (TRAM)**. Any type of reconstruction that changes the length tension relationships of muscle has the potential for short- or long-term musculoskeletal complications.

Women who opt for breast implants should be taught postural exercises prior to this procedure. Depending on the size of the implant, women may adopt a posture of rounded shoulders causing pectoralis tightness and weakness of scapular musculature. In addition, some women will experience pectoralis spasm during the expander phase. Gentle exercises may be employed early to avoid postural changes. A rigorous stretching program is not indicated until the final implant is in place. One should always monitor for areas of erythema, swelling, or necrosis triggering an immediate referral to the plastic surgeon.

The TRAM flap is a **pedicled** flap that uses the transverse rectus abdominis muscle to make a breast mound. The muscle and its blood supply are dissected and tunneled under the skin to the mastectomy site. This procedure can also be performed using a **free flap** by dissecting its blood supply and reconnecting the flap to vessels in the axilla. Surgeons may opt to use either the ipsilateral or contralateral rectus depending on the patency of the blood supply. If the contralateral rectus is used, patients will notice a medial bulge early in their recovery. This bulge is the rectus muscle, which will atrophy over time due to denervation during dissection. Finally, mesh is placed at the donor site to prevent herniation of abdominal contents.

The acute care management of the TRAM reconstruction revolves around maintaining a healthy donor and recipient site. Mobility and lifting is limited by the physician to ensure this goal. Postoperatively, patients are to remain in a flexed posture and limit lifting until the surgeon is comfortable with the health of the flap. This period may last from 3 weeks to a few months depending on healing. The acute care role of the rehabilitation specialist includes teaching proper body mechanics within the limitations prescribed, transfer and bed mobility techniques, and lymphedema precautions. In addition, patients should be taught symptoms that may warrant a physical therapy consultation after the flap has healed.

Patients who develop musculoskeletal complications may begin therapy after 6 to 8 weeks depending on flap viability. Common musculoskeletal consequences include breast and trunk lymphedema, adhesive capsulitis of the shoulder, poor posture, and low back pain. Appropriate therapy interventions may include a back stability program, shoulder ROM, strengthening, myofascial techniques for flexibility deficits, joint mobilization, body mechanics training, and complete decongestive therapy (see Lymphedema).

HEAD AND NECK CANCER

Head and neck cancer includes cancer of the nasal cavity, nasopharynx, oral cavity, hypopharynx, and larynx. Treatment for head and neck cancer may include radiation, chemotherapy, and surgery. These treatments can cause significant dysfunction in mobility, speech, and in the ability to eat and swallow.[10] In addition, the surgeries can be quite disfiguring causing emotional and interpersonal distress.

A proactive stance is important in treating the person with head and neck cancer, as he or she is at risk for radiation induced tissue fibrosis, cancer-related fatigue, deconditioning, lymphedema, and significant cervical and shoulder dysfunction. As the patient is undergoing or recovering from surgery or radiation, he or she is at risk for loss of lean muscle mass due to changes in his or her nutritional intake. Patients are often on modified diets as they go through radiation due to nausea, mucositis, and xerostomia (dry mouth) and may suffer from smell sensitivity. Patients may have temporary or permanent access for enteral nutrition if their treatment has interfered with any part of their gastrointestinal tract.

Surgery for head and neck cancer may include the following procedures:

Radical neck dissection: Removal of all five levels of lymph nodes, sacrifice of spinal accessory nerve (SAN), internal jugular vein, sternocleidomastoid, platysma, and omohyoid musculature. Used for large metastatic tumors and large palpable nodes.

Modified radical neck dissection: Possible removal of sternocleidomastoid and lymph nodes. Preservation of SAN if possible and internal jugular vein.

Selective neck dissection: Removal of the mass and any lymph nodes at highest risk of containing metastasis.

Acute rehabilitation of the person status post (s/p) neck dissection should include a thorough examination of cervical ROM, posture, shoulder function, scapular kinematics, coughing techniques, and lymphedema education.[11] However, therapy should proceed cautiously to allow for proper wound healing. Shoulder flexion should not exceed 90 degrees when drains are present to avoid seroma formation. In addition, conservative cervical ROM should only proceed after initial healing has taken place, usually around postoperative day 6. Patients will often posture with forward head, rounded shoulders, and neck rotation due to pain, tracheostomy, and fear of damaging the surgical site. Posturing in this manner will exacerbate any shoulder dysfunction and decrease the ability to clear secretions. Postural exercises should include pectoralis stretching and strengthening of the trapezius and rhomboids. Neck dissection surgeries alter the venous and lymphatic drainage system of the head, neck, and face. Patient education regarding lymphedema needs to be stressed.

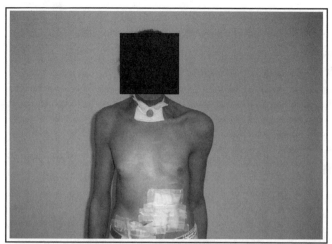

Figure 13–1. SAN palsy. Note left shoulder droop, protracted shoulder.

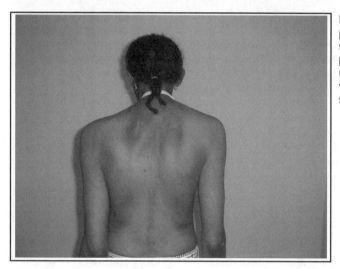

Figure 13–2. SAN palsy. Note left shoulder droop, protracted scapula, and downward rotation of scapula.

Spinal Accessory Nerve

During neck dissection the **SAN** may be sacrificed or suffer a traction injury due to the small surgical area of the posterior cervical triangle.[12–14] The SAN innervates the trapezius, which is an essential element for scapulohumeral rhythm. Statically, the trapezius holds the scapula on the thoracic cage. Dynamically, the trapezius contributes to medial stabilization and upward rotation of the scapula, allowing for full ROM of the humerus for overhead activities. If the SAN was removed or injured during surgery, the patient may demonstrate abnormal scapulohumeral rhythm and the following musculoskeletal abnormalities (Figures 13–1 and 13–2):

- Atrophy of trapezius (chronic denervation)
- Limited shoulder flexion and abduction to 90 degrees or less
- Pain with shoulder flexion and abduction
- Scapular winging and upward rotation
- Scapular protraction and depression
- Subluxation of the humeral head[12]

Altered static and dynamic biomechanics may cause other scapular muscles such as the levator scapula and rhomboids to become strained. It also sets the stage for capsular tightness and chronic pain. Acute care therapy of the patient with SAN palsy should focus on early identification of nerve palsy through testing of the trapezius and educating the patient on supporting the arm during sitting and standing activities.[11] Outpatient physical therapy referrals should be made in the acute care setting to follow through on positioning recommendations and for training of the rhomboids to assist for medial stability of the scapula until there is reinnervation by the SAN.

Head and Neck Reconstruction

Patients who have large head and neck tumors or need resection of the mandible are potential candidates for osseocutaneous or myocutaneous reconstruction. The three most common techniques are **pectoralis flap, fibular flap, and radial forearm flap**. The pectoralis musculature is used when there is a need for muscle bulk due to a large resection. The motion of the pectoralis can be partially compensated for by the latissimus dorsi and subscapularis. However, if the patient has SAN damage, he or she has lost both posterior and anterior stabilization of the shoulder. Acute rehabilitation should focus on postural training and cervical ROM. Once wound healing is achieved, exercises should include scapular retraction and latissimus strengthening for posterior stability.

A fibular osseocutaneous flap can be used to reconstruct the mandible. Up to 10 cm of bone is resected, with preservation of the peroneal nerve.[15] The distal end of the fibula remains intact to allow for ankle stabilization. The long-term functional sequela of a fibular flap is unknown as the fibula serves mostly as a site for muscle attachment and is not a weightbearing bone. In the acute setting, patients are often nonweightbearing for 4 to 7 days. Evaluation of vascular integrity and peroneal nerve function are critical in this time period. Gait training in the early postoperative time should focus on transfers, bed mobility, and pulmonary hygiene. Once the weightbearing status is advanced, gait training will focus on safe household and community ambulation. One should provide verbal feedback to avoid compensatory gait deviations that will increase the energy requirements of walking and potentially lead to long-term postural pain. The surgical team usually evaluates temporal-mandibular joint (TMJ) function after initial healing has taken place and patients may be referred to outpatient physical therapy for treatment.

A radial forearm flap can be used to replace skin lost on the face or in the reconstruction of the oral pharynx. The patient should avoid weightbearing through the donor site during transfers and ADLs. ROM to the wrist, elbow, and shoulder should be taught as well as proper posture. ROM of the shoulder should not exceed 90 degrees until drains are removed to avoid seroma formation.

Table 13–7
STAGES OF HODGKIN'S DISEASE

- Stage I: One area of lymph node involvement
- Stage II: Two or more areas of lymph node involvement above the diaphragm
- Stage III: Two or more areas of involvement both above and below the diaphragm
- Stage IV: Widespread disease

LEUKEMIA AND LYMPHOMA

Leukemia is a hematological disorder that affects leukocytes including neutrophils, basophils, eosinophils, lymphocytes, and monocytes. Leukemia results in proliferation of abnormal, malfunctioning cells. Due to rapid growth, large quantities of these abnormal cells crowd out normal cell lines in the marrow, and the patient will exhibit symptoms of failure of multiple cell lines.

Leukemia is classified according to the cell line that is affected (myeloid or lymphoid) and the stage at which cellular development became abnormal. Acute leukemias are characterized by dysfunction of immature, undifferentiated cells whereas chronic leukemia is characterized by dysfunction of mature, more differentiated cells. The onset of chronic leukemia is more gradual than acute leukemia, and the clinical course is often longer. The mainstay of treatment for leukemia is chemotherapy and/or BMT. Chemotherapy is given in three phases:

- **Induction:** Initial cycle of chemotherapy used to induce remission. The chemotherapy causes bone marrow hypoplasia, allowing normal cells to grow and replenish the marrow.

- **Consolidation:** A second round of chemotherapy aimed to prevent recurrence from resistant or microscopic residual disease.

- **Intensification:** A third round of chemotherapy often given for patients at high risk for recurrence.

Lymphoma is also a hematological disorder that arises from the lymphoreticular system. This system is primarily responsible for the growth and development of B and T lymphocytes. The humoral response to a foreign antigen involves the B cell, which secretes antigen specific antibodies. T cells are a part of cell mediated immunity that develops specifically against a particular antigen (see Chapter 5).

There are two main categories of lymphomas: **Hodgkin's lymphoma** (Hodgkin's disease [HD]) and **Non-Hodgkin's lymphoma (NHL)**. HD peaks in children under 10 and then again between the ages of 20 to 30. The Reed-Sternberg cell, a large multi-nucleated cell, characterizes HD. Treatment for HD includes radiation and/or chemotherapy depending on stage (Table 13–7). Due to advances in detection and treatment, HD has a cure rate in the high 90%s.[16]

NHLs are a heterogeneous group of cancers that can range from indolent tumors, or slow growing, to rapidly progressive tumors. NHL can affect either B or T cells and can appear in any organ of the body. Treatment may include radiation, chemotherapy, or BMT.

The treatments for leukemia and lymphoma can be quite debilitating. The chemotherapy regimens often result in an immunosuppressive state that places the patient at a high risk for infection. Weakness, deconditioning, fatigue, and peripheral neuropathies are all common side effects of treatment. Rehabilitation in the acute setting should focus on prevention of these impairments. All patients undergoing chemotherapy should be provided with a bedside aerobic and strengthening program that accounts for changes in blood values (see Chapter 2), and education regarding the untoward effects of bed rest (see Chapter 4). Home exercise prescription should include a progressive aerobic program to regain endurance and to help mediate fatigue. Please refer to the sections on chemotherapy, radiation, and exercise intervention for more details.

MULTIPLE MYELOMA

Multiple myeloma is a disease of the plasma cell of the immune system. Plasma cells secrete immunoglobulins such as IgG, IgA, IgM, IgD, and IgE (see Chapter 5 [ie, humoral immunity]). If left untreated, survival is approximately 7 months. With therapy, survival may be extended to 2 to 3 years.[1] Average age of onset is 65 years of age and this disease is more common among African-Americans than Caucasians.[1] It is also more common in males, with a male to female ratio of 3:2. Treatment options for multiple myeloma include chemotherapy, radiation, interferon, bisphosphphonates, or BMT.

Myeloma has a significant effect on skeletal stability. As the disease progresses, lytic lesions appear in the bony skeleton, diminishing the structural integrity of bone. It is believed that myeloma cells produce osteoclast activating factors that cause bone destruction, placing the patient at a high risk for fracture, spinal cord compression, and hypercalcemia. Thorough patient history should be taken with an emphasis on radiological evidence of skeletal disease, pain, and functional mobility. Exercise intervention should include weightbearing exercises, if the skeleton is stable, to help prevent osteopenia. Therapy should also include education regarding the signs and symptoms of cord compression and pathologic fracture as noted in Tables 13–12 and 13–13.

If bone disease is present, patients may benefit from surgical intervention, bracing, functional mobility training, ADL training, or education in pain management. Finally, postural training may be beneficial if there is vertebral collapse from lytic disease of the spine. Compression fractures may cause increased thoracic kyphosis due to loss of vertebral height. Kyphotic posture may contribute to pain, poor ventilation, and weakness of the shoulder musculature.

SKIN CANCER

Skin cancer can be separated into **melanoma** and **nonmelanoma skin cancers (NMSC)**. Melanoma has a higher rate of metastasis and poorer survival than NMSC. Treatment for skin cancer includes excision, radiotherapy, immunotherapy, or hormonal therapy. Rehabilitation efforts are focused on the functional sequela of metastasis to brain and bone as well as lymphedema treatment resulting from lymph node excision or radiation to the lymphatic beds.

GYNECOLOGICAL CANCERS

Gynecological cancers include cervical, ovarian, endometrial, vulvar, and vaginal. Treatment for these cancers may include total abdominal hysterectomy (TAH), radical hysterectomy, bilateral salipingo oophorectomy, radiation, and chemotherapy.

TAH: Removal of the body of the uterus and the cervix.

Radical hysterectomy: Removal of the uterus, uterosacral and uterovesical ligaments, pelvic lymph node removal, and removal of upper third of the vagina. Side effects of surgery and radiation may include bladder dysfunction, vaginal stenosis, sexual dysfunction, and lymphedema.

Salipingo oophorectomy: Removal of the ovary and fallopian tube.

Side effects of gynecological cancer treatment including peripheral neuropathy, pelvic pain, urinary incontinence (UI), lymphedema, and sexual dysfunction. Radiation to the pelvic region may result in fibrosis of the muscles and connective tissues in the radiation field. These soft tissue changes can occur both acutely and chronically and lead to decreased flexibility, ROM, and adhesions to nerve fibers. Exercises should focus on the flexibility of hip and abdominal musculature, scar adhesions, and nerve gliding techniques as indicated.

Pelvic pain syndromes, defined as pain in the buttocks, groin, pelvis, upper thighs, or lower abdomen that lasts for more than 3 months after completion of cancer treatments, are common in women being treated for gynecological cancer. Characteristics of pelvic pain include either constant or intermittent pain described as an ache, burn, or "shock-like." Pain may be exacerbated by urination or bowel movements, sexual intercourse, or with extended periods of sitting.

Dyspareunia, or pain with sexual intercourse, may also occur after surgery, radiation, or chemotherapy. Dyspareunia can result from a decrease in vaginal lubrication caused by radiation. In addition, removal or damage to the ovaries decreases circulating estrogen, which can cause dryness and thinning of the vaginal mucosa. Patients may benefit from referral to rehabilitation specialists in women's health for vaginal dilators, lubricants, and pelvic floor re-education.

Another issue surrounding gynecologic cancers and their treatments includes UI or the inability to control urination. Local reflex arcs as well as higher centers in the brain control the act of urination. When the bladder is stretched, a signal is sent to the sacral portion of the spinal cord. A signal from the cord is sent back to the bladder to allow for contraction of the Detruser muscle and concomitant relaxation of the external sphincter. Additionally, a signal is sent to the brain which controls the coordination of bladder emptying and allows for volitional control over the external sphincter.[17] Dysfunction in any one of these areas caused by surgery, radiation, or direct invasion by tumor may affect volitional urination.

Stress incontinence:[17] Incomplete closing of the sphincter due to weakness resulting in incontinence. The primary symptom is leakage during high-impact

---

Table 13–8
KEGEL EXERCISES

1. Contract the pelvic floor muscles during urination and attempt to slow or stop the flow of urine.
2. Hold this contraction for 5 seconds, then release.
3. Rest 10 to 15 seconds between trials.
4. Perform 15 contractions, three to four times per day.
5. Alternate this with trials of a quick hold and release.
6. Once the patient understands her anatomy and can perform the exercises, avoid practicing during urination.

---

exercises, laughing, lifting, coughing, sneezing, and running. Leakage usually ends when the activity stops. Stress incontinence can occur during surgery when there is a neurological insult or when pelvic muscles are stretched. In addition, poor closing of the sphincter can result from treatment induced thinning of the urethra.[1]

Overflow incontinence:[17] Overflow incontinence occurs when urine is blocked from leaving the bladder, limiting effective emptying. A tumor or scar tissue can cause this from surgery. In addition, overflow incontinence can occur when there is nerve damage that decreases the body's ability to determine bladder volume.

Urge incontinence:[17] Urge incontinence occurs when the Detruser muscle surrounding the bladder contracts inappropriately during filling of the bladder. Patients need to urinate frequently and have leakage due to inability to voluntarily stop the urine flow.

Evaluation of the person with incontinence should include the following questions:

- Frequency of urination
- Amount of fluids (water, caffeine, alcohol)
- Frequency of night urination
- Pain or odor with urination
- Ability to stop urine stream
- Describe activity that increases leakage

Treatment for UI can include the following:

- Kegel exercises (stress and urge incontinence, Table 13–8)
- Biofeedback
- Medications (alpha-adrenergic drugs, tricyclics)
- Weighted vaginal cones
- Pelvic floor electrical stimulation
- Change in dietary habits
- Managing hygiene

- Estrogen supplements/creams (controversial in women who have hormone-sensitive cancers such as breast, ovarian, uterine)
- Surgery

LUNG CANCER

Peak incidence of lung cancer for males is between 50 to 60 years of age with poor 5-year survival. Smoking is associated with 90% of cases of lung cancer.[18] Smoking causes chronic irritation to bronchial ciliated epithelial cells. Epithelial cells can regenerate in response to irritation; however, with chronic smoking, they eventually become less differentiated, resulting in cancer.

Lung cancer is separated into **small cell and nonsmall cell cancer (NSCLCA)**. Small cell lung cancer has a high growth rate and a worse prognosis than NSCLCA. The presenting symptoms are often cough, hemoptysis, dyspnea, and wheezing. Patients may also present with shoulder pain and weakness if there is invasion of the brachial plexus. Treatment for lung cancer may include surgical resection, chemotherapy, and radiation. Lung cancer is minimally responsive to the present chemotherapy regimens and, therefore, has a poor survival curve.

Physical therapy interventions should focus on posture, breathing facilitation techniques, and conditioning of the musculoskeletal system. As lung cancer tends to spread to bone and brain, treatment of patients with metastatic disease may focus on gait training, pain control, and cognitive rehabilitation. Patients who undergo surgical resection for lung cancer often develop an acute pain syndrome and altered posture that can lead to diminished vital capacity. Acute care therapy should focus on symmetrical movement of the thoracic cage, splinted coughing, and ROM of the shoulder. In addition, education should be provided for pacing and energy conservation techniques because dyspnea will increase as the disease progresses. Specific treatment interventions can be found in Chapter 7 and the section on bone metastasis in this chapter.

COLORECTAL CANCER

Colon and anal cancers are the third most common types of cancer in the United States.[19] The highest incidence occurs among those older than 50.[20] The natural progression of colorectal cancer begins with benign polyps and then advances to form cancerous lesions. As with most diseases, the earlier the polyp or malignant cell is found, the better the prognosis. Poor prognostic indicators include malignant cells that perforate the bowel, venous or lymph node invasion.[20]

Anal cancer is rare, with the incidence higher among females. The etiology is unclear although associations have been made with HIV, immunosuppression in transplant patients, prior radiation, cigarette smoking, and human papiloma virus (HPV). The most frequent symptom is spontaneous bleeding and complaints of pressure or pain with defecation.[21]

Treatments for colorectal cancers include surgery, radiation, and chemotherapy. Surgery is the primary treatment intervention with adjuvant chemotherapy or radiation for metastatic disease. Patients may undergo a colectomy or removal of part of the rectum. Side effects may include sexual dysfunction due to injury of the sympathetic and parasympathetic nerves that are essential for erectile function. Women may experience a decrease in the size of the vagina if repair is needed after tumor excision. Both men and women may benefit from a referral to a sexual rehabilitation counselor.

PROSTATE CANCER

Possible etiologic factors for **prostate cancer** include infection thorough sexual intercourse, diet, and endocrine factors. Prostate cancer often metastasizes to the bladder, peritoneum, lungs, liver, and kidney. In addition, prostate cancer has a predilection for the bony skeleton, specifically the lumbar spine, pelvis, femur, and ribs.[1,22]

Treatment for prostate cancer may include surgery, radiation, chemotherapy, brachytherapy (implanted radiation seeds), or hormone therapy. Primary surgical intervention can include a **radical prostatectomy**, which involves excision of the prostate, seminal vesicles, and partial excision of the bladder neck. Some patients may undergo an **orchiectomy** or medical castration to decrease circulating androgens that may stimulate cancerous growth. Internal or external beam radiation may be used for local control. Side effects of these treatments may include temporary changes in bowel and bladder function, fascial tightness in the abdominal and pelvic region, and lymphedema. Erectile dysfunction is common after surgery due to disruption of the autonomic nerves that control blood flow to the penis. Incontinence occurs in 8% to 81% of patients for up to 6 months after prostatectomy and 5% to 44.5% in the first year.[23] Patients are often responsive to biofeedback and biobehavioral techniques. See the section on gynecological cancers for more information on UI.

Acute therapy interventions may include mobility training, splinted coughing, and education regarding erectile dysfunction and UI. Therapy may focus on the sequela of bone disease to the spine and pelvis. All patients should be provided with a home aerobic and strengthening program because androgen ablation therapy is associated with osteopenia. Refer to the section on bone metastasis for more information.

TESTICULAR CANCER

The incidence of testicular cancer has been rising over the past 50 years. Peak age is between 20 to 40 years. Possible etiologic factors include having an undescended testicle and the use of exogenous estrogens in birth control by the patient's mother. Most testicular cancers arise from germ tissue and demonstrate a rapid growth pattern. Metastatic testicular cancer often occurs in the lung, liver, brain, and bone.[24]

Treatment for testicular cancer includes orchiectomy, retroperitoneal lymphadenectomy, radiation, or chemotherapy. During surgical intervention, the autonomic nerves involved in ejaculation, erection, and urinary continence may be affected. Radiation therapy in the pelvic region may cause fatigue and bone marrow suppression as well as fascial tightness. Chemotherapy is used for metastatic disease and has a high response rate. However, the agents used in the treatment of testicular cancer are associated with peripheral neuropathies and myalgias.

Acute therapy interventions may include education regarding sexual dysfunction and UI. In addition, patients should be provided with a strengthening program to prevent osteopenia as a result of decreased testosterone levels. Finally, therapy may focus on gait training, transfer training, and strengthening as testicular cancer can spread to the axial skeleton.

GASTRIC, LIVER, AND PANCREATIC CANCER

Gastric, liver, and pancreatic cancer all present with vague symptoms that often lead to late diagnosis and advanced disease at time of diagnosis. Gastric and liver cancers have a tendency to metastasize to bone. Treatments for these cancers include partial or total surgical resection of the involved organ and chemotherapy.[1,22]

Patients undergoing treatment for gastric cancer often develop nutritional deficiencies that can lead to loss of muscle. Therapy interventions should, therefore, focus on a strengthening program to prevent loss of lean tissue. The functional impairments often seen with pancreatic cancer are due in part to pain syndromes associated with this disease. Pain control techniques such as TENS, positioning, or nerve blocks to the lumbo-sacral plexus are often helpful to alleviate pain.

CANCER PAIN

Chronic cancer pain affects up to 50% of patients diagnosed with a solid tumor.[25] In a study by Serlin, patients who rated pain from 1 to 4 on a 10-point scale had minimal impact on function. Pain rated 5 or 6 had a moderate impact on function and seven to 10 had a severe effect on function. All pain levels correlated with a decrease in quality of life.[26] Therapists need to be part of a multidisciplinary pain team due to the functional ramifications of cancer-related pain. This team may include physicians, nurses, social workers, and pastoral care, each of whom provide a different perspective and treatment strategy for cancer-related pain. Adequate control of pain requires frequent reassessment over the course of the disease trajectory. In rehabilitation, pain at rest and with mobility should be clearly documented.

The physical therapy examination of cancer related pain should begin with a thorough evaluation of the characteristics of pain and the patient's goal for pain relief. The questions in Table 13–9 should be part of any comprehensive evaluation.

Cancer pain can be musculoskeletal in origin and may be a result of bone destruction, compression of nerves, collapse of vertebra, nerve inflammation, or altered biomechanics as noted in Table 13–10. Cancer-related pain is often treated with a variety of medications such as tricyclic antidepressants, anticonvulsants, corticosteroids, and Baclofan. These medications can be effective in managing pain, however, fine tuning the dose can be an arduous journey for the patient. There may be periods of oversedation or acute immobilizing pain as medications are titrated to their peak effective dose. During this process, the patient's ability to participate in therapy will vacillate. Patients and families should be taught safety awareness and fall prevention strategies as medications are adjusted.

Table 13-9

EXAMINATION OF CANCER-RELATED PAIN

Temporal	• Is the pain acute or chronic? • When does the pain occur? • How long does it last? • Does it change over the course of a day? • What makes it better? • What makes it worse?
Intensity **(see Table 1–10)**	• On a scale of 0 to 10, what is your pain now? • On a scale of 0 to 10, what is the worst the pain has been in the past 24 hours? • On a scale of 0 to 10, what is the best the pain has been in the past 24 hours?
Topography	• Where is the pain located? (use both patient description and body diagram) • Is the pain focal, multifocal, or referred? • Is the pain deep or superficial?
Quality	• Have the patient describe the pain. Try not to provide patient with descriptive words (eg, burning, throbbing, tingling, shock-like, ache)

Activity should be closely monitored as the patient's perception of pain is dulled and, therefore, at risk for overexertion and injury.

Medications and rehabilitation strategies can be effective in the management of cancer-related pain. Therapy interventions for pain control are listed below. Many of these interventions are based on small case controlled studies so clinical decision making and review of recent literature are paramount to your decision to utilize these modalities. The National Center for Complementary and Alternative Medicine is a well-respected organization that is a good source of information on recent studies in this area.

Transcutaneous electrical nerve stimulation (TENS): TENS uses low-voltage electrical pulses transdermally to help reduce pain as well as nausea.[25] High frequency and low intensity has been shown to be most effective for pain relief. TENS may be effective through blocking the afferent sensory information from higher sensors in the brain (Melzak-Wall Gate Theory). TENS may also be affective by causing local vasodilatation, possibly decreasing local ischemia. Finally, TENS may be effective by stimulating sensory nerves to signal the endogenous opiate release that decrease pain perception. TENS is indicated for postoperative incisional pain, phantom limb pain, visceral pain, and bone pain.

Massage: Massage assists with decreasing muscle spasms that occur from poor positioning or a change in muscle biomechanics. Anecdotal studies reports that massage increases the overall quality of life of those with cancer. Contraindications for massage include acutely irradiated skin, skin breakdown, massage directly over tumor, infection, thrombocytopenia, and coagulopathy.

<u>Table 13-10</u>
CANCER-RELATED PAIN

Type of Pain	Descriptors	Possible Etiology	Exam
Neuropathic pain	• Shock-like • Tingling • Burning • Numbness • Intermittent • Constant	• Tumor adjacent to or adhered to peripheral nerves • Vertebral collapse causing nerve compression • Radiation fibrosis causing tissue adherence to nerve	• Motor weakness • Altered sensation • (+) neural tension tests • Pain along a myotome or dermatome • Numbness/ tingling in distal fingertips and toes
Skeletal pain	• Sharp • Intermittent or constant • Escalating back pain • Pain in supine • Pain with ambulation • Pain in groin with standing	• Altered bone stability from lytic or blastic lesions • Spinal cord compression (SCC) • Avascular necrosis • Tumor increases pressure in periosteum	• Pain with weightbearing • Pain with joint compression (ie, hip scour) • Pain that radiates to groin/anterior thigh with weightbearing • Pain in a band across chest • Pain with coughing
Joint pain	• Pain with functional activity • Ache	• Tumor encroaching joint space • Neupogen pain • Arthralgia syndrome associated with Taxanes	• Possible palpation of tumor • Pain with passive and active ROM
Postsurgical pain	• Pain with coughing • Pain with mobility • Sharp • Constant ache • Intermittent or chronic	• Positioning during surgery • Manipulation of nerves during surgery • Altered biomechanics from nerve palsy • Muscle spasm from positioning	• Pain along surgical site • Tingling along nerve distribution • Pain with deep inspiration

(continued)

Table 13–10   (continued)
CANCER-RELATED PAIN

Type of Pain	Descriptors	Possible Etiology	Exam
Soft-tissue pain	• Ache • Stiffness with movement	• Radiation fibrosis • Soft tissue changes from GVHD • Contracture from immobility • Protective muscle spasm	• Reproduction of symptoms with passive stretching • Decreased skin elasticity • (+) trigger points • Decreased passive or active ROM

Bracing: Bracing can be used to correct deformities caused by the tumor itself, surgery, or from nerve injury. It can also position a joint for maximum comfort. Bracing can also be used to stabilize the spine and prevent rotation that may increase pain.

Assistive devices: Assistive devices allow one to decrease weightbearing over painful or unstable bones.

Superficial heat: Superficial heat can cause local changes in the skin, fascia, and muscle that may affect the sensation of pain. Local heat can increase oxygen and blood supply through vasodilatation to ease local ischemia or to aid in removal of waste products. Heat may also be used to relax muscle spasms, increase flexibility of soft tissue, or aid in relaxation. Heat is contraindicated directly over a tumor site, in the presence of deep vein thrombosis, and in the patient with poor or absent sensation. It is a relative contraindication for any person with cancer.[28]

Cryotherapy: Cryotherapy decreases muscle spindle sensitivity and, therefore, can assist in decreasing muscle spasm. Cryotherapy can also be used to decrease inflammation and may assist in dulling nerve pain by slowing the conduction velocity of nerves thus delaying the transmission of pain impulses. Cryotherapy should not be used over insensate tissue, acutely irradiated tissue, or directly over a tumor site. It is a relative contraindication in those with cancer.[28]

Acupuncture: Acupuncture is beginning to show benefits in the management of cancer-related pain. It may also be beneficial for those who suffer from xerostomia after head and neck irradiation. Caution should be taken in those with bleeding disorders, acutely irradiated tissue, insensate tissue, or at risk for infection.

Exercise: Exercise can be used to assist in pain that result from immobility, joint stiffness, or swelling. Exercise can also address postural changes that occur with pain, surgery, and fatigue.[27]

Relaxation and distraction: Relaxation and distraction may be used to divert attention away from pain. Focused deep breathing, imagery, and progressive relaxation techniques can be effective.[28]

Table 13–11	
LOCATION OF METASTATIC BONE DISEASE	
Vertebrae	69%
Pelvis	40%
Femur	25%
Ribs	25%
Humerus	20%

The use of modalities in the person with cancer is controversial. If certain modalities can increase blood flow to an area, can they potentially increase the chance of metastasis? The present body of literature cannot answer this question. In addition, there is no research to determine if modalities are safe when used at a distant site from the cancer or if they are safe to use once someone is in remission. The preceding list is the present standard of care for the person with cancer. The combination of clinical judgment based on a thorough literature review and consultation with the medical team should assist with your decision to use modalities in this patient population.

BONE METASTASIS

There are approximately 400,000 new cases of bone metastasis per year and the locations of metastatic bone disease is diverse (Table 13–11). Two types of bone lesions can potentially affect the architecture and stability of the skeleton. **Lytic** lesions involve an increase in osteoclastic activity and result in bone destruction and increase the potential for pathological fracture. **Blastic** lesions involve an increase in bone formation.[29] These lesions can cause pain due to a change in the bone structure and from stretching of the periosteum. Metastatic disease to the bone usually consists of a combination of lytic and blastic lesions, although there may be a predominance of one type.[29]

Certain types of cancers such as breast, lung, and prostate are more likely to travel to bone. The mechanism of metastasis and the rationale for this predilection to bone is unknown. The present theoretical framework focuses on the osteoclast as the prime stimulus for the growth of metastatic bone disease.

The first sign of metastatic disease to bone is often subjective complaints of pain. Metastatic bone pain is often described as an ache or sharp pain. Pain can originate from microfractures due to a change in stability, a tumor stimulating C fibers in the periosteum, reactive muscle spasm or nerve root infiltration.[29] Pain may result when there is a disruption of blood flow, causing bone necrosis. Full clinical diagnosis includes subjective complaints, physical exam, and use of various forms of imaging including x-ray, bone scan, magnetic resonance imaging, and CAT scan. It is important for the rehabilitation specialist to be aware of the diseases that have a tendency to spread to bone as well as signs and symptoms of bone disease and impending fracture as noted in Table 13–12.

Table 13–12

PAIN CHARACTERISTICS THAT MAY INDICATE FRACTURE OR IMPENDING FRACTURE

- Pain with weightbearing
- Pain in the groin
- Pain with hip scour
- Pain with hip external rotation and abduction
- Pain with deep inspiration
- Pain in a band around the chest wall
- Increased pain with supine
- Increased pain with valsalva

When a person is diagnosed with bone involvement, multidisciplinary input is critical in determining appropriate treatment. Therapists can provide important information regarding the patient's present functional status, pain with activity, and prognostication for mobility depending on type of treatment chosen.

The team, through subjective and objective assessments, needs to answer several essential questions to determine optimal treatment. The first question that the team needs to address is "What is the likelihood of fracture?" The medical team will use their physical examination in conjunction with imaging to determine the likelihood of pathologic fracture. Second, "What is the patient's expected life span?" If the patient has more than 3 months to live, surgery may be considered. If the patient's life span is short or he or she is not a surgical candidate, radiation and/or limited mobility with bracing may be considered. In addition to the potential to fracture and expected life span, the team needs to consider the patient's present and future quality of life. "What is the likelihood that surgery will decrease pain and increase mobility? What is the patient's goal for pain relief? Can surgery help to attain this level of pain relief?" Finally, "What is the patient's rehabilitation potential?" Rehabilitation specialists play an important role in determining the patient's present functional mobility and potential for rehabilitation after treatment intervention. A thorough examination of strength, coordination, cognition, and social support will help guide the decision for treatment.

Survival of patients after their first long bone pathological fracture has tripled for most cancers in the past 25 years.[30] Goals for surgery include: excision of tumor, cure, stabilization of bone, prevention of sequela from bed rest, and palliation. The method of fixation depends on the location of the fracture and extent of disease. Surgical fixation in oncology patients will usually include a larger area of bone as the area surrounding the primary lesion is usually unhealthy tissue.

If the bone lesion is stable or if the person is not a surgical candidate, radiation therapy is often utilized.

Radiation to the bone causes degeneration and necrosis of tumor cells followed by bone regrowth. Chondrogenesis is initially inhibited, and there are a few reports of acute postradiation fracture. Side effects of radiation to the bone

---

Table 13–13
SIGNS AND SYMPTOMS OF SPINAL CORD COMPRESSION

- Pain that increases when lying supine
- Pain with valsalva
- Escalating back pain
- Motor weakness
- Sensory deficits
- Bowel/bladder dysfunction
- Hyperreactive reflexes

---

include fatigue, skin erythema and hypersensitivity, impaired wound healing, avascular necrosis, and soft tissue fibrosis. Finally, there can be bone marrow suppression if the radiation field includes long bones or iliac wings.

In addition to surgery and radiation, **bisphosphonates** may be used to prevent and treat bone disease.[29] Bisphosphonates bind to areas of increased osteoclastic activity. They disrupt the internal environment of the osteoclast and cause cell death. Bisphosphonates have been shown to reduce skeletal morbidity (pain, fracture, hypercalcemia) in multiple myeloma and breast cancer.[29] Its role in the prevention and treatment of bone disease in other cancer populations is being investigated.

SPINAL CORD COMPRESSION

Spinal cord compression (SCC) occurs when primary or secondary disease spreads to the vertebra and impinges on the spinal column. This can occur by direct invasion into the vertebra and spinal canal, by disruption of the vascular supply to the cord, or when a tumor causes vertebral collapse with bony protrusion into the canal. SCC can lead to demylenation, arterial compromise, and vasogenic edema all of which affect the transmission of motor and sensory signals.[31] Symptoms of SCC are presented in Table 13–13.

Physical therapists play a critical role in the diagnosis and treatment of the person with SCC. The most optimal functional outcomes occur when treatment begins prior to neurological deficits. The neurological deficits at the time of diagnosis are the main determinant of ambulatory function after treatment.[31,32] The longer the patient has had symptoms of SCC before obtaining medical intervention, the worse the functional outcome. Thus, early identification of symptoms that are consistent with SCC and quick referral to the physician can dramatically impact patient outcome.

Treatment determination is dependent upon evaluation of the stability of the spine. Many facilities use the Frankel system or the ASIA system (American Spinal Injury Association), which combine a physical examination of the integrity of the motor and sensory systems at each level of the spinal cord (see Chapter 9 and Table 9–16). These systems are used in conjunction with subjective complaints, radiologic examination, and functional exam. If the images indicate

---

Table 13–14
COMMON LYMPHEDEMA PRECAUTIONS

Lymphedema Prevention	*Signs of Lymphedema*
• Maintain a healthy weight • Prevent any trauma to the area that was affected by lymph node removal or damage to lymph nodes (ie, arm, breast, and trunk for axillary dissection) • No blood pressure on the "affected" arm • No intravenous on the "affected" arm • Keep skin and nails clean, avoid cutting cuticles • Avoid cuts, scrapes, and burns • Avoid tight-fitting clothes/jewelry	• Heaviness in the limb where lymph nodes were removed or damaged • Clothing or jewelry feeling tight • Swelling • Numbness or tingling • Redness/warmth in limb where lymph nodes were removed or damaged

---

spinal instability and the physical exam is consistent with cord compression, surgery is the treatment of choice. The patient should have a life expectancy of at least a few weeks, compression of no more than two to three segments, and progressive paraplegia less than 30 hours duration. If the spine is stable, if the patient is not a surgical candidate, or if paraplegia has been present for several days, radiation therapy with corticosteroids is indicated. Physical therapy focuses on gait training, strengthening, ADL training, transfer training, and bowel/bladder program. Bracing may be an asset to assist with limiting torsion and decreasing pain with mobility.

LYMPHEDEMA

Lymphedema occurs when there is a disruption of the lymphatic system resulting in abnormal accumulation of lymph fluid.[33] People with cancer are at risk for lymphedema after lymph node dissection or radiation or when there is scar tissue or tumor impeding lymph flow. Common areas that can develop lymphedema are as follows: breast, arm, or trunk after axillary node dissection; head and neck after neck dissection; and legs and genitals after groin lymph node dissection.

The lymphatic system consists of lymph vessels that traverse the entire body. These vessels work in conjunction with the venous system to carry lymph fluid that consists of protein, water, cellular waste, and fatty acids. These fluids are transported through the lymph nodes for filtering and returned to the central circulation.

In the acute care setting, patients should be taught about prevention techniques and overt signs of lymphedema. Anyone who receives cancer treatment that has the potential to damage the lymphatic system needs to adopt the lifetime strategies noted in Table 13-14 to prevent the onset of lymphedema.[34]

The present standard for treatment of lymphedema is **complete decongestive therapy (CDT)**.[33] Phase one CDT includes skin care, manual lymph drainage, bandaging, exercise, and a compression garment to maintain the volume of the limb. The second phase, or maintenance phase, consists of wearing a compression garment during the day and bandaging at night. Skin care and exercise are continued and progressed as appropriate. A lymphedema specialist who has extensively studied the anatomy and physiology of the lymphatic system as well as the techniques of lymphatic massage should administer CDT. The National Lymphedema Network (NLN) and the Lymphology Association of North America (LANA) provide guidelines for the education and practice of lymphedema management.

FATIGUE AND DECONDITIONING

Fatigue affects 70% to 100% of people with cancer.[35] **Cancer-related fatigue (CRF)** is a "condition in which a person with cancer experiences an overwhelming and sustained sense of exhaustion and has a decreased capacity for physical and mental work. These situations of fatigue are not relieved by rest."[36] Fatigue is often described as affecting four main areas: sensory, cognitive, physical, and emotional. Common descriptors include a sense of weakness, drowsiness, inability to concentrate, or a feeling of depression.

The etiology of cancer related fatigue is unclear. Potential contributors include the cancer treatment, the cancer itself, anemia, progression of disease, poor nutrition/cancer cachexia, infection, sleep disturbance, medications, electrolyte imbalance, depression, pain, decreased activity, and thyroid dysfunction.[35,37,38] Fatigue occurs when there is an imbalance of energy states. In the healthy individual, there exists an equilibrium in which the energy demands equal the ability of the body to provide this energy. The disease itself places an energy demand on the system, as do the ensuing treatments. This is in addition to the demands of the body's normal metabolic processes and tasks performance (eg, ADLs). The body is expending energy 24 hours a day to fight the cancer and eliminate the waste products produced by cancer treatments. This taxes the body's reserves, possibly resulting in fatigue and deconditioning. Another explanation for cancer-related fatigue includes a gradual shift in muscle energy expenditure.[38] As people change their activity levels due to side effects of cancer treatment, there is a gradual shift from aerobic to anaerobic metabolism. Muscles become less efficient at utilizing oxygen, producing less adenosine triphosphate (ATP) and more lactic acid, causing complaints of fatigue. When activity is decreased over time, the cardiopulmonary system becomes less efficient (see Chapter 4). Finally, a change in sleep patterns, nutritional intake, and emotional stress all contribute to feelings of "tiredness and weakness."

Cancer-related fatigue is often described by patients undergoing radiation therapy.[35,38,39] The fatigue associated with radiation is often cumulative, with maximum levels peaking between the completion of therapy and 4 weeks after treatment has ended. Increased fatigue is often observed with higher doses of radiation and larger fields.

Fatigue is also common during and after chemotherapy.[13,35,38,39] Fatigue during chemotherapy usually peaks 4 to 5 days after infusion, when blood counts begin dropping. Some people report feeling more energy between cycles of chemotherapy, with the fatigue returning with the next cycle.

Due to its pervasiveness, screening for fatigue should occur throughout the trajectory of disease. Medical causes of fatigue should be ruled out prior to the initiation of other treatment modalities. The following questions are guides to help elucidate the unique characteristics of cancer related fatigue.[35]

- What time of day is your fatigue the worst? Best?

- What alleviates your feelings of fatigue?

- What worsens your feelings of fatigue?

- On a scale from 0 to 10 (0 indicating no fatigue/full of energy and 10 indicating worst fatigue and lack of energy), what is your fatigue rating right now?

- At the worst in the past week?

- At its best in the past week?

Fatigue scales have been validated for the cancer population. Some examples include Piper Fatigue Scale, Multidimensional Fatigue Inventory, Brief Fatigue Inventory, SF-36 Fatigue Subscale, Functional Assessment of Cancer Fatigue-Anemia (FACT-An), and the Schwartz Cancer Fatigue Scale.

Exercise interventions have shown consistent results in fatigue management. Many studies report improvements in fatigue levels with the use of an aerobic program such as walking or biking.[5,26,35,40] However, the mode, intensity, duration, and frequency that demonstrate the highest efficacy in fatigue management have yet to be elucidated. Intensity should be modified during active treatment with a return to higher intensity exercise in the recovery and survivorship phases.

In addition to an individualized aerobic program, people with cancer should be taught the principles of pacing and energy conservation. Patients should plan their most important tasks for the period where they feel most energetic and lucid. The tasks that require a lot of energy should be interspersed throughout the day, mixed with periods of simple tasks and rest breaks. Many people report short naps, lasting no more than 20 to 30 minutes, are the most beneficial in restoring some energy and focus.[41]

The combination of exercise, pacing, and relaxation techniques can help minimize cancer-related fatigue. The exercise program should be tailored to the person's individual fitness levels, stage of disease, and stage of cancer treatment. The section below will detail important aspects of exercise prescription for the person with cancer.

EXERCISE FOR THE PERSON WITH CANCER

Exercise plays an important role in prevention and restoration of physical mobility and well-being across the trajectory of disease. It has been shown to elevate mood, decrease anxiety, and improve physical functioning and overall quality of life in people with cancer.[5,6,26,35,40,42–46] The exercise prescription for the person with cancer should be created by a physical therapist who has a keen understanding of cancer and the side effects of cancer treatment. There are many advantages to prescribing and monitoring an exercise program in the acute care environment. Although patients tend to be more tenuous, there is an abundance of monitoring devices such as daily lab values, electrocardiograms, imaging results, and easy access to their primary medical team that can add to the information that influences the exercise prescription..

In addition to blood chemistry, one should consider the type of cancer treatment when prescribing an exercise program. For example, certain chemotherapy agents can cause acute hypotension while others tend to cause hypertension. As mentioned previously, chemotherapy agents may also cause cardiopulmonary dysfunction and peripheral neuropathy. One should also consider the benefits of a weightbearing program in all patients undergoing treatment for cancer. Many diseases affect bone density (such as multiple myeloma) and many cancer treatments may contribute to osteopenia. However, one must be acutely aware of the stability of the skeleton, monitoring for signs of impending fracture. Finally, rehabilitation specialists must consider the stage of disease. As patients' disease progresses, their tolerance to exercise may diminish. It is important to set goals that are appropriate to each patient's disease stage and goals for mobility.

Rehabilitation of the person with cancer has moved to the forefront of cancer care as prevention, identification, and treatments for various diseases improve. Physical therapists have a role in prevention of disease and immobility, restoration of function, and in the palliation of symptoms. We are a critical part of the team whose focus is on improving the quality of life in people with living with cancer.

SUMMARY

Physical therapists play a key role in the prevention and restoration of impairments and functional limitations that result from cancer or its treatments. It is imperative for therapists to understand the basic science of oncology diagnoses with their associated survivorship curves. In addition, therapists must be familiar with treatment strategies and side effects to help provide quality, appropriate interventions that mesh with the patient's goals and stage of disease. Physical therapists are a critical component to the care of the person with cancer at all phases of treatment including palliation. Our goal in the acute care setting are to provide patients with a means to achieve their functional goals within the auspices of improving quality of life.

CASE STUDY

Mr. Emmett is a 38-year-old (y/o) male who is day +32 s/p allogeneic BMT for chronic myelogenous leukemia (CML). His conditioning regimen consisted of Busulfan and Cytarabine as well as total body irradiation. He has acute GVHD—skin, treated with high dose steroids. Physical therapy is consulted to evaluate and treat a patient for "right (R) hip pain."

Patient/Client History

General Demographics/Social History/Living Environment

Mr. Emmett is divorced and has two children, ages 8 and 10. He is presently living with his fiancée in a two-story townhouse outside the city. There is a half bath on the first floor and a full bath on the second floor. He is presently on disability but had previously been working as a chef for a popular restaurant chain.

General Health Status/Family History

Prior to admission for his bone marrow transplant he states he was a "home-body" because of his low energy level. No one else in his family has ever been sick, and he does not know why this happened to him.

Medical/Surgical History

His medical and surgical histories are noncontributory.

Current Conditions/Chief Complaints

Mr. Emmett complains of (c/o) pain in right hip with all movement.

Functional Status and Activity Level

Independent ambulator all surfaces prior to admission for transplant, but states he walked stairs slowly.

Systems Review

Cardiovascular/Pulmonary

Resting vital signs (with head of bed raised 30 degrees) were oxygen saturation (SpO_2) 98% on room air, heart rate (HR) 110, pulse regular, respiratory rate (RR) 16, and BP 150/78. Following manual muscle test (MMT), ROM, bed mobility, transfers, and gait his vital sign response was SpO_2 95%, HR 122, RR 24, and BP 168/76. His cough is weak, dry, and nonproductive. Breath sounds with crackles at his bases, but chest expansion equal bilaterally.

Integumentary

Mr. Emmett has a rash on his upper chest and arms, approximately one-third of his total body surface area.

Musculoskeletal

Mr. Emmett's MMT is within normal limits (WNL), bilateral lower extremity's (BLE) except his right hip flexion 3-/5 limited by pain. His right (R) knee extension is 3/5 and limited by pain. R hip external and internal rotation are also limited by pain. He requires minimal assist for sit to stand from bed, chair and toilet. His ROM is WFL (within functional limit) except for R hip range that is painful mid to end range and, therefore, was not tested to end range.

Neuromuscular

Mr. Emmett's upper (UE) and lower extremity (LE) reflexes are WNL. His sensation is intact to light touch, deep pressure, and temperature.

Communication, Affect, Cognition, Language, and Learning Style

He is alert and oriented, using English as his primary language.

Laboratory Values

Review of the CBC reveals WBC 3.8 thou/uL, HgB 7.8 g/dL, and Plt 21,000/uL.

Tests and Measures

Aerobic Capacity and Endurance

Mr. Emmett is deconditioned as demonstrated by his cardiovascular and pulmonary response to minimal activity. His elevated HR and RR with minimal activity can also be contributed to his anemia (HgB 7.8). Part of the rise in HR, BP, and RR could also be directly related to increase pain with weightbearing.

Assistive and Adaptive Devices

Prior to admission he was independent, but presently uses a rolling walker.

Special Tests

(+) pain with joint compression right hip

Gait, Locomotion, and Balance

Mr. Emmett ambulated with min assist using a rolling walker 10 feel x 1. He demonstrated decreased weightbearing through right LE (RLE) with gait. His RLE was held in external rotation and hip flexion during swing phase, with increased L trunk lateral lean.

Pain

Mr. Emmett rates his pain a 6/10 with rest and 9/10 with activity in right hip.

Diagnosis

Mr. Emmett's differential diagnosis includes muscle strain, hematoma secondary to thrombocytopenia, and avascular necrosis secondary to high dose steroids. Avascular necrosis is less likely due to the short period of high dose steroids given. Recommendation: imaging of right hip to rule out bleed versus AVN.

Imaging revealed (+) hematoma right gluteus medius and R hip joint capsule. Recommend treatment pattern 4E: impaired joint mobility, motor function, muscle performance, and ROM associated with localized inflammation.[47]

Prognosis

Mr. Emmett's prognosis for functional recovery of his right hip is good. It will be tempered by his recovery from bone marrow transplant as well as the speed of his blood count recovery.

Intervention

Recommend ROM to prevent shortening of hip musculature as patient is positioning his hip in external rotation and hip flexion. Recommend cold therapy 10 minutes two to three times/day to help minimize inflammation. Recommend gentle isometrics after initial phase of rest to address strength deficits. This should be progressed slowly, depending on his pain tolerance and levels of thrombocytopenia. Caution should be taken with any aggressive exercises until the patient's platelet level rises sufficiently. Observation of skin appearance, temperature, girth, and pain should be assessed each visit. Aerobic training will include an upper body ergometer (UBE) at a low intensity and no resistance due to anemia and thrombocytopenia. The physical therapist recommended daily therapy to meet goals of increase functional level, endurance level, and decrease pain with weightbearing activities. Mr. Emmett's physical therapy program will be coordinated with the cancer pain team.

Reexamination

Fourteen days after physical therapy was initiated, Mr. Emmett was able to ambulate 50 feet times 2 with the rolling walker and standby assistance, transfer independent from all surfaces, and climb four steps with a handrail and minimal assistance of one. His pain with activity was a 4/10 and at rest 1 to 2/10. Cough fair, nonproductive, and breath sounds clear to auscultation.

Outcomes

Mr. Emmett was discharged to the home setting. Home therapy is scheduled to start 2 days following discharge to continue aerobic training and strength training of his right hip musculature and progress gait and locomotion.

CHAPTER REVIEW QUESTIONS

1. What is the most widely used staging system for cancer?
2. What are three different influences in determining a patient's treatment for cancer?
3. What are three side effects of radiation treatment for cancer?
4. Name two neurologic side effects related to chemotherapy and discuss how these side effects will impact your plan of care.
5. You are treating a patient with multiple myeloma. What are two symptoms that the patient should be educated on that may signify a pathologic fracture during home activities and while performing a home exercise program?

PHARMACOLOGICAL INFORMATION: ONCOLOGICAL DISEASES AND DISORDERS PHARMACOLOGY (ANTINEOPLASTICS)

Alkylating Agents

Action
Alkylating agents cause cross-linking of DNA strands, abnormal base pairing of DNA or DNA strand breaks. The abnormalities inhibit DNA replication and transcription preventing cell division. Cell-cycle nonspecific.

Side Effects
CV: Dysrhythmias, CHF
GI: Nausea and vomiting
GU: Cystisis, sterility
Misc: Myelosuppression (leukopenia, thrombocytopenia), alopecia
Pulm: Pulmonary fibrosis

Common Medications
Nitrogen mustard: Mechlorethamine (Mustargen), Cyclophosphamide (Cytoxan), Chlorambucin, Thiotepa, Busulfan, Melphalan (Alkeran)

Antimetabolites

Action
Antimetabolites are drugs that compete for binding sites on enzymes or mimic and replace natural substances in DNA and RNA. These agents alter cell metabolism and protein synthesis, resulting in altered cell growth and death. Antimetabolites effect cells during the S-phase of cell division.

Side Effects
CNS: Encephelopathy, cerebellum dysfunction (Cytarabine)
GI: Diarrhea, nausea, vomiting
GU: Cystisis, sterility
Misc: Myelosuppression (leukopenia, thrombocytopenia), joint pain, mucositis, alopecia

Common Medications
Fluorouracil (5-FU), Hydrea, Methotrexate, Cytarabine, Gemcitabine

Hormonal and Enzyme Therapy

Action
Hormones may be used as chemotherapeutic agents by binding to specific receptors on cancer cells and inhibiting cell growth. These agents may actively compete with endogenous hormones leading to receptor blockade (eg, Tamoxifen) or augment the effects of a particular hormone (eg, Sandostatin)

Side Effects
CV: Thromboembolism/pulmonary embolism
GI: Nausea, vomiting
GU: Cystisis, sterility
Misc: Hot flashes, weight gain, loss of libido, impotence

Common Medications
Breast cancer: Tamoxifen (Nolvadex), Raloxifene
Prostate cancer: Flutamide (Eulexin), Buserelin (Suprefact), Leuprolide (Lupron)
Pancreatic/metastatic cancer: Octreotide acetate (Sandostatin)
Lymphoma: Corticosteroids (Prednisone, Prednisolone)

Anti-Tumor Antibiotics

Action
Anti-tumor antibiotics bind to DNA preventing DNA and RNA synthesis. Additionally these agents may cause DNA uncoiling and strand breaks. Cell-cycle nonspecific.

Side Effects
CNS: Encephelopathy, cerebellum dysfunction (Cytarabine)
CV: Cardiomyopathy (Daunorubicin, Doxorubicine),
GI: Diarrhea, nausea, vomiting
GU: Renal dysfunction, cystisis
Misc: Myelosuppression (leukopenia, thrombocytopenia), alopecia
Pulm: Pneumonitis/pulmonary toxicity (Bleomycin)

Common Medications
Anthracyclines: Daunorubicin, Idarubicin, Mitoxantrone,
Bleomycins: Bleomycin, Mitomycin

Aromatase Inhibitors

Action
Aromatase inhibitors block the effects of estrogen on estrogen sensitive tumors.

Side Effects
CNS: Headache, weakness, dizziness
CV: Edema
GI: Nausea, vomiting, diarrhea, constipation, abdominal pain
Misc: Hot flashes, back/bone pain
Pulm: Bronchospasm, dyspnea

Common Medications
Anastrozole (Arimidex)

Plant Alkaloids/Antimicrotubules

Action

Plant alkaloids are substances derived from plants that impair the ability of a cell to divide. These agents interfere with cell structure and cell division by binding with tubulin, a necessary protein to form the mitotic spindle during cell division. Plant alkaloids are more effective during S and M phases of cell division.

Side Effects

CNS: Weakness, lethargy
CV: Hypotension, bradycardia
GI: Constipation, abdominal pain
Misc: Peripheral neuropathy (decreased tendon reflexes/parasthesias/weakness), myalgias, myelosuppression (neutropenia, leukopenia, thrombocytopenia)
Pulm: Bronchospasm, dyspnea

Common Medications

Vinca alkaloids: Vincristine, Vinblastine, Vinorelbine
Epipodophyllotoxins: Etoposide
Taxanes: Paclitaxel (Taxol), Docetaxe (Taxotere)

Platinum Compounds

Action

Platinum compounds are believed to produce cross linking of DNA base pairs similar to the alkylating agents as well as binding to various cellular proteins. The result is impaired cell division, growth and promotion of cell death.

Side Effects

CNS: Weakness, tremor
GI: Nausea, vomiting
GU: Renal toxicity
Misc: Peripheral neuropathy, myalgias, myelosuppression (leukopenia, thrombocytopenia), anemia

Common Medications

Cisplatin (Platinol), Carboplatin (Paraplatin)

Monoclonal Antibody Therapy

Action

Monoclonal antibodies are genetically engineered antibodies. An antigen of interest (eg, cancer cells) is infected into an animal (eg, mouse) triggering an immune reaction. The immune reaction generates lymphocytes producing specific antibodies against the antigen of interest.

Side Effects
CNS: Dizziness, depression, fatigue
CV: Cardiomyopathy (Trastuzumab), hypertension, hypotension, tachycardia
GI: Abdominal discomfort, anorexia, constipation, nausea, vomiting
Misc: Fevers, chills, back pain

Common Medications
Alemtuzumab (Campath), Gemtuzumab ozogamacin (Mylotarg), Rituximab,
Trastuzumab

REFERENCES

1. Abeloff. *Clinical Oncology.* 2nd ed. Orlando, Fla: Churchill Livingstone; 2000.
2. Quasthoff S, Hartung HP. Chemotheapy-induced peripheral neuropathy. *J Neurol.* 2002;249:9–17.
3. Su, Chang, Traynor A, Burt RK. Update on stem cell transplantation. *Resident & Staff Physician.* 2001;47(2):44–54.
4. Kelley W, ed. *Textbook of Internal Medicine.* 3rd ed. (Chapter 258.) Philadelphia, Pa: Lippincott-Raven Publishers; 1997.
5. Dimeo F, Stieglitz RD, Novelli-Fischer U, et al. Effects of physical activity on the fatigue and psychologic status of cancer patients during chemotherapy. *Cancer.* 1999;85(10):2273–2277.
6. Dimeo F, Fetscher S, Lange W, et al. Effects of aerobic exercise on the physical performance and incidence of treatment-related complications after high-dose chemotherapy. *Blood.* 1997;90(9):3390–3394.
7. Haid A, Kuehn T, Konstantiniuk P, et al. Shoulder-arm morbidity following axillary dissection and sentinel node only biopsy for breast cancer. *Eur J Surg Oncol.* 2002;28(7):705–710.
8. Schultz I, Barholm M, Grondal S. Delayed shoulder exercises in reducing seroma frequency after modified radical mastectomy: a prospective randomized study. *Ann Surg Oncol.* 1997;4(4):293–297.
9. Harris S, Hugi MR, Olivotto IA, et al. Upper extremity rehabilitation in women with breast cancer after axillary dissection: clinical practice guidelines. *Crit Review Phys Rehabil Med.* 2001;13(2,3):91–103.
10. Campbell B, Marbella A, Layde PM. Quality of life and recurrence concern in survivors of head and neck cancer. *Laryngoscope.* 2000;110:895–906.
11. Cheville A, Packel L. Rehabilitation of the person s/p neck dissection. *Acute Care Perspectives—J Am Phys Ther Assoc.* 2001;10:37–39.
12. Brown H, Burns S, Kaiser CW. The spinal accessory nerve plexus, the trapezius muscle, and shoulder stabilization after radical neck cancer surgery. *Ann Surg.* 1988;208:654–661.
13. Cheng PT, Hao SP, Lin YH, Yeh AR. Objective comparison of shoulder dysfunction after three neck dissection techniques. *Ann Otol Rhinol Laryngol.* 2000;109: 761–766.
14. Thawley SE, Panje WR, Batsakis JG, Lindberg RD. *Comprehensive Management of Head and Neck Tumors.* Vol 1 and 2. 2nd ed. Philadelphia, Pa: WB Saunders Co; 1999.
15. Minami A, Kasashima T, Iwasaki N, et al. Vascularised fibular grafts. An experience of 102 patients. *J Bone Joint Surg Br.* 2000;82(7):1022–1025.
16. American Cancer Society. *Cancer Facts & Figures 2000.* Available at: www. cancer.org. Accessed in June 2004.
17. Curtis LA, Dolan TS, Cespedes RD. Acute urinary retention and urinary incontinence. *Emerg Med Clin North Am.* 2001;19(3):591–619.
18. Alberg AJ, Samet JM. Epidemiology of lung cancer. *Chest.* 2003;123(1 Suppl):21S–49S.
19. American Cancer Society. Colorectoral cancer facts & figures. Special edition 2005. Available at: http://www.cancer.org/downloads/STT/CAFF2005CR4PWSecured.pdf. Accessed in June 2004.
20. American Cancer Society website. Available at: www.cancer.org. Accessed on April 2, 2006.
21. National Cancer Institute - US National Institutes of Health. General information about anal cancer. Available at: www.cancer.gov/cancerinfo/pdq/treatment/anal/patient. Accessed on April 2, 2006.

22. Groenwald S, Frogge MH Goodman M, Yarbro CH. *Cancer Nursing: Principles and Practice.* 4th ed. Sudbury, Mass: Jones and Bartlett Publisher Inc; 1997.
23. Van Kampen W, De Weerdt W, Van Poppel H, et al. Effect of pelvic-floor re-education on duration and degree of incontinence after radical prostatectomy: a randomised controlled trial. *Lancet.* 2000;355:98–102.
24. Oncologychanne: your oncology community. Testicular cancer - overview. Available at: www.oncologychannel.com/testicularcancer/riskfactors.shtml. Accessed on April 2, 2006.
25. Pearl M, Fischer M, McCauley DL, et al. Transcutaneous electrical nerve stimulation as an adjunct for controlling chemotherapy-induced nausea and vomiting in gynecologic oncology patients. *Cancer Nurs.* 1999;22(4):307–311.
26. Schwartz AL. Fatigue mediates the effects of exercise on quality of life. *Qual Life Res.* 1999;8:529–538.
27. Hecox B, Mohrotoab TA, WeisbergJ. *Physical Agents: A Comprehensive Text for Physical Therapists.* Norwalk, Conn: Appleton & Lange; 1994.
28. Portenoy RK. *Pain in Oncologic and AIDS Patients.* 2nd ed. Newtown, Pa: Handbooks in Health Care Co; 1998.
29. Coleman RE. Metastatic bone disease: clinical features, pathophysiology and treatment strategies. *Cancer Treatment Reviews.* 2001;27:165–176.
30. Harrington K. Orthopedic surgical management of skeletal complications of malignancy. *Cancer Supplement.* 1997;80(8):1614–1627.
31. Helweg-Larsen S. Prognostic factors in metastatic spinal cord compression: a prospective study using multivariate analysis of variables influencing survival and gait function in 153 patients. *Int J Radiat Oncol Biol Phys.* 2000;46(5):1163–1169.
32. Lu C, Stomper PC, Drislane FW, et al. Suspected spinal cord compression in breast cancer patients: a multidisciplinary risk assessment. *Breast Cancer Research and Treatment.* 1998;51:121–131.
33. Kelly DG. A Primer on Lymphedema. Upper Saddle River, NJ: Prentice Hall; 2002.
34. National Lymphedema Network Webpage. 18 Steps to Prevention. Available at: www.lymphnet.org. Accessed on April 2, 2006.
35. Marty M, Pecorelli S, eds. *Fatigue and Cancer.* New York, NY: Elsevier Science; 2001.
36. Marien M Jr. Trismus: causes, differential diagnosis, and treatment. *Gen Dent.* 1997;45(4):350–355.
37. Cancer Related Fatigue PDQ. Available at: www.cancer.gov. Accessed on April 2, 2006.
38. Lucia A, Earnest C, Perez M. Cancer-related fatigue: can exercise physiology assist oncologists? *Lancet Oncol.* 2003;4(10):616–625.
39. Manzullo E, Escalante C. Research into fatigue. *Hematol/Oncol Clin North Am.* 2002;16(3):619–628.
40. Mock V, Dow KH, Meares CJ, et al. Effects of exercise on fatigue, physical functioning, and emotional distress during radiation therapy for breast cancer. *Oncol Nurs Forum.* 1997;24(6):991–1000.
41. Berger AM, Farr L. The influence of daytime inactivity and nighttime restlessness on cancer-related fatigue. *Oncol Nurs Forum.* 1999;26(10):1663–1671.
42. Bower JE, Ganz PA, Desmond KA, et al. Fatigue in breast cancer survivors: occurrence, correlates and impact on quality of life. *J Clin Oncol.* 2000;18(4):743–753.
43. Courneya K, Friedenreich C. Physical exercise and quality of life following cancer diagnosis: a literature review. *Ann Behav Med.* 1999;21(2):171–179.
44. Jacobsen PB, Hann DM, Azzarello LM, et al. Fatigue in women receiving adjuvant chemotherapy for breast cancer: characteristics, course and correlates. *J Pain Symptom Manage.* 1999;18(4):233–242.

45. Leddy SK. Incentives and barriers to exercise in women with a history of breast cancer. *Oncology Nurse Forum.* 1997;24(5);885–890.
46. Ream E, Richardson A. From theory to practice: designing interventions to reduce fatigue in patients with cancer. *Oncology Nurse Forum.* 1999;26(8):1295–1303.
47. Guide to Physical Therapist Practice. 2nd ed. *Physical Therapy.* 2001;81(1).

BIBLIOGRAPHY

Barse PM. Issues in the treatment of metastatic breast cancer. *Semin Oncol Nurs.* 2000;16(3):197–205.

Bayley A, Milosevic M, Blend R, et al. A prospective study of factors predicting clinically occult spinal cord compression in patients with metastatic prostate carcinoma. *Cancer.* 2001;92:303–310.

Beers MH, Berkow R. *The Merck Manual of Diagnosis and Therapy.* 17th ed. Available at: http://www.merck.com/mrkshared/mmanual/home.jsp. Accessed in June 2004.

Chen SC, Chen MF. Timing of shoulder exercise after modified radical mastectomy: a prospective study. *Changgeng Yi Xue Za Zhi.* 1999;22(1):37–43.

Coward D, Wilkie D. Metastatic bone pain. *Cancer Nursing.* 2000;23(2):101–108.

Diel I, et al. Bisphosphonates and the prevention of metastasis. *Cancer Suppl.* 2000;88(12):3080–3088.

Craig CR, Stitzel RE. *Modern Pharmacology with Clinical Applications.* New York, NY: Little, Brown, and Co; 1997.

Deglin JH, Vallerand AH. *Davis's Drug Guide for Nurses.* 8th ed. Philadelphia, Pa: FA Davis Co; 2003.

Demirkan F, Chen HC, Wei FC, et al. The versatile anterolateral thigh flap: a musculocutaneous flap in disguise in head and neck reconstruction. *Br J Plast Surg.* 2000;53(1):30–36.

Domchek S. Predictors of skeletal complications in patients with metastatic breast carcinoma. *Cancer.* 2000;89(2):363–368.

Egan M, Barry T. Surgical interventions for bony metastases and implications for physical therapy. San Antonio, Tex: Presentation CSM; 2000.

Egan M. Surgical and physical therapy considerations for patients with bone metastases. *Rehabil Oncol.* 2001;19(2):25–26.

Flombaum CD. Metabolic emergencies in the cancer patient. *Semin Oncol.* 2000;27(3):322–334.

Frassica D, Thurman S, Welsh J. Radiation therapy. *Othop Clin North Am.* 2000; 31(4):557–566.

Futran N, Alsarraf R. Microvascular free-flap reconstruction in the head and neck. *JAMA.* 2000;284:1761–1763.

Giacosa A, Franceschi S, La Vecchia C, et al. Energy intake, overweight, physical exercise and colorectal cancer risk. *Eur J Cancer Prev.* 1999;8:S53–S60.

Goldman L, Bennett J. Cecil *Textbook of Medicine.* 21st ed. Philadelphia, Pa: WB Saunders Co; 2000.

Goldstein M, Maxymiw WG, Cummings BJ, Wood RE. The effects of antitumor irradiation on mandibular opening and mobility. *Oral Surg Oral Med Oral Pathol Oral Radiol Endod.* 1999;88:365–373.

Green R, Brien M. Accessory nerve latency to middle and lower trapezius. *Arch Phys Med Rehabil.* 1985;66:23–25.

Heidenreich A, Hofmann R, Engelmann UH. The use of bisphosphonate for the palliative treatment of painful bone metastasis due to hormone refractory prostate cancer. *J Urol.* 2001;165:136–140.

Hilner BE. American Society of Clinical Oncology guideline on the role of bisphosphonates in breast cancer. *J Clin Oncol.* 2000;18(6):1378–1391.

Hoffmann R, Melcher I, Wichelhaus A, Haas NP. Surgical treatment of bone metastases in breast cancer. *Anticancer Res.* 1998;18:2243–2250.

Karch AM. *Lippincott's Nursing Drug Guide.* Springhouse, Pa: Lippincott Williams & Wilkins; 2004.

Kuhn J, Plancher KD, Hawkins RJ. Scapular winging. *J Am Acad Orthop Surg.* 1995;3:319–325.

Marco R, Sheth DS, Boland PJ, et al. Functional and oncological outcome of acetabular reconstruction for the treatment of metastatic disease. *J Bone Joint Surg.* 2000;82-A(5):642–651.

Manglani H, Marco RA, Picciolo A, Healey JH. Orthopedic emergencies in cancer patients. *Semin Oncol.* 2000;27(3):299–310.

Meraw SJ, Reeve CM. Dental considerations and treatment of the oncology patient receiving radiation therapy. *J Am Dent Assoc.* 1998;129(2):201–205.

Mercadante S. Malignant bone pain: pathophysiology and treatment. *Pain.* 1997;69(1-2):1–18.

Miaskowski C, Lee KA. Pain, fatigue, and sleep disturbances in oncology outpatients receiving radiation therapy for bone metastasis: a pilot study. *J Pain Symptom Manage.* 1999;17(5):320–332.

Nieman D. Exercise and resistance to infection. *J Physol Pharmacol.* 1999;76:573–580.

Paterson A. The potential role of bisphosphonates as adjuvant therapy in the prevention of bone metastases. *Cancer Supplement.* 2000;88(12):3038–3046.

Plunkett TA, Smith P, Rubens RD. Risk of complications from bone metastases in breast cancer: implications for management. *Eur J Cancer.* 2000;36(4):476–482.

Ritter JM, Lewis LD, Mant TG. *Textbook of Clinical Pharmacology.* London, England: Edward Arnold Co; 1995.

Roodman GD. Biology of osteoclast activation in cancer. *Journal of Clinical Oncology.* 2001;19(15): 3562–3571.

Serlin RC, Mendoza TR, Nakamura Y, et al. When is cancer pain mild, moderate or severe? Grading pain severity by its interference with function. *Pain.* 1995;61(2):277–284.

Thiedke CC. Nonhormonal pharmacologic and complementary treatment of menopause. *Clinics in Family Practice.* 2002;4(1):155–171.

Thoma A, Khadaroo R, Grigenas O, et al. Oromandibular reconstruction with the radial-forearm osteocutaneous flap: experience with 60 consecutive cases. *Plast Reconstr Surg.* 1999;104(2):368–377.

Thune I, Brenn T, Lund E, Gaard M. Physical activity and the risk of breast cancer. *N Engl J Med.* 1997;(336):1269–1275.

Verloop J, Rookus MA, van der Kooy K, van Leeuwen FE. Physical activity and breast cancer risk in women aged 20–54 years. *J Natl Cancer Inst.* 2000;92(2):128–135.

Vogelzand N, Breitbart W, Cella D, et al. Patient, caregiver, and oncologist perception of cancer-related fatigue: results of a tripart assessment survey. *Seminars in Hematology.* 1997;34(3[Suppl 2]):S4–S12.

Wax M, Winslow CP, Hansen J, et al. A retrospective analysis of temporomandibular joint reconstruction with free fibula microvascular flap. *Laryngoscope.* 2000;110(6):977–981.

Wedin R, Bauer HC, Rutqvist LE. Surgical treatment for skeletal breast cancer metastases. *Cancer.* 2001;92(2):257–262.

Wright E, Domenech MA, Fischer JR Jr. Usefulness of posture training for patients with temporomandibular disorders. *J Am Dent Assoc.* 2000;131(2):202–210.

Zhau H. Establishment of human prostate carcinoma skeletal metastasis models. *Cancer Suppl.* 2000;88(12):2995–3001.

Chapter 14

TRANSPLANTATION

Daniel J Malone, MPT, CCS
Kathy Lee Bishop Lindsay, MS, PT, CCS

INTRODUCTION

The reality of organ transplantation as a feasible treatment for advanced disease came in the mid 1900s.[1-7] The primary hurdle that the surgical teams faced, which remains the primary challenge, is limited patient survival and limited organ availability. The introduction in 1980 of the immunosuppressive cyclosporin, a calcineurin inhibitor, represented an opportunity to advance organ transplantation.[8-10] Certainly, survival is not the only outcome, but the quality of that survival is important to the team and to the patient and his or her family.[11]

Besides the introduction of cyclosporin into the immunosuppression regime, preservation of the harvested organs, improvements in surgical techniques, and judicious patient selection have dramatically enhanced patient survival over the past 4 decades.[4,6,12] Organ transplantation is no longer considered an experimental procedure. This highly technical and demanding specialty is now considered the standard of care for end-stage organ disease. Although donor organ supply remains the chief limitation to transplantation, survival and quality of life continue to improve.

Therapists are likely to encounter the patient who has undergone organ transplantation regardless of practice setting. Patients may be followed at the transplant medical center during the perioperative and early postoperative periods, but admissions occur at all regional and community hospitals long term. As patients become more active and resume regular activities of daily living (ADLs) including physical exercise, they are susceptible to a variety of medical complications including musculoskeletal injuries. These transplant recipients may be followed for physical therapy in outpatient clinics. Improved understanding of transplant anatomy, physiology, precautions, risk factors, and influences on other systems is key for appropriate care.

Table 14–1
LUNG TRANSPLANTATION, INCLUSION/EXCLUSION CATEGORIES

Inclusion	*Exclusion*
End-stage lung or heart/lung disease	Drug, tobacco (use), or alcohol dependency
Functional limitation	Previous malignant neoplasm
Potential improvement of quality of life and survival	Poor renal/hepatic function
Financial stability	Significant left/right ventricular dysfunction
≥600 feet covered in 6-minute walk test (ambulatory with rehabilitation potential)	HIV positive
Psychosocial support adequate	Noncompliance with medical regime Progressive neuromuscular disorder Untreated coronary artery disease (CAD)
Age ≤65	Advanced connective tissue diseases
Acceptable nutritional status	Active extrapulmonary infection
No systemic disease with nonpulmonary vital organ involvement	

Relative Contraindications

Previous thoracotomy/thoracic surgery
Corticosteroid use >20 mg/day
Pseudomonas Cepacia infections
Pleurodeses
Preoperative evidence of multiresistant organisms

The primary goals of this chapter are to introduce thoracic and abdominal organ transplantation to the therapist working in the acute care setting. The first sections present an overview of the common solid organ transplants and rehabilitation. Recommended goals and precautions will be provided for transplant recipients. Subsequent sections will focus on common concerns in transplantation, a case study, and chapter review questions.

OVERVIEW OF CANDIDATE SELECTION

Who are the potential candidates for organ transplantation? Which patients would best benefit from the limited supply of organs in the United States is a challenging question.[13] Inclusion criteria as well as absolute and relative

Table 14–2
POTENTIAL PREOPERATIVE TESTING FOR TRANSPLANTATION

- Arterial blood gas (ABG) analysis
- Cardiac Catheterization
- Chest x-ray
- CT scan/MRI/multigated acquisition or angiogram imaging (MUGA)
- Echocardiography
- Electrocardiogram
- Exercise stress test
- Financial evaluation
- Laboratory blood work (eg, CBC, electrolyte panel, urinalysis)
- Oxygen saturation
- Posture/functional tests
- Psychosocial evaluation
- Pulmonary function tests
- Quality of life assessment
- Six-minute walk test
- Sputum culture
- Ventilation/perfusion scan

Adapted from:
University of Pennsylvania Health System Lung Transplant Evaluation Tool.
Versluis-Burlis T, Downs AM. Thoracic organ transplantation: heart, lung, and heart-lung. In: *Essentials of Cardiopulmonary Physical Therapy*. 2nd ed. Philadelphia, Pa: WB Saunders Co; 2001.

contraindications for performing the procedure exist, but there is some variability among transplant centers (Table 14–1).[14] Patients with end-stage, single organ disease who have exhausted remaining medical and surgical interventions with reversible nontransplant organ dysfunction are considered for transplant. In addition to primary pathology, comorbidities, age, functional status and quality of life, psychosocial and financial considerations, as well as dependencies on drugs, alcohol, and nicotine must be assessed during the evaluation. Waiting list duration is an important factor, and patients are typically referred for transplantation when life expectancy is limited (eg, lung transplant patients are typically referred when life expectancy is 18 to 24 months). Determination of when to refer is a balancing act among life expectancy, disease progression, and surgical risk, challenging the most experienced medical provider. To optimize candidate selection and donor-recipient match, patients undergo extensive testing, as noted in Table 14–2. Additional information includes medication history and comorbidities. For example, prolonged exposure to corticosteroids impairs wound healing and increases risk for osteopenia/osteoporosis and pathologic fractures.[4,14–17] The negative impact from wound dehiscence, pain, and limited mobility can impair post-transplant outcomes and quality of life. The evaluation process continues to adapt as transplant experience advances.

The team involved in making the decision for appropriate candidacy should be multidisciplinary.[7] The team members include the primary physicians (eg, nephrologist, cardiologist, pulmonologist, hepatologist), nursing coordinators, transplant surgeons, dietitians, social workers, and respiratory, occupational, and physical therapists. Physical therapy evaluates rehabilitative potential, functional limitations, postural deficiencies, enhance airway clearance programs, and identifies fixed versus reversible musculoskeletal pathologies. The physical therapist will work with each team member to support the goals of the team. For example if the patient is at risk prior to transplant for osteoporosis due to low bone mass, poor nutritional status, and previous high levels of corticosteroid exposure, the therapist may focus on a slow progressive resistive training as well as weightbearing exercise. Once the candidate is accepted for transplantation, a rehabilitation program should be designed to optimize the patient's overall exercise capacity, strength, range of motion, and airway clearance to prepare for the rigors of surgery.

Following transplant and discharge from the acute care setting, the accepted practice is that all thoracic transplant recipients will undergo cardiopulmonary rehabilitation to optimize recovery of function, optimize quality of life, and allow the patients to achieve their highest potential exercise capacity. This monitored time also provides ongoing surveillance of infection and rejection.

THORACIC ORGAN TRANSPLANTATION

Lung Transplantation

Introduction/Overview

Lung transplantation encompasses single (SLT), double (DLT), or bilateral single sequential and living-related donor procedures. One-year survival for pediatric thoracic transplants approximates 80%. Survival rates in adults are more diverse with 1-year survival being 73% for lung and 61% for heart-lung;[3,13,17–20] bilateral lung transplant recipients have an improved survival rate after 1 year.[13,19] Improved survival may be attributable to younger age of the recipients and pretransplantation diagnosis. Recipients with primary pulmonary hypertension (HTN), sarcoidosis, and idiopathic pulmonary fibrosis have higher mortality rates during the initial 3- to 6-month period following transplantation.[13]

Indications/Candidate Selection

Table 14–3 highlights a list of diagnoses that are considered for lung transplantation. The type of surgery will depend on the disease process, organ availability, recipient matching, and age. Mechanical ventilation is not an absolute contraindication to transplantation, but ventilator duration, current infectious pathogens, and immobility may adversely affect outcomes. Ventilator-dependent patients account for less than 3% of lung transplantation recipients in the United States and are associated with early mortality.[19,21]

Operative Procedure

The SLT operation is usually performed through a posterolateral thoracotomy via the fourth and fifth intercostal space.[4,17,22] This approach helps to spare the

---

Table 14–3
DIAGNOSTIC GROUPS FOR LUNG TRANSPLANTATION
AND TRANSPLANT TYPE[4,6,7,17,20–23]

- Chronic obstructive pulmonary disease (COPD)/alpha$_1$ antitrypsin (SLT, DLT)
- Asthma (SLT, DLT)
- Cystic fibrosis/bronchiectasis (DLT, HLT)
- Pulmonary fibrosis (SLT, DLT)
- Radiation fibrosis (SLT, DLT)
- Sarcoidosis (SLT, DLT)
- Lymphangiolyomyomatosis (SLT, DLT)
- Connective tissue disorder/scleroderma (SLT, DLT)
- Primary pulmonary HTN (SLT, DLT, HLT)
- Pulmonary veno-occlusive disease (SLT, DLT)
- Eisenmenger's syndrome (HLT, DLT)
- Congenital heart disease (HLT, DLT)
- Bronchiolitis obliterans/retransplantation (SLT, DLT)
- Histiocytosis X (SLT, DLT)
- Pneumoconiosis (SLT, DLT)
- Bronchopulmonary dysplasia (BPD) (SLT, DLT)

SLT: Single lung transplant, DLT: Double lung transplant or single sequential lung transplant, HLT: Heart-lung transplant

---

serratus anterior and latissumus dorsi muscle groups.[17] An anterolateral thoracotomy with transverse sternotomy or "clamshell" has been used in patients who have emphysema and are simultaneously having lung volume reduction on the opposite side.[22] The surgeon dissects the superior and inferior pulmonary veins, the pulmonary artery, and the main stem bronchus. The phrenic nerve and the hilum are exposed when the pericardium is opened and the left atrium is accessed via an extended incision. Some cartilages of the recipient bronchus are removed and shortened to allow telescoping of the donor bronchus within the recipient's optimizing blood supply and healing.[22] The donor and recipient pulmonary arteries are anastomosed along with the left atrial cuff including the pulmonary veins to the recipient's left atrium as noted in Figure 14–1.[4]

The bilateral single sequential lung transplant has replaced the en bloc DLT in the United States. This procedure lessens bronchial anastomosis dehiscence and limits complications associated with cardiopulmonary bypass.[7] The procedure is similar to the single lung transplant except the incision is a median sternotomy or the anterolateral thoracotomy with transverse sternotomy ("clamshell").[17]

Acute Care Management and Complications

Patients are frequently mechanically ventilated 24 to 48 hours following transplantation, but rapid extubation is common. An early goal is to liberate the patient from mechanical ventilation, but potential difficulties with the

Figure 14–1. Lung transplant. Schematic illustrates the three anastomoses: 1) bruncus; 2) pulmonary artery; 3) left atrium with pulmonary veins.

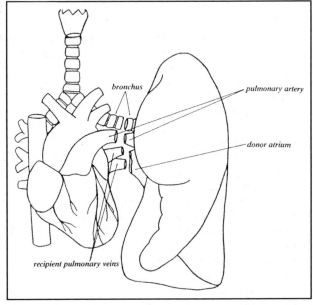

Table 14–4

RISKS FOR PROLONGED MECHANICAL VENTILATION AND EXTENDED LENGTH OF STAY IN THE INTENSIVE CARE UNIT FOLLOWING TRANSPLANTATION

- Advanced age
- Obesity
- Respiratory muscle weakness
- Infection (persistent purulent secretions with donor or aspiration)
- APACHE II score (acute physiology and chronic health evaluation)
- Graft dysfunction/gas-exchange impairment/carbon dioxide retention
- Cardiovascular instability
- Cardiopulmonary bypass duration
- Infiltrates on donor chest x-ray
- Pulmonary hypertensive disorders (Eisenmenger's syndrome, idiopathic pulmonary fibrosis, primary pulmonary HTN)

Adapted from Algar FJ, Alvarez A, Lama R, et al. Lung transplantation in patients under mechanical ventilation. *Transplant Proc.* 2003;35(2):737-738.

weaning process and factors prolonging the intensive care unit (ICU) duration are outlined in Table 14–4.[23,24] Early mobilization and prophylaxis for deep venous thrombosis is an important component of acute care management for any surgical patient. Universal precautions are the standard of care for all patients in a hospital setting, but are fundamental to care of transplant recipients.

Table 14–5

COMMON SIGNS AND SYMPTOMS OF LUNG TRANSPLANT REJECTION

- Low grade temperature
- Lethargy
- Myalgias
- General malaise
- Palpitations
- Increased shortness of breath/dyspnea on exertion
- Decrease in exercise tolerance
- Restrictive pattern on spirometry ($\downarrow$ FVC, $\downarrow$ FEV$_1$)
- Desaturation with activity/exercise, increased oxygen requirements

FVC = forced vital capacity; FEV = forced expiratory volume
Adapted from:
Versluis-Burlis T, Downs AM. Thoracic organ transplantation: heart, lung, and heart-lung. In: *Essentials of Cardiopulmonary Physical Therapy*. 2nd ed. Philadelphia, Pa: WB Saunders Co; 2001.
www.ishlt.org. International Society for Heart & Lung Transplantation.

Table 14–6

PRIMARY CAUSES OF DEATH AND COMPLICATIONS FOLLOWING LUNG TRANSPLANTATION

Early <30 Days	*≥1 Year*
Graft failure	Bronchiolitis obliterans
Noncytomegalovirus infections	Chronic rejection and graft failure
Acute rejection	Lymphoma
Technical (phrenic nerve dysfunction)	Malignancy, other cytomegalovirus
Cardiovascular	(CMV) infections
Pulmonary embolism	

Specific airway complications: malacia, stenosis, dehiscence

Adapted from References 10,13,14,23,40–44.

Risk of infection and rejection are ever present when treating the patient after transplantation. Signs and symptoms of possible lung rejection are outlined in Table 14–5. Complications following lung transplantation can be divided into early and late categories as described in Table 14–6. Rejection falls into both categories but can be further subdivided into acute and chronic conditions. Acute graft dysfunction or primary graft failure has been shown to occur in 11% of the transplant population.[25] Bronchiolitis obliterans reflects chronic rejection and is the leading cause of late morbidity and mortality following lung transplantation and HLT.[26–28] Bronchiolitis obliterans is characterized by fibrosis and scar formation in the smaller airways (see Chapter 7).[29] Improvement in donor lung

---

Table 14–7

POTENTIAL REHABILITATION GOALS BEFORE
AND AFTER TRANSPLANTATION

- Improve cardiovascular and pulmonary endurance and exercise capacity
- Optimize pulmonary hygiene
- Optimize breathing control
- Optimize pain control
- Increase range of motion and strength
- Improve posture and flexibility
- Increase overall functional level and independence with ADLs and IADLs
- Return to work
- Educate on team roles and medication, precautions, signs/symptoms of infection/rejection
- Educate on effective coughing/splinting of incisions/promote effective airway clearance
- Educate on breathing efficiency during ADLs
- Educate on body mechanics for ADLs
- Educate on stress management and relaxation techniques

---

preservation, immunosuppression, surgical techniques, and limiting ischemia-reperfusion injury have led to improved 1-year survival.[29–31] Despite these enhancements, bronchiolitis obliterans remains the nemesis of both lung transplantation and HLT. Upwards of 60% of pulmonary transplant recipients will have bronchiolitis obliterans 5 years after surgery.[31]

Airway anastomotic dehiscence is a complication that occurred early in the development of the surgical lung transplantation procedure. Recipient exposure to corticosteroids, inability to reconnect the bronchial circulation, end-to-end suturing, and immunosuppressives were implicated in impaired wound healing. Telescoping the anastomosis and modifications of the drug regimen have resulted in a reduction of ischemic and stenotic complications of the airway.[10,22,32]

The immunosuppressed patient is at risk for opportunistic infections, but lung transplant and HLT recipients have the added challenge of environmental exposure with every breath. Patient education should incorporate avoidance of unnecessary exposures such as crowded locations, children or adults with active infections, and using a mask when outside during poor air quality times. Patients should be cautioned to avoid gardening and construction projects because of exposure to mold and naturally occurring fungi.

Physical Therapy Implications of Lung Transplantation

Following transplantation, rehabilitation is initiated in the ICU if the patient is hemodynamically stable. Goals during the acute care phase of rehabilitation focus on independence with mobility and ADLs, effective coughing and airway clearance, pain control, and patient education (Table 14–7). The normal cough reflex and lymphatic drainage are absent below the level of the bronchial

Table 14–8

LONG-TERM EXERCISE RESPONSES FOLLOWING LUNG, HEART, AND HEART-LUNG TRANSPLANTATION

Lung	Heart-Lung	Heart
• Exercise capacity and pulmonary function below normal values • $VO_{2\ max.}$ 40% to 50% predicted • DLT VO_2 > SLTx/HLTx • ⇓ in physiologic dead space (V_d/V_T) and alveolar-arterial oxygen gradient ([A-a] PO_2) • Elevated RR, HR, and minute ventilation at rest • Limitations multifactorial but mostly thought to be peripheral (circulation/muscle)	• Exercise capacity and pulmonary function below normal values • $VO_{2\ max.}$ 39% to 62% predicted • Blunted chronotropic/inotropic responses to exercise • Lower anaerobic threshold • Pulmonary function typically restrictive pattern • Limitations multifactorial but mostly thought to be peripheral (circulation/muscle)	• Exercise capacity and pulmonary function below normal values • $VO_{2\ max.}$ 48% to 70% predicted • Lower maximum HR (~25% < controls) • Lower maximum oxygen pulse • Lower anaerobic threshold maximum HR 20% to 25% less than controls • Exaggerated neuroendocrine response • Limitations multifactorial but mostly thought to be peripheral (circulation/muscle)

Adapted from References 11,22,27–40.

anastomosis. Deep breathing exercises and splinted incision coughing should be done every waking hour to assist with prevention of atelectasis and pneumonia. Evaluation of orthostatic hypotension with position change and transfers should be considered a standard precaution during early therapy sessions. The therapist needs to appreciate fluid shifts and effects of immobility, pain, and medications on cardiovascular responsiveness to position changes.

The functional level at time of discharge may be similar to admission level. Physiologic effects of surgery (pain, incision, sleep deficits, limited nutrition, effects of anesthesia, immunosuppressive medications), prior deconditioning, and the native disease continue to limit functional capacity at time of discharge. Patients may frequently complain of dyspnea, and this may or may not be associated with pulmonary impairments. Potential exercise capacity changes following lung transplantation are outlined in Table 14–8. Overall concerns and areas to monitor are outlined in the rehabilitation section for all solid organ transplantations.

Therapists must be cognizant of the signs and symptoms of infection and rejection. Therapy personnel may be the first health care providers to recognize these markers because the therapist is mobilizing the patient and monitoring daily changes in activity levels. Deterioration of the patient's status should be reported to the transplant team. Infection and rejection signs and symptoms are often subtle and early recognition is key to successful treatment. During periods of acute rejection, exercise may be performed cautiously or held due to the increased metabolic demand and pulmonary compromise.

Finally, patients are introduced to hand-held spirometers (microspirometers) to measure daily changes in pulmonary function including the FEV_1 (forced expiratory volume in 1 second) and FVC (forced vital capacity). Patient education focuses on maintaining daily records of weight, temperature, overall perception of well-being, and spirometry.

Living-Related Lung Transplantation

Indications/Candidate Selection

A discrepancy has been described between the availability of potential organs for donation and the increasing demand for lungs for transplantation.[16] Living donor lobar donation has evolved due to this imbalance as a viable option for patients with cystic fibrosis and smaller adults with advanced lung disease (eg, pulmonary fibrosis, bronchopulmonary dysplasia [BPD], pulmonary HTN).[33,34] Living-related lobe donation as an option for transplantation has raised many ethical questions and psychosocial issues especially when there is more than one child in a given family with cystic fibrosis.[16,35]

The procedure involves removing a lower lobe from two donors and transplanting these lobes into the recipient.[4,16] No donor deaths have been documented from complications of the surgery but surgical risk is high.[36] Early and late rejection outcomes are similar to traditional lung transplantations.[35] Interestingly, the primary cause of death is infectious complications versus bronchiolitis obliterans in nonliving related recipients.[37] Questions about improvement in exercise capacity and survival outcomes have yet to be clearly answered.[33]

Heart Transplantation

Introduction/Overview

The 1-year survival rate for heart transplant (Figure 14–2) is 81% to 90%, and is the highest among thoracic transplant recipients.[3,6,13,17–20] The number of transplants performed has plateaued since 1999.[18] This plateau is due to limited donor organ availability promoting advances in surgical techniques and life-saving medications and devices for patients with cardiac disease. Advances include valve repair and coronary artery bypass grafting in higher risk populations, biventricular pacemakers, and ventricular assist devices.[6,38,39] Earlier and more aggressive intervention following cardiac events such as angioplasty for unstable angina or a myocardial infarct is becoming the standard of care.[3]

Indications/Candidate Selection

The indication for heart transplantation is end-stage cardiac disease or heart failure (Table 14–9).[3,4,6,18,20,40] Heart transplant is recommended for patients with maximal oxygen consumption ($VO_{2\ max}$) less than 10 mL/kg/min,

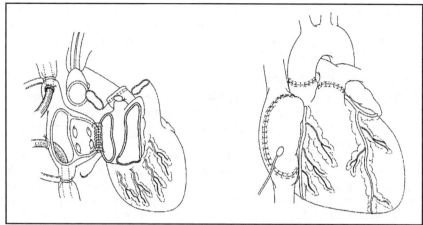

Figure 14–2. Orthotopic heart transplant. Schematic illustrates the biatrial method. Note epicardial pacemaker electrode in place. (Reprinted from Sadowsky HS. Cardiac transplantation: a review. Physical Therapy. 1996;76:498-515. With permission from the American Physical Therapy Association.)

Table 14–9
HEART TRANSPLANTATION, INCLUSION/EXCLUSION CATEGORIES

Inclusion	*Exclusion*
End-stage heart disease congestive heart failure (CHF)	Irreversible extracardiac end-organ dysfunction
Ischemic heart disease/CAD/myocardial infarction (MI)	Recent cancers with uncertain status
Cardiomyopathies	Psychiatric illness with poor medical compliance
Valve disease	Severe irreversible pulmonary HTN
Congenital heart disease	Active infection
Amyloidosis	Cirrhosis of the liver
Retransplantation	High fixed pulmonary vascular resistance

Relative Contraindications	
Diabetes mellitus (DM)	Previous malignancy
Chronic obstructive pulmonary disease	Substance abuse
Peripheral vascular disease	Poor history of compliance with medical regimes
Morbid obesity	Recent pulmonary infarction
Age	

Adapted from References 3,4,6,17,20.

recurrent symptomatic ventricular dysrhythmias refractory to all accepted therapeutic modalities, and severe ischemia which is not treatable with angioplasty or coronary bypass surgery.[6] Candidate evaluation is extensive as previously noted for lung transplantation.

Operative Procedure

Orthotopic heart transplantation, the primary form of cardiac transplant, refers to the removal of the recipient heart followed by replacement with the donor's heart in the same anatomic location. A median sternotomy is made, and the patient is placed on cardiopulmonary bypass. The donor atria are incised to allow anastomosis to the recipient atria. This biatrial method allows for short operative time by anastomosing the donor left and right atria to the recipient's heart at the midatrial level. This method has a higher incidence of mitral and tricuspid insufficiency. An alternative method is the bicaval technique involving individual anastomoses of the inferior and superior vena cavae instead of the right atrial cuff. Additional modifications added an anastomosis of paired pulmonary veins to replace the left atrial cuff anastomosis.[3] This technique has proven effective with fewer electrophysiological complications requiring pacemaker support.[3,6]

Heterotropic heart transplantation is indicated in select cases and is referred to as the "piggyback technique."[6,7] The donor and recipient hearts remains intact, and the right and left atrias are anastomosed to allow the four atria to function as two. The aorta and pulmonary arteries are adjoined to complete the circuit. The two hearts function in parallel sharing the venous return and contributing to the cardiac output (CO). The primary indications for this type of transplant are poor donor heart function, pulmonary HTN, and mismatched size between donor and recipient. The advantage of the technique is to allow the recipient heart to assist during periods of rejection or impaired function. Disadvantages of this technique are dysrhythmias, angina related to the native heart, risk of pulmonary emboli, and long-term use of anticoagulation therapy.

Acute Care Management and Complications

Persistent pulmonary HTN, bleeding, renal dysfunction, rejection, and infection are complications in the initial postoperative phase of heart transplants.[6] Bleeding risk is enhanced in those who have had multiple operations, anticoagulation therapy, and prior liver or renal dysfunction. Perioperative kidney dysfunction may be related to fluid shifts during the surgery, diminished donor heart function, and use of nephrotoxic immunosuppressive medications.[6]

Liberating the patient from mechanical ventilation and aggressive pulmonary hygiene is vital until the patient begins out of bed (OOB) activity. Standard precautions apply for all patients, but in the transplant population, should be overzealously applied.

Rejection of the implanted organ is a life-long challenge, and common signs and symptoms are presented in Table 14–10. Hyperacute rejection occurs within hours of surgery and is considered rare.[6] Acute cellular rejection is more common and occurs within the first 30 days. Identification and treatment of rejection is the most important component of after care for heart transplant patients.

> ## Table 14–10
> ## COMMON SIGNS AND SYMPTOMS OF HEART TRANSPLANT REJECTION
>
> - Low grade temperature
> - Lethargy
> - Myalgias
> - General malaise
> - Palpitations
> - Increased shortness of breath/dyspnea on exertion
> - Decrease in exercise tolerance
> - Soft heart sounds/S3 gallop
> - Increase in resting blood pressure (BP)
> - Hypotension with activity
> - Ventricular dysrhythmias

Patients undergo frequent emdomyocardial biopsies for histologic examination as the standard method to detect rejection. Infection also remains a persistent complication of immunosuppressive treatment. Bacterial infections are more common early while viral infections persist long term as the leading cause of morbidity and mortality in this population.

The primary late complication of heart transplantation is graft CAD also termed cardiac allograft vasculopathy or transplant coronary disease.[3,6,41,42] Transplant vasculopathy is challenging because the stenotic lesion can be diffuse or focal and is often asymptomatic.[42] Focal lesions have been treated with angioplasty, but traditional treatments for CAD like bypass grafting have limited success. Prevention, similar to typical atherosclerosis, may play a role by influencing lipid profiles, diabetes, HTN, and reducing opportunistic infections.[3,6,41,43] Superior vena cava stenosis and tricuspid regurgitation have also been documented as late complications.[3,8]

Physical Therapy Implications of Heart Transplantation

Hemodynamic stability is the number one challenge to the physical therapist in the acute care setting. The transplanted heart is denervated leading to an elevated resting heart rate (HR), blunted HR and BP responses to a given activity, and a prolonged return to baseline of the patient's hemodynamic status with the cessation of activity. Patients rely on venous return to augment end-diastolic volume (eg, Frank-Starling mechanism, see Chapter 6) and circulating catecholamines to elevate HR and stroke volume to increase CO and BP. These physiologic mechanisms take several minutes to activate necessitating the performance of warm-up and cool-down activities with exercise performance. Rating of perceived exertion, HR/pulse, electrocardiograms, BP monitoring, oxygen saturation, observing respiratory rate (RR), pattern, and patient color are all helpful signs of subtle changes in the cardiovascular and pulmonary systems' ability to respond to activity. Tables 14–7 and 14–10 outline some of the more specific issues the physical therapist should be alerted to in patients following heart transplantation.

Heart-Lung Transplantation

Introduction/Overview/Indications/Candidate Selection

The number of HLTs have declined since mid 1990s possibly related to the successful use of lung transplantation for cystic fibrosis and primary pulmonary HTN, as well as donor organ shortage.[17,44] Table 14–3 lists the potential diagnostic groups who have benefited from a HLT.

Operative Procedure

The HLT incision is a median sternotomy or bilateral transverse thoracotomy.[4,7,22] Right and left pneumonectomies are carefully performed to avoid damaging the vagal and phrenic nerves.[4] En bloc implantation involves dissection of the trachea near the carina, and anastomoses of the recipient's aorta, right atria, and trachea.

Acute Care Management and Complications

Management of the patient following HLT is similar to aspects of both post-operative lung and heart transplant care. The challenge for the patient and care team is the denervated heart and lungs. The physical therapist/physical therapist assistant must remember the absence of cough reflex and autonomic nervous system input and the impact these deficits create on physiologic processes. Additionally, the continuous threats of infection and rejection necessitate careful observance for all potential signs and symptoms of untoward events.

ABDOMINAL ORGAN TRANSPLANTATION

Renal Transplant

Introduction/Overview

More than 10,000 renal transplants are performed every year and patient survival 1 year after transplant from a living related donor is >95% and >90% from a cadaver. Transplantation clearly improves the quality and quantity of life compared with other modalities of renal replacement therapy, such as hemodialysis, especially for younger and diabetic patients with end-stage renal disease (ESRD).[45]

There is a diverse array of pathologies that destroy renal function as noted in Chapter 12, but the most common cause of ESRD is DM.[46] Table 14–11 provides a list of the most common renal pathologies leading to transplantation. The patient with ESRD has several treatment options including long-term dialysis, cadaveric kidney transplant, living kidney transplantation, and for those with diabetes and renal failure, simultaneous kidney-pancreas transplantation.

Indications/Candidate Selection

Candidates for renal transplantation undergo an extensive evaluation to identify important medical and psychosocial factors that may lead to adverse effects

Table 14–11

KIDNEY TRANSPLANTATION, INCLUSION/EXCLUSION CATEGORIES

Inclusion/Indications	Exclusion/Contraindications
ESRD (serum creatinine >5mg/dL; BUN >70 mg/dL)	Reversible renal disease
	Recent malignancy
Diabetes	Chronic/active infection
Chronic glomerulonephritis	Active glomerulonephritis
Polycystic kidney disease	Extrarenal complications
Nephrosclerosis	CAD
Interstitial nephritis	Noncompliance
Systemic lupus erythematosussle	Active substance abuse
	Uncontrolled psychiatric disorders
	Advanced age
	Obesity
	Prior renal transplant

on outcome as previously noted for thoracic organ transplantation. Common indications and contraindications to kidney transplantation are listed in Table 14–11. Cardiovascular disease is the most prevalent comorbid condition in patients with ESRD. Several traditional risk factors for atherosclerosis factor into the high incidence of cardiovascular disease in patients with ESRD, including HTN, dyslipidemia, and DM.[45]

Operative Procedure

The surgical approach is a curved incision in the patient's lower quadrant and proceeds through the external oblique to the peritoneum. The transplant site is usually the extra peritoneal space of the right or left lower abdominal quadrant. The surgical technique involves anastomoses of the renal artery and vein and ureter (Figure 14–3). The surgeon performs an end-to-side anastomosis of the donor renal artery to the recipient's external iliac, common iliac, or hypogastric artery. The renal vein is customarily anastomosed to the corresponding vein. The transplant ureter is either placed directly into the bladder wall or anastomosed to the recipient ureter.[45] Precise wound closure is important to prohibit hernia formation and may involve placement of temporary suction drains.[46]

The technique for living donor kidney transplantation is similar to that described for cadaveric donor transplantation.[45]

Acute Care Management and Complications

The incidence of postoperative complications has decreased, but acute rejection and/or infections remain a concern (Table 14–12). The most common complication during the acute care period is allograft dysfunction that may progress to graft loss. Renal failure persisting after transplantation is called delayed graft function (DGF) and is associated with oliguria, diminished urine formation, or the need for dialysis after the operation. DGF is usually due to ATN or

Figure 14–3. Renal transplant. Schematic illustrates three anastomoses: 1) renal artery to hypogastric artery; 2) renal vein; 3) ureter. (Reprinted with permission from Way LW, Doherty GM. Current surgical diagnosis and Treatment. New York, NY: McGraw-Hill; 2003.

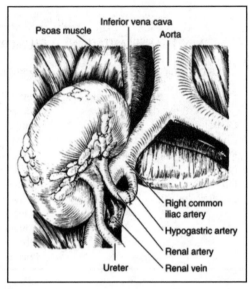

Table 14–12

COMPLICATIONS POST KIDNEY TRANSPLANTATION

- Rejection/infection
- Acute tubular necrosis (ATN)
- Ureteral fistula or obstruction
- Urologic leak
- Renal artery stenosis or thrombosis
- Perirenal hemotoma/abscess, lymphocele formation

Table 14–13

COMMON SIGNS AND SYMPTOMS OF KIDNEY REJECTION

- Decreased renal function, increased serum creatinine/BUN/edema/ decreased urine output
- HTN
- Weight gain
- Tenderness and swelling at graft site
- Fever
- Presence of sediment in urine

---

nephrotoxicity because of the immunosuppressive regimen (especially cyclosporin or tacrolimus). DGF may occur in 20% to 30% of cadaveric transplants and is rare after living donor.[46] Other early but infrequent graft problems include accelerated acute or hyperacute rejection. Common symptoms of rejection are presented in Table 14–13. The diagnosis of rejection is confirmed by ultrasonography to rule out urinary obstruction or anastomotic thrombus or leak followed by biopsy and histologic examination. The most frequent postoperative infections are those similar for all surgical patients and include infections of the urinary tract, indwelling catheters and lines, and postoperative pneumonia. Bacterial infections are more common than fungal and viral infections in the early postoperative period. Opportunistic infections typically occur after the first month and are due to intensive immunosuppression.[45,46] Thirty to 60% of patients suffer some type of infection during the first transplant year, and infectious causes are linked to half of the deaths of transplant recipients. Additional medical management of the acute renal transplant patient emphasizes electrolyte and acid-base management (see Chapter 2).

Physical Therapy Implications of Kidney Transplantation

The acute care physical therapist needs to monitor laboratory values and ascertain potential signs and symptoms of infection or rejection, as well as other patient complaints, to determine safe therapeutic interventions. The physical therapist needs to consider that patients presenting for renal transplantation are physically inactive with reduced exercise capacity and present with multisystem impairments (see Table 12–1).[47] The limited exercise capacity and poor physical functioning has been linked to low quality of life and high mortality in this population. The reason for the debility of patients with ESRD and dialysis is far from clear. The anemias of chronic renal disease, uremic myopathy, and resulting decreased muscle oxygen utilization, and disuse atrophy have a significant impact on the physical functioning of patients.[47,48] Therapeutic interventions are aimed to promote effective airway clearance and restore functional independence with an emphasis on transfers, gait training, and performance of ADLs. Airway clearance is imperative during the initial postoperative period since pulmonary complications are a leading cause of morbidity and prolonged hospitalization for all abdominal surgery patients. Once functional independence has been attained, the exercise prescription can address hobbies, fitness, and sports-related goals.

Exercise training after renal transplant results in higher levels of measured and self-reported physical functioning. Additionally, those who participate in an outlined exercise program demonstrated increased exercise adherence and participation long term.[49] Therefore, the initiation of a home exercise program early in the postoperative rehabilitation course is essential. Close monitoring of hemodynamic status and patient complaints is imperative due to the increased incidence of cardiovascular disease in this population. Brisk diuresis often accompanies successful graft function leading to potential dehydration and signs and symptoms associated with hypovolemia. Alternatively, patients with DGF may exhibit electrolyte and fluid overload secondary to prior uremia.[45] For reasons not entirely clear, but generally attributed to intensive or persistent steroid administration, previously normoglycemic patients may become diabetic in the post-transplant period.[45,46] The colon is especially vulnerable to ischemia and perforation, and all patient complaints of abdominal pain or distress should be forwarded to the medical/surgical team.[45,46]

Table 14–14
LIVER TRANSPLANTATION, INCLUSION/EXCLUSION CATEGORIES

Inclusion/Indications	*Exclusion/Contraindications*
Primary biliary cirrhosis	Active alcohol or drug abuse
Primary sclerosing cholangitis	Active infection
Cryptogenic cirrhosis	HIV positive
Chronic active hepatitis (B, C)	Intrahepatic tumor (>5 mm), extrahepatic
Alcoholic liver disease	malignancy
	Infection outside biliary tract
	Advanced cardiopulmonary disease
	Advanced age (>65 years)
	Hepatopulmonary syndrome

Liver Transplant

Introduction/Overview

Similar to all solid organ transplants, liver transplantation is now a well-established, definitive treatment for irreversible acute and chronic end-stage liver disease (ESLD).[50,51] The procedure is carried out when the patient is well enough to withstand a rigorous operation but significantly ill to warrant consideration for this terminal therapy.[50] The number of liver transplants has grown exponentially for the past two decades, and the list of indications for transplantation has been extended. Common indications for liver transplantation are listed in Table 14–14. Optimally, transplantation should improve both quality and quantity of life. One-year patient survival approaches 90%, and a 3-year survival of 80% is achieved at most major medical centers.[51]

Indications/Candidate Selection

Fulminant liver failure or acute liver failure (ALF) is defined as severe liver injury with the onset of hepatic encephalopathy within 8 to 12 weeks of the first symptoms of liver disease.[52] ALF is associated with 80% to 90% mortality, especially in patients who progress to severe encephalopathy and associated progressive brain swelling and herniation.[46,52] Chronic liver disease leading to cirrhosis arises from two major categories of disease: cholestatic and hepatocellular. The major cholestatic liver diseases include primary biliary cirrhosis, primary sclerosing cholangitis, and cystic fibrosis. Hepatocellular diseases include chronic hepatitis due to hepatitis viral infections (Hepatitis B, C, D), autoimmune reactions, drug toxicity, or alcohol and metabolic abnormalities including hemachromatosis, Wilson's disease, alpha-1 anti-trypsin disease, and the glycogen storage diseases.[46,50]

Operative Procedure

Standard Surgical Procedure

The donor organ is usually procured as part of multiorgan retrieval from a heart-beating, brain-dead donor. The recipient operation consists of the surgical removal of the native organ, a hepatectomy, followed by implantation of the donor liver. **Orthotopic liver transplantation** involves the removal of the native organ where the donor organ is placed in the same anatomic location. The abdominal cavity is entered via a bilateral subcostal incision with a midline extension toward the xiphoid.[53] Hepatectomy in the organ recipient is the most difficult part of the operation because the patient is at risk of developing a serious hemorrhage. Coagulopathy is common in ESLD due to the combination of portal HTN and reduced production of clotting factors leading to defective clotting and fibrinolysis.[54] Prior upper abdominal surgery also complicates the surgical removal of the liver due to potential scar tissue and bleeding risk. Liver implantation involves five end-to-end anastomoses of the bile ducts, the hepatic artery, the portal vein, and an inferior and superior connection of the inferior vena cava, termed the infra- and suprahepatic vena cava.[46,54,55]

Segmental and Lobar Liver Transplantation

The shortage of donor organs and the necessity to maximize the number of liver grafts is the most serious challenge to liver transplantation as with all transplant procedures. Living-donor transplantation and several surgical innovations including the transplantation of "split livers" from cadaveric and living donors has increased organ availability. These procedures, termed **segmental** and **lobar liver transplant**, are possible owing to the unique segmental anatomy of the liver and its potential regenerative capacity. Current methods include the removal of the left lateral segment or the entire right or left lobe from a living donor with subsequent transplantation to a pediatric or adult recipient. Similarly, a cadaveric liver can be split into two parts that can be transplanted into two size-matched recipients. The limitation of segmental liver graft transplantation appears to be related to minimal liver mass necessary for the adequate support of the recipient in the immediate post-transplant period.[53,56] Transplantation of the donated lobe is performed by techniques similar to those developed for whole-liver grafts.[46,53]

The postoperative treatment of the liver transplant patient is complicated by the profound physiologic derangements that accompany ESLD, and complications can generally be divided into hepatic and nonhepatic categories (Table 14–15).[46,56,57] The most serious hepatic complications are graft dysfunction and primary nonfunction (PNF). These complications can range from minor abnormalities in liver functioning to overt graft failure, hemodynamic compromise, multiorgan failure, and death.

Massive fluid shifts, transient renal insufficiency resulting from the surgery, and premorbid liver dysfunction may leave the patient volume overloaded during the postoperative period. This hypervolemia can impair cardiopulmonary function leading to resultant heart failure and pulmonary edema. Pulmonary function may be further compromised due to right hemidiaphragmatic dysfunction associated with incision discomfort limiting ventilation and cough effectiveness.

Rejection is common, with approximately 60% of recipients experiencing one episode in the first 1 to 2 weeks post-transplant. The clinical signs of rejection are listed in Table 14–16. The diagnosis of rejection is confirmed by histologic examination of liver biopsy. Common infectious complications include pneumonia, wound infections, intravenous line infections, and urinary tract infections.[46,56]

Table 14–15

COMPLICATIONS POST LIVER TRANSPLANTATION

Hepatic:
- Primary graft dysfunction
- Vascular compromise
- Portal vein/hepatic artery obstruction or thrombus, anastomotic leak
- Bile duct disorder
- Stenosis/obstruction/leak
- Hemolysis
- Drug toxicity

Nonhepatic:
- Fluid overload
- CHF
- Pneumonia
- Pulmonary vascular permeability
- Renal insufficiency
- Anemia/thrombocytopenia
- Coagolapathy/bleeding
- Seizures/encephalopathy/depression

Table 14–16

COMMON SIGNS AND SYMPTOMS OF LIVER REJECTION

- Right upper quadrant pain
- Fever
- Feeling ill/malaise
- Leukocytosis
- Elevated blood levels of bilirubin and aminotransferase

Physical Therapy Implications of Liver Transplantation

The prolonged waiting times for transplant confers a higher risk for patients with ESLD that impacts the postoperative physical therapy regimen. In addition to the metabolic consequences of liver diseases, patients will frequently present with malnutrition and anorexia, osteoporosis, insulin resistance, fluid imbalances, coagulapathy, variceal bleeding, and encephalopathy leading to physical inactivity (see Tables 11–5 and 11-16).[58,59] This inactivity is due to the disease as well as self-imposed bed rest with resultant muscle atrophy and limited strength and endurance. Studies have revealed that ESLD patients typically present with impairments in exercise capacity, <55% to 70% of age-predicted values, low body mass index, and muscle atrophy.[58,60] The immediate post-transplant period is characterized by a state of hypermetabolism linked to increased protein breakdown associated with glucocorticoid use.

The most common complaints post-transplant include weakness, fatigue, and bone/joint discomfort. As noted previously, pulmonary complications are common following surgery of the abdomen, but distinct diaphragm dysfunction and fluid status increase the risk for complications post-liver transplant. Patients post-liver transplant exhibit impaired peak exercise performance similar to that observed after other solid organ transplants including early anaerobic threshold and decreased age predicted $VO_{2\ max}$.[61] Patients should return to independent ADL and intrumental ADL (IADL) functioning, and many will return to work and leisure pursuits and may even participate in the transplant Olympics. It is important to note, however, that recipients who engage in regular physical activity score higher on quality of life measures providing further credence to the initiation of home exercise programs.[62]

Pancreas and Islet Transplant

Introduction/Overview

Hyperglycemia is the most important factor in the development and progression of the secondary complications of diabetes. Pancreas transplantation has advanced since exogenous insulin cannot prevent the development of the secondary complications of diabetes. Pancreas transplantation is unique among organ transplants in that it is primarily a therapy that attempts to stabilize and prevent the devastating end organ complications associated with Type 1 diabetes as opposed to prolonging life. Indications for pancreas transplant are exceptionally narrow due to the profound organ shortage in relationship to the prevalence of diabetes, the significant surgical risk, and the requirement of lifelong immunosuppression. More than 1200 procedures are performed annually, and 1-year patient survival rate is >90% with 60% to 85% of patients remaining insulin free.[63]

Indications/Candidate Selection

The common indications for pancreas transplantation include patients with Type 1 diabetes that are also candidates for a kidney transplant (85% to 90%), patients with Type 1 diabetes with an adequately functioning kidney transplant who are already prescribed immunosuppression (7% to 10%), and select patients with extremely brittle diabetes that the risks of surgery and immunosuppression are less dangerous than the current health status.[46,63] Additional considerations are similar to other solid organ transplants including freedom from substance abuse, psychiatric disease, malignancy, end organ damage, or disease including CAD and CHF.

Operative Procedure

Most pancreatic transplants are cadaveric, but living related donors who undergo a hemipancreatectomy may be employed. The procedure is heterotopic with the native organ remaining in place, and implantation is through a midline abdominal incision. Surgical techniques vary, but some commonalties exist. The donor graft is explanted with a cuff of duodenum for future buttressing of the exocrine portion of the pancreas. The pancreatic graft's arterial supply is from the patient's right common or external iliac artery and venous outflow is to the

Table 14-17

POTENTIAL POST-TRANSPLANTATION PSYCHOSOCIAL ISSUES

- Donor guilt—guilt over the donor's loss of life to save others
- Stress
- Change in life expectancy, risk of long-term complications, change from sick role to well role leading to social/marital problems
- Finances
- Travel or moving to region of transplant program
- Pre- and postoperative complications and medication side effects
- Coping with disabling or life-threatening illness

Adapted from:
Versluis-Burlis T, Downs AM. Thoracic organ transplantation: heart, lung, and heart-lung. In: Hillegass EA, Sadowsky HS, eds. *Essentials of Cardiopulmonary Physical Therapy.* 2nd ed. Philadelphia, Pa: WB Saunders Co; 2001.
Wrightson N, Blake A, English L. Care of the heart transplant patient. *Nurs Times.* 2002;98(28):34–37.

portal vein, right common, or external iliac veins.[46,64] Exocrine drainage is handled by anastomosis of the duodenal segment to the bladder or to the small intestine.

Acute Care Management and Complications

Most pancreas transplants are simultaneous pancreas-kidney (SPK) transplants from the same cadaver. This allows monitoring of renal allograft function as a surrogate marker for pancreatic functioning. The serum creatinine is monitored and kidney biopsy results allow the diagnosis of rejection. If exocrine secretions are diverted to the bladder, the pancreaticoduodenal with exocrine bladder-drainage procedure allows for the monitoring of urinary amylase as a marker of rejection (amylase decreases 30% <baseline prior to onset of hyperglycemia).[64] Direct biopsy of the pancreas can be performed to provide tissue for histologic examination especially in the pancreas alone transplant procedure.[63]

Complications after pancreas transplant are similar to other abdominal organ procedures and include infection and rejection and vascular thrombosis at the anastomotic sites. Rejection can occur within days or years after the transplant. Urinary tract infections are the most common postoperative infection occurring in >35% of patients. Unique complications for bladder-drained pancreas transplant includes hematuria, cystitis, urethritis, reflux pancreatitis, and metabolic alterations defined below. The most serious complication of the enteric drained-pancreas transplant, exocrine drainage to the small intestine, is enteric leak and abdominal abscess that usually occurs within the first 6 months. Gastrointestinal bleeding and peritonitis have also been noted to occur.[46,64] Additionally, transient hypoglycemia and hyperglycemia may occur.

Physical Therapy Implications of Pancreas Transplantation

The physical therapy regimen post-transplant is similar to that for the renal transplant patient with one notable difference. Postoperative monitoring of laboratory values with special emphasis on electrolytes and fluid status is vital. The normal pancreas secretes vast quantities of bicarbonate and water in addition to the pancreatic enzymes including amylase, lipase, and multiple proteolytic precursors necessary for digestion. However, the transplanted pancreas with bladder attachment allows the urinary loss of extensive volumes of bicarbonate and water with subsequent metabolic acidosis, dehydration, orthostatic hypotension, and cardiac dysrhythmias secondary to electrolyte abnormalities.[64] The physical therapy practitioner must monitor the laboratory values closely until the postoperative medical regimen has stabilized the fluid and metabolic status of the patient.

Successful pancreatic transplant is associated with normalization of blood glucose levels, euglycemia, and glycosolated hemoglobin (Hb A_{1C}) without the need for exogenous insulin. The implications of normal glycemic control includes a slowing and potential reversal of diabetic nephropathy, motor and sensory neuropathy, as well as improved BP control and potential lessening the incidence of cardiac disease.[46,63]

Physically, pancreas-kidney transplant patients are typically younger than renal transplant alone. Similar to renal transplant patients, those who are more active report higher scores on health related quality of life measures.[65]

COMMON CONCERNS POST SOLID ORGAN TRANSPLANTATION

Transplantation and chronic illness is associated with significant psychosocial stressors as noted in Table 14–17. The therapist should be aware of these potential complications and consult with appropriate mental health workers.

INFECTION, REJECTION, AND IMMUNOSUPPRESSION

The allograft, or a transplanted organ, can be rejected acutely or after many years. Rejection is a host-versus-graft immune response and is a major barrier to effective organ transplantation leading to graft dysfunction and tissue destruction. Allograft rejection is typically classified as hyperacute, acute, or chronic, and rejection is either a cell-mediated (innate immunity) or humoral (adaptive immunity) immune event.[46] **Natural or innate immunity** refers to the nonspecific immune events involving macrophages, neutrophils, natural killer cells, complement proteins, and various cytokines. **Adaptive immunity** involves recognition of specific antigens present on the cell membrane from the allograft and activation of specific T and B lymphocytes (see Chapter 5).[66,67]

Hyperacute and accelerated rejection, in which the graft becomes nonfunctional within hours or days, is due largely to ABO blood group or human leukocyte antigen (HLA) incompatibility. HLAs are found on virtually all nucleated cells of the body and platelets, and the placement of an incompatible organ into a recipient with preformed antibodies against the donor antigen stimulates a vigorous immune response. The immune response results in rapid destruction of the graft's vascular endothelium, vessel thrombosis, and organ infarction.

Hyperacute rejection is typically nonresponsive to immunosuppressive therapy and medical care is supportive, but accelerated rejection can sometimes be reversed by vigorous pharmacological therapy.[46,66,67]

Acute rejection of organ allografts is an adaptive response involving T cells mediated by CD8 T cells, by CD4 T cells, or both. Acute rejection is usually treated by bolus intravenous steroid therapy with or without temporary increases in the maintenance immunosuppression. Damaged areas of the allograft heal by fibrosis and the remainder of the graft continues to function.[66,67]

Minimizing the differences between the donor and recipient by verification of ABO compatibility and "crossmatching" decreases the likelihood of acute rejection. Crossmatching refers to testing the recipient's serum antibodies against donor WBCs (lymphocytes). Although HLA matching significantly improves the success rate of clinical organ transplantation, it does not in itself prevent rejection reactions. Chronic rejection describes the late process of graft destruction resulting in graft ischemia and fibrosis.

Chronic rejection is believed to be an antibody mediated process involving the T and B lymphocytes. Other potential factors that have been considered include the initial ischemic insult, the reduced mass of transplanted tissue (especially in the case of kidney and split liver transplants), the denervation of the transplanted organ, the hyperlipidemia and HTN associated with immunosuppressive drugs, the immunosuppressive drugs themselves, and chronic viral injury.[66,67]

Chronic rejection manifests differently in each organ. Chronic rejection in lung transplantation is termed **bronchiolitis obliterans** and results in progressive narrowing of the bronchioles. Chronic rejection in heart transplantation, **cardiac transplant vasculopathy**, is manifested principally as a diffuse myointimal hyperplasia or "accelerated atherosclerosis" proceeding to fibrosis of the coronary arteries and eventual ischemic heart disease and failure.[67,68]

Kidney chronic rejection, **transplant nephropathy/transplant glomerulopathy**, results from vascular thickening and narrowing of the lumen by the accumulation of connective tissue and cellular infiltration. Transplant nephropathy is associated with gradual deterioration of graft function with resultant elevated plasma creatinine, protein in the urine, and worsening HTN.[45,67]

Chronic liver rejection, **ductopenic rejection/vanishing bile duct syndrome**, is also due to progressive parenchymal fibrosis and necrosis, vascular lesions, and cellular infiltration. It is associated with elevated bilirubin and liver function tests (ALP/GGT/ALT) and cholestasis.[46,67]

Immunologic control and suppression is vital to the prevention of allograft rejection and is a critical component of solid organ transplantation. Common immunosuppressive drugs include corticosteroids, azathioprine, mycophenolate mofetil, tacrolimus, cyclosporine, and rapamycin (Table 14–18). Immunosuppression dosing is more intensive immediately post transplant and then gradually diminishes during the first year as the recipient's immune system adapts and the allograft becomes less immunoreactive.[46] Although the immunosuppressive drug regimen suppresses immune function, patients rarely reach a point where the drugs can be discontinued. Acute rejection leading to chronic rejection is almost universally present throughout the postoperative period. The patient's drug regimen is constantly modified, and as new products are introduced, clinical immunosuppression regimens are constantly changed.

Table 14–18
IMMUNOSUPPRESSION MEDICATIONS AND POTENTIAL SIDE EFFECTS

Medication	Impact
Cyclosporin	HTN, lymphocytic proliferative syndrome, nephrotoxicity, neurotoxicity, hepatotoxicity, tremors, increased cholesterol, rare myopathies, hyperkalemia, hemolytic uremic syndrome, gingival hyperplasia
Prednisone	Weight gain, redistribution of body fat, proximal muscle weakness, self-image changes, impaired wound healing, glucose intolerance-diabetes, osteoporosis, bone necrosis, cataracts, HTN
Azathioprine	Increased risk for neoplasm, nausea, vomiting, anorexia, rare myopathies, hepatoxicity
OKT3	Risk for pulmonary edema, bronchospasm, fever, chills, rash pruritus, mental status changes, anaphylaxis, hypokalemia
FK506	Nephrotoxicity, hyperkalemia, neurotoxicity, appetite depression, nausea, headache, insomnia, photophobia, diabetes

Adapted from:
Miniati DN, Robbins RC. Heart transplantation: a thirty-year perspective. *Ann Rev Med.* 2002;53:189–205.
Parekh K, Trulock E, Patterson GA. Use of cyclosporine in lung transplantation. *Transplant Proc.* 2004;36(2 Suppl):S318–S322.
Wrightson N, Blake A, English L. Care of the heart transplant patient. *Nurs Times.* 2002;98(28):34–37.

Immunosuppressive drugs can lead to a myriad of side effects as noted in Table 14–18. Additionally, the physical therapy practitioner must remember that immunosuppression leads to an increase risk of infectious complications, and opportunistic infections can also lead to significant morbidity and mortality. Consistent observation of infection control precautions is central to all physical therapy management of the transplant population (infection control/standard precautions are outlined in Chapter 5).

Patients can participate in physical therapy examinations and therapeutic interventions during active episodes of infection and rejection if stable. However, modifications in the care plan such as reduced exercise intensity and duration and closer vital sign monitoring including perceived exertion are standard. The physical therapist will need to incorporate specific organ issues such as closer observation of laboratory values including electrolytes, blood glucose, and coagulation profiles for the kidney, liver, and pancreas transplant patient; ECG and hemodynamic monitoring for the heart transplant patient; and noting oxygenation (pulse oximetry), sputum production, and airflow in the lung transplant patient.

COMMON LATE COMPLICATIONS

HTN is a common postoperative complication in the transplant patient. The development of HTN is multifactorial and may include nephrotoxic effects of cyclosporin and prednisone, pre-existing or progressive renal insufficiency, and weight gain. **Post-transplant DM** is generally medication related. Corticosteroids increased gluconeogenesis while increasing insulin resistance, and cyclosporin and tacrilimus inhibit insulin release from pancreatic islet cells. **Osteoporosis** is a common bone disorder after solid-organ transplantation, and the majority of bone loss occurs within the first 6 months post-transplant. The principal cause of bone demineralization is the direct inhibition of osteoblastic activity, increased calcium urinary excretion, impaired GI absorption of calcium, and sex hormone inhibition via steroids. The risk of pathologic fracture risk is increased with an increased incidence of extremity fracture as opposed to vertebrae fracture. **Hyperlipidemia** and **hypertriglyceridemia** are also common post-transplant and are believed to be drug side effects. Patients who have undergone transplantation are at an increased risk of **malignancy** development especially lymphomas, skin cancer, and Kaposi's sarcoma.[46,55,56,68]

Other potential late complications of transplantation that the physical therapist should keep in mind include steroid-induced myopathy and skin alterations, aseptic necrosis of bone, gout, visual abnormalities associated with cataracts, heart failure, herpes zoster, and obesity.[46,68,69] Finally, neurotoxicity related to cylcosporin and tacrilimus has been noted and may be manifested as seizures, severe headaches, confusion, and stroke as well as varying levels of delirium.[68]

The role of physical therapy as it relates to the long-term consequences of transplantation is not well developed. Exercise programming has been demonstrated to limit many of the secondary effects of immunosuppression. Specifically, exercise training has been shown to reverse steroid-induced myopathy with improvements noted in strength, muscle cross-sectional area (CSA), and fat-free mass.[70,71] Physical therapy, strengthening, and weightbearing exercise are standard recommendations for patients with osteoporosis.[72] Cardiorespiratory fitness and exercise training have demonstrated positive impacts on patients with diabetes, are an integral aspect of weight control, and have been associated with reduced incidences of cancer.[73,74] Finally, as noted previously, participation in exercise programs leads to enhanced quality of life after transplantation. Although improvements in exercise capacity are noted for each type of transplantation, recipients demonstrate consistent decrements in maximal exercise capacity compared to age-matched individuals (examples shown in Table 14–8). Deconditioning, abnormal mitochondrial functioning, and pulmonary deficits have been proposed to contribute to the reduction in exercise capacity following transplant.[22,27,32]

SUMMARY

Physical therapy consultation and interventions for the patient who has undergone solid organ transplantation is common during the immediate postoperative period. However, patients frequently seek treatment at community and regional hospitals for a myriad of postoperative and general age-related complications. Transplantation is not a cure, but the patient inherits a variety of post-transplant complications, most notably the constant battle between infection and rejection. Exercise plays a large role in maintaining the quality of life for these patients, and it is important for therapists to understand many of the acute and long-term complications of transplantation as they prescribe safe and effective therapeutic interventions. The physical therapist and physical therapist assistant are an integral component to transplant teams. Physical therapy plays a pivotal role in the acute care setting to assist with pain management and observation for infection/rejection, promote pulmonary hygiene and early mobilization, and institute appropriately designed therapeutic programs to reduce functional limitations and return the patient to an independent lifestyle. Common goals for pre- and post-transplantation are summarized on Table 14–7.

CASE STUDY

Mrs. Zema is a 55-year-old (y/o) female who received a left single lung transplant on November second. Mrs. Zema has a history of (h/o) end-stage COPD. Physical therapy was consulted for evaluation and treatment 2 weeks following the transplant.

Patient/Client History

General Demographics/Social History/Living Environment

Mrs. Zema lives with her husband of 34 years in a two-story, older brownstone. She has three daughters who live locally and is expecting her first grandchild any day. Her husband is a truck driver and is on the road 6 days a week. She has five steps to enter the outside of her home, the bathroom and bedroom are on the second floor, and there is no handrail for either stairs. Mrs. Zema is a retired elementary school teacher.

General Health Status/Family History

Previously, Mrs. Zema had been a three-pack-a-day smoker for more than 20 years but stopped 3 years ago. She has been on anti-anxiety medication off and on for 2 years.

Medical/Surgical History

Mrs. Zema is diagnosed with COPD and was dependent on oxygen (O_2) and chronic steroids prior to the surgery. She was cachetic prior to surgery. Her hospital course following transplantation was complicated by failure to wean from mechanical ventilation, and she underwent a tracheotomy 1-week following transplantation. A lung perfusion scan shortly after the surgery showed 46% of blood flow to transplanted lung, but a recent perfusion scan showed a further decline in perfusion to 37%. An open lung biopsy revealed acute lung allograft rejection. Mrs. Zema was treated with a course of high dose steroids and antithymocytoglobulin (ATGAM) that resulted in a 6% increase in perfusion. Mrs. Zema was transferred from the surgical ICU to the medical ICU for continued care 1 month following transplantation. The hospital course continued to be complicated by pseudomonas pneumonia, poorly controlled HTN, positive methicillin resistant staphylococcus aureus (MRSA) and candida in sputum, compression fractures, clostridium difficile associated with severe diarrhea, new onset atrial flutter and diabetes, profound deconditioning, and difficulty in weaning from the mechanical ventilator. Her medications upon transfer from the surgical ICU to the medical ICU were vancomycin, bactrim, nystatin, atrovent, alupent, cyclosporin, imuran, solumedrol, acyclovir, Imodium, digoxin, reglan, vasotec, carafate, haldol, and ativan.

Current Conditions/Chief Complaints

Mrs. Zema is unable to verbalize audibly her complaints but is able to mouth words. She is appears uncomfortable and confirms feeling short of breath (SOB) and very anxious. She is on a mechanical ventilator with the following settings: SIMV (synchronized intermittent mandatory ventilation) 10, pressure support 15, F_iO_2 (fraction of inspired oxygen) 40%, PEEP (positive end expiratory pressure) of 5. She rates her pain on a scale of 0 to 10 a 7, a rating of perceived exertion while in bed at with her head elevated 30 degrees a 9 (on a scale from 0 to 10) by pointing to the scale. Her activity status is fully dependent for all ADLs, bed mobility, and transfers. Her OOB tolerance is less than 45 minutes with a hoyer transfer.

Functional Status and Activity Level

Mrs. Zema did not use an assistive device prior to surgery and was independent with her ADLs but needed additional time to complete tasks due to her SOB. She did attend pulmonary rehabilitation in the outpatient physical therapy department as part of her pre-transplant program. She was able to walk on a treadmill for 17 minutes at 1.7 miles per hour on 3 L of O_2 with an oxygen saturation of 91% and dyspnea score of 4 on the modified Borg scale.

Other Clinical Tests

Recent ABGs revealed: pH 7.40/PCO_2 49/PO_2 80/HCO_3-32. The CBC and electrolyte panel revealed anemia (Hb 8.2 g/dL) and leukocytosis (WBC 22,000 /uL). The electrolyte panel revealed hyponatremia (Na 124 mEq/L) necessitating a free water restriction (ie, no ice chips).

Systems Review

Cardiovascular/Pulmonary

Resting vital signs in supine (head of the bed raised >20 degrees) are oxygen saturation (SpO_2) 94% on F_iO_2 0.50 (50%) and mechanical ventilation settings of synchronized intermittent mandatory ventilation (SIMV) 10, pressure support (PS) 15, positive end expiratory pressure (PEEP) 5, RR 30, BP 140/70, HR 110, sinus tachycardia. ROM, manual muscle test (MMT), and bed mobility examined with a vital response of SpO_2 91%, HR 122, BP 116/74, and RR 36. Mrs. Zema required 4 to 5 minutes of rest for vital signs to return to baseline. Transfer sidelying to sitting was attempted with vital sign change to SpO_2 90%, BP 126/70, RR 40, HR 130. Mrs. Zema complains of (c/o) shortness of breath (SOB) and extreme anxiety. The patient transferred back to supine. Vital signs returned to baseline 5 to 6 minutes post transfer to supine. The patient required suctioning following transfer back to supine.

Integumentary

Mrs. Zema appears cachetic, with purple to blue marks on both forearms, muscle wasting all four extremities, and skin appears grayish, very dry, and scaly. She has a large thoracic incision on left chest wall with multiple smaller incisions from chest tubes in the same chest region. She has a tracheostomy, which appears moist and clean. Knee high pneumatic compression stockings for both LEs are present. With transfer to dangling position a swollen area in her right calf was noted. Palpation revealed warmth in this area and the patient grimaced with knee extension and dorsiflexion. Mrs. Zema has an arterial line in her left radial artery and continues to have a central venous line in the right subclavian vein.

Musculoskeletal

MMT 1–2/5 throughout; ROM decreased bilateral shoulders, hips, knees, and ankles (especially dorsiflexion).

Neuromuscular

Mrs. Zema presented with profound motor weakness, but movement patterns appeared normal. Sensation was intact and reflexes were diminished.

Communication, Affect, Cognition, Language, and Learning Style

Mrs. Zema presently communicates by mouthing words and pointing to sentences on a communication board. She is very expressive with her eye contact. She is alert and awake, but does not follow more than two-step direction at this time.

Tests and Measures

Aerobic Capacity and Endurance

Mrs. Zema demonstrated poor endurance by her vital sign and subjective response to the examination in bed. She presented with a slight drop in BP with transfer and complaints of lightheadedness or dizziness may have been masked by her c/o SOB. Her drop in SpO_2 most likely reflects her limited pulmonary reserve, graft dysfunction, and severe deconditioning, but also her poor breathing pattern with anxiousness and activity. The observed anemia may contribute to her SOB and the ABGs suggest compensated respiratory acidosis.

Assistive and Adaptive Devices

Recommended resting bilateral LE (BLE) splints to limit heel pressure and prevent contractures and a pressure relief mattress cushion for the bed and bedside chair.

Gait, Locomotion, and Balance

Bed mobility was maximal assist of one with bed rails for side-to-side turning. She transferred from sidelying to dangling on the side of the bed with maximum assist of one. She maintained dangling with moderate assist of one and assistance of another staff member for breathing and relaxation techniques. OOB activities (eg, sit<>stand transfers and gait assessment) were not performed at this time.

Pain

Mrs. Zema was able to use a visual analog scale to rate her pain as 6/10 at rest and 8/10 with activity. Recommend coordinating therapy with pain medication delivery. Medical staff was informed of palpation findings in the right LE (RLE).

Diagnosis

The patient presents with severe mobility impairments secondary to motor weakness and atrophy, limited pulmonary reserve, and challenged by SOB and anxiety related to prolonged bed rest and complications of multiple surgeries. Recommended treatment pattern is 6E: impaired ventilation and respiration/gas exchange associated with ventilatory pump dysfunction or failure.[75] RLE findings suggest possible deep vein thrombosis.

Prognosis

Slow, progressive daily therapy will optimize independence with functional activities during the weaning process. Prolonged physical therapy will be necessary to progress to ambulatory independence with appropriate cardiovascular and pulmonary responses. Outcomes are hopeful but guarded due to limited gas-exchanging capabilities of the retransplanted lung, side effects of the pharmacological post-transplant regimen (eg, immunosuppressive medications), deconditioning secondary to prolonged ICU stay and bed rest, and limited pretransplant aerobic capacity, as well as continued airway obstruction associated with the native COPD lung.

Intervention

Recommend daily therapy combined with progression of OOB tolerance. Therapy should focus on therapeutic exercises to improve motor strength, motor control, and ROM; mobility retraining to address functional limitations and enhance OOB abilities; pain management; and integumentary precautions. Breathing retraining and relaxation exercises will be key during progression of functional activities due to patient's profound dyspnea on exertion (DOE) and anxiety. Airway clearance is important to enhance ventilation and gas exchange and reduce the need for suctioning. Careful monitoring of laboratory data, vital signs, and subjective symptoms is important and may provide evidence of infection/rejection in the transplant patient. Mrs. Zema initiated anticoagulation therapy after the physical therapy examination due to doppler findings of a nonocclusive RLE deep vein thrombosis (DVT).

Reexamination

Coordination of pain and anxiety medication was initiated after the initial examination. After 10 days the reexamination status: moderate assistance of one with bed rail for bed mobility and transfer to edge of bed, transfer to chair requires maximum assist of one, supported standing with platform walker moderate assistance of 2 for 30 seconds x 3, and OOB tolerance in supported chair 45 minutes twice a day with hoyer lift back to bed. Mrs. Zema's vital sign responses were BP = 152–164/80–92, RR 26–30, HR 124–128 (sinus tachycardia [ST]), SpO_2 92% to 93% with standing and sitting (F_iO_2 0.4 [40%]), and pain 4-5/10 with activity.

Outcomes

Mrs. Zema developed a compression fracture of L_2 on day 26 resulting in profound LBP and limiting the weaning process, transfers, standing, and gait training. Other complications included frequent pulmonary infections, renal insufficiency, HTN, and gastrointestinal abnormalities (eg, gastroparesis and malabsorption). Her therapy continued slowly, and she progressed to an inpatient rehabilitation unit 2.5 months after initiating physical therapy.

CHAPTER REVIEW QUESTIONS

1. Name at least two early complications of transplantation.

2. What are four potential goals for rehabilitation either prior to or following thoracic transplantation?

3. What is the leading late cause of death following heart, lung, and liver transplantation?

4. List five side effects of immunosuppressive medication that may inhibit rehabilitation in patients following transplantation.

5. Name two of the primary causes of the hemodynamic limitations to exercise in heart transplant recipients.

Pharmacological Information: Transplantation Pharmacology

Calcineurin Inhibitors

Action
Calcineurin inhibitors (eg, cyclosporine) reduce the activity of intracellular calcineurin phosphotase leading to a reduction in the production and release of several cytokines important for the proliferation, differentiation, and recruitment of lymphocytes (eg, interleukin 2, interleukin 3, interleukin 4, tumor necrosis factor). Cyclosporine is highly specific for inactivation of T lymphocytes.

Side Effects
CNS: Headache, dizziness, seizures, visual abnormalities, focal deficits, mild tremor, parasthesias
CV: HTN, dyspnea, leucocytoblatic vasculitis, hyperkalemia, hypertriglycerides, hypercholesterolemia
GI: Nausea, vomiting, epigastric pain, diarrhea, anorexia
GU: Nephrotoxicity
Misc: Malignancy (lymphoproliferative disease, skin neoplasms), myalgia/arthralgia, restless leg syndrome; post transplant infection, hirsutism, gingival hyperplasia

Common Medications
Cyclosporine A (Sandimmune, Neoral)

Purine Synthesis Inhibitors

Action
Purine synthesis inhibitors acts by blocking purine metabolism. The purines, adenine and guanine, are vital components for DNA synthesis. Purine synthesis inhibitors hinder DNA synthesis thereby limiting the proliferation of lymphocytes (eg, T and B cells).

Side Effects
CNS: Headache (insomnia rare)
CV: HTN, anemia (less common with mycofenolate mofetil), peripheral edema
GI: Diarrhea, vomiting, dyspepsia, constipation
Misc: Fever, leukopenia, neutropenia, infection risk

Common Medications
Azathioprine (Imuran); Mycofenolate Mofetil (Cellcept)

Corticosteroids

Action
Corticosteroids primarily inhibit inflammation in addition to suppressing immune responses. Corticosteroids inhibit accumulation of white blood cells (WBCs) at inflammatory sites (eg, sites of rejection) by reducing the release of inflammatory mediators (eg, interleukins, TNF) and inducing cell lysis. Additionally, corticosteroids limit phagocytosis and lysosomal enzyme release impairing leukocyte function. Corticosteroids suppress cell-mediated immune reactions and are the most widely used immunosuppressive agents.

Side Effects
CNS: Insomnia, nervousness, mood swings, hallucinations, depression
CV: Diaphoresis, rare tachycardia
GI: Dyspepsia/heartburn, abdominal distention, increased appetite, diarrhea, constipation, peptic ulcers
Misc: Osteopenia/osteoporosis,acne, facial flushing, delayed wound healing, infection risk, myopathy, muscle wasting, cataracts, amenorrhea

Common Medications
Prednisone, methylprednisolone, prednisolone

FK506 (Tacrolimus)

Action
FK506 is a macrolide antibiotic that functions similarly to cyclosporine by binding intracellular proteins and inhibiting calcium dependant phosphotases. This limits T lymphocyte activation thereby suppressing immune mediated inflammatory responses.

Side Effects
CNS: Headache, dizziness, visual disturbances, decreased hearing, tinnitus, neurotoxicity, photophobia
CV: HTN, dyspnea, leg cramps, hyperglycemia
GI: Nausea, vomiting, epigastric pain
GU: Nephrotoxicity
Misc: Hyperkalemia, infection risk

Common Medications
Tacrolimus (Prograf, Protopic)

Antilymphocyte Preparations

Action
Antilymphocyte preparations include immunoglobulins and antibodies developed from animals against human lymphocytes. The immunoglobulins or antibodies bind to circulating T lymphocytes leading to their inactivation or removal from the circulation, thus producing immunosuppresion.

Side Effects
CNS: Seizures, lethargy, decreased mental function, increased risk of CNS adverse effects with combination of indomethacin
CV: Occasionally dyspnea, apnea, chest pain, phlebitis
GI: Occasionally nausea, vomiting, diarrhea
Misc: Increases incidence of rejection and viral infections (CMV), post-transplantation lymphoproliferative disorder, sensitization/serum sickness and "first-dose effect" (fevers, chills, mild hypotension; arthralgia)

Common Medications
Antithymocyte globulin (ATG, ATGAM), Orthoclone OKT3 (muromonab-CD3)

Proliferation Signal Inhibitors

Action
Proliferation signal inhibitors suppress interleukin 2 (IL-2), a cytokine that promotes the proliferation, differentiation, and recruitment of T-lymphocytes, leading to immunosuppression.

Side Effects
CNS: None, unless combined with other medications
CV: HTN, hypercholesterolemia
GI: Diarrhea
Misc: Acne, arthralgia, fever, weight gain, leucopenia, thrombocytopenia hypokalemia

Common Medications
Everolimus, sirolimus (Rapamycin, Rapamune)

Monoclonal Antibody Interleukin (IL)-2 Receptor Antagonists

Action
Monoclonal antibody interleukin (IL)-2 receptor antagonists prevent activation of the lymphocyte IL-2 receptor reducing proliferation, differentiation and recruitment of this immune response cell type.

Side Effects
CNS: Dizziness, tremor
CV: HTN, cough, dyspnea
GI: Abdominal pain, diarrhea
Misc: Infection, edema

Common Medications
Dacliximab (Daclizumab, Zenapax), basiliximab (Simulect)

REFERENCES

1. Cooper DKC. Christiaan Barnard and his contributions to heart transplantation. *J Heart Lung Transplant*. 2001;20(6):599–610.
2. Dalton ML. The first lung transplant. *Am Surg*. 2004;70(4):364–365.
3. Miniati DN, Robbins RC. Heart transplantation: a thirty-year perspective. *Ann Rev Med*. 2002;53:189–205.
4. Harringer W, Haverich A. Heart and heart-lung transplantation: standards and improvements. *World J Surg*. 2002;26:218–225.
5. Shumway NE. Thoracic transplantation. *World J Surg*. 2000;24(7):811–814.
6. Radovancevic B, Frazier OH. Heart transplantation: approaching a new century. *Tex Heart Inst J*. 1999;26:60–70.
7. Versluis-Burlis T, Downs AM. Thoracic organ transplantation: heart, lung, and heart-lung. In: Hillegass EA, Sadowsky HS, eds. *Essentials of Cardiopulmonary Physical Therapy*. 2nd ed. Philadelphia, Pa: WB Saunders Co; 2001.
8. O'Neill JO, Taylor DO, Starling RC. Immunosuppression for cardiac transplantation: the past, present and future. *Transplant Proc*. 2004;36(2 Suppl): S309–S313.
9. Baran DA, Galin ID, Gass AL. Current practices: immunosuppression induction, maintenance, and rejection regimens in contemporary post-heart transplant patient treatment. *Curr Opin Cardiol*. 2002;17:165–170.
10. Banner NR, Yacoub MH. Cyclosporine in thoracic organ transplantation. *Transplant Proc*. 2004;36(2 Suppl):S302–S308.
11. Braith RW, Edwards DG. Exercise following heart transplantation. *Sports Med*. 2000;30(3):171–192.
12. Scherer S. The transplant patient. In: Frownfelter D, Dean E, eds. *Principles and Practice of Cardiopulmonary Physical Therapy*. 3rd ed. Philadelphia, Pa: Mosby-Year Book, Inc; 1996.
13. Trulock EP, Edwards LB, Taylor DO, et al. The registry of the International Society for Heart and Lung Transplantation: twentieth official adult lung and heart-lung transplant report-2003. *The Journal of Heart and Lung Transplantation*. 2003;22(6):625–635.
14. Levine SM. A survey of clinical practice of lung transplantation in North America. *Chest*. 2004;125(4):1224–1238.
15. Pisani B, Mullen GM. Prevention of osteoporosis in cardiac transplant recipients. *Curr Opin Cardiol*. 2002;17:160–164.
16. Boehler A. Update on cystic fibrosis: selected aspects related to lung transplantation. *Swiss Med Wkly*. 2003;133:111–117.
17. Gilbert S, Dauber JH, Hattler BG, et al. Lung and heart-lung transplantation at the University of Pittsburgh: 1982–2002. In: Cecka, Teraski, eds. *Clinical Transplants* (pp. 253–261). Los Angeles, Calif: UCLA Immunogenetics Center; 2002.
18. Edwards LB, Keck BM. Thoracic organ transplantation in the US. *Clin Transp*. 2002;29–40.
19. www.ishlt.org. International Society for Heart & Lung Transplantation.
20. Taylor DO, Edwards LB, Mohacsi PJ, et al. The registry of the International Society for Heart and Lung Transplantation: twentieth official adult heart transplant report-2003. *The Journal of Heart and Lung Transplantation*. 2003;22(6):616–624.
21. Algar FJ, Alvarez A, Lama R, et al. Lung transplantation in patients under mechanical ventilation. *Transplant Proc*. 2003;35(2):737–738.
22. de Perrot M, Chaparro C, McRae K, et al. Twenty-year experience of lung transplantation at a single center: influence of recipient diagnosis on long-term survival. *J Thorac Cardiovasc Surg*. 2004;127(5):1493–1501.

23. Ferdinande P, Buryninckx F, Van Raemdonck D, Daenen W, Verleden G. Phrenic nerve dysfunction after heart-lung and lung transplantation. *J Heart Lung Transplant.* 2004;23(1):105–109.
24. Burns KE, Iacono AT. Incidence of clinically unsuspected pulmonary embolism in mechanically ventilated lung transplant recipients. *Transplantation.* 2003;76(6):964–968.
25. Christie JD, Kotloff RM, Pochettino A, et al. Clinical risk factors for primary graft failure following lung transplantation. *Chest.* 2003;124(4):1232–1241.
26. Bando K, Paradis IL, Similo S, et al. Obliterative bronchiolitis after lung and heart-lung transplantation: an analysis of risk factors and management. *J Thorac Cardiovasc Surg.* 1995;110:4–14.
27. Sundaresan S, Trulock EP, Mohnaakumar T, Cooper JD, Patterson A. Prevalence and outcome of bronchiolitis obliterans syndrome after lung transplantation. *Ann Thorac Surg.* 1995;60:1341–1346.
28. van den Berg JWK, van Enckevort PJ, TenVergert EM, Postma DS, van der Bij W, Koeter GH. Bronchiolitis obliterans syndrome and additional cost of lung transplantation. *Chest.* 2000;118:1648–1652.
29. Hadjiliadis D, Steele MP, Govert JA, Davis RD, Palmer SM. Outcome of lung transplant patients admitted to the medical ICU. *Chest.* 2004;125(3):1040–1045.
30. Chiang CH, Wu K, Yu CP, Yan HC, Perng WC, Wu CP. Hypothermia and prostaglandin E1 produce synergistic attenuation of ischemia-reperfusion lung injury. *Am J Respir Crit Care Med.* 1999;160(4):1319–1323.
31. Estenne M, Hertz MI. Bronchiolitis obliterans after human lung transplantation. *Am J Respir Crit Care Med.* 2002;166:440–444.
32. Griffith BP, Magee MJ, Gonzalez IF, et al. Anastomotic pitfalls in lung transplantation. *J Thorac Cardiovasc Surg.* 1994;107(3):743–753.
33. Woo MS, MacLaughlin EF, Horn MV, et al. Living donor lobar lung transplantation: the pediatric experience. *Pediatr Transplant.* 1998;2(3):185–190.
34. Starnes VA, Barr ML, Cohen RG, et al. Living-donor lobar lung transplantation experience: intermediate results. *J Thorac Cardiovasc Surg.* 1996;112(5):1284–1290, discussion 1290–1291.
35. Dark JH. Lung: living related transplantation. *Br Med Bull.* 1997;53(4):892–903.
36. Bowdish ME, Barr ML, Starnes VA. Living lobar transplantation. *Chest Surg Clin N Am.* 2003;13(3):505–524.
37. Starnes VA, Bowdish ME, Woo MS, et al. A decade of living lobar lung transplantation: recipient outcomes. *J Thorac Cardiovasc Surg.* 2004;127(1):114–122.
38. De Jonge N, Kirkels H, Lahpor JR, et al. Exercise performance in patients with end-stage heart failure after implantation of a left ventricular assist device and after heart transplantation. *J Am Coll Cardiol.* 2001;37:1794–1799.
39. Frazier OH, Myers TJ, Radovancevic B. The Heartmate left ventricular assist system. *Tex Heart Inst J.* 1998;25:265–271.
40. Deng MC, Smits JM, Packer M. Selecting patients for heart transplantation: which patients are too well for transplant? *Curr Opin Cardiol.* 2002;17(2):137–144.
41. Mehra MR, Ventura HO, Smart FW, et al. New developments in the diagnosis and management of cardiac allograft vasculopathy. *Tex Heart Inst J.* 1995;22:138–144.
42. Valantine H. Cardiac allograft vasculopathy after heart transplantation: risk factors and management. *J Heart Lung Transplant.* 2003;23(Suppl 1):S187–S193.
43. Kobashigawa J. What is the optimal prophylaxis for treatment of cardiac allograft vasculopathy? *Curr Control Trials Cardiovasc Med.* 2000;1(3):166–171.
44. Trulock EP. Lung transplantation for primary pulmonary hypertension. *Clin Chest Med.* 2001;22(3):583–593.

45. Brenner BM, ed. *Brenner & Rector's: The Kidney.* 7th ed. Philadelphia, Pa: Saunders; 2004.
46. Stuart FP, Abecassis, Dixon KB. *Organ Transplantation.* Georgetown, Tex: Landes BioScience; 2000.
47. Sagiv M, Rudoy J, Rotstein A, Fisher N, Ben-Ari J. Exercise tolerance of end-stage renal disease patients. *Nephron.* 1991;57(4):424–427.
48. Painter P, Messer-Rehak D, Hanson P, et al. Exercise capacity in hemodialysis, CAPD, and renal transplant patients. *Nephron.* 1986;42(1):47–51.
49. Painter PL, Hector L, Ray K, et al. A randomized trial of exercise training after renal transplantation. *Transplantation.* 2002;74(1):42–48.
50. Southern PB, Davies MH. Indications and assessment for liver transplantation. *Clinical Med.* 2002;2:313–316.
51. Wiesner RH, Rakela J, Ishitani MB, et al. Recent advances in liver transplantation. *Mayo Clinic Proc.* 2003;78(2):197–210.
52. O'Grady JG, Schalm SW, Williams R. Acute liver failure: redefining the syndromes. *Lancet.* 1993;21:240.
53. Townsend CM. In: Townsend CM, ed. *Sabiston Textbook of Surgery.* 16th ed. Philadelphia, Pa: WB Saunders Co; 2001.
54. Prasad KR, Lodge JPA. Transplantation of the liver and pancreas. *BMJ.* 2001;322:845–847.
55. Martin P, Rosen HG. Liver transplantation. In: Feldman M, Friedman LS, Sleisenger MS, eds. *Sleisenger & Fordtran's Gastrointestinal and Liver Disease.* 7th ed. St. Louis, Mo: WB Saunders Co; 2002.
56. Dienstag JL. Liver transplantation. In: Braunwald E, Fauci S, Isselbacher KJ, et al, eds. *Harrison's Principles of Internal Medicine.* New York, NY: The McGraw-Hill Companies; 2001.
57. McGilvray ID, Greig PD. Critical care of the liver transplant patient: an update. *Curr Opinion Crit Care.* 2002;8:178–182.
58. Vintro AQ, Krasnoff JB, Painter P. Roles of nutrition and physical activity in musculoskeletal complications before and after liver transplantation. *AACN Clin Iss.* 2002;13:333–347.
59. Kelly DA. Managing liver failure. *Postgrad Med J.* 2002;78:660–667.
60. Wong F, Girgrah N, Graba J, et al. The cardiac response to exercise in cirrhosis. *Gut.* 2001;49:268–275.
61. Stephenson AL, Yoshida EM, Abboud RT, et al. Impaired exercise performance after successful liver transplantation. *Transplantation.* 2001;72:1161–1164.
62. Painter P, Krasnoff J, Ascher N. Physical activity and quality of life in long-term liver transplant recipients. *Liver Transplant.* 2001;7:213–219.
63. Robertson RP, Davis C, Larsen J, et al. Pancreas and islet transplantation for patients with diabetes. *Diabetes Care.* 2000;23:112–116.
64. Steen DC. The current state of pancreas transplantation. *AACN Clin Iss.* 1999;10:164–175.
65. Painter P, Tomlanovich L, Hector K, Ray K, Stock P, Melzer J. Cardiorespiratory fitness in pancreas-kidney transplant recipients. *Transplant Proc.* 1998;30:651–652.
66. Janeway CA, Travers P, Walport M, Shlomchik M. *Immunobiology: The Immune System in Health & Disease.* 5th ed. New York, NY: Garland Publishing; 2001.
67. Sykes M. Fundamentals of Transplant Immunology. In: Paul WE, ed. *Fundamental Immunology.* Philadelphia, Pa: Lippincott Williams & Wilkins; 2003.
68. Maurer JR, Zamel N. Lung transplantation. In: Murray JF, Nadel JA, eds. *Textbook of Respiratory Medicine.* Philadelphia, Pa: WB Saunders Co; 2000.

69. Miniati DN, Robbins RC, Reitz, BA. Heart and heart-lung transplantation. In: Braunwald E, ed. *Heart Disease: A Textbook of Cardiovascular Medicine.* 6th ed. Philadelphia, Pa: WB Saunders Co; 2001.
70. Horber FF, Scheidegger JR, Grunig BE, Frey FJ. Evidence that prednisone-induced myopathy is reversed by physical training. *Clin Endocrinol Metab.* 1985;61(1):83–88.
71. Braith RW, Welsch MA, Mills RM Jr, et al. Resistance exercise prevent glucocorticoid-induced myopathy in heart transplant recipients. *Med Sci Sports Exerc.* 1998;30(4):483–489.
72. Scherer SA, Bookstien NA. Clinical perspective: framework and rationale for physical therapy management of lung transplant patients with osteoporosis. *Cardiopulmonary Phys Ther J.* 2001;12:75–82.
73. American Diabetes Association. Diabetes mellitus and exercise: clinical practice recommendations 2002: position statement. *Diabetes Care.* 2002;25(Suppl 1):S64–S68.
74. Lee CD, Blair SN. Cardiorespiratory fitness and smoking-related and total cancer mortality in men. *Medicine & Science in Sports & Exercise.* 2002;34:735–739.
75. Guide to Physical Therapist Practice. 2nd ed. *Physical Therapy.* 2001;81(1).

BIBLIOGRAPHY

Craig CR Stitzel RE. *Modern Pharmacology with Clinical Applications.* New York, NY: Little, Brown, and Co; 1997.

De Bonis M, Reynolds L, Barros J, Madden BP. Tacrolimus as a rescue immunosuppressant after heart transplantation. *Eur J Cardio-Thoracic Surg.* 2001;19(5):690–695.

Deglin, JH, Vallerand AH. *Davis's Drug Guide for Nurses.* 8th ed. Philadelphia, Pa: FA Davis Co; 2003.

Harringer W, Haverich A. Heart and heart-lung transplantation: standards and improvements. *World J Surg.* 2002;26:218–225.

Hodgson BB, Kizior RJ. *Saunders Nursing Drug Handbook 2005.* St. Louis, Mo: Elsevier Saunders; 2005.

Karch AM. *Lippincott's Nursing Drug Guide.* Springhouse, Pa: Lippincott Williams & Wilkins; 2004.

Mignat C. Clinically significant drug interactions with new immunosuppressive agents. *Drug Saf.* 1997;16(4):267–278.

Miniati DN, Robbins RC. Heart transplantation: a thirty-year perspective. *Ann Rev Med.* 2002;53:189–205.

Parekh K, Trulock E, Patterson GA. Use of cyclosporine in lung transplantation. *Transplant Proc.* 2004;36(2 Suppl):S318–S322.

Parizel PM, Snoeck HW, van den Hauwe L, et al. Cerebral complications of murine monoclonal CD3 antibody (OKT3): CT and MR findings. *Am J Neuroradiol.* 1997;18(10):1935–1938.

Physicians' Desk Reference. 57th ed. Montvale, NJ: Thompson PDR; 2003.

Radovancevic B, Frazier OH. Heart transplantation: approaching a new century. *Tex Heart Inst J.* 1999;26:60–70.

Ritter JM, Lewis LD, Mant TG. *Textbook of Clinical Pharmacology.* London, England: Edward Arnold Co; 1995.

Serkova N, Litt L, James TL, et al. Evaluation of individual and combined neurotoxicity of the immunosuppressants cyclosporine and sirolimus by in vitro multinuclear NMR spectroscopy. *J Pharmacol Exp Ther.* 1999;289(2):800–806.

Serkova N, Litt L, Leibfritz D, et al. The novel immunosuppressant SDZ-RAD protects rat brain slices from cyclosporine-induced reduction of high-energy phosphates. *Br J Pharmacol.* 2000;129(3):485–492.

Valantine H. Cardiac allograft vasculopathy after heart transplantation: risk factors and management. *J Heart Lung Trans.* 2004;23(Suppl 1):S187–S193.

Chapter 15

Integumentary Diseases and Disorders/Wound Management

Christy F. Ehlers, PT, CWS

Wounds are defined as any injury to the integumentary system, one of the largest and most complex organs of the body, which involves breaking of the skin and damaging the underlying tissues. The integument not only withstands the abuses of the environment but also is impacted directly and indirectly by other body systems and diseases. The purpose of this chapter is to develop wound care management skills by reviewing the anatomy of the integument, normal wound healing processes, methods of closure, risk factors and etiologies of specific integumentary abnormalities and provide an overview of the therapeutic interventions to achieve a positive outcome, wound healing, or closure. Wound management is complex and may involve a large team of professionals who provide different perspectives and skills to the patient care plan. Throughout the chapter, various professionals are mentioned, but many more exist that play important roles such as the nurse, certified wound nurse, social services, occupational therapist, speech therapist, and even product vendors. Physical therapists have a unique position in the team as professionals who understand and work with the patient/client to improve his or her mobility and quality of life and can determine how these changes impact wounds and overall function. Additionally, therapists are trained in various modalities that can benefit wound management.

Anatomy of the Skin and the Surrounding Tissues

Primary functions of the skin are organ protection, maintenance of fluid status, immune defense (barrier to microorganisms), thermoregulation (conservation and dissipation of heat), production of vitamin D, and provision of sensory feedback (Figure 15–1). Skin is comprised of two layers: the epidermis and dermis. **Epidermis** is the outermost layer and has a uniform depth of 75 to 150 μm,

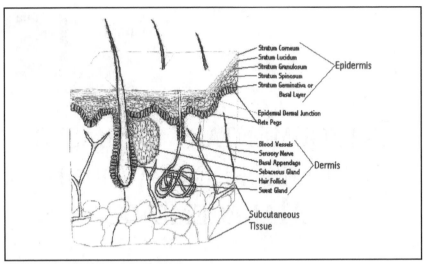

Figure 15–1. Cross section of skin.

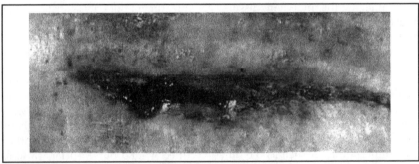

Figure 15–2. Wound in the proliferative phase with significant peripheral reepithelialization.

except in the palms of the feet and hands where it can be up to 0.4 to 0.6 mm to tolerate greater mechanical stress.[1] The epidermis is avascular and comprised of five layers of epithelial cells, from deep to superficial:

1. Stratum Germinotivum (Stratum Basale)

2. Stratum Spinosum

3. Stratum Granulosum

4. Stratum Lucidum

5. Stratum Corneum

The outermost layer, Stratum Corneum, is formed from dead keratinized cells. The deepest layer, the Stratum Germinotivum, is the most physiologically active layer of the epidermis. The Stratum Germinotivum extends into the der-

mis via sweat glands, hair follicles, and sebaceous glands, called basal appendages, and is key to the regeneration of the epidermal layer after partial thickness
injury. The epidermal and dermal layers form peaks and valleys of alternating
depths called **rete pegs**, anchoring the layers together. The dermis is the vascular layer and contains not only blood vessels, but nerves, sweat glands, and
sebaceous glands. This layer gives the skin sensation and the ability to respond
to its environment.

Deeper layers include the subcutaneous layer, or superficial fascia, consisting of adipose tissue, which provides insulation and cushioning. Next are the
muscles, ligaments, and tendons that provide function and movement, and the
deepest layer is bone, the framework of our body.

WOUND HEALING

Wound healing occurs in three separate phases:
1. Inflammation
2. Proliferation
3. Maturation

These phases are defined separately but occur in a cascade of tandem and
simultaneous activity. Wound healing is a complex series of events involving cellular activity facilitated by growth factors and chemotactic substances.
Inflammation occurs immediately at the time of injury and may continue for up
to 10 days. Clinically, the area of injury will be warm to touch and have erythema,
edema, and pain. Wounds in the inflammatory phase should have increased
drainage due to the increase in cellular activity. The presence of necrotic tissue
is a sign that the wound is in the inflammatory phase. The cells of the inflammatory phase are responsible for phagocytosis and cleansing of the wound bed.
Inflammation begins with vasoconstriction to control blood loss followed by
clot formation through platelet aggregation along the endothelium of the injured
vessels. Vasodilation follows allowing the influx of neutrophils and monocytes.
Neutrophils control local bacteria and assist in wound debridement. Monocytes
convert to macrophages and destroy bacteria and remove debris. Macrophages
initiate tissue repair by secretion of growth factors and chemotactic substances.
Chronic wounds are arrested in the inflammatory phase.

Proliferation begins 3 days or less after wounding and the inflammatory
phase. Clinical signs of the proliferative phase are granulation, reepithelialization, and contraction. **Granulation** appears as small pink to red bumps in the
wound that develop because capillary loops have formed within the wound bed.
Reepithelialization is migration of epithelial cells from the basal layer across
the wound bed at the edges. In partial thickness wounds, reepithelialization
can occur in the middle of the wound bed because of the basal appendage that
is attached to hair follicles and sweat glands. New epithelium will be dull pink
to white in color appearing much like waves descending from the shoreline
(Figure 15–2). **Contraction** involves the wound pulling in a drawstring fashion
decreasing the wound size. Fibroblasts arrive to the wound site during the proliferative phase, synthesize and secrete collagen, and can convert to myofibroblasts
that have contractile properties to assist in wound contraction. Endothelial cells

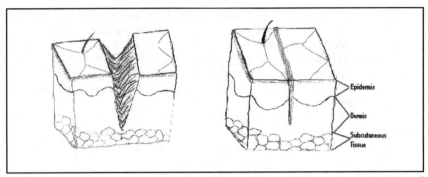

Figure 15–3. Primary intention. Minimal tissue loss with easy approximation of edges.

continue to invade the wound bed forming capillary buds and a new vascular supply. Macrophage activity continues phagocytosis and mediating cellular activities. This dual function makes the macrophage one of the most important cells needed for wound healing. Collagen secretion is completed in the proliferative phase by the fibroblast, and adequate wound tensile strength is dependent on balanced amounts of collagen and collagenase, an endogenous enzyme responsible for collagen degradation secreted by many of the cells present in the proliferative phase. Excessive amounts of collagen in the wound bed create a **hypertrophic** or **keloid scar**. Excessive amounts of collagenase can create a weak and fragile scar that may easily tear or separate.

Maturation defines wound closure. A wound in 100% maturation phase will be completely closed and have adequate tensile strength for the performance of routine activities without rupture. Collagen, secreted during the proliferative phase, remodels from fine, unorganized bundles to thicker, more compact fibers. Soft tissue mobilization and stretching can be performed with mature wounds. Soft tissue mobilization helps organize fibers and obtain greater flexibility of the scar tissue. Stretching or soft tissue mobilization must be started gently and directly on the scar, progressively increasing in intensity. Pulling or distraction of the wound edges may serve to break the scar apart.

METHODS OF WOUND CLOSURE

All three phases of healing must occur for wound closure. It is theorized that inadequate inflammation will lead to deficient succeeding phases and incomplete wound closure. There are three methods closure can be achieved: primary, secondary, and tertiary closure. **Primary closure** (also termed **primary intention**) involves minimal tissue loss. The wound edges are easily approximated and generally close with little difficulty. This method is common in surgical wounds involving exploratory procedures (Figure 15–3). **Secondary closure** (also termed **second intention**) involves significant tissue loss, and closure requires more intensive cellular work to "bridge" the gap via granulation, reepithelialization, and contraction. This method is seen particularly in

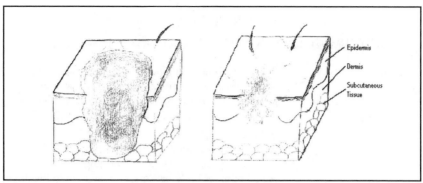

Figure 15–4. Secondary intention with significant tissue loss.

pressure-induced wounds, "pressure sores" (Figure 15–4). **Delayed primary closure** (also termed **third intention**) describes tissue opening as in primary intention, but the wound is left open for a time to be surgically closed later. This occurs with incision and drainage (I&D) procedures for abscesses.

Even with extensive tissue injury, as in secondary intention, closure can occur in different ways and is dependent on the type of tissue lost. **Partial thickness** is the loss of epidermis and a portion of dermis. The remaining dermis contains basal appendages or epithelial cells. These epithelial cells can "roll out" onto the wound bed, not just from the wound edges, but from within the wound bed creating an epidermal (outermost layer of skin) covering over the wound. Partial thickness wounds can close relying mainly on granulation and reepithelialization and need less contraction. Even with extensive tissue damage like burns, partial thickness injuries may not require skin grafts because epidermis is created within the wound. **Full thickness** entails the complete loss of epidermis and dermis. The basal appendages are removed and epithelialization can only occur at the wound's edges. Full thickness wounds must rely more on contraction in addition to granulation and reepithelialization to close.

WOUND EXAMINATION

Table 15–1 outlines specific examination procedures for a variety of wound types, but it is up to the clinician to determine the appropriateness of each procedure.

Wound size can be assessed in many ways. A tape measure provides information on greatest length, width, and depth. Wound tracing is an inexpensive way to measure the wound offering more detail and insight over time. A clean or sterile plastic bag or two pieces of clear plastic and a permanent ink marker is all that is needed for wound tracing. The bag is placed over the wound, and using the ink marker, off to the side of the bag away from the wound, draw a clock reference and label anatomical locations of the patient, then trace the wound edges. Specific wound and periwound details can also be recorded such as erythema, bony prominences, clusters of necrotic or granulation tissue, areas of eschar

Table 15–1
INTEGUMENTARY SYSTEM EXAMINATION (SKIN INSPECTION)

Location	• Use anatomical landmarks • Use clock reference label orientation on body (superior, inferior, medial lateral, foot, head)
Size	• Measure length, width, and depth of wound • Tape measure • Photograph wound/use grid film • Outline using clear wrap or dressing • Full body or body part graphs may help to identify large area wounds like burns **Undermining** (greater tissue damage beneath epidermis) **Tunneling** (cavity with opening on two sides) **Sinus tract** (like tunnel but with only one opening at wound site)
Classification	• Depth: Stage I, II, III, IV (for pressure), partial or full thickness • Phase: Inflammatory, proliferative, maturation • Color: Red, yellow, black • Etiology: Acute/chronic, pressure, vascular, neuropathic
Color	• Observe the color of the area as well as the general appearance of patient • Observe nail beds and lips for any cyanosis
Drainage	• Amount, color, consistency • Exudate: Thicker, creamy appearance, denotes inflammatory phase • Transudate: Thinner, serous, denotes proliferative phase
Skin appearance	• Document any dryness, shininess, drainage, mottling, and/or bruising.
Demarcation	• Present/absent, document in percentages
Tissue types	• Viable/nonviable, eschar/slough, granulation, reepithelialization • Document in percentage or amount
Nail growth	• Observe and describe toenail/fingernail (eg, odor, shape, color, thickness) • Observe for clubbing
Hair growth/loss	• Measure "point" of hair loss from distal extremity, compare side to side

(continued)

Table 15–1 (continued)

INTEGUMENTARY SYSTEM EXAMINATION (SKIN INSPECTION)

Periwound	• Girth measures, compare involve and noninvolved in centimeters • Edema, presence of, pitting, localized/general (see Table 1–3) • Induration, location, with or without pain, indicating abscess or local edema
Temperature	• Don a glove and use the back of the forearm/dorsum of hand to compare side to side
Pulses/vascular studies	• Present/absent, quality (see Table 1–5) • Clinical examination of blood flow (see Table 15–2) (eg, capillary refill, rubor of dependency, venous filling time, Ankle Brachial Index [ABI]), Duplex scans, Doppler studies, angiography
Capillary refill	• Observe the time to "return" to normal color of skin in extremities (usually ~2 seconds)
Orthotics/prosthetics/ ambulatory aids and devices	• Document type of support used • Observe any reddened areas, edema, and calloused areas prior to donning and post doffing device(s)
Pain	• Use pain scale (see Figure 1–11)
Tissue loads	• Note environment/surfaces skin will be in contact—bed surface, chair, wheelchair, air mattress, sheepskin, air-fluidized, low-air loss, alternating air, static flotation (air/water), foam cushions, standard mattress, etc
Type of dressings and number of times/day changed	• Document specific type (eg, wet to dry, dry, alginate, film, foam, gauze, hydrocolloid, hydrogel, pastes/powders/beads)

Adapted from:
Clinical Practice Guideline #15: Treatment of Pressure Ulcers. US Department of Health and Human Services. Public Health Service. Agency for Health Care Policy and Research. AHCPR Publication # 95-0652. December 1994.
Guide to Physical Therapist Practice. 2nd ed. *Physical Therapy.* 2001;(81):1.

versus slough, and locations of tunnels, tracts, or undermining. After removing the plastic, the piece that directly contacted the wound should be removed and discarded appropriately as it will contain body fluids. The plastic with the tracing can be copied or traced onto the individual's medical record (Figure 15–5). Wound pictures should have a measurement scale attached to judge actual size. Photographs will need to have equal lighting, distance, and angle with each follow-up shot to accurately demonstrate wound progress. Weak lighting,

Figure 15–5. Wound tracing.

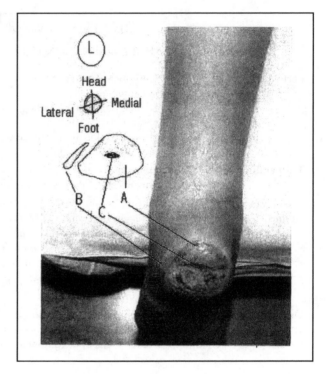

diminished focus, and varying angles give false depictions of the precise wound progression.

Wound assessment should be performed at least weekly for precise documentation of changes. These ongoing measures can detail wound progression, stagnation, or decline. In the situation of wound stagnation or decline, the clinician must first determine if the patient and/or staff is adhering to the care plan. Second, check that all risk factors affecting healing are addressed and determine if risk factor modifications are successful or ineffective. Finally, assess specific wound treatments and determine if the plan of care is addressing all aspects of the wound.

RISK FACTORS FOR IMPAIRED WOUND HEALING

Understanding the etiologies of wounds is important to devise an effective treatment plan. Additional factors (eg, age, nutrition, smoking) can slow or prevent wound healing, and many of these factors can be altered or corrected to significantly improve healing. If all interventions are utilized correctly and appropriately, progress of the wounds should be seen in 2 to 4 weeks.[2] Lack of progression past this time frame may then term the wound as chronic. Chronic wounds likely involve multiple factors contributing to slower healing. Identifying and controlling each factor will lead to greater success in wound management.

The following section will illustrate many of the factors that impact the wound healing process.

Age has an immense impact on wound healing. Older age slows all bodily processes including wound healing. Aging is associated with slower epithelial turnover rate, the number of days it takes for the cells of the basal layer to reach the surface and slough. The turnover rate increases from 28 to 32 days contributing to slower healing times in the elderly. Tissue elasticity declines and the epidermal/dermal junction (rete pegs) flatten reducing their adhesion. This increases the opportunity for skin injury, contusions, and tears. **Nutrition** has many components that can impact wound healing. Components include the food content we take in by mouth, tube feeds (enteral nutrition [TEN]), or intravenously (total parenteral nutrition [TPN]); blood oxygen content; and blood flow to the wound area. Proper nutrition is easily overlooked and many times is a major contributor to poorly healing wounds. Is the patient receiving adequate calories and hydration to heal a wound? Nutritional evaluation can reveal if reduced caloric intake is attributed to loss of appetite, difficulty swallowing, chewing, digesting, or other reasons. Serum protein levels—albumin, prealbumin, and transferrin—can reflect nutritional status (see Chapter 2). These values can be incorrect if the individual is dehydrated or overhydrated leading to false highs and lows respectively. Normal values for albumin are 3.5 to 5.5 g/dL, Prealbumin 15 to 25 mg/dL, and transferrin 200 to 400 mg/dL. Reduced values may indicate malnutrition (except transferrin <100 mg/dL). Vitamins and minerals have also been found to supplement different cells and phases of healing. A nutritionist knowledgeable in the area of wound management may need to be consulted to assess the caloric needs, meal content, and supplements required by an individual to facilitate proper wound healing. Overweight individuals can also be malnourished. Although losing weight is advantageous to the overall health of an individual, weight loss while trying to heal a wound may deplete necessary nutritional elements for wound healing. Chronic open wounds can leave the individual more susceptible to wound infections.

Oxygen is a catalyst for many phases of wound healing. If blood oxygen levels are not adequate, healing will be delayed. Blood gases provide the most accurate measures, but are not feasible on a frequent basis. Pulse oximetry, using fingertip or earlobe probes, can evaluate peripheral oxygen saturation levels (normal SpO_2 = 90% to 98%) (see Chapter 3). Reduced oxygen saturation is seen predominantly in people with pulmonary diseases (eg, chronic obstructive pulmonary disease [COPD], pulmonary fibrosis) and congestive heart failure. When monitoring oxygen saturation, resting levels and levels during activity should be assessed. Oxygen needs increase with activity and the individual may have adequate levels at rest but drop significantly when active. This drop on a repetitive basis can impair wound healing.

Adequate blood supply to the wound is essential to deliver the cells and nutrition needed for healing. See the section on Arterial Insufficiency and Table 15–2 in this chapter for greater detail.

Stress is described in two forms. Mechanical/physical and chemical stresses can significantly impair or be a primary cause of tissue damage.

Mechanical/physical stress involves extended periods of rubbing, pressure, or repeated trauma to an isolated area leading to tissue destruction. Prolonged

Table 15–2

NONINVASIVE, CLINICAL EXAMINATION OF BLOOD FLOW

Capillary refill:
1. Press the finger/toe pad until the blood exits the area and the skin blanches (becomes pale).
2. After removing the pressure, time in seconds how quickly the normal skin color returns. **Normal refill time is <3 seconds**, and **longer times may indicate arterial insufficiency.** This test only assesses the tissues and vessels in the digit and may not be an accurate indication of more proximal disease.

Rubor of dependency:
1. Patient is sitting or the lower extremity (LE) is in a dependent position.
2. Observe the foot, especially the plantar aspect, and note a ruddy or purple-red discoloration, as if it were "blushing."
3. **Discoloration occurs because of arterial occlusion** as blood is shunted to other tissues causing the ruddy discoloration.
4. This test can be difficult to appreciate in individuals with darker skin tones.

Venous filling time:
1. Patient supine.
2. Visualize distended veins on the dorsal aspect of the foot.
3. Elevate the LE above the level of the heart for approximately 1 minute (to drain the blood out of the veins).
4. **Quickly lower the leg having the patient sit bedside with the feet dangling or dependent.**
5. **Time, in seconds, how long it takes until the veins begin to distend on the surface of the foot. Filling times greater than 20 seconds usually indicates severe occlusive disease.**

Ankle brachial index:
1. Apply the cuff to the arm as if taking a brachial blood pressure (BP).
2. Locate by palpation the brachial artery at the elbow.
3. Apply gel over this artery.
4. Hold the Doppler head over the artery at a 45-degree angle in the proximal direction until blood flow can be heard.
5. Holding the Doppler head steady, inflate the BP cuff until the sound disappears, then release the pressure identifying the number when the first sound returns. This will be your brachial number.

Normal: 0.91 to 1.30
Mild obstruction: 0.70 to 0.90
Moderate obstruction: 0.40 to 0.69
Severe obstruction: <0.40
Poorly compressible: >1.30

(continued)

Table 15–2 (continued)

NONINVASIVE, CLINICAL EXAMINATION OF BLOOD FLOW

6. Perform the same procedure placing the cuff around the mid-calf above the ankle area and use either the peroneal (posterior to the lateral malleolus), the posterior tibialis (posterior to the medial malleolus), or the dorsalis pedis (mid dorsal aspect of the foot) arteries. Apply gel to the chosen artery and continue with Steps 4 and 5. This will be your ankle number.

7. The brachial number is divided into the ankle number: **Ankle/Brachial = ABI.**

8. The procedure can also be performed using a stethoscope instead of Doppler ultrasound.

Adapted from:
Bryant R. *Acute & Chronic Wounds, Nursing Management.* 2nd ed. St. Louis, Mo: Mosby, Inc; 2000.
American Diabetes Association. Peripheral arterial disease in people with diabetes. Consensus statement. *Diabetes Care.* 2003:26(12):3333–3341.

---

immobility in one position can lead to pressure ulcers or sores. Pressure is usually greatest at bony prominences, and when external pressure is applied, the blood supply to the tissues between the bone and surface is decreased. If the pressure is not removed, over a period of time, the tissues will perish. Difficulty with mobility can create added shearing to the tissues, especially around bony areas such as the heel, elbow, and sacrum. Weakness causes the individual to drag these parts over surfaces instead of lifting. Erythema occurs initially, as a sign of damage and can be an early indication of pressure ulceration. Rubbing, shearing, and pressure can also be seen in neuropathic patients. Improper fitting shoes can damage tissues, but with insensate neuropathies, this damage will go undetected until extensive destruction has occured.

Chemical stress can cause wounds or impair healing. Caustic chemicals contacted to skin induce extensive damage and are discussed in the burn section of this chapter. Drugs, such as steroids, immunosuppressive agents, and chemotherapeutics, can impair healing. Steroids and immunosuppressive drugs are designed to taper the inflammatory response. A weak inflammatory response will reduce chemotaxis and recruitment of cells that promote more advanced phases of healing. Chemotherapy is utilized to destroy cancerous cells but may not differentiate between cancerous and normal dividing cells. Many wounds are treated with topical agents such as antibacterial creams and pastes (Neosporin, bactroban, silvadene cream, bacitracin), antimicrobial and antiseptic creams and solutions (silvadene cream, acetic acid, chlorpactin, or Dakin's solution), anti-inflammatory creams and ointments (Triamcinolone Acetonide, Temovate, Hydrocortizone), and even skin cleansers and soaps (betadine and chlorhexadine). In some cases, these additives are needed and effective. However, these additives can also destroy cells and slow or arrest healing, and prolonged administration overstresses the body. More cells need to be produced to compensate for the cytotoxic effects of the topical agent. When applying these additives, determine exactly what is happening in the wound. Does the wound need this extra assistance? Is there another method to achieve the same goal without random destruction? For example, wound cleansing can be accomplished with wound cleansers or normal saline instead of skin soaps. If a cytotoxic additive is needed, frequently assess goals such as decreasing bacterial load or wound debridement. Once goals are achieved, immediately discontinue the use of the additive.

Systemic and local **infections** can impair wound healing. First, you must determine if the wound is clinically infected or colonized. Bacteria and microbes exist in all wounds, and four states are used for classification:

1. Contamination
2. Colonization
3. Critically colonized
4. Infection

Contamination means bacteria are present but are not proliferating. **Colonization** is when bacteria are present and proliferating but not disrupting or destroying the surrounding tissues. **Critically colonized** describes the presence of proliferating bacteria that are disrupting only the local wound bed, prohibiting wound healing but not yet clinically infected. **Infection** exists when the bacteria are destroying the host and $\geq 100,000$ organisms per gram of tissue is identified by culture. Critically colonized and infected wounds may benefit from the use of systemic and/or topical medications. It is debated if colonized wounds will benefit or be hampered by further measures. Using only clinical observation, inflammation can indicate a normal healing response or signs of an infection. Clinical judgment is needed to determine what treatment course works best. Patient compliance, environment, and history of wound complications may need to be considered. Infections differ from normal inflammation by a significant increase in white blood cells on serum lab values, causing general malaise and possibly systemic elevation in temperature (ie, fever). The gold standard for diagnosing a wound infection is needle aspiration or ulcer biopsy of the viable tissue near the wound bed.[2]

Carcinomas can cause open wounds. Tissue biopsies are essential for accurate diagnosis. See the dermatological section under Etiologies in this chapter for more discussion.

Diabetes does not cause wounds but increases risk and impairs wound healing (see Chapter 10). Elevated blood glucose, >110 mg/dL, increases the risk for atherosclerotic changes in the vasculature and decreases blood flow especially to the LEs. Blood flow may be reduced to tendons, ligaments, and bone, contributing to Charcot deformation and hammertoes (Figure 15–6). Peripheral

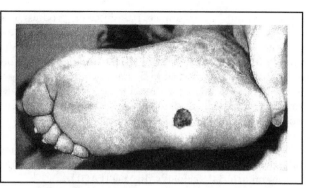

Figure 15–6. Charcot foot with ulcer.

neuropathy leads to sensory and motor alterations that increase the risk for repetitive trauma in the feet and legs. Repetitive trauma causes callous formation that easily split or crack leading to small open wounds and opportunity for infection. Once tissue damage has occurred, impaired sensation prevents the individual from properly protecting and off loading the wound, obstructing its contraction. Blood glucose levels consistently above 200 mg/dL halt macrophage migration and suppress normal wound healing. Nutritional status can be impaired by gastroparesis leading to abdominal discomfort, emesis, and reduction of oral intake. Retinopathy limits visual inspections of the feet for trauma and the capacity to change their own wound dressings. Blood glucose control between 70 to 110 mg/dL is a major goal for wound healing. Proper blood glucose control should be coupled with patient education and therapeutic interventions to significantly improve wound healing.

ETIOLOGIES—DISEASES/CONDITIONS THAT CAN CAUSE WOUNDS

Common processes that cause and increase risk for wounds include: arterial insufficiency, venous insufficiency, pressure, neuropathies, dermatological disease, burns, and surgery, including amputation. These abnormalities may occur singularly or in combination. The physical therapist must prioritize the patient's problems and determine the first and safest measures to employ. For example, in the case of arterial and venous insufficiency, it is important to obtain accurate blood flow measures. Compression is a treatment of choice for venous insufficiency but can lead to disastrous outcomes if compression occludes arterial flow.

Arterial Insufficiency

Wounds occur due to a lack of blood supply. The common cause of these ulcers is atherosclerotic disease or arteriosclerosis obliterans or, less frequently, trauma, entrapment syndromes, or acute embolic syndromes.[1] Wounds are commonly observed in the LEs on or below the ankle and over bony prominences particularly in areas of greater trauma like tips of toes and malleoli. Clinically, ischemic wounds look punched out in appearance, pale in color, produce less discharge, and are painful, especially to touch. On interview, the patient may complain of pain that interferes with sleep. LE elevation will increase the pain and dangling the extremity off the bed may provide relief. Ambulation may be limited because of pain, **claudication,** after certain distances that increase with further walking (see Table 1–2). Ischemia or an inability to provide adequate blood flow to the tissues during increasing demand causes claudication pain. Observation of the involved leg will reveal a limb pale in color, lacking hair growth, and the feet and toes may be cool to the touch. Check for the peroneal (posterior to the lateral malleolus), the posterior tibialis (posterior to the medial malleolus), or the dorsalis pedis (mid dorsal aspect of the foot) pulses; absence of these can indicate **peripheral arterial occlusive disease (PAOD).**

Noninvasive, clinical assessments to gain objective data on blood flow are the **Rubor of Dependency, Venous Filling Time,** and **Capillary Refill** tests as noted in Table 15–2. Clinically, these tests provide objective data in suspected arterial insufficiency but provides no specific measures on the severity of the problem. **ABI** can provide quantifiable data. A Doppler unit for assessing peripheral blood flow, conductive gel, and a BP cuff are needed. Stethoscopes can be used, but may not give accurate results. To perform an ABI measurement, review Table 15–2. The ABI number should be near or equal to 1.0. If the ABI is <0.8, mild to moderate peripheral arterial disease is present, and <0.5 is considered severe arterial insufficiency. Toe cuff pressures can also be performed but require a specialized toe cuff. Normal flow is considered >0.6.[1] More extensive tests to measure arterial blood flow are available and include pulse volume readings, segmental pressure recordings, transcutaneous oxygen pressure recordings, and color duplex imaging.

Restoration of blood flow is the first priority in arterial insufficiency, especially if severe enough to cause open wounds. This is typically accomplished surgically. Nonsurgical treatments include appropriate dressings, off loading and protecting the wound where needed, exercise, and patient/family education. The severity of the disease will dictate the dressings needed. ABIs of 0.4 to 0.5 may be left dry or antimicrobial solutions used to discourage bacteria growth. The goal is to contain the wound. Amputation of digits or the limb may be necessary if limb salvage is not possible or the wound poses a threat to the peripheral tissues or overall patient health. Wounds present in areas with an ABI >0.5 can utilize dressings that provide moisture. These dressings will facilitate autolysis (self-debridement) of any necrotic tissue while supporting granulation, reepithelialization, and contraction. Exercise such as ankle pumps, LE range of motion (ROM), and progressive resistive exercises and walking or biking to the claudication threshold are activity choices. These activities may help increase the flow of lesser used collateral arteries over time. Proper skin cleansing with mild, nonirritating soaps or skin cleansers and use of moisturizers can help prevent further ulceration due to cracking, dry skin. Off loading and protection of the wound area using proper fitting shoes may delay further wound damage and allow enhanced patient mobility by decreasing pressure and pain. Off loading splints like the multipodus or custom made splints can help prevent and protect wounds especially in the heels and toes with proper fit and usage patterns. Assistive devices, walker, and canes and weightbearing restrictions may decrease or eliminate pressure on the foot or leg. Consider the patient's abilities, skills, comfort, safety, and possible limb salvage. A wheelchair might be needed if the patient is unable to be safely mobile. Wheelchairs offer more options in pressure relief and provide the patient greater independence and self-esteem than being bed bound.

Venous Insufficiency

Venous insufficiency is caused by ineffective return of blood flow from the LEs to the heart. Visual observation will show swelling of the legs with the presence of varicose and/or spider veins. Edema will increase when the legs are in a dependant position and decrease with elevation. A brown discoloration or staining called **hemosiderin deposits** can be seen in a splotched or circumferential pattern around the area between the malleoli and calf termed "gaiter area." Staining results from spilling and breakdown of red blood cells in the interstitial tissues. Venous insufficiency wounds are typically below the knee and above or around the ankles, irregular in shape, and may produce excessive discharge. The discharge will decrease with better control of the edema either through elevation or compression.

The underlying pathology for venous insufficiency is venous hypertension. Venous hypertension can be caused by obstruction, valve incompetence, or muscle pump failure. The common cause of venous obstruction is deep vein thrombosis (DVT). Other causes include pregnancy, obesity, congestive heart failure, edema, ascites, tumors, or severe trauma to the leg. Obstruction blocks the flow of the blood causing venous distention and leakage of deoxygenated blood into the interstitial tissues. Valvular incompetency is not fully understood. It is believed that venous distention, venous hypertension, or DVT damages the vein leaflets. The insufficient valves allow blood to flow retrograde and pool in the distal veins and tissues. Muscle pump failure describes inadequate removal of blood during activity. Residual blood accumulates resulting in venous hypertension. Muscle pump failure is poorly understood but may include inactivity, neuromuscular abnormalities, or musculoskeletal changes resulting from aging, arthritis, or a sedentary lifestyle.[1]

The most recommended treatment option is compression in the 30 to 40 mmHg range to control edema. Chronic edema leads to skin breakdown and, in the presence of an existing wound, impairs wound healing. The pressure of the accumulated fluids flowing out of the wound plus the force of the excess fluid expanding the tissues keep the wound bed from closing or contracting. First, it must be established that the patient has adequate arterial circulation under compression (an ABI $\geq$0.8). Compression used in a limb with inadequate arterial flow can lead to limb ischemia and amputation. Second, patient compliance and ability to return for follow-up care must be known before embarking on compression. Three and four layer wrap systems are available to use with venous insufficiency in the presence of wounds, offering both compression and absorption. These systems must be applied properly and are generally changed within 3 to 4 days after the first application and weekly thereafter until wound closure is achieved. Wound dressings may need to be absorptive, and if used under compression, dressings will need to be of uniform depth to prevent pressure areas because of sporadic bulky spots. Venous insufficiency is a lifelong problem for most patients and requires ongoing treatment. Custom and

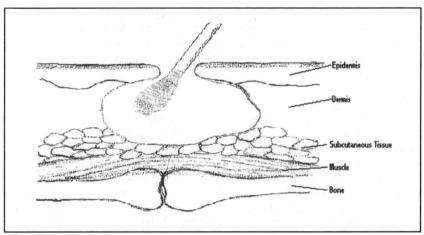

Figure 15–7. Cross section of undermining.

off-the-shelf compression garments (socks and stockings) are available and must be utilized anytime the patient's legs are in the dependent position. Two, new stockings should be purchased every 6 to 12 months to allow one pair to be cleaned while wearing the other. Inelastic compression (Circaid) has also proven helpful in edema management. Inelastic compression is a series of stiff Velcro straps that cover from the metatarsal heads to the upper calf and offer rigid support. Mechanical sequential pump systems are available but can only be used at rest. Weight loss and LE elevation coupled with exercise will also help decrease LE edema. For patients with arterial flow less than 0.8, frequent elevation with exercise may be the safest option.

Pressure

Pressure ulcers are any lesion caused by unrelieved pressure resulting in damage of underlying tissue and are frequently observed in the mobility challenged.[2] Wounds are found over bony prominences, as tissue compression is greatest in these areas. Pressure ulcers are characterized by undermining with damage nearest to bone. A cross section view of undermining would look like a vase with the wider portion in the muscle and subcutaneous area and the narrow opening at the epidermis (Figure 15–7). Shearing of the tissues from dragging the skin can be an early signal of an area predisposed to pressure breakdown. The skin will be red, a stage one ulcer. The pressure ulcer staging system was developed to classify the degree of tissue damage observed and can be found in Figure 15–8.[2] Pressure ulcers can occur in bed bound patients, but may also be observed in ambulatory patients with neuropathy.

The optimal treatment for pressure ulcers is off loading or pressure removal from the wound region with redistribution to the largest possible area. Two aspects of off loading will be reviewed: supine and sitting. Frequent position changes greatly decrease pressure. Supine patients should be turned every 2 hours with utilization of multiple positions. Options include supine, side lying, prone (if tolerable), one-fourth side lying and one-fourth prone. If a wound is

Pressure Wound Classification Guidelines

Stage I	Nonblanchable erythema of intact skin, the heralding lesion of skin ulceration. In individuals with darker skin pigmentation, discoloration of skin, warmth, induration, or hardness may also be indicators.
Stage II	Partial thickness skin loss involving epidermis, dermis, or both. The ulcer is superficial and presents clinically as an abrasion, blister, or shallow crater.
Stage III	Full thickness skin loss involving damage or necrosis of subcutaneous tissue that may extend down to, but not through, underlying fascia. The ulcer presents clinically as a deep crater with or without undermining of adjacent tissue.
Stage IIII	Full thickness skin loss with extensive destruction, tissue necrosis, or damage to muscle with exposed bone or supporting structures (such as tendon, joint capsule). Undermining and sinus tracts also may be associated with Stage IV pressure ulcers.

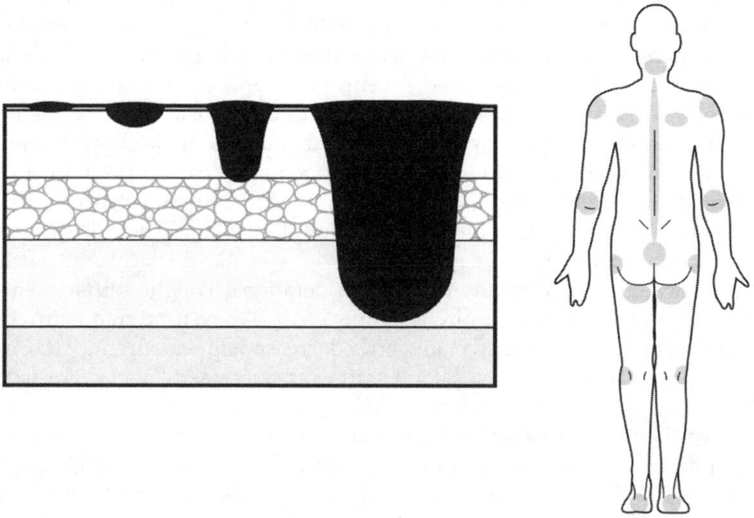

Figure 15–8. Pressure ulcer staging system. (Images reprinted from Irion G. *Comprehensive Wound Management.* Thorofare, NJ: SLACK Incorporated; 2002:93.)

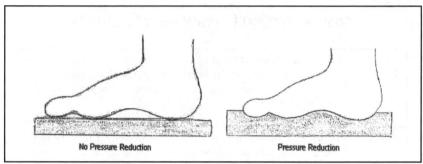

Figure 15-9. Comparison of weightbearing with and without pressure reduction.

present, the patient should be positioned off the sore at all times. Assess the patient for any other problems that may prohibit certain positions and create a positioning program that will include all permissible options. Pillows and wedges can be used to maintain positions and to separate and cushion bony prominences, such as knees. Specialized beds, mattresses, and overlays come in multiple varieties. Many of these are pressure reducing or decreasing overall pressure, not relieving. One feature these offer is pressure distribution by conforming to all the body curves and surfaces as demonstrated in Figure 15-9. These pressure reductions are not a replacement for good turning practices but can help prevent further ulceration. Special need beds are also available such as bariatric beds that convert to a sitting position to promote upright in a potentially mobility challenged population (see Chapter 11, Surgical Information). Even with good turning practices and pressure-reducing devices, heels can still breakdown. Heels are susceptible to breakdown because they carry large amounts of the LEs' weight on one small bony area, and if neuropathy and/or arterial insufficiency are present, heel breakdown is highly probable. Pillows placed under the entire length of the calf leaving the heel suspended are an easy method of off loading, but in the more mobile individual, it is hard to maintain correct position. Splints can be made or purchased that will relieve all heel pressures by suspension; of these, some will also position the ankle in neutral to help prevent foot drop and plantar flexion contracture.

Sitting positions require additional considerations. Weight shifts in sitting should be performed every 15 minutes. If the chair is to be used frequently, does it fit the patient well? Oversized chairs offer decreased upper extremity (UE) and trunk support causing dramatic lateral shifts and decreased leverage for weight shifts. Small chairs create additional pressure areas and can complicate transfers out of the chair. A wheelchair or seat cushion that provides good weight distribution without added pressures to bony prominences is ideal. Assess the patient's wound locations, and determine in what position the wound experiences the greatest pressure, and completely avoid that posture or position. Sacral wounds are frequently mistaken for being acquired in sitting. Assess the patient in sitting and determine if the wound is being compressed. If so, can alterations to the chair for proper fit and positioning be made and wound pressure relief met? If not, should the patient be sentenced to bed until the ulcers heal?

Wheelchair-dependent patients will need to have the chair, the cushion, and the patient in the chair assessed to make adjustments as needed to prevent repeat breakdown. Computerized pressure mapping systems are available to located pressure areas and measure the effectiveness of the cushion and chair. This can be performed as a single treatment assessment or data recorded over time to help pinpoint ongoing problems.

Additional tips to reduce pressure wounds are as follows:

- Avoid dragging the patient for repositioning; lift and use draw sheets.

- Good hygiene, cleaning stool and urine from the skin as soon as possible, using appropriate cleansers to reduce rubbing time, and barrier ointments to protect the skin can prevent skin breakdown.

- Strengthening and transfer training can help the patient increase mobility and provides him or her the opportunity to independently manage his or her own turning and weight shifts.

Neuropathies

Neuropathic wounds are most common in patients with diabetes mellitus. Other causes of peripheral neuropathies include Hansen's disease, chronic alcoholism, spinal cord injury, peripheral trauma, and critical illness (see Chapter 4). This section will focus on diabetic neuropathies. The section in this chapter on Risk Factors in Diabetes describes many of the additional complications these patients face. Peripheral neuropathies cause the patient to experience pain or the absence of sensation, which may go undetected. Wounds are usually located around the nail beds, tips of toes, bony prominences, and the plantar surfaces of the feet. Wounds may appear punched out, pale in color, and surrounded by callous in areas of repeated trauma.

Clinical assessments may include ABIs, but results are limited because small vessel disease is not detected and inaccuracies are associated with artherosclerotic changes in the vessels. Toe cuff pressures may offer more accurate information. Blood glucose and glycosolated hemoglobin (HbA1c) monitoring are important measures (see Chapters 2 and 10). For the diabetic patient, blood glucose control can be the most important factor to wound healing. Sensation testing is imperative to identify the location and extent of the neuropathy. Monofilament testing will offer objective and specific assessments of peripheral sensation. The monofilament size used is 5.07 and this applies 10 grams of pressure to the skin surface. A 5.07 monofilament assesses protective sensation, the ability to detect contact with other objects and react to protect skin before tissue damage can occur. Testing is done only on intact skin, not the wound or over the callous. The filament should contact the skin at a 90-degree angle, buckle slightly on impact, then be quickly removed as noted in Figure 15–10. The patient should be asked to close his or her eyes or look away from the LE. Ask him or her to identify the location of the contact. Use an alternating rhythm and occasional fake contact to gain a genuine assessment. Figure 15–11 identifies specific testing sites. Keep in mind this does not mean the patient can feel nothing. Many times, patients can detect deep pressure, which fools the individual into believing he or she has no sensation loss. A tuning fork can be used to assess protective sensation as well, using the same locations as noted in Figure 15–11. Manual muscle testing (MMT)

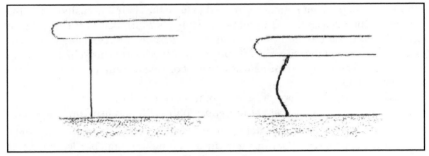

Figure 15-10. Technique for monofilament testing.

Figure 15-11. Foot assessment sites for monofilament or tuning fork sensation tests.

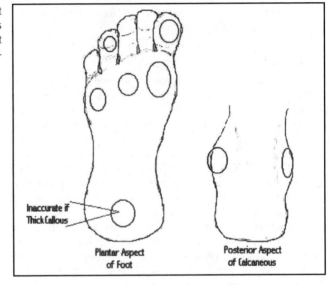

Inaccurate if Thick Callous

Plantar Aspect of Foot

Posterior Aspect of Calcaneous

of the LE and reflex testing of the patellar tendon and Achilles tendon can be helpful in assessing muscular involvement (see Table 1–6 for reflex testing).

The second most important factor is off loading of the immediate wound area. Standing or weightbearing off load devices range from splints, adapted postoperative shoes, cast walkers, and custom fit shoes with custom fit inserts. These devices use materials that reduce pressure at and around the wound site and conform to the curves and varying depths of the foot to distribute the weight over the largest possible area. The "gold standard" is total contact casting or total contact splints. This technique requires special clinician training. It offers optimal off loading of the wound area with contouring of the entire foot and leg and added stability at the ankle. Part of the superiority of casting over splinting involves removal of the device. Cast compliance can be 100%, but weekly assessments are necessary to ensure proper fit and wound management. Orthotist and podiatrists can create custom shoes and inserts, but often prefer to wait for wound closure prior to provision of the devices because they are permanent long-term devices that require an exact fit. Walkers, crutches, and wheelchairs assist the patient in off loading the LEs. The patient will need to be evaluated and trained in the proper use of the device on the specific terrain he or she will encounter. Proper footgear and assist devices may provide the optimal conditions to allow patient safety, stability, and wound closure. Many diabetics can develop nephropathy, kidney insufficiency, leading to variable LE edema. Additionally, peripheral neuropathies can cause foot drop that can be controlled with the use of an ankle foot orthotic (AFO). Many AFOs are made of hard plastic and will not adjust to varying leg circumferences. Variable edema with lack of peripheral sensation can significantly increase risk for pressure ulcer development with use of an AFO. Consultation with an orthotist clarifying these specific problems can yield a safe, custom-molded device. Patient and caregiver education in proper skin inspections and appropriate care plans can prove vital to the prevention of foot ulcers. It has been said, "If I treat you, I help you today. If I teach you, I help you for a lifetime." Finally, callous must be kept trimmed and pliable to prevent interference with wound contraction and further opportunities for infection. Wound dressings may need to provide moisture, unless infected or in the inflammatory state, then absorptive dressings will be more effective.

Dermatological Disease

Dermatological lesions comprise a large number of diseases that are difficult to classify and may include cancers, allergic reactions, immunological complications, or insect bites to factitious (self-inflicted) wounds. These lesions are usually diagnosed using skin and tissue biopsy and require proper management by specific medical professionals trained to manage the individual disease such as a dermatologist, oncologist, or psychiatrist. Treatments for these wounds vary, but correction of the primary problem may require medications including steroids, antibacterial agents, or chemotherapy.

Treatment options of open wounds may involve odor control, simple protection, or maintenance until the primary etiology can be controlled. An example is Pyoderma Gangrenosum, a diagnosis more commonly seen in patients using steroids within the past year. Characterized by a blue gray or battleship gray periwound, these lesions are typically painful and begin after a local trauma such as an ant bite, bee sting, or simple local abrasion. The wound quickly progresses to a larger, necrotic wound. Localized trauma to the area initiates the destructive process and may be exacerbated by repeated trauma. Debridement or debriding agents may worsen the problem. Like pyoderma, other dermatologic lesions will have their own unique presentations and interventions. It is important to understand the specific etiology and proper treatment in order to select the most efficacious intervention.

Burns

Burn wounds are caused by three main sources:
1. Thermal
2. Chemical
3. Electrical

The damage can be minor or encompass enormous body surface areas. Two classification systems exist for evaluating burn wounds. The Rule of Nines divides the entire body in percentages to calculate the area affected but only accounts for second- and three-degree wounds. The Lund and Bower chart defines all severities of wound damage and is calculated as a percentage of affected body surfaces.

Initial treatment begins with medical stabilization of the patient. Topical antimicrobials (eg, Silvadene cream) may be used upon admission to prevent additional infections. Once the patient is stable, other treatment options are initiated including skin grafting. Moist wound dressings may be utilized and some are designed especially for large body coverage. Clinicians may continue to use antimicrobial creams until wound closure, even though these creams can slow healing. Antimicrobial care is warranted due to the cost of special dressings, adhesive properties that are too aggressive to the peripheral tissues, or limited product availability. Newly closed wounds can easily dry and crack. Regular moisturizing with an appropriate cream or ointment can prevent cracking. Hypertrophic scarring can be functionally limiting and cosmetically unappealing. Compression garments at 30 to 40 mmHg worn from the time of closure and throughout the maturation phase of healing can help shape and correct hypertrophic scarring. Adhesive scar management sheets (eg, Cicacare) help apply local, direct pressure to smaller or difficult areas (eg, cervical region). Compression must be continued over a 1- to 2-year period, the duration of the maturation phase, for maximal effectiveness. Physical therapy assessment of ROM and strength are important to discover areas of limitation. Working with the patient throughout the wound healing phases may be imperative to maximize functional mobility once healing has occurred.

Surgical Incisions and Amputations

Routine surgical incisions were discussed in the Methods of Closure section under primary and tertiary intention. Most surgical incisions will close with minimal intervention. Stitches or staples are typically removed in 10 to 14 days or less. Surgeons will often leave stitches and staples in place longer to accommodate slower healing times for patients with diabetes mellitus (DM), the elderly, and those prescribed corticosteroids. Skin glues and steristrips are alternatives to sutures and staples. New incisions should be kept clean and protected. Wound contraction may be impaired with excessive strain or pulling at or around the incision site and should be avoided at all times. If bone, ligament, or tendons were incised, healing time duration is prolonged to 4 to 8 weeks to allow repair of these structures. Using clinical skills, discern which movements and ADLs may need to be altered or avoided to allow proper healing to occur. One example is the sternotomy approach used for many cardiac and thoracic surgeries. Patients who are overweight, have diagnosed DM, or have experienced prolonged mechanical ventilation or a perioperative infection are at risk for sternotomy dehiscence. It is prudent to limit UE weightbearing to afford proper bone healing in this population. Patients who require extensive UE function and weightbearing for mobility may have to find alternative or adaptive solutions. Each case should be individually assessed.

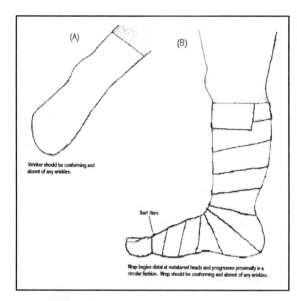

Figure 15-12. Types of compression.

Amputations involve the partial or complete loss of a limb. The amputated region includes all involved damaged and nonviable tissue and may include adjoining viable tissue but should provide residual limb length to support a prosthesis if possible. Amputations of the leg include below knee (BKA), where the foot and ankle are removed; above knee (AKA), where the foot, ankle, and knee joints are removed; and hip disarticulation, where the entire leg is removed up to the hip joint. Several approaches have been applied to the foot from individual digits, transmetatarsal amputation (TMA); removal of the metatarsal heads, mid-foot; and ankle disarticulation, removal of the foot at the tibial-calcaneaous joint.

Common therapeutic interventions for the amputee include ROM to joints around the amputation to ensure functional movement, strengthening exercises of the involved and uninvolved limb and UEs secondary to mobility needs, and balance assessment in sitting and standing. Limb loss alters the center of gravity and may require extensive balance retraining. Surgeons will have different protocols regarding prosthetic fitting and wearing schedules, and the therapist must be familiar with physician preferences prior to initiating patient education or prosthetic training. Usual treatment includes waiting until the staples are removed, good wound tensile strength is established, and there is stable limb circumference. Stump shrinkers or ace wraps conform to the residual limb and apply greater pressure distally to decrease edema and shape the residual limb in preparation for the prosthesis as noted in Figure 15-12. Incorrect ace wrapping techniques can damage the limb. Wraps will need to be changed up to three times a day to prevent wrinkling and tissue damage.

DEBRIDEMENT AND WOUND HEALING

Necrotic tissue is dead matter within the wound bed, provides a medium for bacteria to survive and thrive, and increases the opportunity for local and systemic infections. Additionally, necrotic tissue creates a physical barrier to the cells and mediators encouraging wound closure. Necrotic tissue is not viable and appears yellow, gray, green, or black. Eschar is thick, tough dead tissue that cannot be hydrated. Slough is dead tissue that remains moist or can be penetrated by moisture if dried. Clinically, debridement of necrotic tissue enhances wound closure. Factors that need to be assessed to determine the safest, most effective debridement methods are:

- Is the patient prescribed anticoagulants?
- Is the blood supply adequate to support wound healing?
- Do the institution policy and procedures and state practice acts support me in sharp debridement?
- Is further training needed before performing certain types of debridement?
- What is the difference between viable and nonviable tissue?
- What structures lie in and around the wound that need to be protected and avoided?
- Are the instruments sterile and suitable for the job?
- How can bleeding be stopped?

Mechanical debridement includes hydrotherapy and wound scrubbing using gauze-type dressings. This method is nonspecific and can also damage viable tissues.

Autolytic debridement is the selective removal of necrotic tissue by the body's endogenous enzymes. It can be achieved by using moist wound dressings that support cell function. The process is slow and, in certain patient populations (eg, geriatric, malnourished, and immune-suppressed individuals), difficult to achieve because of reduced production of enzymatic cells.

Sharp debridement uses sharp, sterile instruments (eg, scissors, hemostats, tweezers, scalpels) to remove dead necrotic tissue and reduce or shave callous. It can be very specific to the removal of necrotic tissue, but requires an appropriately trained health professional. Each profession is governed by its own State Practice Act, and individuals need to determine their institution's policies and procedures prior to performance of sharp debridement. Sharp debridement can be contraindicated in patients on anticoagulation therapy as bleeding control can be difficult. Should bleeding occur, apply direct pressure and elevation. Silver nitrate sticks or the application of alginates or collagen can help stop bleeding. Knowledge of the surrounding anatomy and recognizing the difference between viable and nonviable tissues are keys to performing efficacious debridement to avoid damaging key structures. Viable tissue bleeds, senses pain, and contracts (ie, moves when stimulated). Nonviable tissue is avascular, aneural, and is immobile. Only nonviable, necrotic soft tissue can be removed by the physical therapist.

Enzymatic or chemical debridement involves topical exogenous enzymes or chemical solutions to break down necrotic tissue. Products may be specific to the substrates they affect (eg, collagenase) or more broad (eg, papain-urea compounds). Wound environment must also be considered. For example, collagenase works best in moist environments, and dry eschar may need to be incised or cross-hatched to the moist base to be most effective. Manufacturer's instructions will guide you in the safest way to utilize each product.

DRESSINGS AND WOUND HEALING

There is a large variety of wound dressings, and this section will review general considerations and provide clinical tips to aid the decision-making process. However, prior to reviewing the myriad of dressings available, it must be established that moist wound healing is the optimal environment.[2] The cells necessary for wound closure normally thrive in moisture. A common concern with moist dressings is an increase in bacterial growth and wound infections. However, a study comparing moist wound environments to conventional gauze demonstrated reduced infection rates using the moist wound environment (2.6% versus 7.1%).[3] The wound bed does best moist, not sloppy wet. Too much moisture, superhydration of the epidermis, leads to **peripheral maceration**. Moisture inhibits cell anchoring and stability allowing cells to float away from the wound surface. Peripheral maceration appears as a white rim around the wound edge. The wound characteristics and established goals determine wound dressing selection. Instruction on application and appropriate dressing change times can be found in the individual package inserts. Specialized dressings initially appear to cost more than the traditional gauze dressings. However, the physical therapist must calculate the cost of the dressing needed over a week's time and include accurate number of dressing changes per day. Additionally, it is assumed that moist wound environments heal faster requiring fewer dressings over the wound closure time period. The specialized dressings over the entire course of wound care may actually cost less and deliver desired outcomes faster. Finally, patient preferences, patient and/or caregiver ability to appropriately apply the desired dressing, and product availability must be considered in the decision-making process.

MODALITIES AND WOUND HEALING

Modalities in wound care offer additional benefits to wound healing. Many are used, but only electrical stimulation has substantial evidence proving its efficacy. Listed below are several modalities and the understood impact on wound healing.

Ultrasound can stimulate fibroblasts and macrophages, promote angiogenesis, and reduce the inflammatory phase of wound healing.

Pulsatile lavage is a fluid-based modality combined with suction applied within the wound bed. The fluid softens and loosens necrotic tissues to assist with debridement, and the negative pressure pulls the debris away from the wound surface. Water pressure delivery is controlled at 15 psi or less. Greater pressures may drive bacteria into the tissues enhancing infection risk.

Hydrotherapy helps to debride devitalized tissue, remove surface contaminants, and promote circulation. It is contraindicated in dry gangrenous wounds and in limbs with an ABI <0.4. It is a nonselective form of mechanical debridement and works best in patients with extensive necrotic tissue. Once the necrotic tissue is removed, whirlpool should be discontinued and other appropriate treatments that will augment wound healing chosen. Other concerns are venous insufficiency (dangling the extremity in warm water can increase edema), neuropathic wounds (possible thermal injury), intact skin that is dry and cracking, which will worsen if moisturizers are not applied soon after removal from the water, and burns (especially in the presence of large surface area wounds (the water must remain mobile to reduce bacterial colonization).

Electrical stimulation can have multiple effects on the wound. It can augment circulation, wound contraction, epidermal migration, reduce edema, increase tensile strength, and has bactericidal effects. This is achieved through the use of negative and positive polarities to attract cells to the wound. It can be used with clean or necrotic wounds.

Hyperbaric oxygen increases tissue oxygen levels and enhances cellular activity. The patient must breathe 100% oxygen while being exposed to pressures greater than 1 atmosphere. This requires full body chambers such as used with divers for decompression sickness. Topical applications such as single extremity units do not offer the same benefits and are not considered in this category.

Vacuum-assisted closure utilizes negative pressure to pull excess fluids away from the wound. The negative pressure at the wound surface stimulates cellular activity and supports wound contraction. The wound should be at least 75% clean before using this modality.

GOAL SETTING AND WOUND HEALING

Goal setting for wound care can be a difficult process. The physical therapist should have a thorough comprehension of the phases of wound healing and specifically understand the clinical appearance of the wounds at each stage. To set goals, determine the current stage of the wound and the presumed next phase with progressive healing. Recall that wounds in the inflammatory stage are erythematous, contain necrotic tissue, and the edges may not be well defined or demarcated because of recent injury. Granulation, reepithelialization, and contraction characterize the proliferative phase. Possible goals for the wound in the inflammatory phase might be clear definition or demarcation of wound edges, a reduction in necrotic tissue, a decrease in wound size, or the emergence of granulation tissue or peripheral reepithelialization, all signs of the proliferative phase. To determine a time frame, evaluate risk factors. If this individual has multiple risk factors and is noncompliant with risk factor modification and/or the care plan, progress will be delayed. Two weeks or more may be needed to accomplish small increments of change. If there are few risk factors and the patient adheres to the care plan, then significant progress can be made each week. These measures can be defined using percentages.

A key element to wound healing that is often overlooked is wound contraction. The edges need to approximate and adhere for complete closure. Challenges to contraction occur in many forms and may include direct pressure (weightbearing on the wound), trauma (heel wounds dragged over the sheets, bed, or with pushing the heel into a shoe), or indirect forces that manipulate the wound edges (wounds in edematous extremities will expand in size as the edema increases and decrease in size as the edema decreases). Another example of indirect forces impacting wound healing is calf area wounds. These wounds tend to close faster when the patient is sitting and ambulating compared to prolonged supine positioning. Calf pressure is reduced in sitting and standing, but increased lying down. The supine position applying direct calf pressure leads to calf tissue spread and expansion, disrupting wound contraction.

CASE STUDY

Mr. Preston is a 65-year-old (y/o) black male who has been admitted from a nursing home with fevers and altered mental status of unknown etiology. Physical therapy is consulted to evaluate and treat per wound clinical pathway.

Patient/Client History
General Demographics/Social History/Living Environment

Mr. Preston has been living in the nursing home for the past 6 years. He has a wife who visits him regularly and four children who live locally who visit once a month.

General Health Status/Family History

Prior to his admission to the hospital he was in his usual state of health per chart review.

Medical/Surgical History

Mr. Preston has a history of type 2 DM with good oral medication control and Alzheimer's disease. He requires full-time supervision.

Current Conditions/Chief Complaints

Mr. Preston has a condom catheter with little urine production. He has a small necrotic wound over his sacrum measuring 2.0 cm in diameter and 1.0 cm deep with undermining up to 2.0 cm around the entire distal one half of the wound bed.

Functional Status and Activity Level

One-week prior to admission, Mr. Preston was getting out of bed (OOB) to the chair with minimal assistance. He would attend the group activity classes by ambulating with a rolling walker and minimal assistance of one. He had been participating in a lightweight training program 3 days a week utilizing sand bag weights.

Systems Review
Cardiovascular/Pulmonary

Resting vital signs in left sidelying are oxygen saturation (SpO_2) 96% on room air, heart rate (HR) 94, pulse regular, respiratory rate (RR) 20, BP 140/84, patient unable to use pain scale, breath sounds diminished but clear to auscultation. A "distinct" odor was picked up with auscultating his breath sounds. Following ROM, MMT, bed mobility, transfers, and wound assessment his vital signs were SpO$_2$ 98%, HR 102, RR 24, BP 146/82. Highlights of his laboratory results include elevated white blood cell count 13,500, decreased albumin 2.9 mg/dL, prealbumin 12 mg/dL, an elevated creatinine 2.2 mg/dL, and a hemoglobin A$_1$c of 11.4%.

Integumentary

Mr. Preston appears malnourished and possibly dehydrated. His condom catheter is intact with low urine output. He has a small necrotic wound over his sacrum measuring 2.0 cm in diameter and 1.0 cm deep with undermining up to 2.0 cm around the entire distal one half of the wound bed. A tracing was made of the wound and subsequent "clean" tracing was taped into his chart. He has an intravenous (IV) line in his left antecubital space.

Musculoskeletal

MMT/ROM results for all extremities were within functional limits (WFL). He was unable to follow specific directions, but was able to move his UE/LE against gravity. He required moderate assistance for transfer OOB to standing to avoid "shearing" of sacral dressing. Mr. Preston was able to stand for 30 seconds with moderate assist of one. A standard walker was used to assist patient in maintaining standing.

Neuromuscular

Balance was poor for static and dynamic in standing. Did not test seated at edge of bed because of dressing area. Myofilament was not tested because the patient could not consistently follow one- or two-step directions or questions.

Communication, Affect, Cognition, Language, and Learning Style

Mr. Preston is awake but not oriented or able to consistently follow one- or two-step directions. He recognizes his wife and son who are in the room but is unable to carry a conversation in the present tense with his family. His primary language is English.

Tests and Measures

Aerobic Capacity and Endurance

Mr. Preston demonstrated a normal vital sign response with mobilization OOB. His "distinct" breath odor may be directly related to his poorly controlled diabetes at this time.

Assistive and Adaptive Devices

Presently Mr. Preston required a standard walker for standing activities today but may ambulate less encumbered with a rolling walker due to his inability to follow multiple steps/directions.

Gait, Locomotion, and Balance

Mr. Preston is unsafe to ambulate without assistance. His static/dynamic standing balance was poor and he ambulated 25 feet with moderate assistance of one to prevent him from falling and advance the walker appropriately.

Pain

Unable to assess via an analog scale, but patient grimaces with palpation around the immediate external area of the wound borders.

Diagnosis

This man has several risk factors that have contributed to the development of this sacral lesion. They include fevers or possible infection, poorly controlled diabetes, decreased urinary output either from dehydration or kidney failure, and Alzheimer's disease with limited mobility. The source of the fevers needs to be determined and a wound infection must be considered. The decreased urinary output can be a nutritional issue, dehydration or inadequate oral intake, and needs to be resolved to maximize wound healing. Limited urinary output may also reflect renal insufficiency and may indicate more advanced effects of the patient's diabetes (nephropathy). Review of laboratory values should include blood glucose and glycosolated hemoglobin. His elevated hemoglobin A_1c reinforces the poor diabetic control, and the increased creatinine may also reflect the renal consequences of his diabetes. His declining nutritional state may also be related to the worsening diabetes. Subtle skin changes such as erythema from pressure, shearing, or infection are difficult to appreciate in dark-skinned individuals. This wound could possibly have been developing over a period of time. Recommend treatment pattern 7D: impaired integumentary integrity associated with full-thickness skin involvement and scar formation.[4]

Prognosis

Alzheimer's disease and wound location will prevent this patient from being independent with his wound care, and family/caregiver education and consultation with the nursing home staff will optimize the wound care plan.

Intervention

A strict turning schedule needs to be implemented with the restriction of the supine position. Mr. Preston should be assessed in sitting to determine if he can maintain a posture that keeps the sacrum free from pressure. A pressure reduction bed mattress and wheelchair or seat cushion will also be needed, and these measures will need to be continued after discharge. Electrical stimulation may be helpful in promoting wound sterilization and closure. The physical examination and subsequent therapeutic interventions must address strength, ROM, transfer status, gait abilities, and balance. Patient independence or minimal to standby assistance with bed mobility, transfers, and ambulation will increase his activity level and decrease time in bed. A nutrition consult is recommended to address potential dietary deficiencies. If the wound is infected, topical antibiotics and a dressing that will adhere and protect the sacral wound from shear and fecal contamination should be applied. IV or oral antibiotics will also be necessary and prescribed by the medical staff. If the nursing home is unable to continue this additional care, other facilities may need to be considered with the help of social workers and discharge planners.

Reexamination

Mr. Preston's medical regiment included adding insulin injections two to three times per day per sliding scale algorithm in addition to his oral medication to improve his glucose control. He was also put on topical and IV antibiotics. Day 4 of his hospital admission, his urine output increased, the "distinct" odor from his breath had diminished, and the wound was being aggressively treated with dressings and topical antibiotics. He was ambulating with minimal assistance with a rolling walker 40 feet x 3.

Outcomes

Mr. Preston was transferred back to the nursing home with full instructions of wound care program and activity progression. The acute care physical therapist's contact number was provided for questions and follow-up.

CHAPTER REVIEW QUESTIONS

1. What are the primary functions of the skin?
2. What are the three phases of wound healing?
3. What is the difference between a full thickness and partial thickness wound?
4. Name at least three risk factors for poor healing.
5. Describe three noninvasive, clinical assessments of blood flow.

REFERENCES

1. Bryant R. Acute & chronic wounds. *Nursing Management*. 2nd ed. St. Louis, Mo: Mosby, Inc; 2000.
2. US Department of Health and Human Resources. *Treatment of Pressure Ulcers, Clinical Practice Guideline*, Number 15. Rockdale, Md: AHCPR Pub; 1994.
3. Kerstein MD. Moist wound healing: the clinical perspective. *Ostomy Wound Management*. 1995;41(7A Supp);37S–44S.
4. Guide to Physical Therapist Practice. 2nd ed. *Physical Therapy*. 2001;81(1).

BIBLIOGRAPHY

Baker LL, Chambers R, Demuth SK, Villar F. Effects of electrical stimulation on wound healing in patients with diabetic ulcers. *Diabetes Care*. 1997;20(3):405–412.
Burton CS. Venous ulcers. *Am J Surg*. 1994;167(1A Suppl):37S–41S.
Feedar JA, Kloth LC, Gentzkow G. Chronic dermal ulcer healing enhance with monophasic pulsed electrical stimulation. *Phys Ther*. 1991;71(9):639–649.

Field FK, Kerstein MD. Overview of wound healing in a moist environment. *Am J Surg.* 1994;167(1A):2S–6S.

Gates JL, Holloway GA. A comparison of wound environments. *Ostomy Wound Manage.* 1992;38(8):34–37.

Gentzkow GD. Electrical stimulation to heal dermal wounds. *J Dermatol Surg Oncol.* 1993;19:753–758.

Glover JL, Weingarten MS, Buchbinder DS. A 4-year outcome-based retrospective study of wound healing and limb salvage in patients with chronic wounds. *Adv Wound Care.* 1997;10(1):33–38.

Gogia PP, Marquez RR, Minerbo GM. Effects of high voltage galvanic stimulation on wound healing. *Ostomy Wound Manage.* 1992;38(1):29–35.

Haisfield-Wolfe ME, Rund C. Malignant cutaneous wounds: a management protocol. *Ostomy Wound Manage.* 1997;43(1):56–66.

Laing P. Diabetic foot ulcers. *Am J Surg.* 1994;167(1A Suppl): 31S–36S.

Lavery LA, Arnstrong DG, Harkless LB. Classification of diabetic foot wounds. *Ostomy Wound Manage.* 1997;43(2):44–53.

Leigh IH, Bennett G. Pressure ulcers: prevalence, etiology and treatment modalities: a review. *Am J Surg.* 1994;167(1A Suppl):25S–30S.

McCulloch J. Physical modalities in wound management: ultrasound, vasopneumatic devices and hydrotherapy. *Ostomy Wound Manage.* 1995;41(5):30–32.

McCulloch JM, Kloth LC, Feeder JA. *Wound Healing Alternatives in Management.* 2nd ed. Philadelphia, Pa: FA Davis Co; 1990.

Michlovitz SL, Wolf SL. *Therapeutic Ultrasound; Thermal Agents in Rehabilitation.* FA Davis Co; 1986: 141–173.

Nelson EA. Compression bandaging for venous leg ulcers. *Prof Nurse.* 1997;12(7 Suppl):S7–S9.

Nelzen O, Bergqvist D, Lindhagen A. Long-term prognosis for patients with chronic leg ulcers: a prospective study. *Eur J Vasc Endovasc Surg.* 1997;13(5):500–508.

Ryan TJ. Wound dressing. *Dermatol Clin.* 1993;11(1):207–213.

Sheffet A, Cytryn AS, Louria DB. Applying electric and electromagnetic energy as adjuvant treatment for pressure ulcers: a critical review. *Ostomy Wound Manage.* 2000;46(2):29.

Staley M, Richard R. Management of the acute burn wound: an overview. *Adv Wound Care.* 1997;10(2):39–44.

Surman MW. An introduction to hyperbaric oxygen therapy for the ET nurse. *J Wound, Ostomy, Continence Nurs.* 1996;23(2):80–89.

Tompach PC, Lew D, Stoll JL. Cell response to hyperbaric oxygen treatment. *Int J Maxillofac Surg.* 1997;26(2):82–86.

Wiley TL. *A Dressing Application Guide for the Care of Wounds Using Moist Healing Principles.* London, England: Smith & Nephew; 1989.

Willey T. Use a decision tree to choose wound dressings. *Am J Nurs.* 1992;92(2):43–46.

ABBREVIATIONS

"	inches
(A-a) PO$_2$	alveolar to arterial oxygen gradient
+	plus
<	greater than
>	less than
6 MWT or MWD	six minute walk test or distance
ASPEN	American Society for Parental & Enteral Nutrition
A1AD	alpha-1 antitrypsin deficiency
AAA	abdominal aortic aneurysms
AACVPR	American Association of Cardiovascular and Pulmonary Rehabilitation
AAOS	American Academy of Orthopedic Surgeons
AAROM	active assistive range of motion
AAT	alpha-1 antitrypsin
ABG	arterial blood gas
ABI	ankle brachial index
AC	assist control (ie, mode of mechanical ventilations)
ACA	anterior cerebral artery
ACB	active cycle of breathing
ACDF	anterior cervical discectomy and fusion
ACE	angiotensin converting enzyme
Ach	acetylcholine
ACSM	American College of Sports Medicine
ACT	airway clearance technique
AD	autogenic drainage
ADH	antidiuretic hormone
ADLs	activities of daily living
ADP	adenosine diphsophate
AF	atrial fibrillation
AFO	ankle foot orthosis
AHI	apnea-hypopnea index
AI	aortic insufficiency
AICA	anterior inferior cerebellar artery
AICD	automatic implanted cardiac defibrillator

AIDS	acquired immunodeficiency syndrome/ autoimmune deficiency syndrome
AKA	above knee amputation
ALB	albumin
ALF	acute liver failure
ALI	acute lung injury
ALIF	anterior lumbar interbody fusion
ALL	anterior longitudinal ligament
ALS	amyotrophic lateral sclerosis
ALT	alanine aminotransferase
AMS	acute myopathy syndrome
ANF	atrial natriuretic factor
ANP	atrial natriuretic peptide
AoV	aortic valves
AP	action potential
A-P	anterior-posterior
APACHE II score	acute physiology and chronic health evaluation
APTA	American Physical Therapy Association
APTT	activated partial thromboplastin time
AR	aortic regurgitation
ARDS	adult respiratory distress syndrome/acute respiratory distress syndrome
ARF	acute renal failure
AROM	active range of motion
AS	aortic stenosis
ASD	atrial septal defect
ASIA	American Spinal Injury Association (ie, ASIA Impairment Scale)
AST	aspartate aminotrasnferase
AT	atrial tachycardia
ATCH	adrenocorticotropin hormone
ATN	acute tubular necrosis
ATP	adensoine triphosphate
ATPase	an enzyme that catalyzes the hydrolysis of ATP to ADP
ATPS	ambient temperature, pressure, saturated
A-V fistula	arterio-venous fistula
AV junction	atrioventricular junction

AV node	atrioventricular node
AVM	arteriovenous malformation
AVN	avascular necrosis
AVR	aortic valve replacement
AZT	azidothymidine
BCAA	branch chain amino acids
BD	bronchial drainage
BETS	blind endotracheal suctioning
BID	twice a day
BKA	below knee amputation
BLT	bilateral lung transplant
BMD	bone mineral density
BMI	body mass index
BMT	bone marrow transplantation
BO	bronchiolitis obliterans
BOOP	bronchiolitis obliterans organizing pneumonia
BP	blood pressure
BPD	bronchopulmonary dysplasia
BPH	benign prostate hypertrophy
bpm	breaths per minute or beats per minute
BSA	body surface area
BUN	blood urea nitrogen
C/D/I	clean, dry and intact
CA	cancer
Ca^{++}	calcium
CABG	coronary artery bypass grafting
CAD	coronary artery disease
CAM	complimentary alternative medicine
cAMP	cyclic adenosine monophosphate
CAPD	continuous ambulatory peritoneal dialysis
CAT scan	computerized axial tomography
CAVH	continous arteriovenous hemofiltration
CBC	complete blood count
CCB	calcium channel blocker
CD	cluster designation: cell surface proteins that characterize cell types (eg, CD4 T cells; CD8 T cells)
CDC	Centers for Disease Control and Prevention
CDT	complete decongestive therapy

CF	cystic fibrosis
cGMP	cyclic guanosine monophosphate
CHD	congenital heart disease
CHF	congestive heart failure
CHO	carbohydrates
CI	cardiac index
CIDP	chronic idiopathic demyelinating polyradiculo-neuropathy
CIDP	chronic inflammatory demyelinating polyneuropathy
CIP	critical illness polyneuropathy
CJD	Creutzfeldt-Jakob disease
CK	creatine kinase
CK-BB	CK bands specific to brain and neural tissue
CK-MB	CK bands specific to heart muscle
CK-MM	CK bands primarily found in skeletal muscle
CL	cutaneous leishmaniasis
Cl-	chloride
cm	centimeters
cm H_2O	centimeters of water pressure
CMD	cardiac muscle dysfunction
CMV	controlled mechanical ventilation
CMV	cytomegalovirus
CNS	central nervous system
CO	cardiac output
CO	carbon monoxide
CO_2	carbon dioxide
COAD	chronic obstructive airway disease
COLD	chronic obstructive lung disease
COMT inhibitors	catechol-o-methyl transferase inhibitors
COP	cryptogenic organizing pneumonia
COPD	chronic obstructive pulmonary disease
COTA	certified occupational therapist assistant
CP	chest pain
CPAP	continuous positive airway pressure
CPK	creatine phosphokinase
CPM	continuous passive motion machine
CPR	cardiopulmonary resuscitation

CPT	chest physical therapy
CRF	chronic renal failure
CRF	cancer-related fatigue
CRH	corticotropin-releasing hormone
crp	c-reactive protein
CRRT	continuous renal replacement therapy
CSF	cerebrospinal fluid
CSII	continous subcutaneous insulin infusion
CT scan	computed tomography scan
CTLO	cervical thoracic lumbar orthosis
CTLs	cytotoxic T lymphocytes (also called CD_8 T Cells)
CTO	cervical thoracic orthosis
CTSIB	clinical test of sensory interaction on balance
CVA	cerebral vascular accident
CVAHD	continuous arterio-venous hemodialyis
CVC	central venous catheters
CVD	cardiovascular disease
CVP	central venous pressure
CVS	cardiovascular system
CVVHD	continuous veno-venous hemodialysis
CWS	certified wound specialist
CXR	chest roentogram or x-ray
DAD	diffuse alveolar damage
DAI	diffuse axonal injury
DBP	diastolic blood pressure
DCL	diffuse cutaneous leishmaniasis
DGF	delayed graft function
DHS	dynamic hip screw
DHT	dihydrotestosterone
DI	diabetes insipidus
DIC	disseminating intravascular coagulopathy or coagulation
DIP	desquamative interstitial pneumonia
DKA	diabetic ketoacidosis
DLCO	diffusing capacity of carbon monoxide
DM	diabetes mellitus
DM	dermatomyositis

DMARD	disease modifying antirheumatic drugs
DNA	deoxyribonucleic acid
DOE	dyspnea on exertion
DPG	diphosphoglycerate
DSA	digital subtraction angiography
DVT	deep vein thrombosis
eg	for example
EC	extracellular
$ECCO_2 R$	extracorporeal CO_2 removal
ECF	extracellular fluid
ECG	electrocardiogram
ECMO	extracorporeal membranous oxygenation
ed.	edition
EDH	epidural hematoma, also called an extradural hematoma
EDP	endiastolic pressure
EDV	endiastolic volume
EEG	electroencephalogram
EF	ejection fraction
EGD	esophagogastroduodensocopy
EMG	electromyography
EMT	emergency medical technician
EP	electrophysiology
EP	evoked potentials
EPS	electrophysiology studies
ERCP	endoscopic retrograde cholangiopancreatography
ERV	expiratory reserve volume
ESLD	end-stage liver disease
ESR	erythrocyte sedimentation rate
ESRD	endstage renal disease
etc.	ecetera
ETOH	ethanol (alcohol)
ETT	endotracheal tube
ETT	exercise tolerance test
Ex Fix	external fixation
exam	examination
Fe^{3+}	iron

FEF$_{25-75}$	mid expiratory flow rates
FEV$_1$	forced expiratory volume in one second
FFA	free fatty acid
FFP	fresh frozen plasma
FIM	functional independence measure
F$_i$O$_2$	fraction of inspired oxygen
FK506	Tacrolimus—trade name
FOS	flight of stairs
FRC	functional residual capacity
FSH	follicle stimulating hormone
FVC	forced vital capacity
g/dl	grams per decileter
GABA	gamma-aminobutyric acid
GBS	Guillain Barre syndrome
GCS	Glascow coma scale
GERD	gastroespohageal reflux disease
GFR	glomerular filtration rate
GGT	gamma glutamyl transferase
GH	growth hormone
GI	gastrointestinal
Glut4	glucose transporter protein 4
GnRH	gonadotrophin releasing hormone
GU	genitourinary
GVHD	graft vs host disease
GYN	gynecological
H$^+$	hydrogen ion
H$_2$O	water
HA	headaches
Hb A1c	hemoglobin A1C
HBV	hepatitis B virus
HCO$_3$-	bicarbonate
hct or HCT	hematocrit
HCV	hepatitis C virus
HD	hemodialysis
HD	Hodgkin disease (Hodgkin's lymphoma)
HDL	high density lipoprotein
HF	heart failure

HFCWC or HFCWO	high frequency chest wall compression or oscillation
Hgb or Hb	hemoglobin
HH	hiatal hernia
HHNK	hyperosmolar hyperglycemic nonketotic
HIV	human immunodeficiency virus
HLA	human leukocyte antigen
HLT or H-L Tx	heart lung transplant
HMG CoA	3-hydroxy-3 methyl glutaryl-coenzyme A or hydroxy-methylglutaryl coenzyme A
HPI	history of present illness
HPTX	hemopneumothorax
HPV	human papilloma virus
HR	heart rate
HRCT	high resolution computerized tomography
HTN	hypertension
Hz	hertz
I & D	incision and drainage
ie	that is
IABP	intra-aortic ballon pump
IADL	instrumental activities of daily living
IBM	inclusion body myositis
IBS	irritable bowel syndrome
IBW	ideal body weight
IC	inspiratory capacity
IC	intracellular
ICA	internal carotid arteries
ICD	implantable cardiac defibrillator
ICH	intracranial hematomas
ICH	intracerebral hemorrhage
ICP	intracranial pressure
ICU	intensive care unit
IDDM	insulin dependent diabetes mellitus (type 1)
IFN	interferons (IFNα, IFNβ, IFNγ)
IgG, IgA, IgM, IgD and IgE	immunoglobulins (antibodies)
IHSS	idiopathic hypertrophic subaortic stenosis
ILD	interstitial lung disease

IMN	intermedullary nail
IMR	intermedullary rod
IMT	inspiratory muscle training
IMV	intermittent mandatory ventilation
INH	isoniazid
INR	International Normalization Ratio
IPF	idiopathic pulmonary fibrosis
IRV	inspiratory reserve volume
IS	incentive spirometry
IV	intravenous
IVC	inferior vena cava
IVP	intravenous pyelogram
JP drain	Jackson-Pratt drain
JVD	jugular venous distention
K^+	potassium
kg/m^2	kilograms per meter squared
L/min	liters per minute
L4 to L5	lumbar segments 4 through 5
LA	left atrium
LAD	left anterior descending
LAM	lymphangioleiomyomatosis
LANA	Lymphology Association of North America
LAP	left atrial pressures
LBBB	left bundle branch block
LCx	left circumflex artery
LD or LDH	lactate dehydrogenase
LDL	low density lipoprotein
LE or L/E	lower extremity
LES	lower esophogeal sphincter
LGI	lower gastrointestinal
LH	luteinizing hormone
LLE	left lower extremity
LOC	loss of consciousness
LOCF	level of cognitive functioning
Lpa	lipoprotein (A) (Lpa1 = lipoprotein particle A1)
LPN	licensed practical nurse
LSO	lumbar sacral orthosis

LUE	left upper extremity
LUQ	left upper quadrant
LV	left ventricle
LVAD	left ventricular assist devices
LVEDP	left ventricular end diastolic pressure
LVESP	left ventricular end systolic pressure
LVH	left ventricular hypertrophy
LVRS	lung volume reduction surgery
MA	medical assistant
MAFO	molded ankle foot orthosis
MALTs	muocosal-associated lymphoid tissues
MAP	mean arterial pressure
MCA	middle cerebral artery
MCH	mean cell hemoglobin or mean corpuscular hemoglobin
MCHC	mean cell hemoglobin concentration or mean cellular hemoglobin content
MCL	mucocutaneous leishmaniasis (also called espundia)
MCV	mean corpuscular volume
MD	physician/medical doctor
MD	muscular dystrophy
MDI	meter dose inhalers
mEq/L	milli-equivalents per liter
METS	metabolic equivalents
Mg	magnesium
MG	myasthenia gravis
μg/dL	micrograms per deciliter
mg/dL	milligram per deciliter
MI	myocardial infarction
MIP	maximum inspiratory pressure (also called NIF)
Misc	miscellaneous
mL	milliliters
mm	millimeter
mmol/L	millimoles per liter
MMSE	mini-mental state examination
MMT	manual muscle test
mNIHSS	modified NIH stroke scale

MOD	multiple organ dysfunction
MOF	multiple organ failure
MRA	magnetic resonance angiography
MRCP	MRI retrograde cholangiopancreatography
MRI	magnetic resonance imaging
MR	mitral regurgitation
MRM	modified radical mastectomy
MRSA	methicillin resistant staphylococcus aureus
MS	multiple sclerosis
MS	mitral stenosis
MS	mental status
MS04	morphine
MUD	matched unrelated donor
MUGA	multigated acquisition or angiogram imaging
MV	mechanical ventilation
MV	mitral valve
MV	minute ventilation
MVA	motor vehicle accident
MVC	motor vehicle crash
mVe	minute ventilation (RR x V_T)
MVR	mitral valve replacement
N/V	nausea/vomiting
Na+	sodium
NCV	nerve conduction studies
NG	naso-gastric (suction or tube)
NH_3	ammonia
NHL	non-Hodgkin's lymphoma
NIDDM	noninsulin dependent diabetes mellitus (type 2)
NIF	negative inspiratory force (also called MIP)
NIH	National Institutes of Health
NLN	National Lymphedema Network
NMSC	nonmelanoma skin cancers
NPO	nothing per os, nothing by mouth
NPPV	noninvasive positive pressure ventilation
NS	normal saline
NSAID	nonsteroidal anti-inflammatory drugs
NSCLCA	nonsmall cell lung cancer

NSR	normal sinus rhythm
NTG	nitroglycerin
NTS	nasal tracheal suctioning
NWB	nonweightbearing
NYHA	New York Heart Association
O_2	oxygen
OA	osteoarthritis
OB	obliterative bronchiolitis
OGTT	oral glucose tolerance test
OHT	orthotopic heart transplant
OOB	out of bed
ORIF	open reduction internal fixation
OSA	obstructive sleep apnea
OT	occupational therapy
P	phosphate
PA	physician assistant
PAB	prealbumin
PAC	pulmonary artery catheter
PAC	premature atrial contraction or complex
PAD	premature atrial depolarization
$PACO_2$	partial pressure of carbon dioxide in alveolar gas
$PaCO_2$	partial pressure of carbon dioxide in arterial blood
PAD	peripheral arterial disease
PAOD	peripheral arterial occlusive disease
PAP	pulmonary artery pressure
PAT	paroxysmal atrial tachycardia
PAWP/ PAOP	pulmonary artery wedge or occlusion pressure
PBC	primary biliary cirrhosis
PCA	patient controlled analgesia
PCA	posterior communicating arteries
PCA	posterior cerebral artery
PCO_2	partial pressure of carbon dioxide
PCP	pneumocystis carinii pneumonia
PCP	primary care physician
PCR	polymerase chain reaction
PCWP	pulmonary capillary wedge pressure
PD	postural drainage

PD	Parkinson's disease
PD	peritoneal dialysis
PDGF	platelet-derived growth factor
PDQ 39	Parkinson's disease quality of life questionnaire
PE	pulmonary emboli
PEEP	positive end expiratory pressure
PEFR	peak expiratory flow rate
PEG	percutaneous endoscopic gastrostomy (tube)
PEJ	percutaneous endoscopic jejunostomy (tube)
PEP	positive expiratory pressure
PET	positron emission tomography
pH	hydrogen ion concentration
PH	pulmonary hypertension
PPH	primary pulmonary hypertension
PHR	peak heart rate
PICA	posterior inferior cerebellar artery
PLB	pursed lip breathing
PLF	posterolateral lumbar fusion
PLIF	posterior lumbar interbody fusion
PLL	posterior longitudinal ligament
PLT	platelets
PM	polymyositis
PM	pacemaker
PPM	permanent pacemaker
PMD	primary medical doctor
PMH/PMHx	past medical history
PMI	point of maximal impulse
PND	paroxysmal nocturnal dyspnea
PNF	primary nonfunction
PO_2	partial pressure of oxygen
PPD	pack per day
PPE	personal protective equipment
PPH	primary pulmonary hypertension
PPI	proton pump inhibitors
PRBC	packed red blood cells
PRE	progressive resistive exercise
PRI	PR interval of an ECG

PROM	passive range of motion
PRV	post residual void
PS	pressure support (ie, mode of mechanical ventilation)
PS	Parkinsonism syndrome
PSA	prostate specific antigens
PSC	primary sclerosing cholangitis
PSV	pressure support ventilation
PT	physical therapist
PT	prothrombin time
PTA	physical therapist assistant
PTCA	percutaneous transluminal coronary angioplasty
PTFE	polytetrafluoroethylene
PTH	parathyroid hormone
PTT	partial thromboplastin time
PTX	pneumothorax
PUD	peptic ulcer disease
PV	pulmonic valve
PVC	pulmonary vascular congestion
PVC	premature ventricular contraction/complex
PVD	peripheral vascular disease
PVR	pulmonary vascular resistance
PWB	partial weight bearing
QOL	quality of life
QRS	QRS interval of an ECG
QT	QT segment of an ECG
RA	rheumatoid arthritis
RA	right atrium
RAP	right atrial pressure
RAS	reticular activating system
RBBB	right bundle branch block
RBC	red blood cell
RCA	right coronary artery
RHR	resting heart rate
RLE	right lower extremity
RN	registered nurse
RNA	ribonucleic acid

ROM	range of motion
RPE	rating of perceived exertion
RR	respiratory rate
RSV	respiratory syncytial virsus
RT	respiratory therapist
RUE	right upper extremity
RUQ	right upper quadrant
RV	right ventricle
RV	residual volume
RVAD	right ventricular assist device
RVEDP	right-ventricular end-diastolic pressure
Rx	treatment or prescription
SA node or SAN	sinoatrial node
SAH	subarachnoid hemorrhage
SAN	spinal accessory nerve
SaO_2	arterial oxygen saturation
SBO	small bowel obstruction
SBP	systolic blood pressure
SBS	short bowel syndrome
SCC	spinal cord compression
SCI	spinal cord injury
SDH	subdural hematoma
SDH	subdural hemorrhage
SGOT	serum glutamic-oxaloacetic transaminase
SIADH	syndrome of inappropriate anti-diuretic hormone
SIMV	synchronized intermittent mandatory ventilation
SIRS	systemic inflammatory response syndrome
sit<>stand	transfer sitting to stand and return to sitting position
SLE	systemic lupus erhythematosus
SLT	single lung transplant
SOB	shortness of breath
SOMI	sternal occipito mandibular immobilizer
SpO_2	oxygen saturation measured via the pulse
SPECT	single photon emission computed tomography
spiral CT	spiral computerized tomography scan ("corkscrew" scan pattern)
supine>sitting	supine transfer to sitting

SV	stroke volume
SVC	superior vena cava
S_VO_2	mixed venous oxygen saturation
SVR	systemic vascular resistance
SVT	supraventricular tachycardia
T lymphocytes or T cells	precursors arise in bone marrow and mature in thymus, a primary lymphoid organs
T10 to T12	thoracic segments 10 through 12
T3	triiodothyronine
T4	thyroxine
TAA	thoracic aortic aneurysm
TAH	total abdominal hysterectomy
TB	mycobacterium tuberculosis
TBI	traumatic brain injury
TBW	total body water
TCA	tricarboxylic acid cycle (Kreb's cycle)
TCD	transcranial doppler
TEE	transesophageal echocardiography
TEN	total enteral nutrition
TENS	transcutaneoous electric nerve stimulation
TH	thyroid hormone
THA	total hip arthroplasty
TIA	transient ischemic attack
TID	three times a day
TKA	total knee arthroplasty
TLC	total lung capacity
TLSO	thoracic lumbosacral orthosis
TMA	transmetatarsal amputation
TMJ	temporal mandibular joint
TMR	transmyocardial revascularization
TNF	tumor necrosis factor
TNM	tumor/nodal/metastasis
tPA	tissue plasminogen activator/alteplase recombinant
TPN	total parenteral nutrition
TPR	total peripheral resistance
TR	tricuspid regurgitation
TRAM	transverse rectus abdominus myocutaneous flaps
TRH	thyroid releasing hormone

TSA	total shoulder arthroplasty
TSH	thyroid stimulating hormone
TTE	transthoracic echocardiography
TTP	thrombotic thrombocytopenic purpura
TUIP	transurethral incision of the prostate
TUMT	transurethral microwave thermotherapy
TUNA	transurethral needle ablation
TURP	transurethral resection of the prostate
TV	tricuspid valve or tidal volume
Tx	transplant
UA	urinalysis
UBE	upper body ergometer
UBW	usual body weight
UC	ulcerative colitis
UE or U/E	upper extremity
UES	upper esophageal sphincter
UGI	upper gastrointestinal
UI	urinary incontinence
UIP	usual interstitial pneumonitis
UNOS	United Network of Organ Sharing
UPDRS scale	unified Parkinson's disease rating scale
US	United States
US	ultrasound
UTIs	urinary tract infections
V/Q	ventilation/perfusion
VAD	ventricular assist devices
VAS	visual analog scale
VATS	video-assisted thoracostomy
(Vdf/VT)	physiologic dead space/tidal volume
VF	ventricular fibrillation
VHD	valvular heart disease
VLDL	very low density lipoproteins
VO_2	oxygen consumption
$VO_{2\,max}$	maximal oxygen uptake
VOR	vestibulo-ocular reflex
VRE	vancomycin resistant enterococci
VS	vital signs

VSD	ventricular septal defect
VT	ventricular tachycardia, ventricular tachyarrhythmia
V_T	tidal volume
WBC	white blood cell
WFL	within functional limits
WHO	World Health Organization
WNL	within normal limits
WPW Syndrome	Wolff-Parkinson-White syndrome
XRT	radiation therapy
Δ	change

APPENDIX

Example of Acute Care Competency Check-Off Sheet
Adapted from University of Pennsylvania Health System/Division of
Occupational and Physical Therapy/Department of Rehabilitation Medicine

	The following are categories from the written competency for the entry level evaluation and treatment in the ICU.	Review of Written Material	Discussed/ Asked Questions	Practiced Competency (practice test)	Pass/Date/ Initials of Tester (demonstrated ≥85% understanding)
I.	**Written competency**				
A.	Examination				
B.	Line identification				
C.	Electrocardiogram (ECG) identification				
D.	Ventilation/ oxygenation				
E.	Intervention/ methods for progression				
F.	Tests and procedures				
G.	Common diseases/disorders				
II.	**Practical**				
A.	Examination skills: look/listen/ feel				
1.	Therapist describes universal precautions and infection control				
2.	Therapist reviews medical record and documents per department policy				

3.	Therapist checks with shift or charge nurse prior to examination and intervention of patient				
4.	Therapist assesses breathing pattern and describes				
5.	Therapist assesses respiratory rate (RR) and cough				
6.	Therapist assesses pulse and describes 3 ways to check heart rate (HR)				
7.	Therapist assesses level of alertness, cognition, and ability to communicate				
8.	Therapist assesses skin color, temperature, nail beds/clubbing				
9.	Therapist assesses blood pressure (BP)				
10.	Therapist assesses orthopnea				
11.	Therapist assesses shortness of breath (SOB)				
12.	Therapist assesses rating of perceived exertion (RPE)				
13.	Therapist assesses oxygen saturation (SpO_2)				

14.	Therapist auscultates for breath sounds (BS) or interprets documented BS				
15.	Therapist assesses endurance				
16.	Therapist assesses orthostatic signs				
17.	Therapist identifies primary diagnosis during a cotreatment and at least 3 comorbidities with ability to define and describe impact on treatment				
B.	Line/tube identification				
	(Name line/tube and describes two precautions for examination and intervention				
1.	Arterial line				
2.	Central venous line (ie, Swann-Ganz)				
3.	Peripheral intravenous line (IV)				
4.	Therapist identifies two types of dialysis ports (hemodialyis and peritoneal dialysis)				
5.	Therapist identifies foley catheter				

6.	Therapist identifies peripherally inserted cardiac catheter (PICC)				
7.	Therapist identifies intracranial pressure device				
8.	Therapist identifies nasogastric tube, gastronomy tube, jejunostomy tube				
9.	Therapist identifies rectal catheter/bag				
10.	Therapist identifies Jackson-Pratt drain and/or hemovac				
11.	Therapist identifies left ventricular or right ventricular assist device (LVAD/RVAD)				
12.	Therapist identifies aortic balloon pump (IABP)				
13.	Therapist identifies Hickman or port-a cath				
14.	Therapist identifies an epidural catheter				
15.	Therapist describes patient controlled analgesia)				
16.	Therapist identifies a lumbar drain				
17.	Therapist identifies and describes two types of pacemakers				

18.	Therapist identifies ECG and electrodes				
19.	Chest tube and suction unit				
C.	ECG identification and impact on therapy				
1.	Therapist identifies sinus rhythms:				
a.	Normal sinus rhythm				
b.	Sinus arrhythmia				
c.	Sinus bradycardia				
d.	Sinus tachycardia				
2.	Therapist identifies other sinus rhythms and describes any impact on evaluation and treatment				
a.	Sinus bradycardia				
b.	Sinus tachycardia				
3.	Therapist identifies atrial rhythms:				
a.	Premature atrial contraction				
b.	Paroxysmal atrial tachycardia and atrial tachycardia				
c.	Atrial flutter				
d.	Atrial fibrillation				
4.	Therapist identifies different types of heart blocks				
a.	First degree heart block				

b.	Two types of second degree heart block				
c.	Complete or third degree heart block				
5.	Therapist identifies ventricular rhythms:				
a.	Premature ventricular contraction (unifocal versus multifocal premature ventricular contractions)				
b.	Couplets, bigeminy and trigeminy				
c.	Ventricular tachycardia				
d.	Ventricular fibrillation				
e.	Idioventricular rhythm				
5.	Therapist identifies asystole				
6.	Therapist describes three possible reasons for irregular heart beat				
7.	Therapist describes possible causes of artifact on ECG during examination and intervention				
8.	Therapist describes two ways to validate SpO_2 value from pulse oximeter				
D.	Ventilation/ oxygenation				

1.	Therapist identifies nasal canula and oxygen prescription				
2.	Therapist identifies trach/face mask and oxygen prescription				
3.	Therapist identifies venturi set up for trach or face mask and prescribed oxygen L/minute				
4.	Therapist identifies mechanical ventilator and current ventilator setting (ie, assist control, pressure support, intermittent mandatory ventilation, continuous positive airway pressure, oxygen prescription, PEEP)				
5.	Therapist demonstrates four precautions for mobilizing a patient with an artificial airway (eg, ETT, trach)				
6.	Therapist demonstrates where mechanical ventilator alarms are located and what the alarms mean (list four and describe purpose)				

7.	Therapist describes and demonstrates two ways of assessing patient tolerance to activity with a patient on supplemental oxygen or on a mechanical ventilator				
8.	Therapist is able to describe manual ventilator (ambu) and purpose				
9.	Therapist describes proper technique for turning on and shutting off oxygen cylinders ('e or h tank')				
10.	Therapist describes purpose of extracorporeal membrane oxygenation (ECMO) and precautions				
E.	Physical therapy: interventions/ methods for progression				
1.	Therapist describes rationale and lists four precautions for bed exercises				
2.	Therapist demonstrates different types of bed exercises and describes hemodynamic monitoring for patient response response to exercises				

3.	Therapist describes rationale and lists four precautions for progression to semifowler position				
4.	Therapist describes rationale, precautions, and hemodynamic monitoring progression to dangling, supported and then unsupported				
5.	Therapist describes rationale, precautions, and hemodynamic monitoring while progressing transfers, standing, and OOB activities				
6.	Therapist describes rationale, precautions, and hemodynamic monitoring for progression to gait training and OOB exercise				
7.	Therapist describes physical therapy examination proceedures to determine patient tolerance to transfers, gait, and OOB exercises in context of progressing intervention intensity, duration, and frequency				

8.	Therapist describes progression of activity with change in supplemental oxygen and progression of oxygen delivery devices: (ie, MV, trach, button, face mask, nasal cannula, etc)				
9.	Therapist describes progression of activity level with change in device and therapist assist (ie, tilt table, rolling platform walker, rolling walker, walker, multi-prong cane, single point cane, etc) (maximum assist, moderate assist, contact guard, standby assist, etc)				
10.	Therapist reviews with care team activity progression and documents progress and hemodynamic responses in medical record				
11.	Therapist describes and demonstrates two assisted cough positions and techniques				
12.	Therapist describes two precautions pre/post-suctioning for a patient				

F.	Tests and Procedures				
1.	CABG				
2.	Angioplasty percutaneous transluminal coronary angioplasty (PTCA)/stents (coated and non-coated)				
3.	Orthotopic heart transplant				
4.	Pneumonectomy				
5.	Thoracotomy				
6.	Mean arterial pressure				
7.	SVO_2, SaO_2, SpO_2				
8.	Cardiac index				
9.	Ventriculotomy				
10.	Cardiac catheterization/coronary angiography				
11.	Positron Emission Tomography (PET) scan				
12	Thallium scan (pharmacologic/exercise)				
13.	Echocardiogram (transthoracic, transesophogeal); stress or dobutamine				
14.	Ankle brachial index (ABI)				
15.	Ventilation perfusion scan				

16.	Implantable car-dioverter defibril-lators (ICD's) and pacemakers				
17.	Holter monitor				
18.	Chest roetenogram (x-ray)				
19.	Exercise tolerance test				
20.	Computed tomog-raphy (CT) scan				
21.	Magnetic reso-nance angiography (MRI)/magnetic resonance imaging (MRA)				
22.	Electrophysiology studies				
23.	Electomyography				
24.	Thoracentesis				
25.	Valvuloplasty				
26.	Pulmonary function tests, spirometry				
27.	Arterial blood gases				
28.	Dialysis: hemo/peritoneal/con-tinuous				
29.	ORIF, external fix-ators, partial/total joint replacements				
G.	Common Diseases/Disorders				
30.	Therapist should describe the fol-lowing pathophysi-ologies and impact on treatment:				
a.	Adult respiratory distress syndrome				

b.	Pneumonia				
c.	Heart failure				
d.	Chronic obstructive pulmonary disease (chronic bronchitis, asthma, emphysema)				
e.	Coronary artery disease/atherosclerosis				
f.	Obesity				
g.	Describe effects of bed rest on cardiovascular and pulmonary, neurologic, integumentary, and musculoskeletal system				
h.	Diabetes mellitus (DM)				
i.	Hypertension				
j.	Respiratory failure/respiratory distress				
k.	Myocardial infarction (MI), myocardial ischemia (angina and angina equivalents				
l.	Pleural effusion				
m.	Pneumothorax (tension)				
n.	Pulmonary emboli				
o.	Pulmonary edema				
p.	Coronary artery bypass graft (CABG)				
q.	Percutaneous transluminal coronary angioplasty (PTCA)				

r.	Flail chest				
s.	Atelectasis				
t.	Deep vein thrombosis (DVT)				
u.	Compartment syndrome				
v.	Cerebral vascular accident (CVA)				
w.	Pulmonary fibrosis (interstitial)				
x.	Pulmonary hypertension/cor pulmonale				
y.	Orthostatic hypotension				
z.	Pericarditis				
aa.	Peripheral vascular disease/intermittent claudication (PVD/IC)				
bb.	Cardiac tamponade				
cc.	Tuberculosis				

Sample Test: Written Competency

To pass the written competency section the therapist must correctly answer >85% of the questions. The questions are multiple choice. Circle the most appropriate answer(s).

A. Assessment

1. Which of the following is (are) the best way(s) to assess HR?
    a. Palpate radial pulse and external jugular vein
    b. Palpate pulse and read from ECG*
    c. Observe and read the rate off mechanical ventilator
    d. Observe arterial BP tracing on monitor

2. Which of the following is (are) the best way(s) to validate oxygen saturation?
    a. Palpate pulse and compare to pulse rate on saturation monitor*
    b. Palpate pulse and compare to rate on mechanical ventilator
    c. Observe ECG on monitor and compare with central venous pressure
    d. All of the above

3. Which of the following is the best way to assess patient tolerance to evaluation or a treatment session?
    a. A change in mental status
    b. A change in lip color or nail polish color
    c. A change in baseline to activity vital signs
    d. a, c*

4. A patient has developed the following changes during the examination: new onset S_3, rales >one-third up bilateral posterior lung regions, increased RR, positive accessory muscle use. Which of the following is most likely to be the diagnosis?
    a. Interstitial pulmonary fibrosis
    b. Congestive heart failure*
    c. Cystic fibrosis
    d. Chronic bronchitis

5. Which of the following is the best possible diagnosis given these findings on assessment: patient status post (s/p) motor vehicle accident (MVA) with flail chest on the left confirmed by x-ray: tracheal deviation to the right, hyperresonant left chest to right with mediate percussion, distant BS on auscultation left to right, decreased chest wall movement left to right, pale, and rapid RR with accessory muscle use.
    a. Adult respiratory distress syndrome
    b. Pneumothorax*
    c. Pneumonia
    d. Pleural effusion

B. Line Identification

1. Which of the following is not a precaution when mobilizing a patient with a dorsalis pedis arterial line?
    a. avoid weight bearing on the extremity with the arterial line

     b. keep the transducer at heart level

     c. avoid trunk flexion >90 degrees*

     d. allow extra tubing to avoid dislodging arterial line when mobilizing

2. Which of the follow represents the only contraindication when mobilizing a patient with a PICC line?

     a. avoid any type of range of motion (ROM) on the extremity 7 days after placement

     b. allow the patient to have his/her BP measured in that extremity*

     c. allow the patient to perform activities of daily living as tolerated

     d. avoid OOB activities for 24 hours after placement

3. Which of the following is the best precaution for moving a patient OOB with a foley catheter?

     a. maintain the foley catheter bag below the bladder*

     b. drain the foley catheter prior to transferring back to bed

     c. allow extra tubing to be added to the catheter before transfers out of bed

     d. all of the above

4. Which of the following best represents a precaution for mobilizing a patient with chest tubes?

     a. check placement of tubes, security of tubes sutured to skin, move pleurovac out from under bed, do not open up foot rest on bottom of pleurovac, check for last dosage of pain medication

     b. check placement of tubes, security of tubes sutured to skin, do not move pleurovac out from under bed, do not open up foot rest on bottom of pleurovac, and check for last dosage of pain medication

     c. check placement of tubes, security of tubes sutured to skin, move pleurovac out from under bed, open up foot rest on bottom of pleurovac, and check for last dosage of pain medication*

     d. check placement of tubes, loosen sutures on skin, move pleurovac out from under bed, open up foot rest on bottom of pleurovac, check for last dosage of pain medication

5. Which of the following is (are) the most reasonable precaution(s) during examination and intervention of a patient with a central venous catheter?

     a. avoid moving the joint closest to the central line

     b. avoid dislodging the central line by checking for tautness on line

     c. avoid dislodging the central line by checking the level of the transducer

     d. a, b*

C. ECG Identification

1. Which of the following is most likely the rhythm described: regular rate, unable to determine if P wave present in any form, rate >100, QRS complex <.12 seconds?

     a. sinus tachycardia*

     b. ventricular tachycardia

     c. idioventricular rhythm

     d. none of the above

2. Which of the following best represents this rhythm: p wave in front of QRS complexes, QRS complex <.12 seconds, 2 p waves appear different then others, rhythm is slightly irregular?
   a. sinus rhythm with first degree heart block
   b. sinus rhythm with bigerminy
   c. sinus rhythm with premature ventricular contractions
   d. sinus rhythm with premature form atrial contractions*

3. Which of the following best represents the rhythm that is likely to have an irregularly irregular pulse and negetively impact exercise tolerance?
   a. atrial tachycardia
   b. atrial fibrillation*
   c. sinus arrhythmia
   d. sinus bradycardia

4. Which of the following rhythms is most likely to have a slightly irregular pulse, but the pattern repeats with the patient's RR?
   a. sinus arrhythmia*
   b. atrial flutter
   c. sinus tachycardia
   d. ventricular tachycardia

5. Which of the following diagnoses is most likely to lead to a blunted response to an increase in activity?
   a. Adult Respiratory Distress Syndrome
   b. Orthotopic Heart Transplant*
   c. New Onset DM
   d. Subcutaneous Emphysema

D. Ventilation/Oxygenation

1. Which of the following is the most likely reason for the high pressure alarm to go off on the mechanical ventilator?
   a. disconnection
   b. water in the humidifier
   c. coughing*
   d. bronchodilation

2. Which of the following is most likely to be used as a supplemental oxygen device when the patient with a tracheostomy is progressed for the first time off the mechanical ventilator (mv) for 1 hour?
   a. nasal canula
   b. trach mask and collar*
   c. ambu bag (manual ventilator)
   d. nonrebreather mask

3. Which of the following best describes the reason to use 100% oxygen before, during, and following suctioning?
   a. to prevent pneumothorax
   b. to prevent dysrhythmias
   c. to prevent hypoxemia
   d. b, c*

4. Which of the following best represents how an assistive cough should be taught when the patient just had a right chest tube placed and a gastronomy tube placed yesterday?
   a. cross one arm across the anterior chest and one arm across abdomen without a blanket or pillow
   b. cross one arm across anterior chest and one arm across abdomen with a blanket or pillow*
   c. perform abdominal thrusts with pain medication prior to treatment
   d. none of the above

5. Which of the following statements is the most true?
   a. a patient can breath over and above an intermittent mandatory ventilation setting on a mechanical ventilator*
   b. a patient can set off a low pressure alarm on a mechanical ventilator by coughing
   c. a patient can set off a high pressure alarm on a mechanical ventilator by a disconnection
   d. a patient can not breath over and above an intermittent mandatory ventilation setting on a mechanical ventilator

E. Methods for Progression

1. Mr. Jones is awake, alert, and has rested on the ventilator overnight. This is your first time in to evaluate or treat Mr. Jones. The nurse tells you he has just been suctioned for a moderate amount of secretions and took a few minutes to stop coughing. Which of the following will be the most likely reason you choose to go ahead and evaluate his functional status today?
   a. his RR, breathing pattern, and HR have returned to his baseline prior to suctioning*
   b. his oxygen saturation is 89% compared to 100% during suctioning
   c. his BP is 20 mmHg above his baseline from the RN flow sheet and he has a headache
   d. his heart rhythm has changed to a rapid atrial fibrillation and he is complaining of light headedness

2. Mr. Jones is awake, alert, and has rested on the ventilator overnight. This is your third time treating Mr. Jones. The nurse tells you he has just been suctioned for a moderate amount of secretions and took a few minutes to stop coughing following the suction by the respiratory care personnel. Which of the following will be the most likely reason(s) you choose not to progress his functional status today?
   a. he is having difficulty following 2-step directions during his ROM and bed mobility exercises (SpO_2 89% on 40% trach mask)
   b. he is not coughing during this ROM and bed mobility exercises (SpO_2 95% on 40% trach mask)
   c. he is having difficulty communicating and you notice accessory muscle use during his ROM and bed mobility exercises (SpO_2 89% on 40% trach mask)
   d. a, c*

3. Mr. Jones is awake, alert, and has rested on the ventilator overnight. This is your third time treating Mr. Jones. The nurse tells you he has just been suctioned for a moderate amount of secretions and took a few minutes to stop coughing following the suction by the respiratory care personnel. Which of the following will be the most likely reason(s) you choose to progress his functional status and activity level today?
   a. he is able to follow multi-step directions during his ROM warm up exercises and his BP, SpO_2, RR, and breathing pattern have not varied from baseline*
   b. he reports feeling rested and his RR is 10 bpm above resting, his Systolic BP is 20 points above resting, and his HR is 20 beats above the resting value
   c. he is not able to follow more then 1 step commands, which is a change from his second treatment session and his vital signs are deteriorating since he was suctioned
   d. his ECG shows new onset multifocal premature ventricular beats, and he is now complaining of sharp pain on inhalation

4. While transferring Mr. Jones OOB, water enters his endotracheal tube via the ventilator tubing. Which of the following is most likely the best scenario for you to follow?
   a. complete the transfer out of the bed to place Mr. Jones safely in the chair, shut the ventilator alarm off, and then continue therapy if vital signs are stable
   b. complete the transfer OOB to place Mr. Jones safely in the chair, let the nurse or respiratory care personnel who helped you with the transfer go ahead and repeat the suction of Mr. Jones, and then continue therapy immediately
   c. immediately transfer Mr. Jones back to bed, calm him down, shut off the ventilator alarm, inform the nurse, and then continue therapy if vital signs are stable
   d. immediately calm Mr. Jones down, complete the transfer to the chair, suction Mr. Jones again, and continue the therapy if his vital signs are stable*

5. Of the following scenarios which most likely represents how a therapist would determine "positive" progression in functional activity for Mr. Jones?
   a. vital sign response to activity, continued need for endotracheal suctioning, paradoxical breathing pattern during a 3 hour wean session, and lack of sleep
   b. vital sign response to activity, decrease need for endotracheal suctioning, no paradoxical breathing pattern during a 3 hour wean session, and adequate sleep*
   c. vital sign response to activity, continued need for endotracheal suctioning, paradoxical breathing pattern during any attempt to wean, and new crackles in right lower lung field
   d. vital sign response to activity, decreased need for endotracheal suctioning, no paradoxical breathing pattern during the first hour of the wean session, development of crackles in bilateral lower lung fields, and resting tachypnea

Sample Answer Sheet: Written Competency

Staff Member Name: _____ Score: _____

A. Assessment

    1. a.   b.   c.   d.

    2. a.   b.   c.   d.

    3. a.   b.   c.   d.

    4. a.   b.   c.   d.

    5. a.   b.   c.   d.

B. Line Identification

    1. a.   b.   c.   d.

    2. a.   b.   c.   d.

    3. a.   b.   c.   d.

    4. a.   b.   c.   d.

    5. a.   b.   c.   d.

C. ECG Identification

    1. a.   b.   c.   d.

    2. a.   b.   c.   d.

    3. a.   b.   c.   d.

    4. a.   b.   c.   d.

    5. a.   b.   c.   d.

D. Ventilation/Oxygenation

    1. a.   b.   c.   d.

    2. a.   b.   c.   d.

    3. a.   b.   c.   d.

    4. a.   b.   c.   d.

    5. a.   b.   c.   d.

E. Methods for Progression

    1. a.   b.   c.   d.

    2. a.   b.   c.   d.

    3. a.   b.   c.   d.

    4. a.   b.   c.   d.

    5. a.   b.   c.   d.

INDEX